Clinical Aspects of Dental Materials

Theory, Practice, and Cases

Third Edition

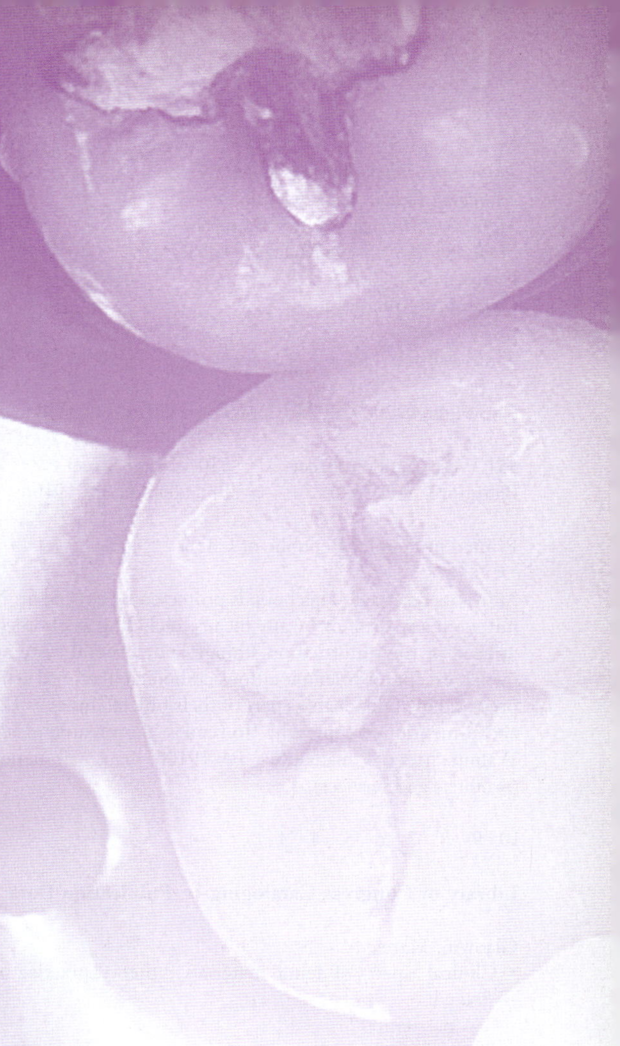

Clinical Aspects of Dental Materials

Theory, Practice, and Cases

Third Edition

Marcia Gladwin, R.D.H., Ed.D.
Professor
Department of Periodontics
Division of Dental Hygiene
West Virginia University
School of Dentistry
Morgantown, West Virginia

Michael Bagby, D.D.S., Ph.D.
Professor
Division of Pediatric Dentistry
West Virginia University
School of Dentistry
Morgantown, West Virginia

Wolters Kluwer Health | Lippincott Williams & Wilkins
Philadelphia • Baltimore • New York • London
Buenos Aires • Hong Kong • Sydney • Tokyo

Acquisitions Editor: Barrett Koger
Managing Editor: Andrea Klingler
Marketing Manager: Nancy Bradshaw
Production Editor: Eve Malakoff-Klein
Designer: Risa Clow
Compositor: Aptara, Inc.

Third Edition

351 West Camden Street
Baltimore, MD 21201

530 Walnut Street
Philadelphia, PA 19106

Printed in Peoples Republic of China

10 9 8 7 6 5 4 3

Library of Congress Cataloging-in-Publication Data

Gladwin, Marcia A.
Clinical aspects of dental materials : theory, practice, and cases / Marcia Gladwin, Michael Bagby. — 3rd ed.
p. ; cm.
Rev. ed. of: Clinical aspects of dental materials / [edited by] Marcia Gladwin, Michael Bagby. 2nd ed. c2004.
ISBN 978-0-7817-6489-6
1. Dental materials. 2. Dental casting. I. Bagby, Michael D. II. Title.
[DNLM: 1. Dental Materials—Case Reports. 2. Dental Casting Technique—Case Reports. 3. Dental Impression Technique—Case Reports. WU 190 G543ca 2009]
RK652.5.G56 2009
617.6'95—dc22

2007043567

To those teachers who have influenced us as educators

General McLane High School, Edinboro, Pennsylvania
Mr. Hap Holowach
Mr. Ralph Zindel

University of Pittsburgh, Dental Assisting-Oral Hygiene Program
Dr. Herman Langkamp (deceased)
Dr. Joanne Nicoll
Dr. Margaret Pipko (deceased)

West Virginia University, Morgantown, West Virginia
Ms. Catherine Graves
Dr. Mark Wicclair
Dr. Richard Walls
Dr. John Carline

— *MG*

Tinley Park High School, Tinley Park, Illinois
Mr. Leo Kaiser
Ms. Tish Kirk
Mr. William VanWyhe

Augustana College, Rock Island, Illinois
Dr. Robert Berntsen
Dr. Robert Johnson
Dr. Robert Troll
Dr. Anna Wartman

Loyola Dental School, Maywood, Illinois
Dr. Ted Quilitz
Dr. Marshall Smulson
Dr. William Stoffel (deceased)

Northwestern University, Chicago, Illinois
Dr. Jerome Cohen (deceased)
Dr. Evan Greener
Drs. Bill and Sally Marshall

— *MB*

Preface

The third edition of *Clinical Aspects of Dental Materials: Theory, Practice, and Cases* continues to provide a dental materials background that emphasizes the clinical aspects of dental materials. Hopefully, the student will become more familiar with the practice of dentistry through the use of this textbook.

Organization

The text is divided into three distinct parts: Theoretical Perspectives, Laboratory and Clinical Applications, and Case Studies. Chapters have been updated throughout the book and a few have been reorganized for easier understanding. Five chapters reflect significant revisions, including Chapter 4, Adhesive Materials; Chapter 5, Direct Polymeric Restorative Materials; Chapter 16, Polishing Materials and Abrasion; Chapter 17, Tooth Whitening; and Chapter 31, Clinical and Laboratory Aspects of a Whitening Tray.

Two new chapters have also been added to Part II. Chapter 36, "Finishing and Polishing Composite Restorations," provides a step-by-step technique and suggests a variety of instruments that will achieve the desired result. It has been presented in this format because there are many finishing and polishing instruments and abrasives, and each dentist has a preference in performing this procedure. Chapter 37, "Tips for the New Hygienist," is written by a contributing author who wanted to share some valuable information for the future dental hygiene practitioner. The text authors wholeheartedly agreed, so this short chapter is added at the end of this section. Part III, which highlights clinical case studies, has had two new cases added, for a total of six.

Some sections of many chapters are labeled as optional. The instructor should feel free to designate other sections as optional as well. The outline format is designed to provide a clear organization of the topic and to facilitate the reading of both the theory and laboratory chapters.

Features

Part I, which includes Chapters 1 through 22, now has more Review Questions. Part II chapters—those addressing laboratory and clinical applications, and specifically 23 through 36—have had Review Questions added. These are designed for not only course review, but for review for national boards as well.

"Tips for the Clinician" and "Precaution" boxes are included in almost all of the chapters in Part II. Summaries of procedures are also highlighted in boxes to provide easy review.

This new edition of *Clinical Aspects of Dental Materials* has a 4-page color insert that contains several photographs with descriptive captions. Being able to see color in certain dental materials, matching restorations, and differences after tooth whitening will provide for better understanding.

Answers and Justifications for *all* chapter and clinical case review questions are provided in Appendix 1. At the end of the chapters in Part II, the text refers the reader to Appendix 2, where the Skill Performance Evaluation Sheets are located. They are perforated for easy removal and can be folded for separate evaluations by the student and instructor. The instructor can use this section as a dental materials and/or expanded functions lab manual for the course being taught.

Ancillaries

Instructors' materials are available to adopting instructors and include an image bank, PowerPoint lecture outlines, and answers to the review questions (Appendix 1). These items are also available on the book's website, at http://thepoint.lww.com/gladwin3e.

We hope that the third edition of *Clinical Aspects of Dental Materials* is user-friendly, appropriately updated, and instrumental in helping students gain a basic understanding of the clinical aspects of dental materials. We wish the instructor and students a very successful academic year!

Acknowledgments

The authors wish to express their thanks to the following individuals for their contributions to this edition:

To the twelve contributing authors for their cooperation and dedication to this effort in the midst of their busy schedules. Their acceptance of our suggestions and editing has been most appreciated.

To Drs. Daniel Della-Giustina and Thomas Razmus for their comments and assistance with specific chapters. Their contributions improved our final manuscript.

To Ms. Marilyn Powley for preparation of some of the manuscript. Her time, patience, skills, and pleasant attitude were not only appreciated, but made a large project seem smaller.

To the many clinicians, dental materials scientists, and dental products manufacturer representatives who contributed photographs, text, and artwork.

To the patients used in Part III: Clinical Cases.

And lastly, to the team at Lippincott Williams & Wilkins: John, Kevin, Barrett, Andrea, and the production staff for their guidance and assistance in making our efforts suitable for the dental hygiene student.

Contributors

Linda Bagby, B.A., B.S.
Safety Consultant
Morgantown, West Virginia

Michael Bagby, D.D.S., Ph.D.
Professor
Division of Pediatric Dentistry
West Virginia University
School of Dentistry
Morgantown, West Virginia

Cathryn Frere, B.S.D.H., M.S.Ed.
Associate Professor
Division of Dental Hygiene
West Virginia University
School of Dentistry
Morgantown, West Virginia

Joan Gibson-Howell, R.D.H., Ed.D.
Assistant Professor
Dental Hygiene Program
The Ohio State University
College of Dentistry
Columbus, Ohio

Marcia Gladwin, R.D.H., Ed.D.
Professor
Division of Dental Hygiene
West Virginia University
School of Dentistry
Morgantown, West Virginia

Marylou Gutmann, R.D.H., M.A.
Professor and Graduate Program Director
Department of Dental Hygiene
The Texas A&M University
Dallas, Texas

Jacqueline Harper, R.D.H., M.S.
Staff Hygienist
Departments of Orthodontics and Periodontics
West Virginia University
School of Dentistry
Morgantown, West Virginia

Christine Nathe, R.D.H., M.S.
Professor and Graduate Program Director
Division of Dental Hygiene
University of New Mexico
Albuquerque, New Mexico

James Overberger, D.D.S., M.S.
Professor Emeritus
Department of Restorative Dentistry
West Virginia University
School of Dentistry
Morgantown, West Virginia

Carol Spear, R.D.H., M.S.
Professor
Division of Dental Hygiene
West Virginia University
School of Dentistry
Morgantown, West Virginia

Michele R. Sweeney, R.D.H, M.S.D.H.
Associate Professor
Dental Hygiene Program
West Liberty State College
West Liberty, West Virginia

Rebecca Thomas, B.S.D.H.
Public Health Hygienist
Mount Morris, Pennsylvania

John H. Tucker, D.M.D.
General Practice
Erie, Pennsylvania

A. Todd Walls, D.D.S.
Assistant Professor
Department of Restorative Dentistry
West Virginia University
School of Dentistry
Morgantown, West Virginia

Meg Zayan, R.D.H., M.P.H.
Associate Professor and Director
Fones School of Dental Hygiene
University of Bridgeport
Bridgeport, Connecticut

Reviewers

Debra Jennings, D.M.D.
Department of Dental Services
Trident Technical College
Charleston, South Carolina

Diana Sullivan, M.Ed.
Program Director
Dental Department
Dakota County Technical College
Rosemount, Minnesota

Donna Warren, R.D.H., M.Ed.
Associate Professor
Department of Periodontics
School of Dental Hygiene
University of Texas—Houston
Houston, Texas

Contents

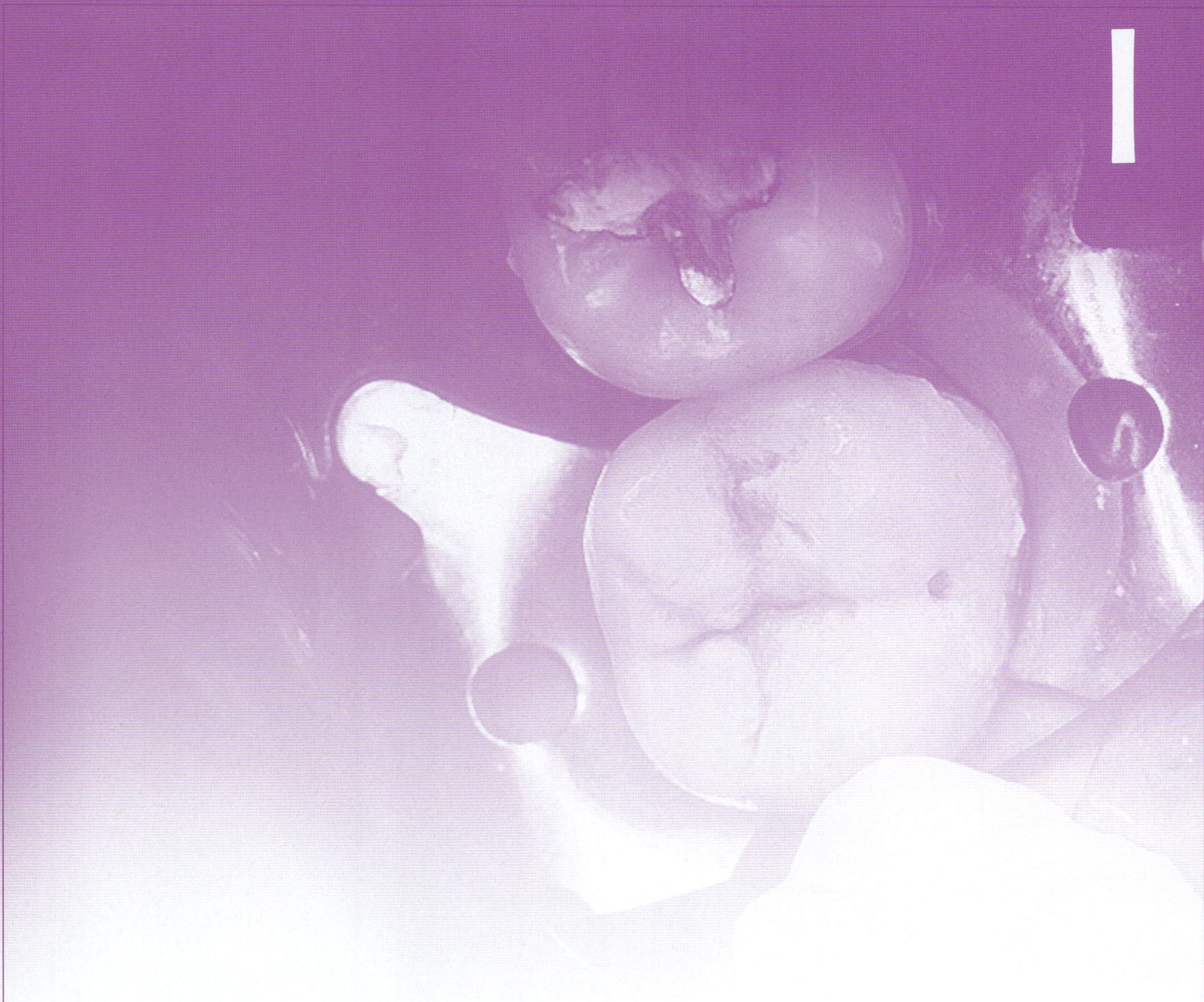

I

Theoretical Perspectives

Introduction

1

Objectives

After studying this chapter, the student will be able to do the following:

1. Summarize the reasons why a dental hygienist should be knowledgeable in the science of dental materials.
2. Discuss some of the conditions that make the oral cavity a hostile environment.
3. Identify four characteristics or properties a dental material must possess to survive in the oral environment.
4. Explain how the following organizations evaluate and/or classify dental drugs, materials, instruments, and equipment:
   - American Dental Association (ADA)
   - U.S. Food and Drug Administration (FDA)
   - International Standards Organization (ISO)
5. Name three ways dental materials may be classified, and discuss each.
6. Specifically discuss the locations of all six cavity classifications and the appropriate restorative material to be used for each. Include the following in your discussion:
   - Anterior and/or posterior
   - Involvement of incisal angle
   - Involvement of proximal surface
   - Smooth surfaces versus pit and fissures

Key Words/Phrases

abutment
base
biocompatibility
biomaterials
bridge
cast
cavity preparation
dental implants
dental materials
denture
diagnostic cast
direct restorative materials
esthetic materials
fixed partial denture
impression
indirect restorative material
liner
luting agents
maxillofacial prosthesis
polishing
pontic
prosthesis
removable partial denture
restorations
restorative materials
retainer
specifications
study model

INTRODUCTION

Courses in basic science and dental hygiene science must be studied and integrated with each other to provide students with the knowledge and skills necessary to ensure that quality dental hygiene care is provided to their patients. This care includes assessing and diagnosing the patient's oral needs. To fulfill these needs, the dental hygienist must establish, implement, and evaluate goals specified for the patient.

I. Rationale for Studying Dental Materials

"Dental materials" is one of many required courses in the dental hygiene curriculum and focuses on those items and products used in the prevention and treatment of oral disease and the promotion of health. The scope of practice of a dental hygienist includes the delivery of therapeutic, educational, and preventive patient services. Materials used in the practice of dental hygiene include instruments made from common industrial materials, therapeutic agents, and dental biomaterials to prevent disease. At times, therapeutic dental products and preventive materials overlap.

The preventive aspects of dental hygiene include primary prevention, which attempts to impede the development of disease, and secondary prevention, which attempts to limit the destruction caused by disease. Both aspects of preventive dentistry involve the use of instruments (made from materials) and dental materials.

A dental hygienist should be knowledgeable in the science of dental materials for the following four reasons:

A. To Understand the Behavior of Materials

This will aid in the delivery of quality patient care. The dental hygienist must understand why specific materials behave as they do and why they are used for certain functions in certain locations to replace missing oral tissues. For example, the proper placement of sealants will prevent dental caries. The proper restoration of teeth and maintenance of restorations will limit the destructive effects of caries and periodontal disease. The proper care and maintenance of instruments (prevention of corrosion) are important when sterilizing and disinfecting. The proper use of all dental materials is fundamental to the art and science of dentistry.

B. To Handle Materials Properly

Both preventive and restorative dentistry rely heavily on the proper use of biomaterials. **Biomaterials** are man-made materials that are used to replace tissues or that function in intimate contact with living tissues. **Dental materials** are biomaterials used in or around the oral cavity. The hygienist may or may not be involved in the placement of restorations, but he or she plays a significant role in the placement of preventive materials and the maintenance of restorations. The proper handling of dental materials is important because improper handling could affect their physical, chemical, and mechanical properties. In turn, this could affect the overall service to the patient.

Therefore, handling a dental material properly is a primary factor in the success or failure of its use. The goal of this text is to present dental materials and their manipulation from a clinical perspective. If materials are properly mixed and placed, improved patient care will result.

C. To Assess and Treat the Patient

The dental hygienist must be able to recognize all dental materials placed in the mouth. These may be visible clinically and/or radiographically. Proper identification is important so that they are not mistaken for caries (radiographically) or another similar-looking restoration that should be maintained in a different manner. An example would be the clinical recognition of an all-ceramic crown. Acidulated phosphate-fluoride (APF) gels can etch the surface of some ceramic materials. Using an APF gel is contraindicated for patients with ceramic restorations; instead, a neutral fluoride gel should be used.

D. To Educate the Patient

In many instances, patients may ask the dental hygienist to discuss the characteristics and properties of one dental material compared to another, both of which may be a reasonable option for the patient. Patients may also ask the hygienist to describe the steps involved in the fabrication of a certain type of restoration, or they may also inquire about home care regimens ("Will I need to do anything more than brushing or flossing?"). Knowledge of dental materials is critical so that the patient is given professional, complete, and correct answers.

II. Biomaterials and the Oral Environment

A. Oral Tissues as Biologic Materials

Whether a material is used for preventive or restorative purposes, the oral environment places great restrictions on which materials can be used and the manner in which those materials are used. When one realizes that oral tissues are biologic materials, a variety of properties and functions are evident. All oral tissues must function in the hostile environment of the oral cavity.

1. **Enamel**

Enamel is a hard, wear-resistant surface material. It is able to resist the compressive forces of biting, but it is weak in its resistance to bending and other forces that occur when food is ground by molars. Enamel is well supported by dentin. Enamel will dissolve in oral fluids if the pH is too acidic; dental caries is the result of such an acidic attack.

2. **Dentin**

Dentin makes up the bulk of the tooth. It acts as a cushion for the brittle enamel, and it provides strength to resist the complex forces that occur when biting. Dentin is more susceptible than enamel to acidic attack.

3. **Pulp**

Pulp provides nutrients to the dentin and responds to stimuli with pain.

4. **Periodontium**

Periodontium supports the tooth in a stable but dynamic position, and it provides feedback regarding the force placed on the tooth. Periodontium includes the periodontal ligament, cementum, and alveolar bone.

5. **Gingival Tissue**

A very important function of gingival tissue is to seal out the many noxious agents of the oral cavity, which include chemicals and microbes, from gaining access to the periodontium and deeper tissues in the body. Gingival tissues surround and attach to teeth, forming a barrier. Although the oral cavity is considered to be inside the body, in many ways it is more like the outside. Biomaterials placed in the oral cavity have very different requirements from those of devices implanted inside the body.

B. Replacement Materials for Oral Tissues

1. **Restriction on Materials Use**

When oral tissue is lost, dental professionals attempt to replace it with a dental material. The replacement material mimics the function of the oral tissue, and it must withstand the same harsh environment. The biologic nature of the oral environment and the size of the oral cavity restrict the use of materials. These restrictions include:

a) Biting forces that may fracture teeth and replacement material
b) Degradation of:
- Materials, such as corrosion of metal
- Teeth, such as dental caries

c) Temperature changes that cause restorations to contract and expand differently than teeth, causing leakage around the restoration as well as tooth sensitivity
d) **Biocompatibility** (the lack of harmful effects to the patient)
e) Esthetic demands of the patient

2. **Effects of Dental Materials and the Oral Environment on Each Other**

The dental hygienist must understand the characteristics and properties of dental materials. This knowledge will provide insight regarding how a dental material may affect the oral environment. An orthodontic appliance makes oral hygiene difficult and increases the patient's susceptibility to gingival inflammation and caries. The oral environment affects the dental materials as well. Yeast or other microbes may colonize a denture, causing it to become foul-smelling. These characteristics and properties may also limit the selection and use of a dental material.

III. History and Selection of Dental Materials

A. History

1. **Ancient Times to the 1700s**

Why are certain materials chosen instead of others to serve as dental restorative materials? Actually, much has been learned throughout history by trial and error. In ancient times, gold was used not only for its corrosion resistance but also for its "workability" or ease of processing. Long ago, artists learned to form gold into many shapes. The relationship between the art and science of dentistry dates back to the infancy of the profession. Remember that for centuries humans have attempted to improve their appearance with adornments, such as jewelry and makeup. The replacement of lost teeth is also an ancient practice. At that time, it was more likely for esthetics than for function. As dentistry developed throughout the ages, more and more materials were used. Some of these included:

a) Ivory, which was carved
b) Porcelain, which was fired into tooth shapes
c) Wax and gypsum, which were used for impressions and models
d) Zinc oxide–eugenol and zinc phosphate, which evolved as fillings and cements to "glue" the restoration to the tooth

2. **The 1800s**

By this time, dentistry was becoming a scientifically based discipline. The pace of development of new materials quickened. Amalgam, a silver filling material, was widely accepted and frequently used. Porcelain was also used for inlays and crowns.

3. The 20th Century

a) Dental materials science had now developed into its own discipline. New materials and techniques were constantly being developed.

b) A variety of cast metals were used. Alloys were made of gold, chromium and nickel, chromium and cobalt, and titanium. Cast metals were used for crowns, bridges, and partial dentures.

c) Polymers and composites were alternatives for nearly every dental materials need.

4. The 21st Century

a) New ceramic materials and processing technologies have been adapted by dentistry.

b) The pace of dental materials development is so fast, some of this text will be outdated before it is published.

c) Luckily, the basic concepts of materials science and their use do not change. Both the student and the practitioner need to understand the behavior of the materials they use. After all, they are the ones who must select a product from a rather long list of possibilities.

B. Selection of Dental Materials and Products

The knowledge gained in a dental materials course will aid in the selection of products. Manufacturers readily provide data regarding strength and a variety of other properties. At times, they also provide the results of short-term clinical trials. How reliable is that information? More importantly, how useful is that information? It has been a goal of dental materials scientists to predict the performance of a material from its strength and other mechanical properties. Unfortunately, success has been elusive. Clinical trials are the most reliable source of information for most products. The clinician must evaluate the product information, but he or she must also consider the source of that information.

IV. Standards for Dental Materials

Standards for dental materials have been developed in dentistry in the same manner as in other industries. Standards describe the properties of a product so that a user may select the proper material for a particular use. Standards are common in everyday life. Examples include the octane rating of gasoline, film speed, the size of nuts and bolts, computer communications protocols, and low-fat foods. In the United States, standards are published and administered by the American National Standards Institute (ANSI). Many industries have organizations that work under the guidance of ANSI to develop and administer the standards for the products of that industry.

FIGURE 1.1 Seal of Acceptance of the American Dental Association. (Courtesy of the American Dental Association, Chicago, IL.)

A. Council on Scientific Affairs of the American Dental Association

In the United States, standards and guidelines for evaluating dental products are developed and administered by the Council on Scientific Affairs of the ADA. The Council evaluates dental drugs, materials, instruments, and equipment. A successful evaluation culminates in awarding of the ADA's Seal of Acceptance. The applicant (e.g., a toothpaste company or any manufacturer of a dentally related product) submits data for their product following the ADA guidelines. On approval of the product, the applicant is permitted to use the ADA's Seal of Acceptance. The Seal is illustrated in Figure 1.1. It is commonly seen on accepted brands of toothpaste and toothbrushes. The ADA Seal is awarded for a period of 3 years, after which the applicant must resubmit the product. In addition, advertising for products that have been awarded the ADA Seal is reviewed by the ADA.

Some of the ADA guidelines have very specific requirements for physical and mechanical properties that are measured in the laboratory and are called **specifications.** Specifications have been developed for many (but not for all) dental materials. Unfortunately, researchers have not been able to develop a series of tests that adequately predict the clinical performance of many dental materials. As a result, the Acceptance Program relies on clinical data for the evaluation of certain dental products. If a product is shown to be safe and effective, it can be given the Seal of Acceptance.

The Acceptance Program of the ADA is voluntary. Manufacturers are not required to have the Seal to market dental products in the United States. Although products might be approved for sale by the U.S. FDA, some products fail the ADA specifications when tested.

B. Medical Device Amendments of 1976

The federal government, under the auspices of the U.S. FDA, has the authority under the Medical Device Amendments of 1976 to ensure the safety of all medical devices. The U.S. FDA considers dental materials to be devices, and medical devices are grouped into three categories:

1. **Class I**

   These devices are the least regulated. Only good manufacturing practices are required. Prophy paste or brushes are two examples of such products.

2. **Class II**

   Class II devices gain approval from the FDA after being shown to be equivalent to products currently in use. Equivalency is demonstrated by meeting performance standards, such as the ADA's Seal of Acceptance Program. Some dental products have been "grandfathered in," because they were marketed before 1976. Composite and amalgam restorative materials are two examples of Class II products.

3. **Class III**

   These devices are the most regulated; they require premarket approval. Clinical data must be submitted to the U.S. FDA for evaluation before Class III devices are sold. If safety and efficacy of the device is supported by the data, the U.S. FDA then gives approval to market the product. Bone graft materials are common example of such products.

C. International Standards Organization

Many other countries have dental specifications or standards and governmental regulations. To simplify the mass of regulations, the International Standards Organization (ISO) attempts to unify standards throughout its member countries. The ISO standards for many dental materials have been developed (and continue to be developed) under the guidance of the Fédération Dentaire Internationale, the international equivalent of the ADA.

Many dental products carry the CE marking symbol of the European Union on their packaging, as shown in Figure 1.2. CE stands for Conformite Europeene, and the marking is required for sales in most of Europe. The CE symbol indicates compliance with ISO standards and European Union marketing requirements for dental products.

D. Selecting Products

Dentists are fortunate because several products usually will meet the needs of a particular clinical situation. It is important to select and use materials that result in quality service to the patient. The same product may not do so for all practitioners. It is acceptable to select products based on handling characteristics, a company's reputation and service,

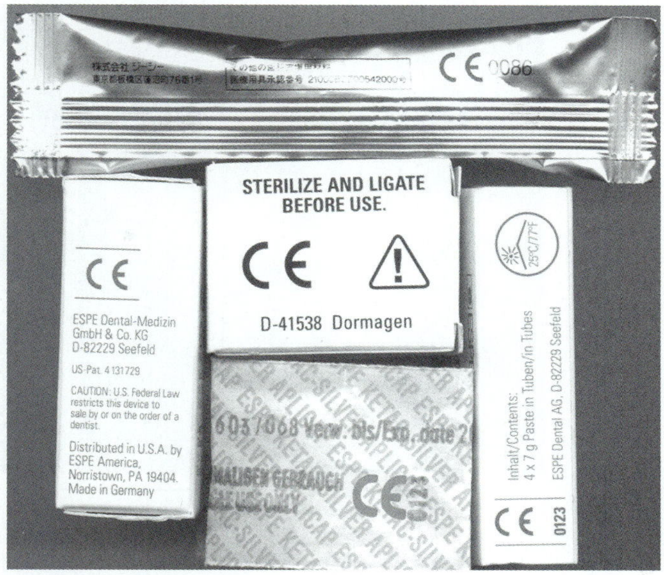

FIGURE 1.2 Photograph of dental products from American, Asian, and European companies displaying the CE marking symbol.

or packaging. If two products have been shown to be excellent, the ill-defined characteristics of "feel" or "looks" may be the final criteria that result in its selection. It is important to realize that most products require some time to learn to use them properly. If the clinician is always changing products to have the latest and greatest "widget bonder," he or she may be spending so much time learning to use new products that patient care may be affected. Of less consequence, that clinician will also have drawers, closets, and refrigerators filled with expensive, partially used dental products.

V. Classifications of Dental Materials

Like oral tissues, dental materials serve a variety of functions. Some materials replace lost tooth structure and restore the function of the teeth. These materials must withstand biting forces and therefore be strong and wear resistant. Other materials are used to make impressions of oral tissues from which replicas are made. Many impression materials are soft and can be distorted and stretched when removed from the mouth. In dentistry, as in other disciplines, use of a material must be matched to the properties of that material. Dental materials can be classified in a variety of ways but typically are classified by their use or function. Restorative materials are also classified by the location of fabrication or by the longevity of use.

A. Classification by Use

Materials used to replace lost oral tissues are called **restorative materials.** As mentioned earlier, those that replace lost tooth structure and restore the function of the teeth must be strong and hard

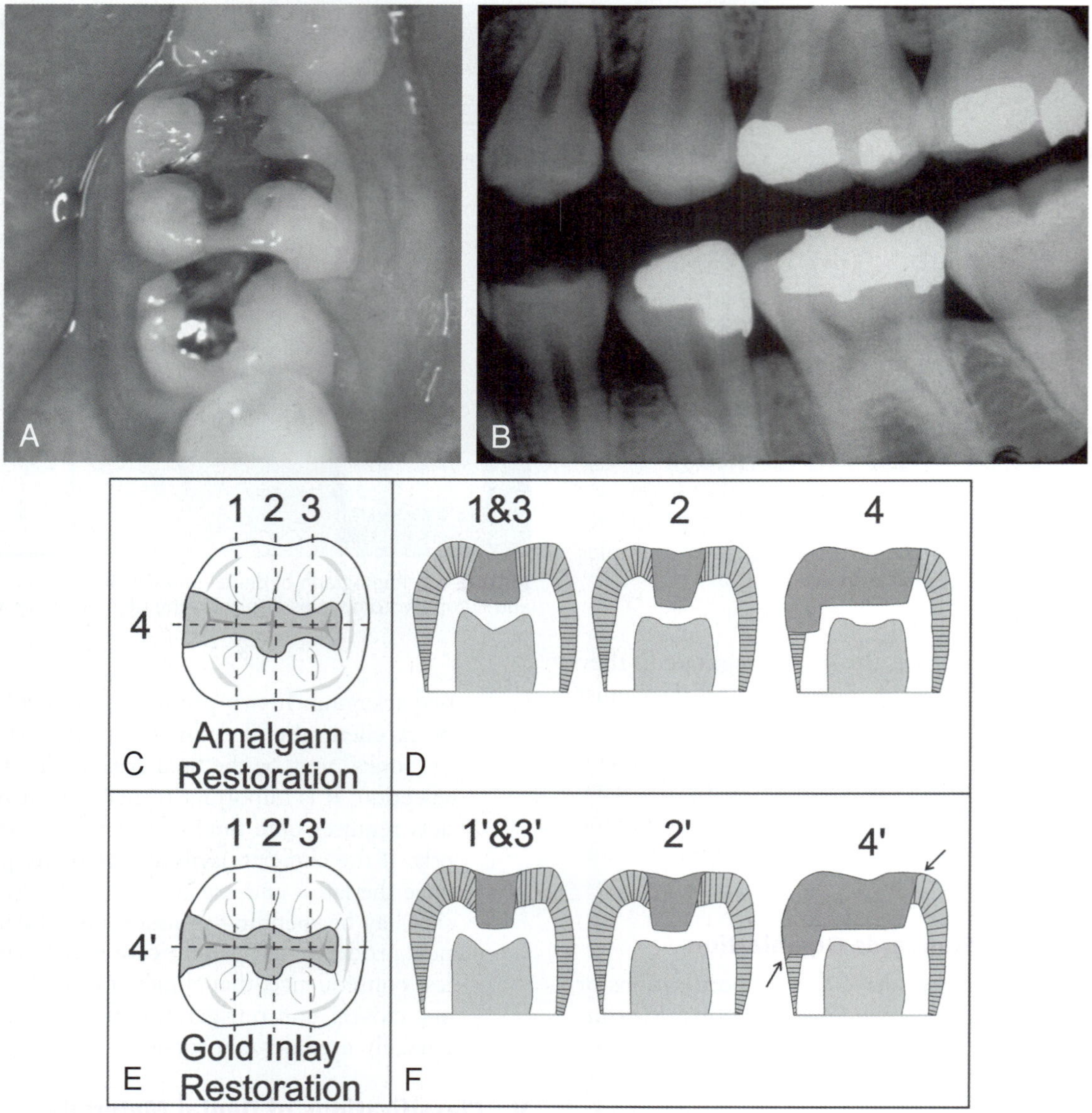

FIGURE 1.3 Photograph **(A)** and radiograph **(B)** of inlay (tooth #20) and amalgam (tooth #19) restorations. Drawings (**C–F**) show the convergence and divergence of preparations for the two materials. The amalgam (**C** and **D**) has several convergent walls (undercuts) at 1 and 3. The inlay (**E** and **F**) has only divergent walls at 1′, 2′, and 3′. *Arrows* indicate bevels for the inlay.

(Figs. 1.3, 1.4, and 1.5). Some restorative materials simulate the appearance of the tissues that are being replaced (see Figs. 1.10 and 5.9). Tissues simulated by restorative materials include the enamel of teeth (fillings and crowns), the mucosa of the periodontium (dentures), and even the skin of the face (maxillofacial prostheses). Materials that are tooth-colored are often called **esthetic materials.**

1. Restorations

Depending on the degree of destruction of a tooth, different restorations or fillings are used to replace lost tooth structure. Some **restorations** replace a small to moderate amount of tooth structure and are supported by the remaining tooth structure. Such restorations are held in the tooth by undercuts (mechanical locks), adhesion, or both. An inlay is a restoration that is made outside the mouth, usually in a dental laboratory. Inlays do not have undercuts and are cemented or "luted" into the tooth (Fig. 1.3).

Restorations are restricted to the physical size of the missing tooth structure. Excessively large restorations could affect speech or the patient's bite, or overwork the chewing muscles.

2. Crowns

Crowns are used to restore teeth when a substantial amount of tooth structure is missing.

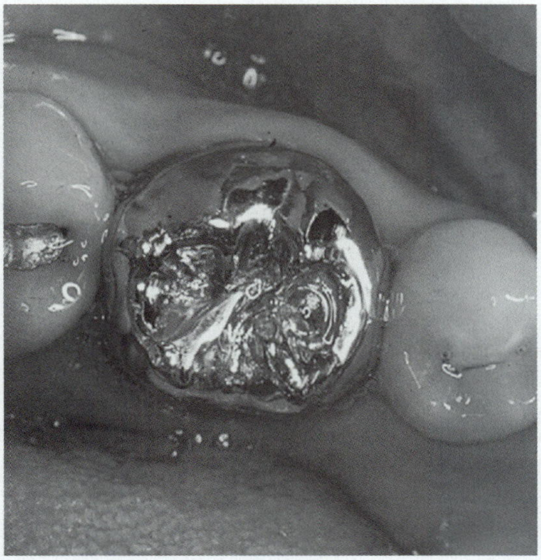

FIGURE 1.4 Photograph of a full gold crown.

Crowns encircle and support the remaining tooth structure (Fig. 1.4). Crowns are cemented in place similar to an inlay. If a crown or filling is too large or overcontoured, it will be detrimental to the health of the gingival tissues.

3. **Bridges**

A dental **bridge** replaces a lost tooth or teeth (Fig. 1.5). A typical dental bridge is much like a bridge over a river. At each end, the dental bridge is supported by a tooth called an **abutment.** Each abutment is prepared and then restored with a crown called a **retainer.** The missing tooth is replaced with a false tooth called a **pontic.** A pontic is a replacement tooth, but only the crown portion of the tooth is replaced. The pontic and abutments are strongly joined together so that biting forces will not break the bridge. The dental bridge is cemented onto the prepared teeth in the same manner as a crown or an inlay. Like all restorations, the physical size of a bridge is limited by the physiology and anatomy of the mouth.

4. **Complete and Partial Dentures**

Because of the ravages of caries or periodontal disease, some people lose many or all of their teeth. If all the teeth of an arch are missing, the teeth are replaced by a prosthesis called a complete denture, as shown in Figure 1.6. A **prosthesis** is an artificial device that replaces a lost organ or tissues. A **denture** replaces missing teeth, bone, and gingiva after the teeth have been lost or extracted. A complete denture is supported by and precisely rests on the mucosal tissue covering the maxilla or mandible. The functions of a complete denture include chewing

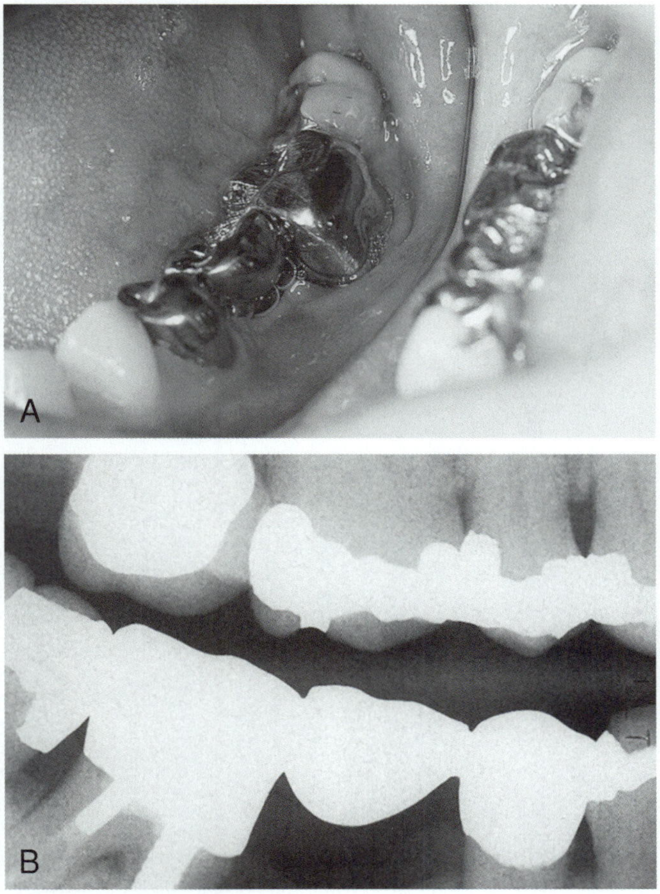

FIGURE 1.5 Photograph **(A)** and radiograph **(B)** of a gold bridge.

food (mastication), proper speech, and esthetics. Frequently, dentures improve a patient's self-esteem, appearance, and oral function. The supporting tissues are replaced with a pink plastic that simulates the appearance of gingiva.

If some teeth are present in an arch, the replacement prosthesis is called a partial denture (Fig. 1.7) . A bridge is often called a **fixed partial denture because** it is cemented into place. A **removable partial denture** is sometimes referred to as a "partial" and replaces a few to many teeth. A removable partial denture is placed and removed by the patient in the same manner as a full denture. Typically, a removable partial denture has several metal clasps that are designed to encircle several remaining teeth so that the prosthesis is stabilized, somewhat like the abutments of a fixed bridge. The replacement teeth of a removable partial denture are much like a section of a full denture. As with a complete denture, the teeth and gingival tissues are simulated to make an esthetically pleasing prosthesis for the patient. The remaining natural teeth greatly stabilize the partial denture and significantly improve function.

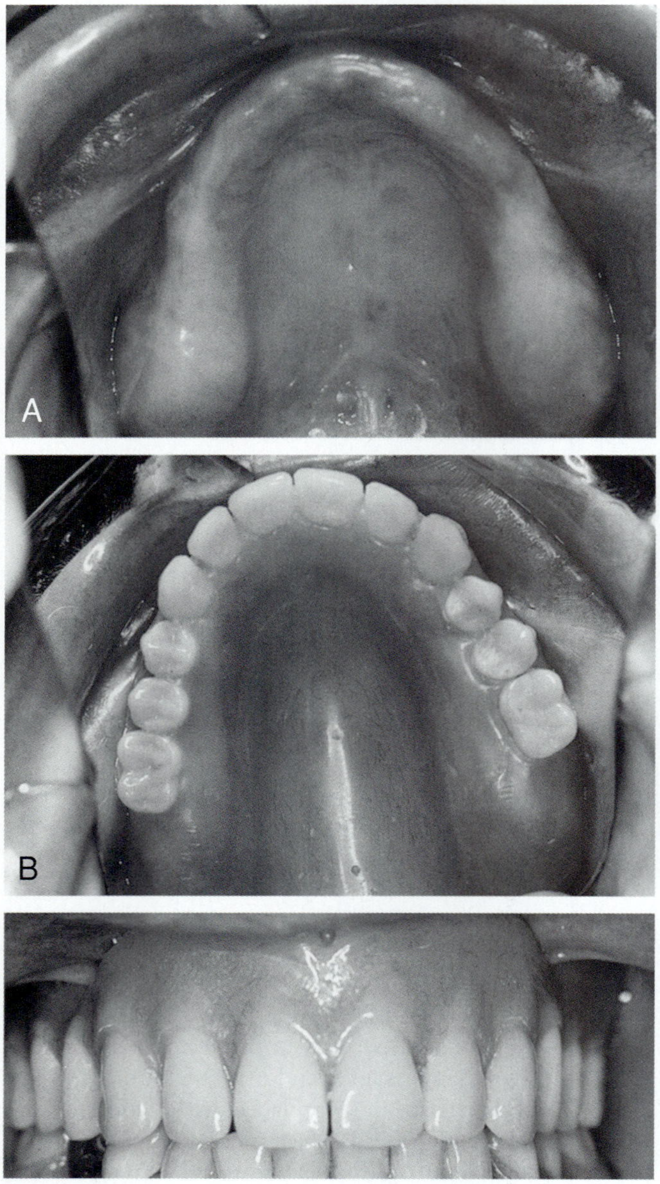

FIGURE 1.6 Photographs of an edentulous maxillary ridge **(A)** and denture in place (**B** and **C**). (Courtesy of Dr. Henry Miller, Morgantown, WV.)

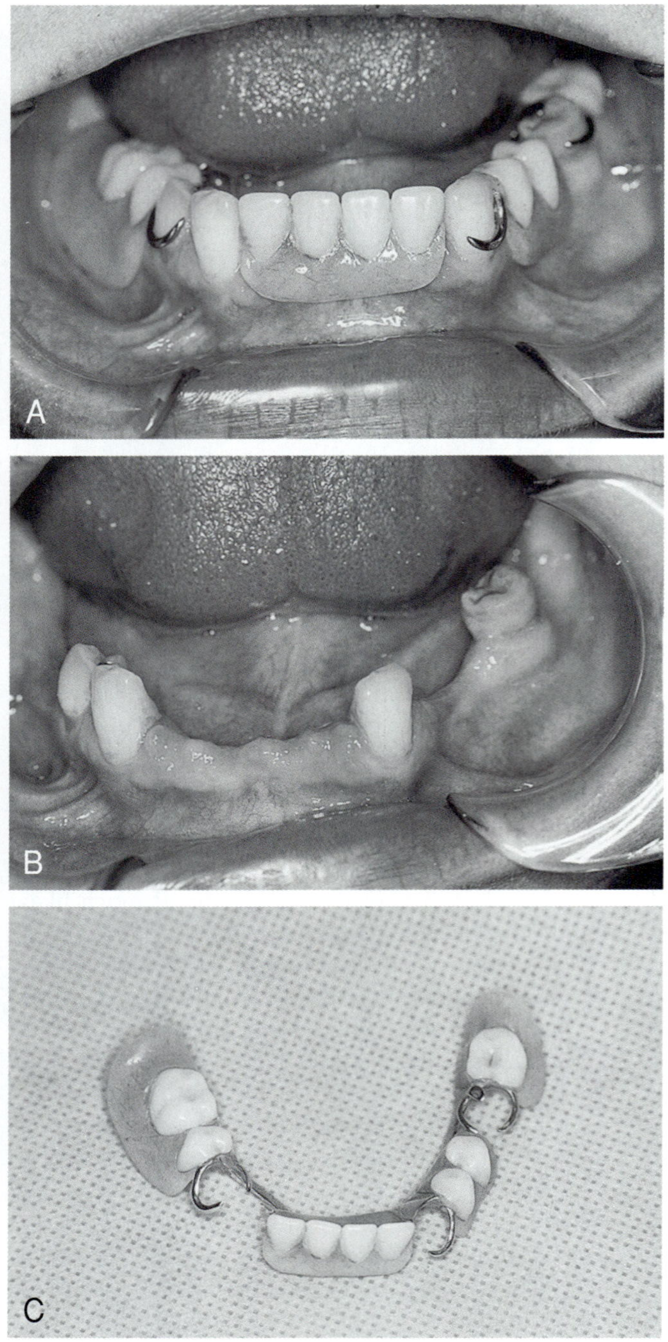

FIGURE 1.7 Photographs of a patient with **(A)** and without **(B)** a removable partial denture in place and the removable partial denture **(C)**. (See color images.)

5. Impressions, Casts, and Models

When a restoration or prosthesis is constructed in a dental laboratory, a precise replica of the supporting tissues of the patient is required. To produce the replica (or positive copy), an impression is made of the prepared tooth or remaining alveolar ridge. The dental **impression** (or negative copy) is then filled with a material that solidifies to form the replica, as shown in Figure 1.8.

If a restoration is constructed on the replica, it is called a **cast.** If the resulting replica is used to study the size and position of the oral tissues, it is called a **study model** or **diagnostic cast.** A replica of the patient's oral tissues is frequently used for both functions. First, it would be used to study the position of teeth and other oral tissues. Second, it would serve as an opposing cast to aid in the construction of a restoration.

A variety of impression materials are used in dentistry. Most models and casts are made with gypsum materials, which are very similar to plaster of Paris.

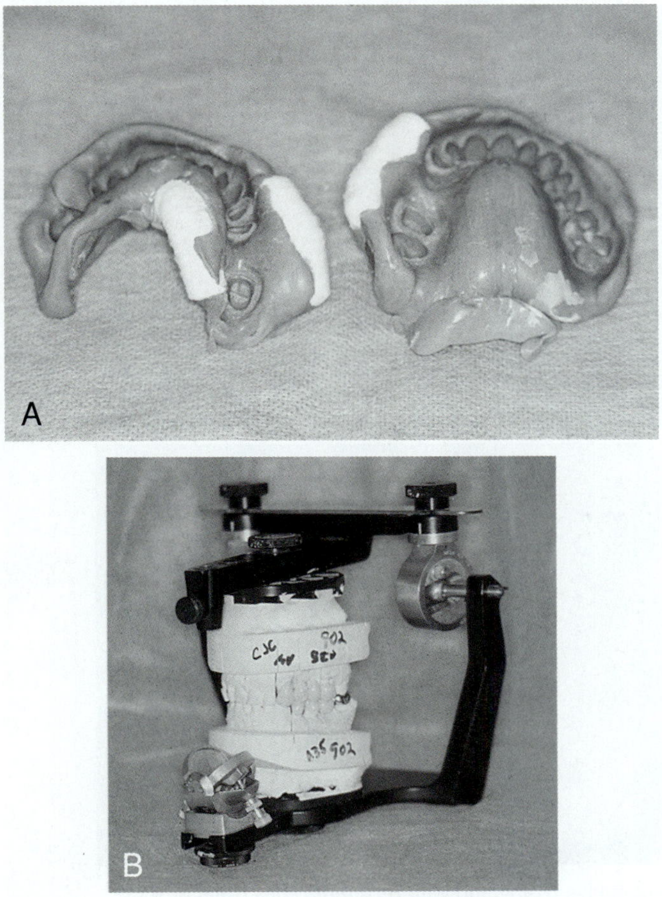

FIGURE 1.8 Photographs of impressions **(A)** and of casts mounted on an articulator **(B)**.

6. Cements

a) As Luting Agents

After a crown has been made, it must be held in place (or "luted") to the prepared tooth. Luting is the same as gluing two objects together, and it is also called cementing. **Luting agents** are frequently called dental cements. The cement holds the crown onto the prepared tooth and fills in the microscopic gaps between the tooth and the crown. After mixing, cements must flow like a thin liquid so that a precisely made crown will fit properly. Several minutes after setting, the cement is expected to be strong and insoluble in oral fluids. Requirements of dental cements are quite rigorous. Proper handling of all materials, especially dental cements, is critical to successful patient care.

b) As Bases and Liners

Many of the materials used for luting crowns, bridges, or inlays may also serve other purposes. These include protecting the pulp from irritating materials, such as acids, or serving as insulating layers under metal restorations. Metals conduct hot and cold much more quickly than dentin and enamel. Using a base or liner under a metal restoration (between the pulp and the filling) can reduce or eliminate sensitivity to cold and hot foods and beverages (Fig. 1.9) The term **base** implies a degree of strength and thermal insulation, whereas the term **liner** does not. Historically, bases and liners were distinct groups, but now much overlap exists. The use of both terms best describes the function of these materials. A liner would be a relatively thin layer of material painted on to protect the underlying dentin from chemical irritation. A base has greater bulk, which serves to restore part of the missing tooth structure and to provide thermal insulation.

7. Temporary Materials

a) Temporary Crowns

When a crown is made in the dental laboratory, the dentist and patient must wait days or weeks before it can be cemented into place. What happens to the tooth that has been prepared for a crown? Such preparation requires that a surface layer be removed from the tooth. The thickness of the layer to be removed depends on the material that will be used to replace the missing tooth structure. Frequently, most of the enamel not already destroyed by decay is removed. If the tooth is vital (the pulp is alive), the patient will likely experience pain when eating, drinking, and, at times, breathing if the crown preparation is not protected in some manner. Many times, the appearance of a front tooth that is prepared for a crown also is not esthetically acceptable. What is done to solve this problem? A temporary crown is made before the patient leaves the office (Fig. 1.10).

The temporary crown is constructed and luted during the same appointment in which the crown preparation is performed. Temporary crowns are not as strong or esthetically pleasing as permanent restorations, but they provide adequate service while the permanent crown is being made. Temporary crowns are typically made from plastics that are formed in the mouth. These replicate the missing tooth structure very closely. Other types of temporary crowns consist of metal or plastic shells (shaped like crowns of teeth) that are lined with the same plastic materials. Construction of temporary crowns is presented in Chapter 35.

Temporary crowns must be removed when it is time to cement the permanent crown. Temporary crowns are cemented with

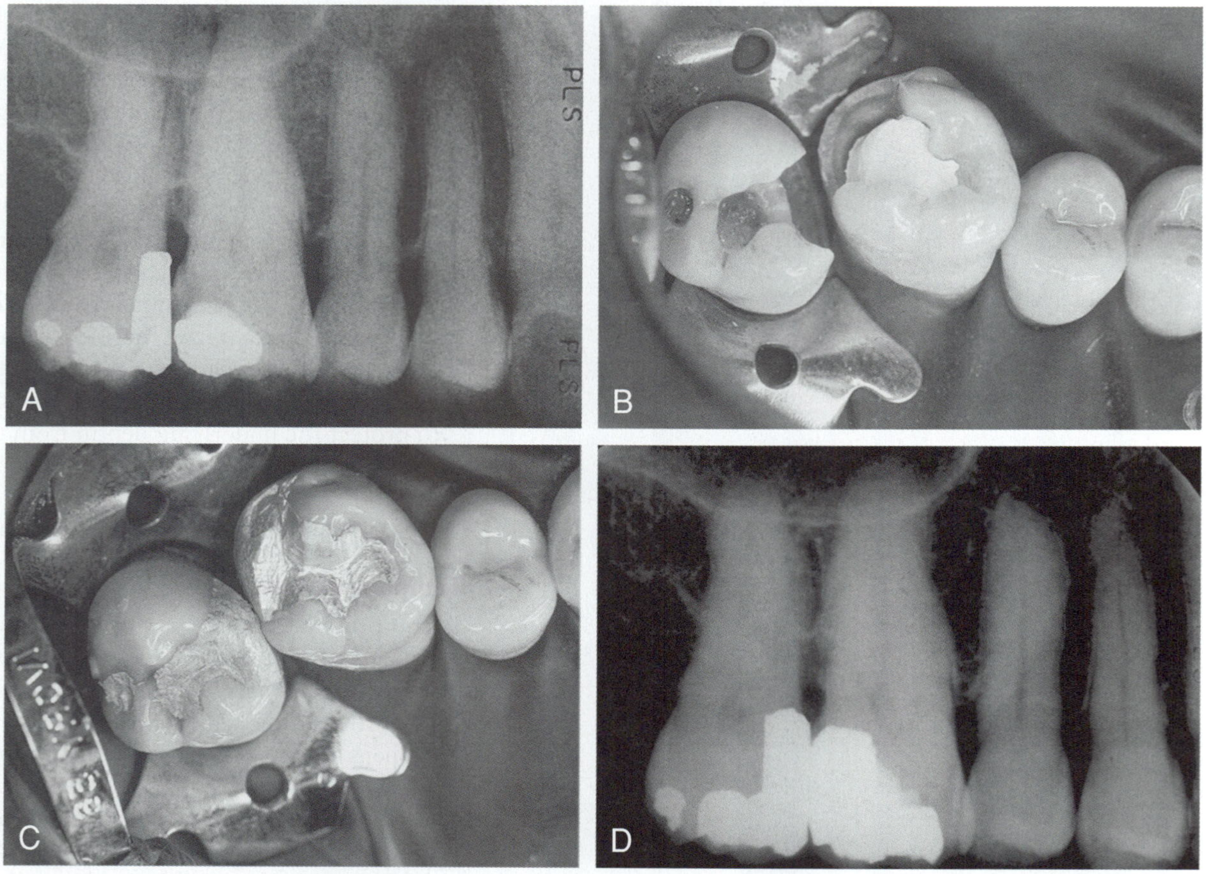

FIGURE 1.9 Example of a base and amalgam restoration. **A.** Preoperative radiograph with recurrent caries distal of #3. **B.** Photograph of cavity preparations in teeth #2 and #3. Tooth #3 has a base. **C.** Completed amalgam restorations. **D.** Postoperative radiograph. (See color images.) (Courtesy of Dr. Henry Miller, Morgantown, WV.)

"weak" temporary cements so that they may be easily removed.

b) Temporary Restorations

At times, a dentist is unsure of the best treatment for a patient or a particular tooth. The exact condition of the pulp may not be obvious from the patient's symptoms. A dentist may remove all or part of the decay from a tooth and then place a temporary restoration to give the pulp time to heal before determining the specific treatment that is needed. Treating biologic tissues, especially the pulp, is not as predictable as both the dentist and the patient would like it to be, so a temporary restoration is placed.

8. Preventive Materials

Several materials are used predominantly to prevent disease or trauma. These include:

a) Pit and fissure sealants, to prevent decay (Fig. 1.11)

b) Mouthguards, to prevent injury during athletic activities (Fig. 1.12).

c) Fluoride trays, custom and stock, which fit over the teeth to apply topical treatments. Custom fluoride trays look very much like custom mouthguards or bleaching trays (see Fig. 1.12 and Chapter 18).

9. Polishing Materials

A tremendous amount of time in a dental practice is spent polishing teeth, restorations, and appliances. Use of a rubber cup with an abrasive agent is termed **polishing,** but the predominant function is to remove stain, plaque, and debris from the tooth surface. True polishing involves moving an abrasive over the surface of an object to remove a thin layer of material. This action results in a surface that is clean, smooth, and lustrous. Dental professionals use many different devices and materials to polish teeth and restorations. Understanding the polishing process is important to achieving the desired result and is presented in Chapter 16.

10. Implants

Dental implants are considered to be part of restorative dentistry, but because of their specialized nature, they are segregated from other materials. **Dental implants** are typically screws

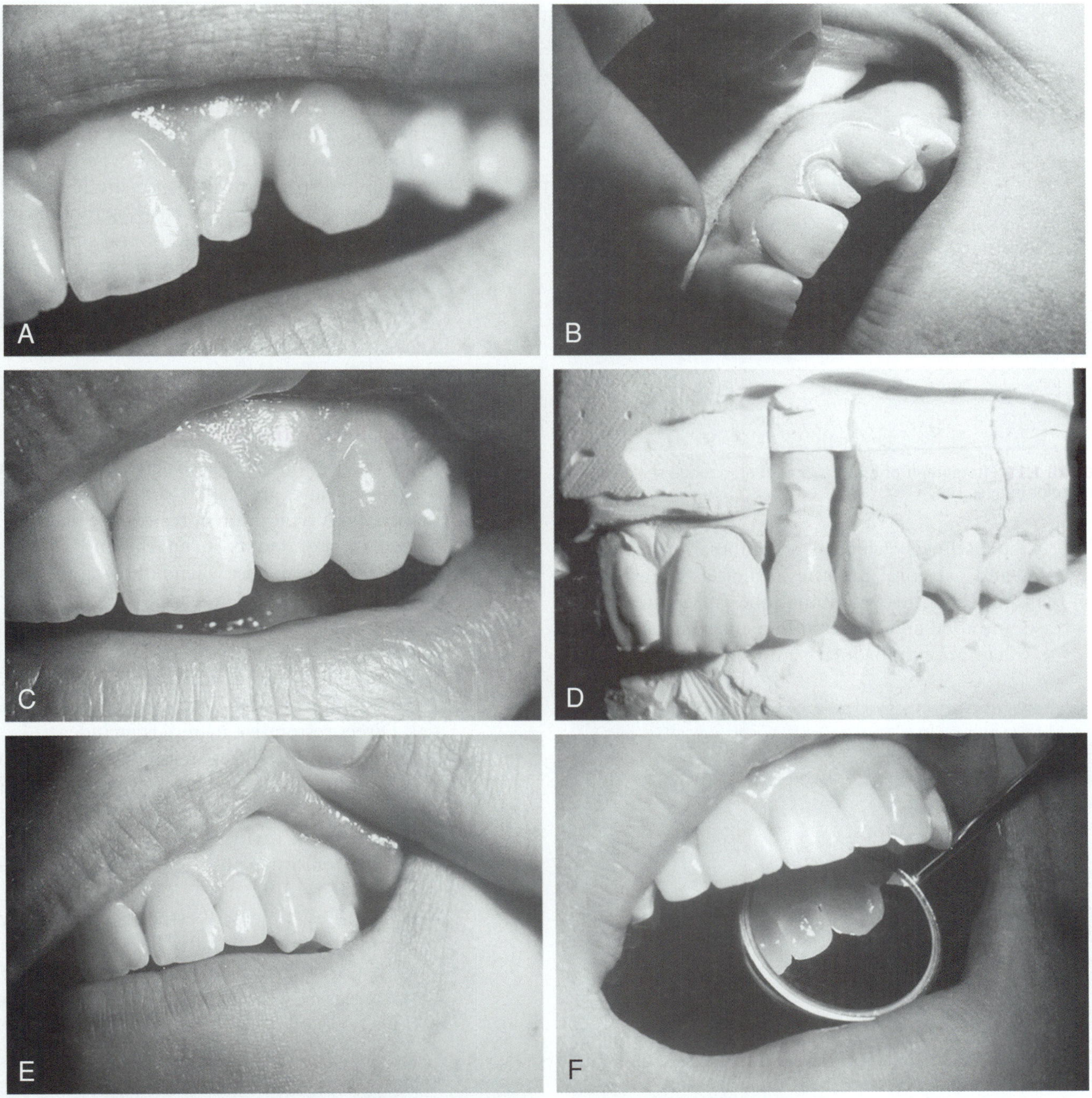

FIGURE 1.10 Restorative photographic series. **A.** Preoperative "peg-shaped" lateral incisor. **B.** Crown preparation. **C.** Temporary crown. **D.** Articulated casts with a permanent all-ceramic crown. **E** and **F.** Cemented crown in place. (See color images.)

or posts that are anchored into alveolar bone and that protrude through the gingiva into the oral cavity. An illustration of a dental implant is shown in Chapter 12. Implants are used to replace the root portion of lost teeth. Implants are unique in that they are both inside the body (in the alveolar bone) and outside the body (exposed in the oral cavity). Keeping the contents of the oral cavity from seeping along the surface of the implant into the supporting bone has been a very difficult problem. Luckily, this may be accomplished with the use of several materials if they are manufactured and handled properly.

Dental implants are used to support a great variety of restorations or prostheses. Single crowns, bridges, and dentures can be supported by dental implants. Often, a **maxillofacial**

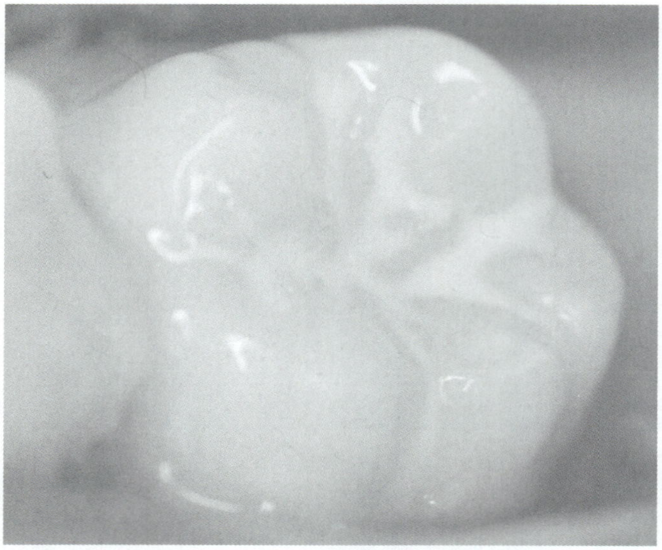

FIGURE 1.11 Photograph of tooth #19 with an opaque sealant. (See color images.)

prosthesis, which is a combination intraoral and extraoral prosthesis such as an artificial nose/denture combination, is retained with intraoral and extraoral implants. Implants have had an extraordinary impact on patient care when traditional restorative treatments have failed to provide adequate function.

11. Specialty Materials

Many specialties in dentistry have products and materials unique to that field. At times, these products overlap (e.g., sutures), whereas others are limited strictly to that specialty (e.g., "rubber bands" or elastics used in orthodontics). Many times, the specialties of oral surgery and periodontics use the same (or very similar) materials for bone regeneration. These materials that are used in the dental specialties are discussed further in Chapter 13.

B. Classification by Location of Fabrication

1. Direct Restorative Materials

Some restorations are constructed directly in the oral cavity and are called **direct restorative materials.** A typical direct restorative material is placed in the **"cavity preparation"** that was "drilled" by the dentist when removing the decay (see Fig. 1.9).

Each material has its own requirements for the design of the cavity preparation. When initially placed, a direct material is a putty-like material that sets to become a hard, strong material. Direct restorative materials include:

a) Amalgam, a metallic material that is formed by combining liquid mercury with powdered metals. The freshly mixed amalgam is placed directly in the cavity, is carved to resemble the missing tooth structure, and then hardens (see Figs. 1.3 and 1.9).

b) Composites, which are esthetic materials that polymerize in the mouth. These are supplied as pastes that are placed into the preparation and are set by a specific chemical reaction (Fig. 1.13).

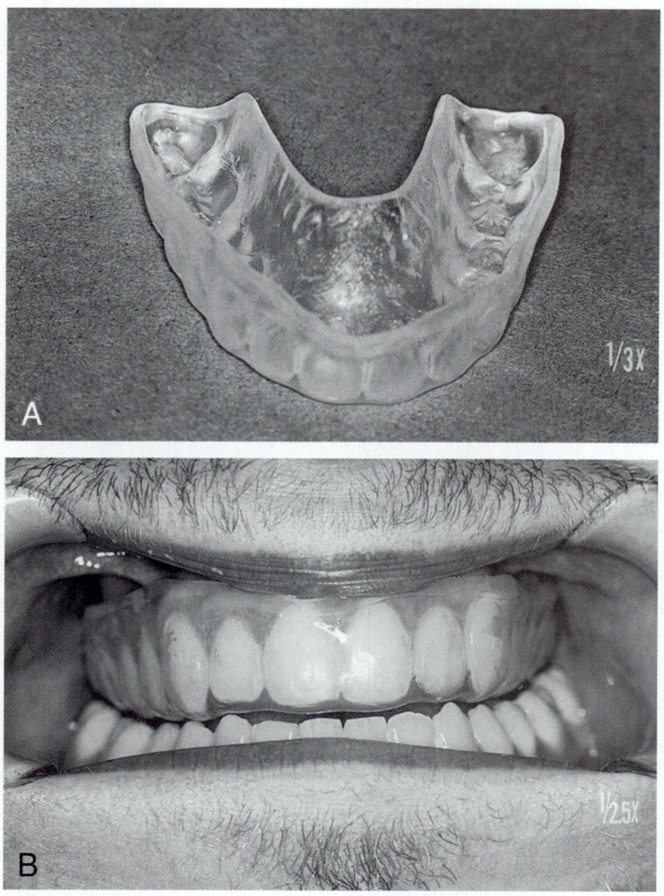

FIGURE 1.12 Photographs of a mouthguard **(A)** and of the mouthguard in place **(B)**.

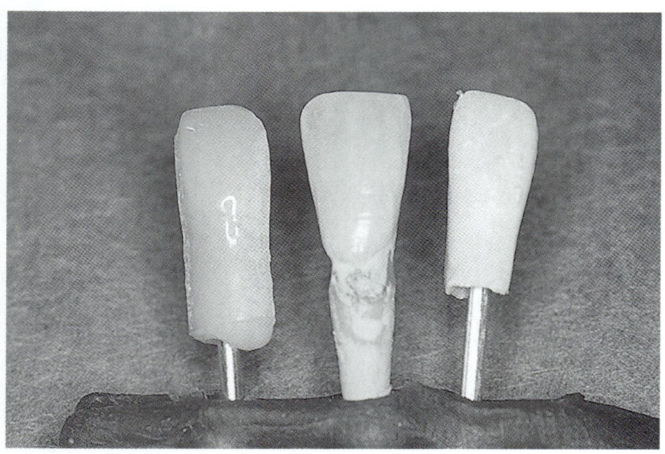

FIGURE 1.13 Photograph of, from *left* to *right*, a composite sample, an extracted tooth, and a glass ionomer sample.

c) Glass ionomers and other cements, which are mortar-like materials that set by an acid-base chemical reaction in the mouth (see Fig. 1.13) and resemble tooth material.

2. Indirect Restorative Materials

Other materials must be fabricated outside the mouth because the processing conditions of many materials would harm oral tissues. Such materials are called **indirect restorative materials** because they are made indirectly on a replica of the patient's oral tissues. Indirect materials include:

a) "Gold" crowns and inlays, which are restorations that are made by melting metals and pouring (forcing) them into molds of the exact size and shape needed for each patient (see Figs. 1.3 and 1.4).

b) Ceramic materials, which are processed by a number of techniques. Many times, a ceramic powder is fired at a very high temperature and becomes a solid object (just as a clay pot is fired). An example would be a porcelain crown (see Fig. 1.10).

c) Indirect restorative polymers, which are plastics typically processed or cured at elevated temperatures and under high pressures. An example would be the pink "gingival" portion of a denture (see Figs. 1.6 and 1.7).

C. Classification by Longevity of Use

1. Permanent Restorations

Permanent restorations are those restorations that are not planned to be replaced in a particular time period. Although they are referred to as permanent, they are not. Fillings, crowns, bridges, and dentures do not last forever. All restorative dentistry wears out and fails! Quality restorative dentistry in a well-maintained oral cavity, however, will give the patient years and years of service. It is best to prevent the need for restoration and replacement of teeth by aggressive preventive dentistry. The cycle of restoration and re-restoration of teeth is becoming an important factor in the practice of dentistry. What is best for the patient for a lifetime of oral health must be considered along with the immediate dental needs of the patient.

2. Temporary Restorations

Temporary restorations are restorations that are planned to be replaced in a short time (e.g., a week or a month). As discussed earlier, temporary crowns are placed after the tooth is prepared for a permanent crown and are used to protect the tooth while the final restoration is being made at the dental laboratory (see Fig. 1.10*C*).

3. Interim Restoration

At times, dental treatment requires "long-term" temporary restorations or "interim" restorations. An example would be a patient who has a fractured front tooth and needs a crown but is presently undergoing orthodontic treatment. A large composite restoration may be adequate until orthodontic treatment is completed or the tooth is close to its final position, and a permanent crown may then be fabricated.

VI. Classification of Dental Caries and Restorations

Dental caries are not evenly distributed throughout the mouth. Certain surfaces of the teeth are particularly susceptible to carious lesions; others are nearly immune. In the late 1800s, Dr. G.V. Black classified the most common sites for dental caries. His classification system adequately describes most simple carious lesions. In high-caries patients, a single tooth may have more than one lesion. These lesions may be of the same class or of different classes. At times, extensive lesions could be described as being a combination of two classes.

A. Class I

The pits and fissures of teeth, particularly posterior teeth, are the most susceptible to dental caries. Pit and fissure caries are called Class I lesions, and the associated restorations are called Class I restorations. Figures 1.14 and 5.10 show Class I caries and restorations in a molar.

B. Class II

The area of the tooth just below the interproximal contact is also susceptible to caries. If such a lesion occurs in a posterior tooth, it is called a Class II lesion. Dental radiographs are commonly used to diagnose Class II caries. Figures 1.3, 1.9, 1.14, 6.10, and 15.6 show Class II caries and restorations in molars and premolars.

C. Class III

If interproximal caries occur in an anterior tooth, it is called a Class III lesion. Dental radiographs and clinical examination are commonly used to diagnose Class III lesions. Figures 1.14 and 1.15 show Class III caries and restorations.

D. Class IV

If a Class III lesion is left untreated, it may progress and involve the incisal angle of an anterior tooth. A

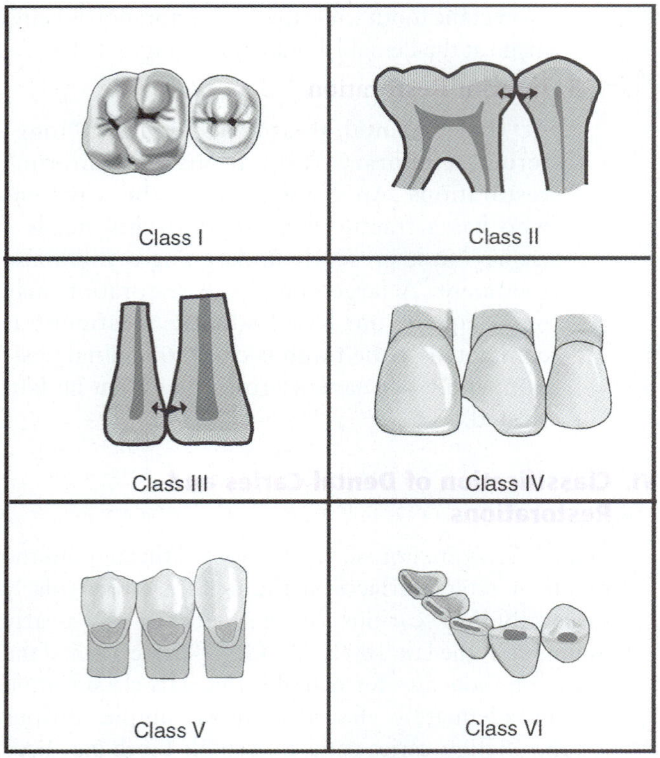

FIGURE 1.14 Drawing depicting the Dr. G.V. Black classification of caries.

lesion that involves the incisal angle of an anterior tooth is called a Class IV lesion (see Fig 1.14). Class IV restorations are also used to restore the incisal angle of an anterior tooth that has been fractured as the result of trauma, as shown in Figures 5.9 and 13.1*B*.

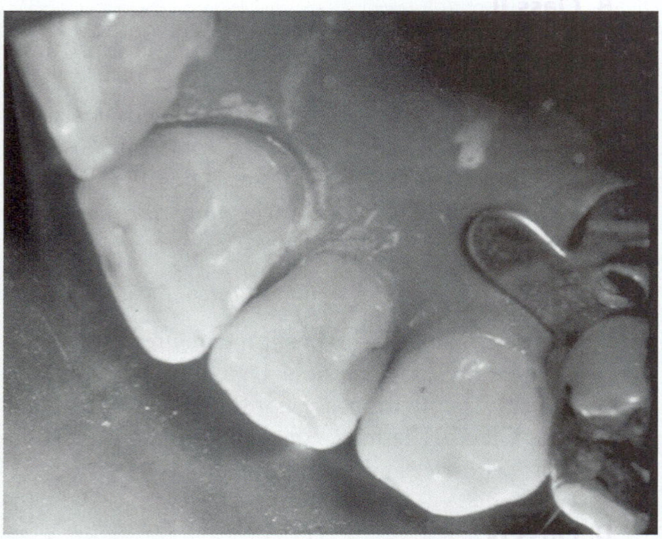

FIGURE 1.15 Photograph showing a Class III stained composite in the distal of tooth #7 and a Class III lesion (white chalky area) on the distal of tooth #8. (Courtesy of Dr. Birgitta Brown, Morgantown, WV.)

E. Class V

The gingival third of the facial and lingual surfaces of both anterior and posterior teeth is susceptible to caries when patients have poor oral hygiene or a high-sugar diet. Class V caries and restorations are shown in Figures 1.14, 5.12, and 6.13.

F. Class VI

The Class VI lesion was a later addition to Black's classification. As shown in Figure 1.14, a Class VI lesion involves the cusp tip or incisal edge of a tooth. Actually, a Class VI carious lesion is quite rare. For most people retaining a large number of teeth later in life, however, wear of cusp tips and incisal edges is not uncommon. When attrition causes dentin to become exposed, it wears much faster than the surrounding enamel because enamel is much harder than dentin. The result is a "dished out" area of worn dentin (Fig. 1.16) . Some clinicians call these restorations of such worn cusp tips and incisal edges Class VI restorations.

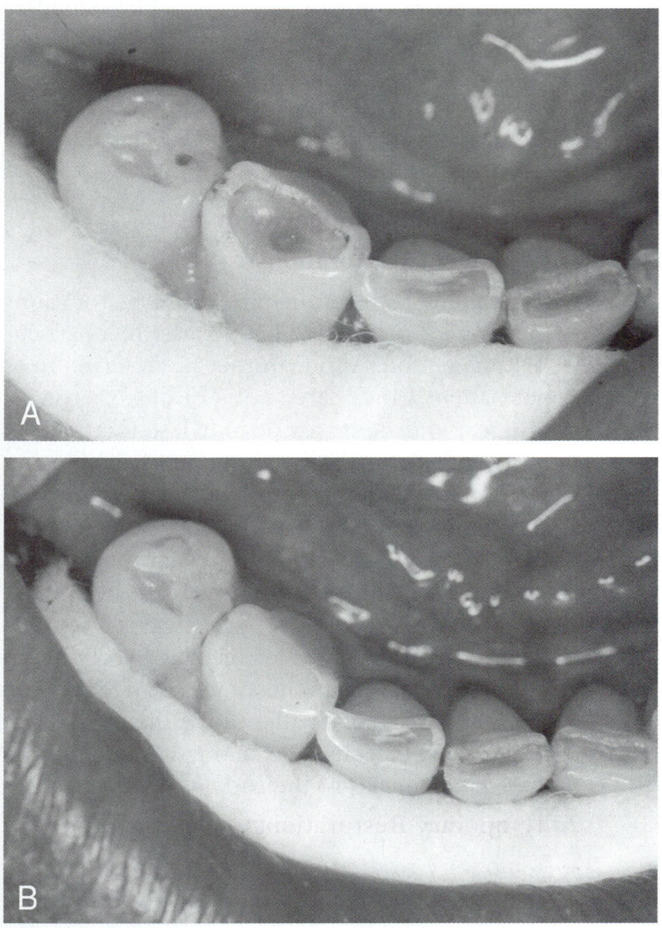

FIGURE 1.16 Photographs of severely worn teeth **(A)** and a composite restoration protecting the dentin of tooth #27 **(B)**. (Courtesy of Dr. Birgitta Brown, Morgantown, WV.)

SUMMARY

The dental hygienist should be knowledgeable in the science of dental materials for several reasons. It should be clear why a restorative material is prescribed for one restoration rather than for another. The best material is selected based on its behavior for providing function and service to the patient. Handling materials properly will enhance the function and longevity of the material that is placed into the patient's mouth. The hygienist must be able to recognize all dental materials so that they can be maintained in the proper manner. The ability to educate patients and answer their questions about the characteristics and properties of dental materials is yet another reason.

Dental professionals must remember that oral tissues, such as enamel, dentin, pulp, periodontium, and gingival tissues, are biologic materials and that they function in the hostile environment of the oral cavity. This environment places restrictions on which materials may be used to replace oral tissue. These restrictions include biting forces, degradation of teeth and materials, temperature changes, biocompatibility, and esthetics.

In the United States, standards are published and administered by ANSI. Other organizations work under their guidance to develop and administer standards for products of their industry. The ADA's Council on Scientific Affairs is one such organization that sets the standards and guidelines for evaluating dental products. The Medical Device Amendment of 1976 ensures the safety of all medical devices. The U.S. FDA considers dental materials to be devices, of which there are three classes. The ISO attempts to unify the standards of its member countries throughout the world.

Dental materials can be classified in three ways: by use, by location of fabrication, or by longevity. When classifying by use, a dental material would be listed under one of the following categories: restorations, crowns, bridges, complete and partial dentures; impressions, casts and models, cements; temporary materials; preventive materials; polishing materials; implants; and specialty materials. When classifying by location of fabrication, a dental material would be listed under one of two categories: direct restorative materials, which are fabricated directly in the mouth and include materials such as amalgam, composites, and glass ionomer; and indirect restorative materials, which are fabricated outside the mouth and include materials such as gold, ceramics, and special polymers. When classifying by longevity of use, a dental material would be listed under one of three categories: permanent, temporary, and interim restorations.

Dental caries and restorations are also classified into categories. The categories were developed by Dr. G.V. Black during the late 1800s and are still used today.

Learning Activities

1. Discuss other examples of products used in everyday life that have standards on which we rely for their safety and effectiveness.
2. In the clinic, divide into pairs and, with the use of hand and/or mouth mirrors, look for different kinds of dental materials, such as restorations, sealants, orthodontic retainers, and temporary restorations.
3. Classify the restorations that you found in activity 2 using Black's classification system.
4. Classify five of the restorations found in activity 2 by the location of fabrication (direct or indirect).
5. Pull patient charts and radiographs, and look for restorations and other dental materials.
6. In a drug store, see how many different kinds of over-the-counter dental products are available that carry the ADA Seal of Acceptance.
7. Referring to the following list of restorations, briefly discuss the specific home care instructions that would be necessary for your patient to maintain optimal oral health:
   - A four-unit, fixed partial denture
   - An implant
   - A removable partial denture
   - A porcelain-fused-to-metal crown.

Review Questions

1. In the United States, standards for dental materials are developed and administered by the:
a) FDA (Food and Drug Administration)
b) ADA (American Dental Association)
c) AADR (American Association for Dental Research)
d) OSHA (Occupational Safety and Health Administration)

2. All of the following are reasons for a dental hygienist to have a knowledge and understanding of dental materials EXCEPT:
a) Explaining the different types of restorative materials available to the patient
b) Assessing the patient's oral condition
c) Deciding which material is best for the patient's restoration
d) Understanding the behavior of dental materials

3. An amalgam restoration located on the gingival third of tooth #3 would be a Class _____ restoration.
a) I
b) II
c) III
d) IV
e) V
f) VI

4. The biologic nature of the oral environment and the size of the oral cavity restrict the use of dental materials. One restriction is the degradation of restorations.
a) The first statement is true; the second statement is false.
b) The first statement is false; the second statement is true.
c) Both statements are true.
d) Both statements are false.

5. When the temperature changes in the mouth, the teeth and most restorative materials expand and contract by the same amount. No leakage occurs around the restoration.
a) The first statement is true; the second statement is false.
b) The first statement is false; the second statement is true.
c) Both statements are true.
d) Both statements are false.

6. Which of the following oral tissues provides feedback to the individual regarding the forces placed on the tooth?
a) Pulp
b) Dentin
c) Periodontium
d) Gingival tissue

7. Which of the following restorations are utilized when a substantial amount of a tooth is missing?
a) Crown
b) Pontic
c) Implant
d) Fixed partial denture

8. The design of a cavity preparation aids in the retention of a restoration. The walls of an amalgam preparation diverge while the walls of an inlay converge.
a) The first statement is true; the second statement is false.
b) The first statement is false; the second statement is true.
c) Both statements are true.
d) Both statements are false.

9. If a restoration is fabricated on a replica (positive reproduction) of a patient's teeth, it is referred to as a:
a) Student model
b) Cast
c) Diagnostic cast
d) Any of the above terms may be used

10. An example of an indirect restorative material would be:
a) Amalgam
b) Glass ionomer cement
c) Composite
d) Ceramic (porcelain)

Supplemental Readings

Anusavice KJ. Phillips' Science of Dental Materials. 11th ed. Philadelphia: Saunders, 2003, Chapter 1.

Powers JM & Sakaguchi RL, eds. Craig's Restorative Dental Materials. 12th ed. St. Louis: Mosby, 2006, Chapter 1.

Jablonski S. Illustrated Dictionary of Dentistry. Philadelphia: Saunders, 1982.

Stedman's Medical Dictionary for the Dental Professions. Baltimore: Lippincott Williams & Wilkins, 2006.

Wilkins EM. Clinical Practice of the Dental Hygienist. 9th ed. Baltimore: Lippincott Williams & Wilkins, 2008, Chapter 1.

Materials Science and Dentistry

2

Objectives

After studying this chapter, the student will be able to do the following:

1. List the phases into which materials are classified. Discuss the varying amounts of attraction between the molecules and atoms of each phase. Recall the differentiating characteristics of each phase.
2. Explain the basic difference between primary and secondary bonds.
3. Name the three types of primary bonds, and describe the differences between them.
4. Summarize the similarities and differences of secondary bonds, which include permanent dipoles, hydrogen bonds, and fluctuating dipoles.
5. Contrast the bonding characteristics of metals, ceramics, plastics, and composites.

Key Words/Phrases

amorphous
ceramic
colloids
composites
covalent bonds
cross-linking
crystalline
dental materials
emulsions
fluctuating dipole
hydrogen bonds
ionic bonds
long-range order
materials science
metallic bonds
metals
permanent dipole
polymers
primary bonds
secondary bonds
short-range order
valence electrons

INTRODUCTION

Many different kinds of materials are used to make the products we use in everyday life and in the profession of dentistry. Understanding the behavior of materials is important in the selection, placement, and maintenance of dental materials. The behavior of any given material is based on the atomic bonds in that material. Many will think the material covered in this chapter is too theoretical for dental hygiene students. If so, the authors urge you to skip this chapter and read only the summary at the end.

I. Materials Science

Materials science is the part of the physical sciences that seeks to explain the properties and performance of materials by examining their internal structure. Materials science is a combination of chemistry, physics, and engineering rather than a separate scientific domain. Materials science tries to explain why materials behave as they do, based on the atoms and molecules in materials and the bonds that exist between these atoms and molecules. Materials science also tries to understand the effects of manufacturing processes on materials and any changes in materials that may occur during the useful life of a product. In dentistry, a subgroup of materials science has developed. This subgroup, called **dental materials,** is part of the larger field of biomaterials and, at times, is called dental biomaterials. Whatever term we use, however, the goal is to understand why materials behave the way they do and how the clinician can maximize the performance of these materials.

In this book, the handling (processing) of dental materials will be stressed, and a discussion of the underlying materials science will be included as well. At times, simply memorizing step-by-step procedures will seem to be much easier, but understanding their nature will simplify the use of the vast number of materials currently on the market. No other branch of scientific inquiry has a greater impact on our day-to-day lives than the development of new materials and the innovative ways in which these materials are being used.

II. Atomic Bonding

How do teeth withstand the forces that occur when we bite and grind food? To understand the strength of teeth, we need to understand the nature of atomic bonds. Teeth and restorative materials need to be stronger—and to have stronger atomic bonds—than the food we eat.

A. Phases

We commonly classify materials into one of three phases: solid, liquid, or gas. Familiarity with these phases will provide a foundation for understanding the nature of the forces that hold atoms together in materials. Later in this chapter, we will discuss colloids, which are a mixture of two of these phases.

1. Gases

The atomic bonds between gas molecules are very weak. These bonds are easily broken by the normal microscopic vibrations of atoms at room temperature. These atomic vibrations are the result of the thermal energy of the material. Gases have no molecular organization and will take on the three-dimensional shape of any container that they fill. If thermal energy is removed by cooling, gases condense into liquids. An example is the condensation of water vapor on the outside of a mug of ice-cold root beer on a hot, humid day.

2. Liquids

Liquids have stronger attraction between molecules than gases do, but this attraction is not strong enough to carry a load or to maintain a shape without support. The attraction between molecules results in short-range order. **Short-range order** is a consistent spatial relationship among atoms or molecules 5 to 10 neighbors apart. Liquids lack long-range order. Molecular attraction keeps liquids from boiling, but not always from evaporating. Other characteristics of a liquid are vapor pressure, boiling temperature, viscosity, and surface tension.

3. Solids

Solids exhibit the strongest attraction between atoms and molecules. The atomic bonds of solids maintain the shape of objects and resist external forces placed on them. Solids can be classified as crystalline or amorphous. **Crystalline** solids have a consistent spatial relationship of atoms or molecules repeated hundreds to thousands to millions of times that is called **long-range order** (Fig. 2.1*A*). The distances and angles among such atoms or molecules are uniform, much like rooms in a dormitory or hotel. Table salt, diamonds, and the hydroxyapatite of teeth are crystalline solids. Crystalline solids have both short-range and long-range order of their atoms or molecules.

Amorphous solids (Fig. 2.1*B*) have the same strong atomic bonds but only short-range order, much like liquids. The glass in a window or a dental mirror is an amorphous solid. Some solid objects are stronger than others. The difference is determined by the type of atoms that make up the material and the strength of the atomic bonds that hold the material together. Some materials can be amorphous or

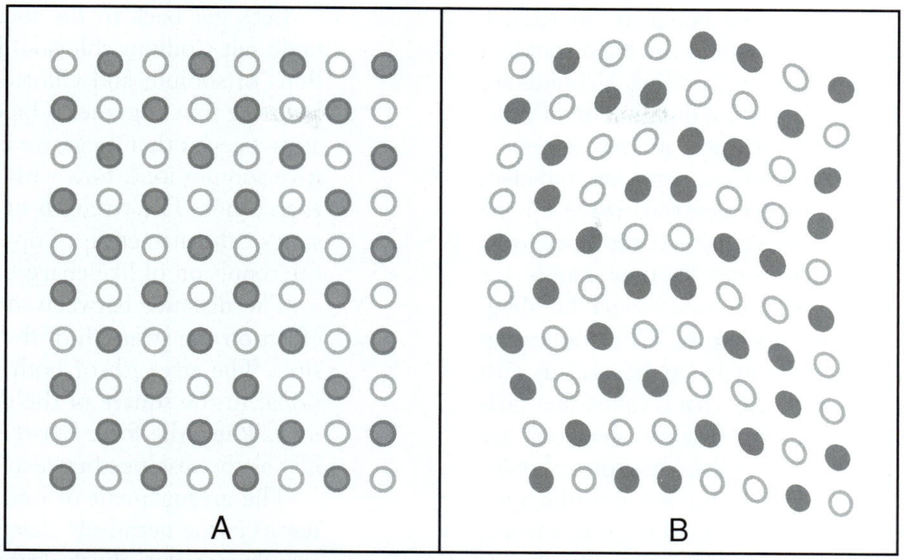

FIGURE 2.1 A two-dimensional depiction of the arrangement of atoms in a crystal **(A)** and an amorphous solid **(B)**.

crystalline. They tend to be stronger if they are crystalline, but making them so can be difficult.

B. Atomic Bonds in Solids

How does a strong solid object know how much force it needs to resist the load of an object resting on its surface? If you place a 2-pound book on a table, the table pushes up with 2 pounds of force, just enough to support the book—not too little, and not too much. How does the table know to push up with 2 pounds of force? This "smart" behavior is a characteristic of solid objects and a function of the nature of atomic bonds in materials.

Atomic bonds are a result of electromagnetic (EM) force. For this discussion, we will focus on the electronic part of the EM force. The electronic force causes positive charges to attract negative charges and negative charges to attract positive charges. Positive charges are repelled by positive charges, and negative charges are repelled by negative charges. The magnetic force exhibits similar attraction and repulsion and is easily demonstrated with two magnets. We will use the familiar magnetic force to help us understand attraction and repulsion. The north pole of a magnet attracts the south pole and repels the north pole. It takes force to bring the north poles of two magnets into proximity. The closer they get, the harder you have to push, much like a spring. In fact, the atomic bonds between atoms act much like the springs of a mattress or a car.

To compress a spring, it must be pushed. To stretch a spring, it must be pulled. When no force is applied to a spring, it is said to be unloaded and has an equilibrium length. When force is applied, the spring changes length and resists the applied force by developing an equal and opposite force. Solids can be thought of as a collection of millions and millions of springs or atomic bonds. When you place a book on a table, the atomic bonds of the table are compressed and oppose the force of the book. The heavier the book, the more the bonds are compressed and the greater the force that is developed in the table. Is this really true? We do not see the table change height when we put the book on it. We must remember that the table has millions and millions of atoms and, therefore, millions and millions of atomic bonds. Each bond is compressed a submicroscopic distance. The total of the change in length of these bonds is still microscopic, too small to be seen by the unaided eye, but the change in height of the table can be measured with specialized equipment. Again, the atomic bonds of the table are compressed when a book is placed on it, and these bonds act like springs. When one stretches a rubber band, the same phenomenon occurs, but it can be seen by the unaided eye. Different kinds of internal atomic bonds respond to external forces in different manners.

The change in the height of the table when a book is placed on it is an example of something that happens but that we cannot see happen. These changes may be microscopic, or they may occur very slowly and, thus, may not be noticed. Such changes occur in dentistry: Teeth compress when biting, erupt into the mouth, change color during a person's lifetime, wear, and dissolve in acids, forming caries.

C. Primary Bonds—Optional

Primary bonds are the strong bonds between atoms that involve the transfer or sharing of electrons between atoms. In high-school and college chemistry classes, the ionic and covalent bonds are presented. Another bond that is important to the understanding of certain materials is the metallic bond. All bonds are a result of the EM force and the distribution of positive and negative charges of atoms and molecules.

The atom is made of protons, neutrons, and electrons. The protons and the neutrons make up the nucleus; the electrons move around the nucleus in shells. Electrons in the outer shell of atoms are involved in chemical reactions and atomic bonding. They are called **valence electrons.** When discussing atomic bonding, it is easier to group the nucleus with the nonvalence electrons into what is called the "positive core." The remaining valence electrons are those that are principally involved in atomic bonds. We can therefore restrict our discussion to the positive core of the atom and the valence electrons. Explaining why some elements form metallic bonds and others form covalent bonds is beyond the scope of this text (and its authors' understanding of the subject). However, understanding how atoms fill up their outer shell with electrons from other atoms will help us to understand the nature of atomic bonds and give us some insight regarding why materials behave as they do.

1. Ionic Bonds

Ionic bonds are the result of an electron being given up by one atom and being accepted by another. Why does an atom give up or accept an electron? Atoms are "content" when their outer shell of electrons is full; in this situation, they have a lower state of energy. An element like sodium has one valence electron in its outer shell, and it will readily give up this valence electron. If a sodium atom gives up this valence electron, the next inner shell becomes the outer shell and is a full shell. The atom then becomes an ion with a charge of +1. An element such as chlorine, however, is one electron short of filling its outer shell. Therefore, chlorine readily accepts an electron and becomes an ion with a charge of –1. When sodium and chlorine bond to each other, both will have full outer shells. The opposite electrical charges of these ions attract each other, and atomic bonding results.

Chemical reactions, in which atoms fill their outer shells with electrons and form bonds, are examples of nature lowering the energy of a system. Other examples of systems lowering their energy include a ball rolling downhill, water flowing over a waterfall, a candle burning, and a battery powering a flashlight. The conversion of energy from one form to another (whether chemical, electrical, mechanical, or thermal) is governed by the laws of thermodynamics. Again, such forbidding subjects are beyond the scope of this text.

Let's get back to the ionic bond. A grain of table salt (sodium chloride) has billions and billions of sodium and chloride ions. Ionic bonds hold the ions together. Oppositely charged ions attract each other (negative chloride ion and positive sodium ion). Ions with like charges repulse each other. The strength of the salt grain is the sum of the attraction of opposite charges minus the repulsion of like charges.

The distance between ions has an important effect on the strength of the attraction or repulsion. The strength of both is inversely proportional to the square of the distance between the ions. Thus, the force between the ions falls rapidly as the distance between the pair increases.

The arrangement of ions in sodium chloride results in the negatively charged chloride ions surrounding each positively charged sodium ion. Likewise, each negative ion is surrounded by positive ions. The familiar checkerboard pattern is a two-dimensional example of such an arrangement. As a result, the attraction between oppositely charged "next-door neighbors" is strong because they are close together. The repulsion of similarly charged ion pairs is weaker because they are farther apart (Fig. 2.2). The attraction forces overpower the repulsive forces, and the result is a strong material.

2. Covalent Bonds

Covalent bonds between two atoms are the result of two atoms sharing a pair of electrons (Fig. 2.3). Sharing electrons with other atoms allows an atom

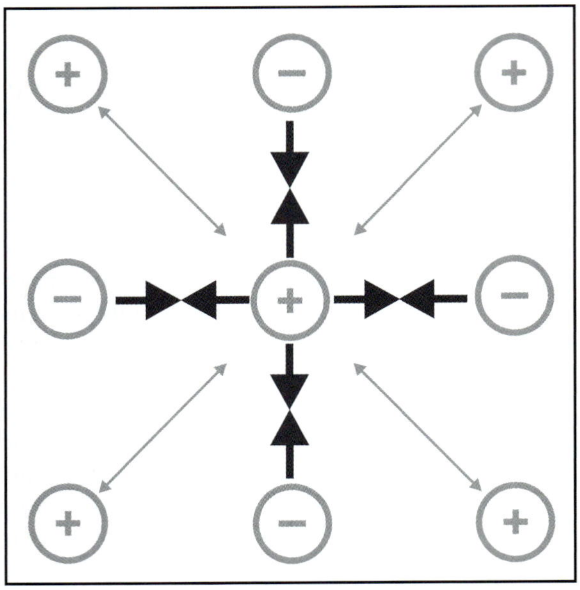

FIGURE 2.2 A two-dimensional depiction of an ionic material. The *black arrows* pointing toward each other represent the attraction of unlike-charged ions. These ions are closer; therefore, the force is stronger. The *gray arrows* pointing away represent repulsion of like-charged ions. The like-charged ions are farther apart; therefore, the force is weaker.

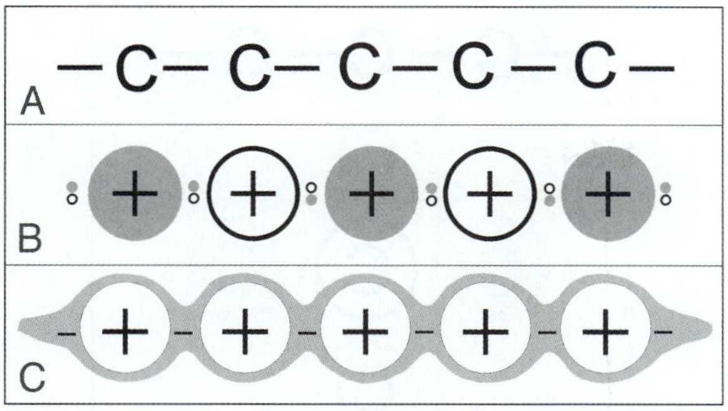

FIGURE 2.3 Three representations of covalent bonds between carbon atoms. In **A,** *lines* represent the bonds. In **B,** pairs of shared electrons represent the bonds. In **C,** the distribution of the electrons is shown. Note in **C** the alternating negative charges of the electrons and positive charges of the cores.

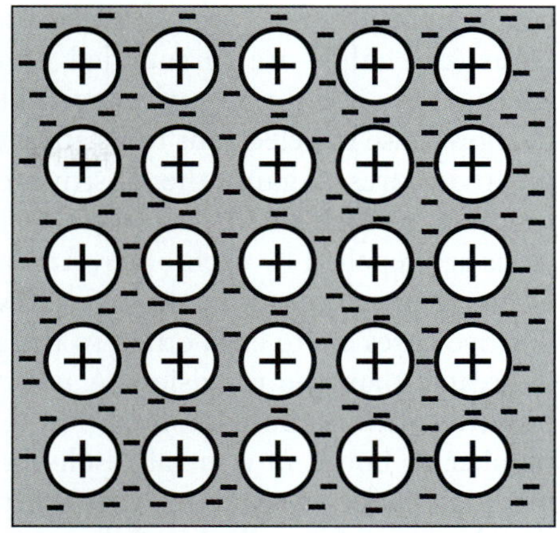

FIGURE 2.4 A two-dimensional representation of the metallic bond. Note that the positive cores (nuclei and nonvalence electrons) are surrounded by an electron "cloud."

to fill its outer shell with electrons and, thus, to lower its energy. How does sharing a pair of electrons bond two atoms together?

The physical space that an electron occupies around the nucleus is called an orbital, and it is centered around the nucleus when not involved in an atomic bond. When two atoms share an electron, the shape of the orbital changes. When a pair of electrons is shared and forms a covalent bond, the orbital surrounds both atoms. Now the electrons spend some time in the physical space between the two atoms. By spending time between the two atoms, bonding of the two atoms occurs. A partial negative charge is created by the presence of the electron pair between the two atoms. The partial negative charge of the bond is attracted to the positive cores of the two atoms that are sharing the electron pair. The positive core of the first atom is attracted to the relatively close partial negative charge (because of the electron pair spending time there) between the atoms. The same is true for the second atom that shares the electron pair.

The attraction of the partial negative charge to the two positive cores is greater than the repulsion between the positive cores because the distance between the two positive cores is greater. We have probably set organic chemistry back a century with this simplistic description of the covalent bond, but it will serve our purposes and help to explain the behavior of polymers (and it's the best the authors can do).

Covalent bonds between the two atoms sharing the electron pair are strong and very directional. However, few materials are bonded with only covalent bonds. One well-known material that is covalently bonded is diamond. Each carbon atom is bonded to four other carbon atoms via a covalent bond. One of the hardest materials known results from this bonding. Many materials are the result of long chains of covalently bonded atoms. The chains are strong, but the materials are not always strong. This is because their properties are determined by the manner in which the long chains are bonded to each other. Polymers are long chains of covalently bonded carbon atoms. Examples of polymers include man-made plastics and rubbers as well as many biologic macromolecules, such as proteins and DNA. The varied properties of polymers and plastics will be better explained in the discussion of secondary bonds.

3. Metallic Bonds

Metals have characteristic properties that allow us to easily identify a material as being a metal. Metals are typically dense, heavy materials. They are good conductors of both electricity and heat, are cold to the touch at room temperature, and, if shaped properly, will ring like a bell if struck. All these properties of metals are a result of metallic bonds. **Metallic bonds** are similar to covalent bonds in that valence electrons are shared between atoms. The difference is that the electrons in a metal object are not shared by two atoms; instead, they are shared by all the atoms that make up that object (Fig. 2.4). We can illustrate this difference by comparing a marriage to students in a school. In a marriage, the relationship is between two people, and the sharing is between those two. Within a school, however, all students are part of the student body. They have a less intense relationship, but they all share the feeling of being part of the school.

Metals can be thought of as positive cores in a cloud of negative mobile valence electrons, much like chocolate chips in ice cream. The chocolate chips are the positive cores, and the ice cream is the electron cloud. Because the positive cores (the chips) are surrounded by electrons (the ice cream), the negative–positive electric charges cause the electrons to be attracted to the positive cores. Again, the positive cores are repelled by each other, and the negative electrons are repelled by each other. And again, the electrons are closer to the positive cores than the positive cores are to each other, so the attraction is greater than the repulsion. A weak primary bond in all directions results. The enormous number of bonds in a metal results in a strong material. Later, we will see that the nondirectional nature of metallic bonds has an important effect on the properties and use of metals.

D. Secondary Bonds—Optional

Secondary bonds, or van der Waals forces, are the result of partial charges from an uneven distribution of electrons around an atom or a molecule. The partial charges can be temporary or permanent, very weak or somewhat strong. Secondary bonds are important in determining the properties of polymers because they determine the interaction of the polymer chains and, thus, the properties of the polymer itself.

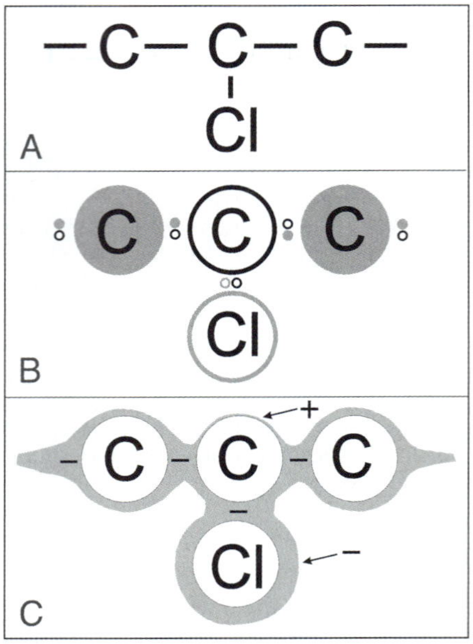

FIGURE 2.5 Three representations of a permanent dipole. In **A,** *lines* represent the bonds. In **B,** pairs of shared electrons are shown. In **C,** the distribution of the electrons is seen. The electron density is greater around the chlorine atom and less around the middle carbon atom. Note in **C** the uneven distribution of the electron density that results in partial charges or dipoles.

1. Permanent Dipoles

Depending on the type of atoms bonded by a covalent bond, the shared electrons may not be shared equally. Some atoms are "greedy" and pull the shared electrons more strongly toward themselves. The result is an uneven distribution of the electron pair around the atoms involved in the covalent bond. One atom involved in the bond is partially positive, and the other is partially negative. A permanent partial charge, or a **permanent dipole,** thus occurs (Fig. 2.5). When one molecule with such partial charges encounters another, the negative attracts the positive, and vice versa. Permanent dipoles result in weak bonds, but they have a significant effect on the behavior of many materials.

The dipoles that result from the chlorine atoms on the chain of a polyvinyl chloride (PVC) molecule make PVC a strong and stiff material. The bond between the carbon atom and the chlorine atom is not an equal sharing of electrons. Electrons are pulled toward the chlorine atoms, making it partially negative. The carbon atom is partially positive. The interaction of these partial charges reduces the slippage of the carbon chains against one another in molecules of PVC. A strong, stiff plastic (commonly used for drainpipes in houses) results. When electrons are more evenly distributed, the dipoles are much smaller, and the material is much weaker and much less stiff. An example of such a material is polyethylene, which is commonly used as a plastic wrap for food.

2. Hydrogen Bonds

Hydrogen bonds are a special case of a permanent dipole. The hydrogen atom contains only one electron. When this single electron is pulled away from the hydrogen nucleus by a "greedy" atom, such as oxygen, the nucleus is left partially unshielded, but to a much greater extent than in other elements with multiple electrons. The resulting interaction between molecules results in a bond that is much stronger than other secondary bonds.

We can understand the significance of unshielding the hydrogen nucleus if we consider four children in two beds during the cold of winter. Two children in one bed have one blanket, and the other two children have three blankets. If the blankets of both pairs of children were shared equally, then the partners in each pair would be equally comfortable. Each pair of children in a bed would have two blankets. However, our story has one bed with one blanket and one bed with three blankets. What happens if one child of the pair with three blankets gets cold and pulls one of the blankets completely over to his or her side of the bed? The other child is left with two shared blankets and might not notice much difference. What if the same thing happens with the other pair of children, the two with only one blanket? When the single blanket is pulled away, one child will get cold while the other child stays warm.

So is the case of the hydrogen atom: when its partner pulls away its only electron, its nucleus is more unshielded than the nucleus of other elements with multiple electrons in the same situation. A strong dipole occurs, and significant bonding between molecules results. Hydrogen bonding is important in biologic polymers, such as proteins and DNA. The three-dimensional structure of enzymes is determined by hydrogen bonding as the protein chain folds back on itself. In DNA, it is the hydrogen bonds that pair thymine with adenine and cytosine with guanine in the cross-links of the double helix.

3. Fluctuating Dipole

What about atoms or molecules without a permanent dipole (partial charges)? How do they stay together as solids or liquids? The noble gases, such as helium (He), have a symmetrical charge distribution; they have no dipole. Molecules of two of the same atoms, such as nitrogen gas, theoretically have a symmetrical charge distribution. Such atoms and molecules with a symmetrical charge distribution have very weak bonds between molecules. These gases need to be cooled to very low temperatures to liquefy. Their bonds are the result of an intermittent, uneven distribution of electrons around the atoms or molecules. These weak bonds are called a **fluctuating dipole** (Fig. 2.6). Although this uneven distribution lasts only for an extremely short time and is always changing, positive and negative charges result, as does a very weak attraction between these atoms or molecules.

If one thinks of an outside light at night during the summer, one can get a feeling for this ever-changing distribution. The insects flying around the light can be thought of as electrons, and the light is the positive core. The insects seem to fly around the light as if attracted by some unseen force. They are unable to escape the close proximity of the light, similar to the relationship of an electron and a positive core. If one observes the insects and the light for a few seconds, one sees that the insects are not always evenly spread out around the light. Sometimes, for a just a second or so, they congregate more to one side than to the other. The unevenness then quickly changes.

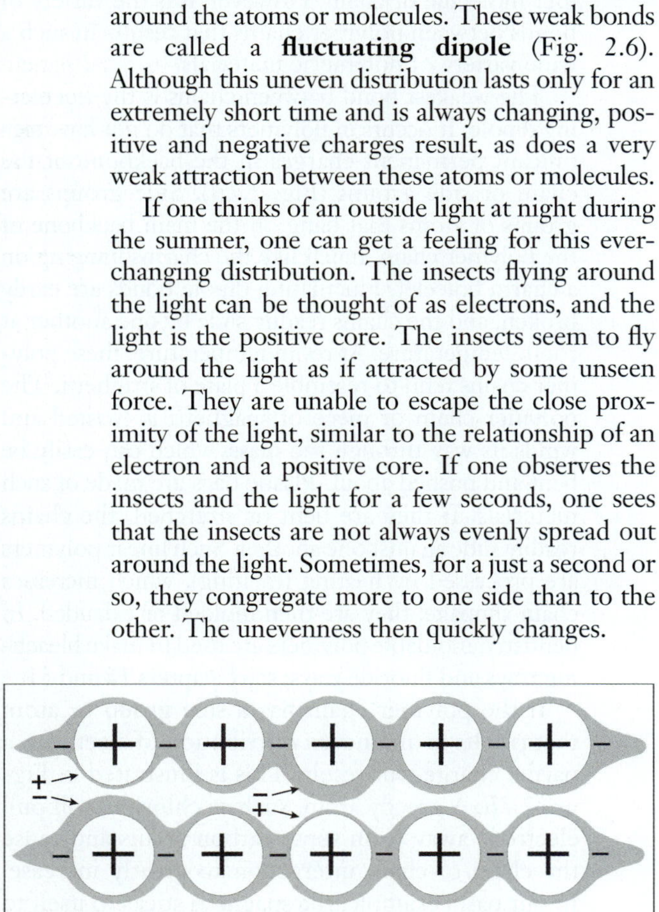

FIGURE 2.6 A fluctuating dipole. The intermittent, uneven distribution of the electron density (*gray-shaded area*) results in a constantly changing, or fluctuating, dipole.

Electrons around uncharged atoms and molecules behave in the same way. (Of course, the physical size of their orbits and the duration of the unevenness are millions and millions of times smaller than those of the insects and the light.) The result is a constantly changing, very weak attraction that allows uncharged atoms and molecules to be cooled down and liquefied, but only at very low temperatures.

4. Summary

Secondary bonds are the result of uneven electron distribution around atoms and molecules. The more uneven the distribution is, the stronger the charge, the greater the attraction, and the stronger the bond. Secondary bonding in materials is most important when combined with covalent bonding, as in polymers.

III. Materials and Their Atomic Bonds

The atoms that make up a material and how these atoms are bonded determine the properties of that material. Weak bonds make for weak materials, and vice versa. Materials can be classified into three categories based on their primary atomic bonds: metals, ceramics, and polymers. A fourth category is composites. Composites are "mixtures" of two materials from two different categories. Dental composites are a combination of a ceramic and a polymeric material.

A. Metals

Metals are held together with metallic bonds. Few metals, however, have pure metallic bonds. Most metals have bonds that are predominantly metallic but that also show some covalent or ionic tendency. The broad range of mixtures of metallic and other primary bonds results in metallic materials with a range of properties. In this chapter, we will focus on metals in which the metallic bond predominates. A good example is 24-carat gold, which is pure gold. Gold is ductile, meaning that it can easily be bent without breaking yet retains its strength. Gold behaves differently than a ceramic material, such as porcelain or plastic. This mechanical behavior is a result of the metallic bond.

What happens when an object is bent? Some atoms are pushed together. Others are pulled apart. Still others slide past one another. We will focus on the atoms' ability to slide by one another because this is an important determinant of mechanical properties. In a metal, each positive core is surrounded by an electron cloud. The positive core "feels" the attraction and repulsion of all the charges that make up the object, but what the core feels is greatly dominated by the electron cloud. What happens if an atom slides by another atom? Does the atom feel any difference in its surrounding? The electron cloud is still there and has not changed. Thus, the atom feels little (if any) difference. The surroundings (or the atomic bonding) have not changed, so the properties do not change. The ease with which metals can be bent and shaped enabled early humans to make strong tools that were tough and resisted fracture. What would happen if you tried to make a hammer out of a ceramic or a polymeric material rather than a metal?

In dentistry, we bend orthodontic wires and clasps of partial dentures. We also use instruments to adapt (marginate) the edges of a gold restoration closely to the tooth. All are examples of bending metals, a process that forces the atoms to slide against each other. It is the metallic bond that enables metals to have such useful properties.

B. Ceramics

The atoms of a **ceramic** material are bonded with ionic bonds. Table salt (sodium chloride) is a good example. Salt is strong but brittle. If enough force is applied to a grain of salt, it can be crushed. Why is salt so brittle? What happens if a sodium ion slides away from its original position next to a chloride ion? Because the chloride ion is surrounded by sodium ions, the next ion over is a sodium ion. Therefore, as a sodium ion slides past a chloride ion, it approaches another sodium ion, and now there is repulsion where there once was attraction. The sodium ions push away from each other, and the material breaks or fractures.

Many ceramic materials used in everyday life, such as dishes, concrete, china, and bricks, are bonded by both ionic and covalent bonds. The ionic bond dominates the behavior of the material, resulting in strong, brittle materials. The strong nature of the bonds of these materials is reflected in the high temperatures needed to process many ceramic materials and their chemical stability.

In dentistry, the notable advantage of ceramic materials is the range of colors that can be produced. Crowns made of ceramic materials are colored to match the appearance of the patient's natural teeth. These materials are also translucent, meaning that some light passes through, as in natural teeth. This translucency gives the ceramic crown a more natural appearance that other materials cannot provide (see Fig. 1.10*F*).

Some ceramic materials, such as glass, are transparent. There are actually many different kinds of glass, each with somewhat different compositions and manufacturing techniques. Glass is a general term for an amorphous or noncrystalline ceramic material. Many ceramic materials are strong and chemically inert, and they are used to make stain-resistant pots and baking dishes.

In summary, ceramic materials are strong when compressed, because the atoms are forced together. However, ceramic materials are weak and brittle when pulled or bent.

C. Polymers or Plastics

Polymers are composed of long chains of covalently bonded, repeating units. The chains are thousands of units long and consist of carbon, hydrogen, and other elements. A wide variety of polymers are used in everyday life. Some are soft, weak, and flexible; these are called "plastics." They make good toys, garbage bags, and fabrics. Others are hard, stiff, and fairly strong; these are called glassy polymers or resins. Such plastics are used to make parts for cars, outdoor furniture, plumbing pipes, and dishes. Another important group can be stretched out a great deal and still return to their original shape; these are called rubber materials. Where would we be without elastic waistbands or latex (rubber) gloves?

Why do polymers exhibit such a wide range of properties? Some properties of polymers are dependent on the covalent bonds between the carbon atoms that make up the backbone of the polymer molecule or chain. However, it is the variety of bonds between polymer chains that results in such a wide variety of polymeric materials.

The weakest bond between chains is the fluctuating dipole. It occurs in polymers that do not have significant permanent charges in the backbone of the chain or side groups (Fig. 2.7*A*). Side groups are groups of atoms that hang on the main backbone of the polymer chain, much like the charms hanging on a charm bracelet. Fluctuating dipole bonds are easily broken, and the chains readily slide by one another at room temperature. At room temperature, these polymer chains tend to resemble a plate of spaghetti. The polymer chain or piece of spaghetti is twisted and winds its way through the mass, which can easily be bent and pushed about. Plastic bags are made of such materials. If they are bent or stretched, the chains readily slide against one another. Such linear polymers are processed by heating (melting), which increases chain slippage; they are then molded or extruded. In dentistry, moldable polymers are used to make bleaching trays and fluoride trays; see Chapters 18 and 31.

If the polymer chain has a side group or atom that results in an uneven distribution of electrons, a partial charge will result. This is illustrated in Figure 2.7*B*. A greedy atom, such as chloride, will pull electrons away from some carbon atoms and cause the chain-to-chain interaction to greatly increase. In our pasta example, the spaghetti sticks to itself to a small extent. The previously discussed PVC is a good example. As the number and intensity of the charges increase, the strength and stiffness of the

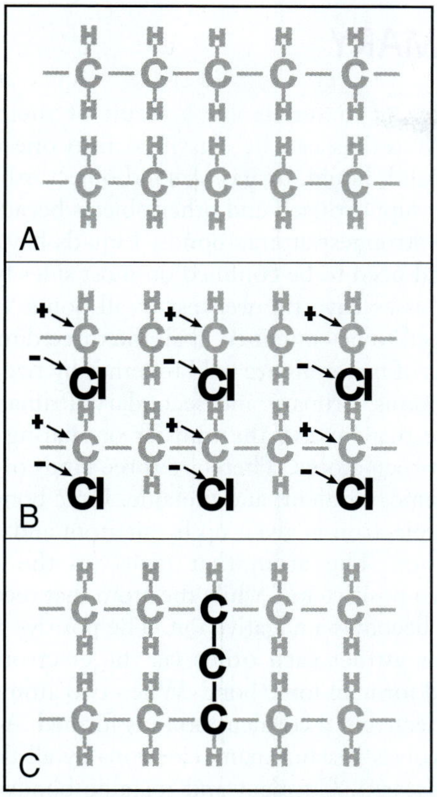

FIGURE 2.7 Three kinds of chain-to-chain interaction in a polymer. **A.** Linear polymer has weak secondary forces, as in Figure 2.6. **B.** Polymer with a permanent dipole is stronger. **C.** Cross-linking covalent bonds result in an even stronger polymeric material.

polymer increase. Also, higher temperatures are required to melt these polymers when they are processed. Some dental instruments are made from these stiff, plastic materials.

Polymers have been developed that go beyond the weak bonding of secondary bonds and incorporate primary atomic bonds between the chains in their polymeric structure. These polymers have cross-links between the chains (Fig. 2.7*C*). The chains are linked by covalently bonded atoms to form a three-dimensional structure and can no longer slide past each other, resulting in stiff, strong material. The structural biologic polymers, such as collagen fiber in animals and wood fiber in plants, fit into this group. Dental composite filling materials use cross-linked polymeric materials. Heat will not melt these polymers; the chains cannot slip by each other. If these materials are heated to a high-enough temperature, however, decomposition results, such as the burning of wood.

A few man-made polymers have charged groups hanging off the polymer backbone that result in ionic bonds between chains. Such polymers are not widely used in everyday life, but one is used in dentistry: polyacrylic acid, which will be discussed later. In biology, several amino acids have groups that ionize. These charged groups are the part of a protein that greatly affects its three-dimensional structure and function. The three-dimensional structure of protein is critical if an enzyme is to function properly.

Why do we keep using examples from biochemistry? The typical dental hygiene student has a good background in biology. Man-made polymers follow the same "rules" as those of the biologic polymers with which the student is familiar. Biologic polymers, such as collagen and DNA, form helical structures. It is the stretching of these helixes (coils) that enables biologic polymers to stretch when we bend our joints. Man-made polymers have the same coiled three-dimensional structures. However, what keeps the coils from sliding by each other when they are stretched? A few covalent cross-links along the polymer chain keep the coils in place and prevent their movement. Depending on the interaction of the coils, some man-made polymeric materials can also stretch and return to their original shape.

Just like biologic rubbery materials, man-made rubber materials have polymeric coils that stretch out and recoil, similar to the spring-like toy called a "Slinky." Rubber bands and polymeric impression materials are examples of materials that stretch and return to their original shape. A better description of a rubber material is a pile of Slinkies tangled together, with a few wired together. The linking of one coil (or polymer chain) across to another with wire (or a covalent bond) is called **cross-linking.** The mass can be stretched, but it cannot be untangled. The more cross-links that a rubber material has, the stiffer it will be. If too many cross-links are present, the rubber is too strong and hard, and it behaves more like a stiff plastic.

D. Composites

Composites are materials that are made of two or more different materials. Common composites are mixtures of a polymer and a ceramic, such as fiberglass. Each material that makes up a composite is called a phase. Materials or phases are chosen and combined so that the resulting composite has properties better than those of either individual material. A composite is a kind of "team" of materials and is usually best appreciated on a microscopic level. The properties lacking in one material are compensated for by those of the other material. Strong, lightweight materials and products result. Sporting goods, such as skis, rackets, and golf clubs, are made from composite materials to minimize weight while retaining strength and flexibility. In dentistry, composites were first used as an esthetic restorative material, but today, they are commonly used for a variety of purposes. Enamel is a composite of apatite (a ceramic material) and protein (a polymer).

E. Colloids

Colloids are also two-phase materials. Colloids are mixtures of gases, liquids, or solids at the microscopic level. Colloids are not true solutions of one material dissolved in another, such as saltwater. Colloids are suspensions of one material in another, such as fog (a suspension of water droplets in air). Properties of composite materials are a result of the properties of the component materials. Properties of colloids, however, are a result of the properties of the components but are also greatly affected by the properties of the surfaces of the component phases. It is the large amount of surface area around the small particles that gives colloids their properties. When we discuss adhesion and bonding, we will again discuss the subject of surface science. Common colloids are Jell-O, foam, milk, smoke, and emulsions. Several dental impression materials are also colloids, as are fluoride foams.

Emulsions are a type of colloid composed of two liquids that do not blend together to form one liquid. When the two liquids are vigorously mixed, tiny droplets of each liquid are formed and dispersed among droplets of the other liquid. Oil-and-vinegar salad dressing is a good example. The oil and vinegar do not blend, but when they are vigorously shaken, a new liquid seemingly results. This new liquid is an emulsion of oil and vinegar. The surfaces of the two liquids are temporarily stable, and the dressing is neither vinegar nor oil. The resulting dressing, however, combines the taste of both and the spices dissolved in each. Milk as well as liquid soaps and lotions are emulsions.

The transformation from a liquid to a gel is the important feature of other colloid materials. Jell-O and jellies are good examples. If warmed, these materials become liquid. If cooled, they become a semisolid gel. In dentistry, hydrocolloid impression material behaves in this manner.

F. Teeth and Food

One of the main functions of teeth is to start the digestion of food. Food varies a great deal in texture, from mashed potatoes to rock candy. Teeth chop, tear, and grind a variety of materials to allow the digestive fluids to access the greater surface area that is inherent in smaller pieces of food. Teeth, jaws, and muscles are able to apply a great amount of force to food to crush it. The teeth must withstand these forces for a lifetime. Luckily, teeth are made from materials that are able to resist these forces. Teeth are stronger than the food we eat. The dental restorative materials that are used to replace tooth structure must have these same characteristics. In the next chapter, we will discuss the mechanical and physical properties of materials. We will compare dentin and enamel to restorative and other materials used in dentistry.

SUMMARY

Properties of materials are a result of their atomic bonds. Materials can be classified into one of three phases: solid, liquid, or gas. A solid object exhibits the ability to support itself and other objects because solids have the strongest atomic bonds. Liquids have weaker bonds and need to be confined on most sides by a container. Gasses have the weakest of all bonds and their atoms need to be contained in all the three dimensions.

Atoms of materials are held together by two types of atomic bonds: primary and secondary. Primary bonds are those that involve the transfer or sharing of electrons between atoms. There are three kinds of primary bonds: ionic, covalent, and metallic. Ionic bonds result when an electron is given up by an atom and accepted by another. The atom that gives up the electron becomes a positive ion, while the atom that receives the electron becomes a negative ion. The positive and negative ions attract each other via the electromagnetic force and form an ionic bond. When two atoms share a pair of electrons, a covalent bond is formed. A metallic bond involves sharing many electrons by all the atoms in the material. Covalent and metallic bonds are also the result of positive and negative electromagnetic attraction of atoms and their electrons.

Secondary bonds occur when a partial charge is created from an uneven distribution of electrons. The three types of secondary bonds are: hydrogen bonds, permanent dipoles, and the fluctuating dipole. Of the three, the hydrogen bond is the strongest, and the fluctuating dipole is the weakest. The hydrogen bond is important in biologic molecules such as DNA and proteins, and biologic materials such as ligaments and cartilage.

Materials can be classified into three categories based on their primary atomic bonds: metals, ceramics, and polymers. Composites are a combination of two solid materials and may be considered a fourth category. Metals are ductile, yet retain strength when bent because the metallic bond allows atoms to slide by one another and not disrupt the bonds in the metal. Ceramic materials are strong when compressed, but weak and brittle when pulled or bent. When the arrangement of the positive and negative ions in a ceramic material is changed, attraction may change to repulsion and a break or fracture is likely. Polymers or plastics have a range of properties because they have covalent bonds and a range of secondary bonds in their atomic structure. Many different polymers are used to make everyday products. Those that are soft, weak, and flexible are termed plastics or rubber. Those that are hard, stiff, and strong are called resins or glassy polymers. Composites are a mixture of two or more distinct materials. An example is fiberglass, made of both a polymer and a ceramic.

Learning Activities

1. Pick out several objects in the room. Discuss the type of materials used to manufacture those objects, the kind of atomic bonds in the materials used, and the properties that result.
2. Describe the advantages and disadvantages of using a metal, a ceramic, or a polymer as a restorative material.

Review Questions

1. The molecules found in a pane of glass can be best described as:
   a) Crystalline solid, having short-range order only
   b) Crystalline solid, having both short-range and long-range order
   c) Amorphous solid, having long-range order
   d) Amorphous solid, having short-range order
2. A partial charge resulting from an uneven distribution of electrons around an atom forms a bond known as:
   a) Metallic
   b) Secondary
   c) Covalent
   d) Ionic
3. What type of bond is it when the electrons are shared by all the atoms that make up that object and may be thought of as "positive cores" in a "cloud of negative mobile valence electrons"?
   a) Metallic
   b) Secondary
   c) Covalent
   d) Ionic
4. A notable advantage of using ceramic materials in dentistry is the property of:
   a) Transparency
   b) Translucency
   c) Opacity
   d) Brittleness
5. A dental polymer with many cross-links as compared to one with no cross-links would be a dental material that is:
   a) Flexible but strong
   b) Flexible and weak
   c) Stiff and strong
   d) Stiff but weak
6. All of the following are examples of a composite except:
   a) Set Jell-O with sliced peaches
   b) Enamel
   c) Fiberglass
   d) Tin foil
7. When the shared electrons of a covalent bond are not shared equally, and one of the bonded atoms is partially positive and the other is partially negative, a ___________ is formed.
   a) Permanent dipole
   b) Fluctuating dipole
   c) Hydrogen bond
   d) Primary bond
8. The sliding of atoms past each other allows this material to bend, not fracture, and maintain its strength. This material is an example of a:
   a) Metal
   b) Ceramic
   c) Polymer
9. A mixture of two liquids that do not blend together to form one liquid is termed a (an):
   a) Composite
   b) Emulsion
   c) Colloid
   d) Solution
10. When two atoms share a pair of electrons, the resulting atomic bond is termed a (an) ___________ bond.
    a) Secondary
    b) Ionic
    c) Covalent
    d) Metallic

Supplemental Readings

Anusavice KJ. Phillips' Science of Dental Materials. 11th ed. Philadelphia: Saunders, 2003:22–26.

Callister WD. Materials Science and Engineering: An Introduction. 7th ed. New York: Wiley, 2007: Chapter 2.

Park JB, Lake RS. Biomaterials: An Introduction. 2nd ed. New York: Plenum, 1992, Chapters 1 and 2.

Van Vlack LH. Elements of Materials Science and Engineering. 6th ed. Redding, MA: Addison-Wesley, 1990, Chapters 1 and 2.

3

Physical and Mechanical Properties of Dental Materials

Key Words/Phrases

abrasion resistance
bending
biologic properties
chemical properties
coefficient of thermal expansion
color
compression
creep
density
elasticity
elastic deformation
elastic limit
fatigue
force
fracture toughness
Goldilocks principle
galvanic shock
hardness
heat capacity
heat of fusion
heat of vaporization
load
mechanical properties
modulus of elasticity
percolation
permanent dentition
physical properties
plastic deformation
Poisson's ratio
proportional limit
resilience
shear
shade guide
solubility
specific heat capacity
strain
stress
stress concentration
stress relaxation
tension
thermal conductivity
torsion
toughness
ultimate compressive strength
ultimate strength
ultimate tensile strength
vapor pressure
viscosity
yield point
water sorption
wetting

Objectives

After studying this chapter, the student will be able to do the following:

1. Describe or define the key words and phrases.
2. Relate the physical properties of materials discussed in this chapter to their use in dentistry.
3. Define wetting. Include in the definition a drop of liquid and the contact angle formed with the surface.
4. Name the units of measure for the following properties:
    - Density
    - Heat capacity
    - Stress
    - Strain
    - Modulus of elasticity
5. Define "proportional limit," and name two other nearly equivalent terms.
6. Name the four types of stress, and provide an example of each found in everyday life.
7. Describe two situations in which dental materials are subjected to bending stresses when in function.
8. Compare the properties of "toughness" and "hardness," and provide examples.
9. Explain the difference between stress relaxation and creep.
10. Discuss the phenomenon of stress concentration, and compare its effects on a poorly placed amalgam restoration as well as on a properly placed one.

INTRODUCTION

When substituting one material for another, as in the restoration of teeth, we must be aware of the requirements for the new material. It seems obvious that the replacement material should have the same characteristics as enamel, which is very hard and strong. Should dentists restore teeth with the strongest and hardest material? In certain situations, the replacement material should have the same appearance as teeth for proper esthetics. Several other questions also need to be addressed: Is the material as good a thermal insulator as enamel and dentin are? Is the material "kind" to the pulp of the tooth? Does the material break down and release toxic chemicals?

We should also consider the cost of materials and labor when selecting restorative materials. As the list of requirements grows, we begin to realize that the criteria for an ideal restorative material are many and varied. Unfortunately, no ideal material exists, so we are always compromising in one way or another. The only sure way to eliminate this difficult dilemma is through prevention.

The important question is, what are the requirements for a particular restoration for a particular tooth and patient? Determining what is required and what will best meet the clinical situation are complex questions. Typically, a compromise is made among the many factors being considered. This chapter will discuss many of these factors or properties of materials. In addition, this chapter will describe the relationship between these properties and the materials science concepts previously discussed.

In everyday life, we notice that different materials have different properties. When we pick up an object, we feel its weight, which is an indication of its density. We also feel its temperature, which is an indication of its thermal "content" and its ability to transmit heat. Some objects feel strong and hard; others feel weak and flexible. Engineers have devised a variety of laboratory tests to quantify the properties of materials. Dental materials scientists use the same tests (as well as several others) to describe the physical properties of materials used in dentistry.

I. Properties of Materials

Properties of materials can be divided into three categories: physical, chemical, and biologic. **Physical properties** are based on the laws of physics that describe mass, energy, force, light, heat, electricity, and other physical phenomena. Examples are color, density, and thermal conductivity. **Mechanical properties** are a subgroup of physical properties. Mechanical properties describe a material's ability to resist forces. Mechanical properties are dependent on the amount of material and on the size and shape of the object. Examples are strength and stiffness. **Chemical properties** describe the setting reactions as well as the decay or degradation of materials. For example, gypsum products (used to make study models) set via a precipitation process, whereas dental composites polymerize. **Biologic properties** of materials are the effects the materials have on living tissue. For example, a crown should not irritate the gingiva, tongue, or buccal mucosa.

The chemical and biologic properties of dental materials will be discussed with each group of materials presented in the chapters that follow. This chapter will focus on the physical and mechanical properties.

II. Physical Properties

A. Density

The amount or mass of a material in a given volume is the **density** of the material. A common unit of density is gm/cm^3. Density depends on the type of atoms that are present (as the atomic number increases, so does the density), the packing together of atoms and molecules, and the voids in the material. The high density of most metal objects makes them feel heavy. Most metals have high atomic numbers, and their atoms are packed closely together into solids. A metal maxillary partial denture will feel heavy and have a tendency to become "unseated" if it is not designed to adapt to the remaining teeth.

B. Boiling and Melting Points

Boiling and melting points are physical properties of materials. In analytical laboratories, they can be used to help identify chemicals. Mixtures often have a melting or boiling range rather than a specific melting or boiling point. Dental waxes are an example of mixtures with a melting range. When an object melts or boils, the atomic bonds between the atoms or molecules are broken by the thermal energy of the material. Some dental metals melt at very high temperatures and are difficult to cast. Other materials do not boil or melt; instead, they decompose if heated sufficiently. Wood and cookie dough are common examples of materials that decompose.

C. Vapor Pressure

Vapor pressure is a measure of a liquid's tendency to evaporate and become a gas. As the temperature of a liquid increases, the vapor pressure also increases. We notice that steam rises from a pot of water more and more as it is heated because the increased thermal energy allows more atoms or molecules to escape from the liquid and become vapor. Materials with a low vapor pressure, such as cooking oil, do not evaporate quickly. Materials with a high vapor pressure, such as rubbing alcohol, evaporate readily at room temperature.

Materials with a high vapor pressure are very useful as solvents in the application of viscous (syrupy) liquids, such as glue or paint. The viscous liquid is "thinned" by mixing it with a solvent. The "more runny" mixture is then applied to a surface. As the solvent evaporates, it leaves behind a thin layer of the viscous liquid. In dentistry, we use solvents to apply a thin layer of a thick liquid, such as copal varnish or a dentinal adhesive. Rubber cement, oil-based paints, and perfumes use the same process: A mixture is applied, and the solvent evaporates, leaving behind a thin film of the desired substance.

Methyl methacrylate, a component of dental acrylic resins (plastics), has a high vapor pressure and can evaporate easily when a denture is processed. Porosity may result, weakening the denture. Denture processing techniques are designed to minimize the evaporation of methyl methacrylate and the resulting porosity, see Figure 11.3.

D. Thermal Conductivity

In the kitchen, we use a wooden spoon to stir hot liquids. We do not use a metal spoon because it conducts heat well and would quickly become too hot to hold. In dentistry, we are also interested in the thermal conductivity of materials. **Thermal conductivity** is the rate of heat flow through a material. Measurement of thermal conductivity depends on the distance the heat travels, the area in which the heat travels (much like the size of the pipe through which water travels), and the difference in temperature between the source and destination. Because thermal conductivity is a rate, it is measured as heat flow over time. Thermal conductivity is measured as calories/second·meter·degree. Pulpal sensitivity is likely if conductive materials, such as metals, are placed in close proximity to the pulp. If caries are deep and a metal restoration is planned, an insulating base is placed beneath the metal restoration to insulate the pulp from hot and cold stimuli, see Figure 1.9.

E. Heat Capacity

Some objects, such as a "microwave trivet," can store a lot of heat. The **heat capacity** of a material is a measure of the amount of thermal energy that a material can hoard. Some materials require more energy than others to heat. The **specific heat capacity** of a material is the amount of energy needed to raise the temperature of one unit of mass of that material by 1°C. Specific heat capacity is measured as calories/gram·degree. The heat capacity of water is 1 calorie/gram·degree.

F. Heat of Fusion and Vaporization

The **heat of fusion** is the amount of energy required to melt a material. Conversely, the **heat of vaporization** is the amount of energy required to boil a material. Both are typically large in relation to the heat capacity. It requires 80 times more energy to melt a given quantity of ice than to increase the temperature of the same amount of water by 1°. It takes 540 times more energy to boil that same quantity of water. The high heat of fusion allows a small amount of ice to effectively cool a much larger amount of beverage without excessive dilution as it melts. We shall see that the heat of fusion of metals must be overcome when gold is cast. The solid metal must be heated to the melting temperature, and then a significant amount of energy must be added to melt the metal.

G. Coefficient of Thermal Expansion

If a balloon filled with room temperature air is brought outside on a cold January day in West Virginia, the balloon shrinks. This is a visible example of what happens to nearly all materials when cooled: They shrink or contract. On the other hand, most materials expand when heated. The **coefficient of thermal expansion** is a measure of this change in volume in relation to the change in temperature. This concept, however, is slightly more complicated than that explanation suggests.

The coefficient of thermal expansion is a fractional change in volume or length. In Figure 3.1, several examples of expansion are illustrated. In Figure 3.1*A*, the 10-unit-long bar is extended by 1 unit (or 10%). The new bar is now 1.1 times the original length. In Figure 3.1*B*, the 5-unit-long bar is extended by 0.5 unit, becoming 5.5 units long. It is also 10% longer (or 1.1 times the original length).

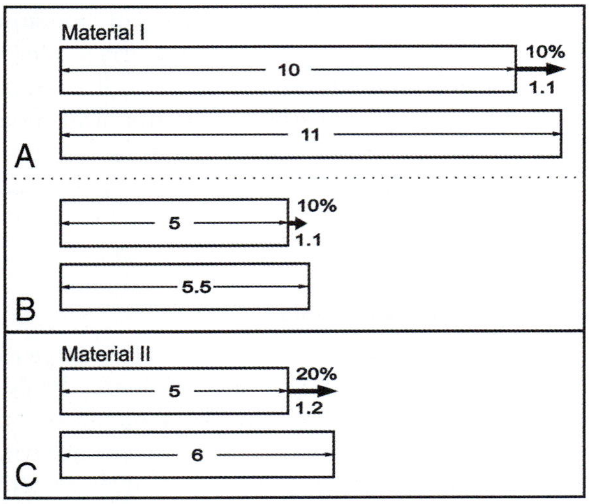

FIGURE 3.1 Three examples of expansion of a material in terms of percentage or fractional change in length.

Therefore, larger objects of the same material expand more in quantity than smaller objects do, but larger objects expand by an equal amount in terms of the percentage or fractional change. In Figure 3.1*C*, a different material expands more, and the result is a 20% change in length. We shall look at fractional change of length again later in this chapter, when strain is discussed.

Our interest in the coefficient of thermal expansion of dental materials is in relationship to those of enamel and dentin. A polymeric material, such as polymethyl methacrylate (an early tooth-colored restorative material of the 1950s), shrinks and expands 7 times more than tooth structures. Compared with those used, the restorative materials of today more closely match the coefficient of thermal expansion of teeth. When the mismatch is great, the restoration will shrink with cold beverages, opening gaps between the restoration and the tooth. When the tooth heats up again and expands, the gap is closed. The process of heating and cooling, and the accompanying opening and closing of the gap, is called **percolation.** Percolation results in microleakage, tooth sensitivity, and recurrent decay. Microleakage will be discussed in Chapter 4.

H. Electrical Conductivity

Electrical conductivity is not typically thought of as an important property, but we should know which materials are conductive. Metals are good electrical conductors. Polymers and ceramics are poor conductors and are termed insulators. During electrosurgery or electronic pulp testing, it is important to know which restorations are conductive and which are not. Electrical conductivity also affects corrosion, which will be discussed in the section on instruments. Occasionally, a new amalgam filling will hurt when it is touched with a metal fork. This **galvanic shock** is the result of electricity flowing from the fork to the amalgam and through the pulp.

I. Viscosity

When placing materials, the handling characteristics of those materials are important. Some materials should flow easily and wet the surface. Other materials need to be more like putty, which can be adapted or formed into a desired shape. The **viscosity** of a material is its ability to flow. Thick or viscous liquids flow poorly, whereas thin liquids flow easily. Viscosity is a temperature-dependent property. For example, pancake syrup pours much more easily when it is warmed. Viscosity is measured as grams/meter·second, or as poise (P). Water at 20°C has a viscosity of 0.01 P, or 1 centipoise (cP). Impression materials have viscosities between 100,000 and 1,000,000 cP.

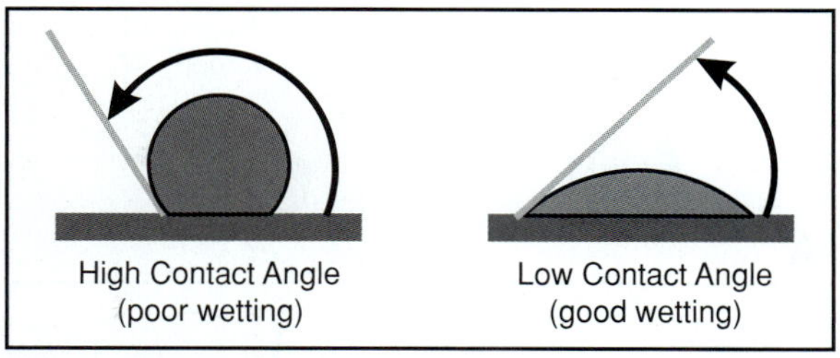

FIGURE 3.2 Contact angle measurements demonstrate a liquid's ability to wet a surface.

A low viscosity and the ability to wet a surface are important in the use of many dental materials. **Wetting** a surface with an adhesive material, such as a sealant, brings the material into intimate association with the surface so that chemical and micromechanical bonding can occur. Wetting is measured by determining the contact angle of a liquid on a solid, as shown in Figure 3.2. A low contact angle, such as that of a drop of water on a piece of ice, indicates good wetting. A high contact angle, such as that of a drop of water on most plastics, indicates poor wetting. Another example of wetting in dentistry occurs when a gypsum product (plaster) is poured into an impression. If the mixed material wets the surface of the impression material, the fine details of the impression will be reproduced in the cast. If poor wetting occurs, bubbles will likely result in insufficient detail and an unusable cast.

J. Hardness

Enamel is the hardest biologic tissue in the human body. Hard materials resist scratching and indenting by soft materials. **Hardness** is a property that is measured by scientific instruments that press a special tip into the surface of the test material. The tip has a characteristic shape made of a very hard material, such as steel or diamond, as shown in Figure 3.3. The size of the indentation created is then measured. Hardness is calculated based on the size of this indentation. Several different methods can be used to measure hardness. The Brinell and Knoop methods are illustrated in Figure 3.3. Two other methods are called the Rockwell and Vickers hardness tests. The Knoop hardness number (KHN) of enamel is 350, whereas the KHN of dentin is 70. Some dental materials are harder than enamel. Porcelain has a KHN of 400 to 500. Other materials are not as hard as enamel. For example, acrylic denture teeth have a KHN of 20.

K. Durometer Measurements

Some materials are soft and even spongy. One example would be the rubber grip sometimes used on an instrument's shaft. A different kind of hardness test is used for these materials because a sur-

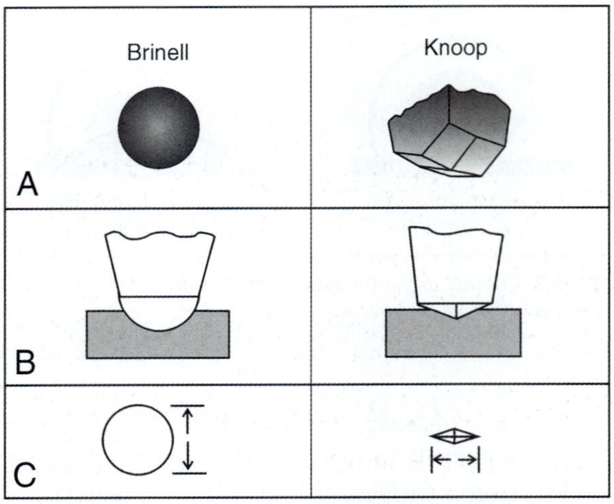

FIGURE 3.3 Comparison of two hardness indenter tips, the Brinell and the Knoop. **A.** Perspective views of the two tips. **B.** Cross section of the tips in contact with test samples. **C.** Test material showing the indentation that is measured to calculate hardness.

face hardness indentation will not occur. A durometer measures how deep a steel ball will sink when pressed into the surface of a material. Durometers are used to measure the hardness of impression materials and other elastic polymers.

L. Abrasion Resistance

Harder materials tend to be more resistant to abrasion than softer materials. In dentistry, we are interested in the **abrasion resistance** (wear resistance) of dental restorations to food and opposing teeth. We are also interested in the wear of natural teeth opposing dental restorations. If a restorative material is too hard, it will wear the opposing teeth at an unacceptably accelerated pace. An example is the excessive wear of natural teeth that oppose a denture with porcelain teeth. Therefore, a restoration must be hard enough so that the restoration does not wear away, but not so hard as to excessively wear away the opposing teeth. This is a good example of what has been called the **Goldilocks principle:** not too hard; not too soft; just right. More often than not, a material's properties need to fit within a particular range of values, not the maximum value, to be the material of choice.

M. Solubility

Materials placed in the oral cavity are exposed to various aqueous fluids. The solubility of materials in water is an important consideration. **Solubility** is the amount of a material that dissolves in a liquid, such as water. Sugar is a highly soluble material, but enamel is not. Restorative materials should not appreciably dissolve in the mouth. Additionally, some materials tend to dissolve faster in acidic environments. To measure solubility, a test sample is immersed in water. The weight of the material dissolved into the water is the solubility of that material. The solubility of some dental cements is measurable and clinically significant. Excessive solubility leads to loss of material and increases the risk of recurrent decay.

N. Water Sorption

Some materials absorb water. This property is termed **water sorption.** Water sorption is measured much like solubility. A test sample is immersed in water, and the weight that is gained by that sample is the water sorption. A cookie dunked in milk is an example of milk sorption. When materials absorb water, they tend to swell. Some materials both dissolve and absorb water at the same time, making measurement of one of these properties difficult.

O. Color

The appearance of a restoration for an anterior tooth can be a factor when choosing materials. The color and surface luster of the restoration are important. In addition, the shape and health of gingival tissues adjacent to a restoration are also noticed.

Color is a complex phenomenon that is a psychological response to a physical stimulus. The physical stimulus is the light reaching the rods and cones of the eye. Because processing of that stimulus by the brain is a psychological phenomenon, the perception of color varies between individuals. Two people may agree that two objects match in color, while a third person disagrees. In addition, the color of an object depends on the light in which the object is viewed. For all these reasons, matching restorative materials to a patient's teeth can be difficult.

Two types of systems are used to measure color. Both use three numbers to describe a color. One system involves matching the test object to color tabs resembling those available in a paint store. It is called the Munsell color system. Each tab has hue, chroma, and value numbers assigned. Hue is the fundamental color of an object, as in red, green, or blue. Chroma is the strength or color saturation of the hue, as in pink versus red. Value is the light or darkness of the color, as in shades of gray. In dentistry, esthetic materials have their own set of color tabs or shades, called a **shade guide.** Some manufacturers use a standard set, such as the Vita shade guide, which is shown in Figure 3.4. Recently, handheld devices have been developed that measure the color of teeth via a digital camera. These devices provide maps of the various shades of a tooth.

The other system involves measurement of color with a spectrophotometer or a colorimeter. A spectrophotometer measures the intensity of light that is reflected by an object at numerous wavelengths of visible light. The colorimeter measures light at

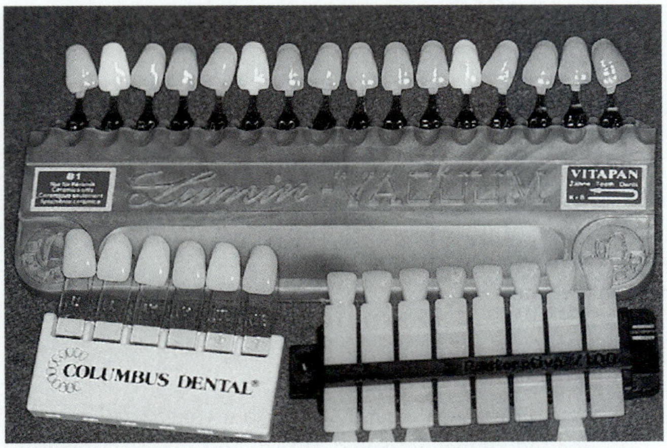

FIGURE 3.4 Photograph of several shade guides, including a Vita shade guide. (See the color insert for a color version of this image.)

several wavelengths, much like the human eye. For both devices, the data are mathematically manipulated by a computer to reduce the information to three numbers: L*, a*, and b*. The number L* is very similar to value. The number a* is a measure of the red–green character of a color. The number b* is a measure of the blue–yellow character of a color. The measurement of color with spectrophotometers is common in dental research, but it has not proven to be useful clinically. Several colorimeters have been marketed for clinical use (see Fig. 31.2).

The interaction of teeth and dental materials with ultraviolet light causes fluorescence and affects their appearance. Fluorescence of restorations is important when fluorescent lighting or "black" lights are present. Inadequate fluorescence will make a crown or a filling appear dark in certain lighting, but excess fluorescence will make a tooth "glow" in the same lighting.

P. Interaction of Materials With X-rays

It is important for the clinical interpretation of radiographs to know how dental materials interact with x-rays. Some materials are radiolucent and are not seen on radiographs. Examples are some ceramic materials and denture acrylic resin. Other materials, such as metal restorations, are radiopaque and are evident on radiographs. Some dental restorative materials have been formulated by the manufacturer to match the radiopacity of enamel to facilitate the diagnosis of recurrent decay. Dental materials and their radiographic appearance will be discussed further in Chapter 15.

III. Mechanical Properties

Because teeth are used to tear and grind food, they must be strong, and so must the materials that are used to replace missing tooth structure. Luckily, engineers and materials scientists have studied materials and their use for centuries. Dentistry has used this information along with trial and error.

What happens to a tooth or restoration when we bite on it? A external force (biting) is placed on the tooth. A **force** is a weight or **load** applied to an object. Inside the tooth, an internal stress develops to resist the applied external force. The **stress** is the force divided by the area on which the force has been applied. The internal stress that develops in the tooth is equal to the external force applied; however, they are opposite in direction.

Why don't teeth break when we use them to grind our food? Teeth are composed of strong materials with strong atomic bonds. Teeth and their atomic bonds are stronger than the stresses that develop as a result of biting. On the other hand, food cannot resist these forces and breaks because the strength of the weak atomic bonds of the food morsel is exceeded.

A. Elasticity

Just like the atoms of the table on which we placed a book in Chapter 2, the atomic bonds of teeth can be thought of as microscopic springs. These springs are compressed each time we bite. When we relax our bite and our teeth are no longer in contact, the springs return to their original length.

Let's use the example of a common spring to help us understand how atomic bonds and materials respond to forces. If we take a typical spring from a hardware store and hang an object, such as a monkey charm, from it, we can see the coils separate as the spring stretches out (Fig. 3.5). As we increase the number of charms hanging from the spring, the length of the spring increases. If the weight of

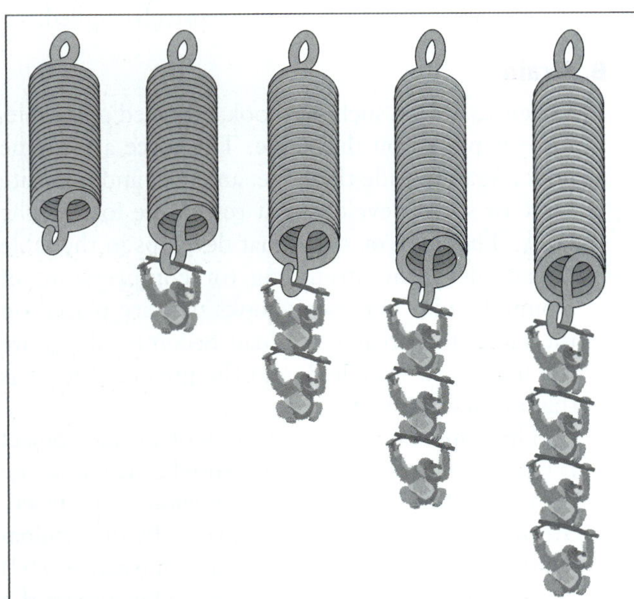

FIGURE 3.5 An illustration of elasticity: As the load increases, so does the elongation.

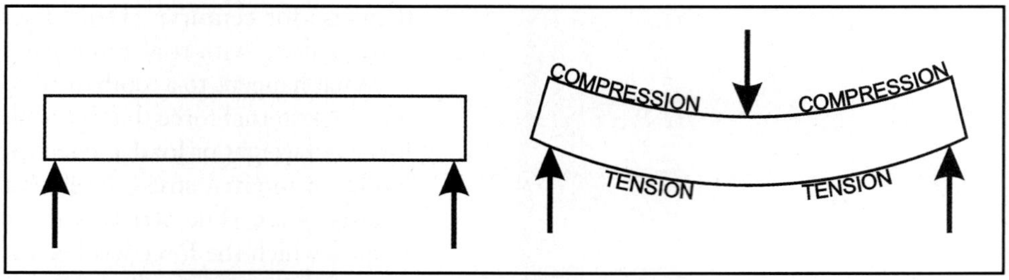

FIGURE 3.6 Bending is a combination of tension and compression.

charms is not too great, we find that the length increases by the same amount with each additional charm. Fishermen use this same concept when they use a fisherman's scale to weigh fish (so they know how big a lie to tell). As the size of the fish increases, the spring is stretched out more, and a greater weight is read on the scale. This is how atomic bonds are stretched when we use our teeth. If the charms are removed from the spring, the spring returns to its original length. In other words, the atomic bonds that were stretched return to their original length.

In everyday life, we tend to see more examples of objects that are bent than we do of objects that are stretched. When an object is bent, the same stretching of atomic bonds occurs in some parts of that object. In other parts, however, compression of atomic bonds occurs, as shown in Figure 3.6. When the force is removed, the object returns to its original shape because the atoms return to their original position. Scientists and engineers have extensively investigated this phenomenon of change in shape and return to the original shape. This phenomenon is called **elasticity.** Force (a measure of push or pull), stress, and change in shape have been quantified, and their relationships have been extensively studied.

B. Strain

When an object, such as a book, is placed on a table, force is placed on that table. The force affects the table. Again, inside the table, an equal and opposite force or stress develops that resists the load of the book. The force or stress that develops in the table is caused by the stretching (or compression) of atomic bonds. The more books that are placed on the table, the greater the load becomes, the more the bonds are stretched, and the greater the stress that occurs in the table.

The compression or elongation of a loaded object is typically very small. It is measured in terms of the fractional change in length, as previously discussed. **Strain** is the change in length divided by the original length. Strain is measured as a fraction (such as 0.02) or as a percentage (such as 2%). The longer the object is, the more it must be stretched to have the same strain (compare Fig. 3.1*A* and Fig. 3.1*B*).

C. Stress

As mentioned earlier, the force that develops in a loaded object is called stress, and stress is proportional to the applied force or load. Stress is also related to the size of the object. In Figure 3.7, the number of charms hanging from a spring is increased, but the size of the spring is increased at the same time. The change in length or strain remains constant, as does the stress in the spring. Stress is the load (force) divided by the cross-sectional area of the object:

stress = load/area

When a load or a force is applied to an object, the stress occurs throughout the object's entire length. The expression "a chain is only as strong as its weakest link" is based on this principle. Each link of the chain must bear the load.

Stress is measured as pounds per square inch (psi). In the metric system, stress is measured as pascals. Typical stresses are large, and the megapascal unit is used to reduce the number of zeros (nonsignificant figures).

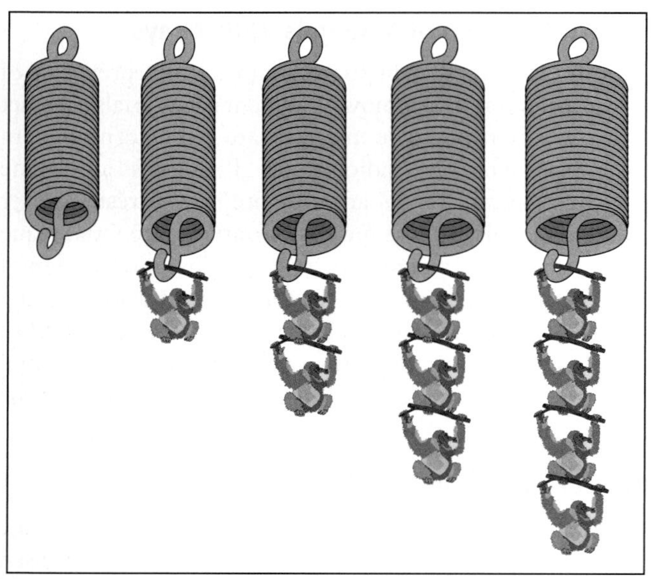

FIGURE 3.7 Larger springs can support larger loads without additional elongation.

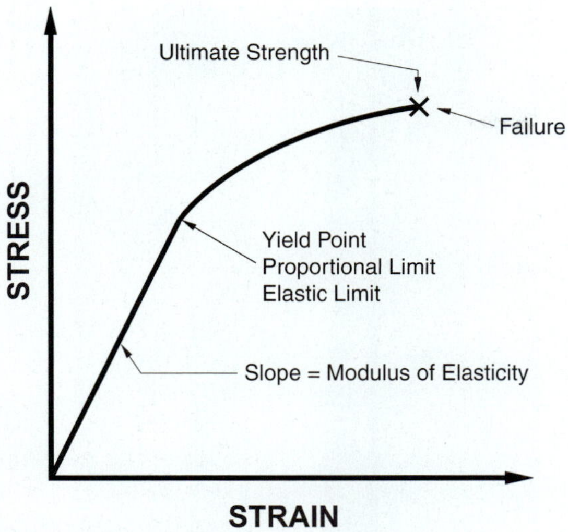

FIGURE 3.8 Typical stress–strain plot.

D. Relationship of Stress and Strain

The load (stress) and the change in length (strain) are proportional. They always occur together; you cannot have one without the other (like love and marriage?). If the load is small, the change in length may be difficult to measure. The proportionality constant, or the slope of a graph of stress versus strain, is called the **modulus of elasticity,** or Young's modulus:

modulus of elasticity = stress/strain

The stress–strain relationship is graphed in Figure 3.8.

The modulus of elasticity (or, more simply, the modulus) is characteristic of a material and its atomic bonds. It is the scientific term for the stiffness of a material. The higher the modulus of elasticity is, the stiffer the material. Enamel has a high modulus of elasticity. A rubber band has a low modulus of elasticity. As with stress, the modulus is measured as psi or pascals; however, the numbers are much larger. When a large number (a stress) is divided by a small number (a strain), a very large number results. Thus, the modulus of a material is often given in psi $\times 10^6$, or gigapascals.

E. Stress–Strain Plot

If we were to continue adding charms to the spring of Figure 3.5, we could graph the number of charms and the length of the spring (or the change in length of the spring). Initially, we would get a straight line, as shown in Figure 3.8, with the slope being equal to the modulus of elasticity. Also, if we take all the charms off the spring, the spring should return to its original length. When a stress is removed and the object returns to its original length, the initial change in length is called **elastic deformation.** If we continue adding charms, however, at some point the line on the graph begins to curve, which means stress is no longer proportional to strain. At this point, if we take all the charms off the spring, the spring does not return to its original length. It has become permanently stretched out. This condition is termed **plastic deformation** or **permanent deformation.** Plastic deformation occurs when an orthodontic wire is bent to fit a patient's arch. Force is placed on the wire and it bends. If the force is great enough, the wire will not return to its original shape; it has been plastically deformed. The point on the stress–strain plot at which the line starts to curve and plastic deformation begins is called either the **elastic limit,** the **proportional limit,** or the **yield point,** as shown in Figure 3.8. These three terms are different mostly in method of measurement, not in concept.

If we could keep loading on more and more charms, at some point the spring breaks (or failure occurs). We have exceeded the strength of the spring. The stress at that point is called the **ultimate strength.** If the test is a tensile test, it is then called the **ultimate tensile strength.** Likewise, if the test is a compressive test, it is then called the **ultimate compressive strength.** The load (charms) on the spring has caused a stress (force) to develop in the spring that is greater than the strength of the atomic bonds that hold the material together; as a result, the object breaks. This is bad for bridges, whether they are in someone's mouth or underneath someone's car.

F. Types of Stress

We have discussed compression and tension, but other types of stress exist. It is important to remember that in the real world, a single kind of stress rarely occurs. Combinations of several kinds of stresses are most common.

1. **Compression** is a pushing or crushing stress.
2. **Tension** is a pulling stress.
3. **Shear** (slip) stress occurs when parts of an object slide by one another. For example, if the front and back covers of a book are pushed in opposite directions, the pages slide or "shear" by each other.
4. **Torsion** stress is a twisting force. Turning a doorknob is an example of a torsional stress.
5. **Bending** is a common stress and is actually a combination of several types of stresses, as illustrated in Figure 3.6. When an object is bent, one side is compressed, but the opposite side is stretched. In addition to these compressive and tensile forces, shear forces also occur inside the object. A variety of bending tests are used to examine the ability of materials to resist bending.

G. Mechanical Properties of Dental Materials

Each use of a dental material has its own set of physical and mechanical requirements (Fig. 3.9). These requirements will be discussed along with each cate-

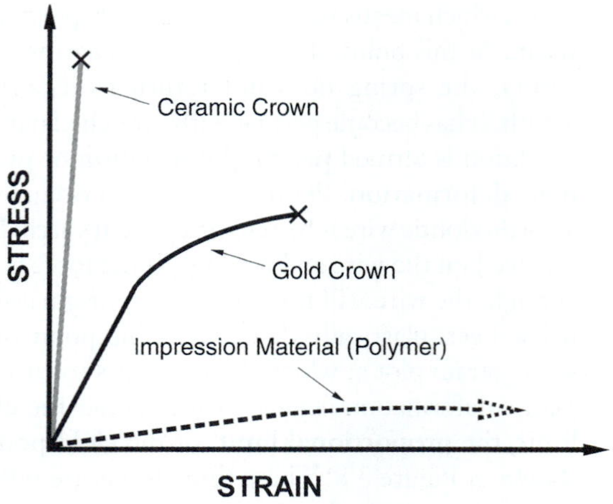

FIGURE 3.9 Stress–strain plots of several dental materials. Note that the *x* axis for the impression material has been compressed.

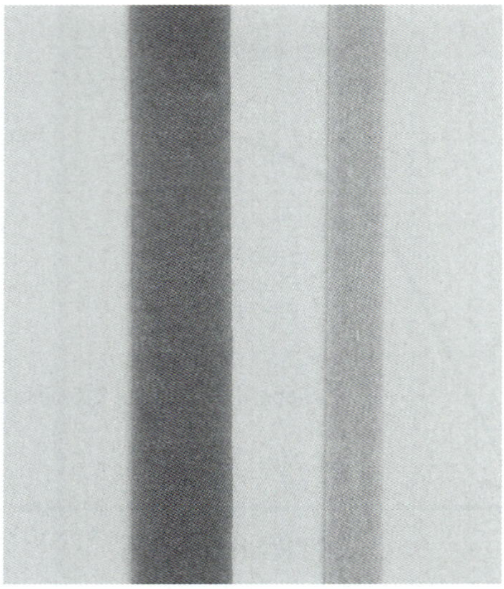

FIGURE 3.10 A rubber band at rest (*left*) and the same rubber band stretched approximately 100% (*right*).

gory of dental materials in the chapters that follow. In restorative dentistry, the materials that we use for fillings and crowns need to be stiff and strong. The materials that we use for taking impressions are much less stiff than restorative materials. Some impression materials are quite flexible and stretch a great deal.

To function properly, a restoration must be hard (hardness), strong (yield strength), and stiff (modulus) enough to withstand the forces of mastication. For many uses of materials, the yield strength is more important than the ultimate strength. If a gold crown yields or plastically deforms (changes shape) when one bites down, it is no longer the same shape and is not likely to fit the preparation precisely. Recurrent caries is then likely. Thus, we are much more concerned with the fit of a restoration in service (not exceeding the yield strength) than we are with a restoration breaking (ultimate strength). For brittle materials, such as a ceramic crown (see Fig. 1.10*E*), yield strength and ultimate strength are essentially one and the same (Fig. 3.9).

The concept of plastic and elastic deformation needs a little more attention. Elastic deformation occurs whenever force is applied to an object. As the force increases, plastic deformation may occur. However, plastic deformation may or may not be a bad thing. Most of the time, we do not want a restoration or an impression to be plastically deformed (permanently distorted) when force is applied. We want the restoration and the teeth to be elastically deformed and return to their original shape when the biting force is removed. The same is true for impressions. Impressions should return to their original shape after they have been removed from the mouth. If not, the resulting stone cast will not be the same size as the teeth or cavity preparation. For most uses of materials, plastic deformation is not a good thing, but exceptions do exist. One is the bending of an orthodontic wire.

H. Other Mechanical Properties of Interest—Optional

1. Poisson's Ratio

Solid objects deform a little differently than our spring with the monkey charms. Stretch a rubber band, and notice how the width of the rubber band narrows as it is stretched, as shown in Figure 3.10. All materials change shape in three dimensions, even if the stress is only in one direction. **Poisson's ratio** is a mechanical property that is the ratio of the strain in the direction of the stress to the strain in a direction perpendicular to the stress. So, when we bite on a filling and apply compressive force in the occlusalapical direction, the filling becomes wider in the mesial-distal and the buccal-lingual directions (but only to a microscopic degree). If a dental restoration is distorted in one direction, it will likely be distorted in the other two directions as well.

2. Resilience and Toughness

Anyone watching televised college football games sees the players wearing brightly colored mouthguards. The plastic mouthguard material is chosen for its ability to absorb energy. The energy of a blow to the mouth will not cause trauma if the energy is absorbed by the mouthguard rather than by the teeth and the other facial structures. Such an ability to absorb energy and not become deformed is called **resilience.** Resilience is measured as the area under the stress–strain curve up to the yield point.

Other safety devices are designed to absorb energy while distorting or fracturing. A crash helmet is successful if the wearer is not injured; whether the helmet is broken does not matter.

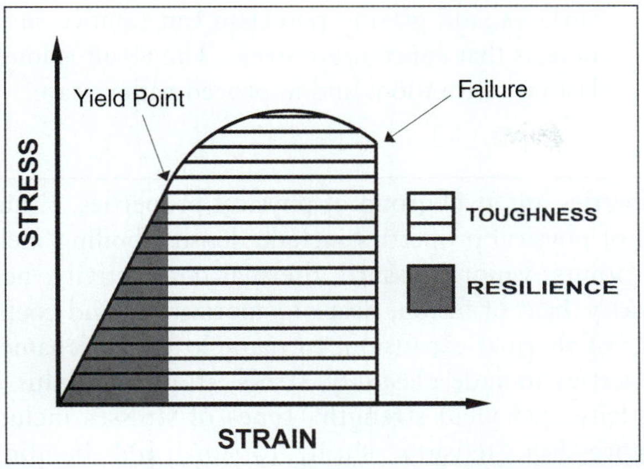

FIGURE 3.11 Resilience and toughness are measured from different areas on the stress–strain plot.

The energy absorbed (as by the helmet) up to the failure point on the stress–strain diagram is the **toughness** of the material. The helmet can be replaced; a person's head cannot (except in Frankenstein movies).

Both resilience and toughness are illustrated in Figure 3.11. Plastics in general have high resilience and toughness values.

3. Fracture Toughness

Some materials do not plastically deform easily. They just fracture. Such materials are susceptible to cracks and defects. **Fracture toughness** is a measure of the energy required to fracture a material when a crack is present. Fracture toughness is measured in units that are quite odd: megapascals times the square root of meters (Mpa· √m). Glass and dental porcelain have a low fracture toughness value, whereas metals have high fracture toughness values. Many researchers have sought to improve dental composites by improving their fracture toughness.

4. Fatigue

We use our teeth over and over again to grind food. The mechanical properties that we have discussed in this chapter are tested by compressing or pulling materials until the specimen breaks during a one-time test. This type of testing may be good for disposable items, such as baby diapers and patient napkins, but most things used in dentistry are used multiple times, such as restorations, scalers, and perio probes. Many things fail after being stressed repetitively for a long time, and such failure is called **fatigue.** An example of fatigue is when a scaler breaks. Fatigue testing more closely replicates such real-world use. A test specimen is cyclically compressed, pulled, or bent with a given amount of force, and the number of cycles needed to break the specimen is recorded. Increasing levels of force are plotted against the number of cycles that it takes to break the test specimen. Based on these data, researchers can predict the amount of stress (the fatigue strength) that the material can endure without breaking. Isn't it good to know that you can drive over that bridge forever and it will not collapse (assuming the metal reinforcements do not corrode and the concrete does not deteriorate)?

I. Time-Dependent Properties–Optional

Changes that occur too slowly to be easily observed were discussed in Chapter 2. Some slow changes reflect mechanical properties of interest. Just as glaciers flow and continents drift, certain dental materials change too slowly to be easily observed but fast enough to affect the use of the material and the resulting patient care. Two of these changes follow:

1. **Creep** is the small change in shape that results when an object is under continuous compression. It can be thought of as very slow flow. Creep was once considered to be an important factor in the selection of an amalgam. However, it only grossly differentiates between products. Amalgam and composite restorations can slowly change shape (creep) as the result of continuous stress. It is important to note that although we typically think of viscosity and flow only as properties of liquids, solids also flow. We cannot observe this flow, however, because it takes place over a long period of time (the same way that bureaucracies change).
2. Stress relaxation is similar to creep. Both occur slowly, over time. Creep is a slow change in shape, but **stress relaxation** is a slow decrease in force over time. If a rubber band is stretched to a constant length, the pull of the rubber decreases (or relaxes) over time. The loss of pull (decrease in stress or force) by the rubber band over time is called stress relaxation. The same loss of force or stress relaxation occurs with orthodontic elastics or rubber bands. As a result, orthodontic patients must frequently change their rubber bands to apply the proper force to their teeth. Both creep and stress relaxation increase as temperature increases.

J. Stress Concentration

Previously in this chapter, it was stated that loads applied in one direction result in stress along all three dimensions. The real world is even more complex. It is difficult to make objects without holes, scratches, cracks, bubbles (voids), or other defects, but defects do not simply require the rest of the object to carry a greater load. Stress increases around defects. This phenomenon is called **stress concentration.** Fracture becomes more likely because cracks can develop around a defect and spread throughout the object. A glass cutter makes a scratch that concentrates stress at a single location. When a bending stress is applied to the glass, fracture occurs along the scratch, where stress is concentrated, resulting in the shape the cutter desired. Controlling defects in objects is important to reduce stress concentration and produce stronger products.

In dentistry, it is important to mix and handle materials properly to reduce the occurrence of voids and defects. Designing restorations properly, polishing surfaces, and glazing porcelain can remove surface defects that concentrate stress. The result is longer-lasting restorations and improved patient care.

SUMMARY

The dental materials used to replace tooth structure will vary depending on the type of restoration and the specific tooth. No restorative material has characteristics identical to those of the natural tooth structure. Usually, a compromise regarding one or more of the properties must be made. This chapter discussed these properties and the extent to which these properties can be compromised. Properties of materials may be divided into three categories: physical, chemical, and biologic. Mechanical properties are a subgroup of physical properties. Examples of physical properties include density, boiling/melting points, vapor pressure, thermal conductivity, heat capacity, heat of fusion, heat of vaporization, and coefficient of thermal expansion, to name a few. Mechanical properties include elasticity, stress, strain, modulus of elasticity, and yield strength. Types of stresses include compression, tension, shear, torsion, and bending. Resilience, toughness, fatigue, creep, stress relaxation, and stress concentration are other mechanical properties that affect the practice of dentistry.

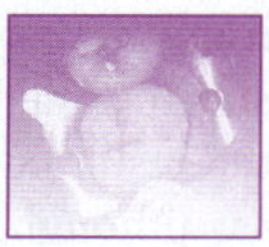

Learning Activities

1. In the library, look up the specific heat and the heat of fusion for gold. Calculate the energy required to melt 1 kg of gold, and compare this with the energy required to raise the temperature of 1 kg of gold by 1°C.
2. Bring several objects that are an off-white color to a paint store or the paint section of a hardware store. Have different people match the color of the objects with the store's "paint tabs." Compare the results. Some paint stores have color-measuring devices. Compare your results to the results of the device (if available).
3. Compare the color of several students' teeth to a shade guide. Did each student pick the same shade for each test tooth?
4. Using a spring and several metal pipe fittings purchased at a hardware store, plot the length of the spring versus the number of fittings hanging from the spring. Calculate the spring constant in terms of fittings per meter of stretch.
5. Stretch a rubber band while noting the change in its width and length. Are there other objects that show the same changes?

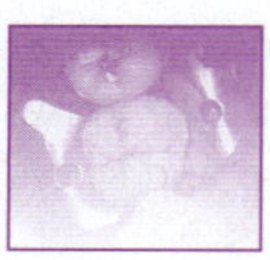

Review Questions

1. A drop of water on a Popsicle is an example of:
   a) Poor wetting (low contact angle)
   b) Good wetting (high contact angle)
   c) Good wetting (low contact angle)
   d) Poor wetting (high contact angle)
2. The tightening of a guitar string is an example of which of the following stresses?
   a) Compression
   b) Torsion
   c) Shear
   d) Toughness
3. The modulus of elasticity is an indication of what property of a material?
   a) Resilience
   b) Strength
   c) Stiffness
   d) Tension
4. Cooled materials will contract, and heated materials will expand. A measurement of this change in volume in relation to change in temperature is called the coefficient of thermal expansion.
   a) The first statement is true; the second statement is false.
   b) The first statement is false; the second statement is true.
   c) Both statements are true.
   d) Both statements are false.
5. When a stress is induced in a material that is greater than the material's yield strength, the stress is ________________ proportional to the strain, and the material does not return to its original shape.
   a) Always
   b) No longer
   c) Equally
   d) None of the above

6. Which formula defines the modulus of elasticity?
a) *stress/strain*
b) $stress^2/strain$
c) *strain/stress*
d) $2 \times stress/strain$

7. An example of a physical property is:
a) Density
b) Strength
c) Stiffness
d) Setting reaction

8. A twisting force is termed:
a) Compression
b) Shear
c) Tension
d) Torsion
e) Bending

9. The ability of a material to dissolve in liquid is termed:
a) Viscosity
b) Water sorption
c) Solubility
d) Wetting

10. Elasticity is an example of which of the following properties?
a) Physical
b) Mechanical
c) Chemical
d) Biologic

11. The rate of heat flow through a material is referred to as:
a) Heat of fusion
b) Coefficient of thermal expansion
c) Heat capacity
d) Thermal conductivity

12. Jennifer is a practicing hygienist who goes to a nearby restaurant each day for lunch. She often orders a cola with ice and a bowl of homemade soup. As she eats and drinks, her composite restorations (tooth colored) and tooth structure are expanding and contracting at different rates. This change in volume or length of these materials due to the hot food and cold drinks is referred to as:
a) Heat of fusion
b) Coefficient of thermal expansion
c) Heat capacity
d) Thermal conductivity

13. Fingernail polish remover has "solvent" properties, as it will remove the polish from our fingernails. Another property polish remover has is its tendency to evaporate. Fingernail polish remover can be said to have:
a) A high vapor pressure
b) A low vapor pressure
c) No vapor pressure
d) An intermittent vapor pressure

14-16. Match the properties listed below with the procedures or situations in questions 14, 15, and 16.
a) Solubility
b) Compression
c) Stress concentration
d) Viscosity

14. _________ is the force used to condense an amalgam in a preparation.

15. Low _________ of a hardened cement can firmly hold a patient's gold crown in place for years in a wet environment.

16. _________ is the term given to the increase of stress around defects within an object.

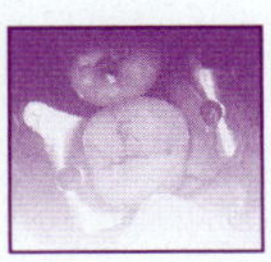

Supplemental Readings

Anusavice KJ. Phillips' Science of Dental Materials. 11th ed. Philadelphia: Saunders, 2003, Chapters 3 and 4.

Callister WD. Materials Science and Engineering: An Introduction. 7th ed. New York: Wiley, 2007, Chapter 6.

Park JB, Lake RS. Biomaterials: An Introduction. 2nd ed. New York: Plenum, 1992, Chapters 3 and 4.

Powers JM, Sakaguchi RL, eds. Craig's Restorative Dental Materials. 12th ed. St. Louis: Mosby, 2006, Chapter 3 and 4.

4

Adhesive Materials

Key Words/Phrases

acid etching
adherend
adhesive
adhesive failure
biofilm
cohesive failure
dentinal bonding
enamel bonding resin
enamel tags
glass ionomer cements
hybrid layer
interface
macromechanical bonding
microleakage
micropores
micromechanical bonding
margins
orthophosphoric acid
percolation
polycarboxylate cements
postoperative sensitivity
primers
resin tags
smear layer

Objectives

After studying this chapter, the student will be able to do the following:

1. Describe an "adhesive."
2. Explain the difference between micromechanical bonding and macromechanical bonding, and provide an example of each type.
3. Recall three benefits the patient receives from restorations that are bonded to tooth structure.
4. Compare the differences of the microanatomy of enamel and of dentin regarding etching and bonding. The comparison should include the following terms:
   - Orthophosphoric acid
   - Enamel tags
   - Smear layer
   - Hybrid layer
   - Primer
   - Adhesive
5. Discuss two of the earlier fallacies about dentinal bonding and how research has changed current practice.
6. Summarize the main differences between glass ionomer cements and dentinal bonding.

INTRODUCTION

Adhesion, or bonding, is the joining together of two objects, using a glue or cement. It is common in everyday life, and it is used in manufacturing, repairs, and dentistry. It is also important when a protective layer is applied to an object, such as when a metal surface is painted to prevent rust or when a pit and fissure sealant is applied to prevent decay.

The definition of adhesion or bonding in dentistry is not concise. A material that can stick to a flat surface or bond two flat surfaces together is typically called an **"adhesive."** Most dental materials that are adhesive involve micromechanical adhesion or bonding. Remember that all dental materials must function in a wet, hostile environment for an extended period of time to be useful. Therefore, the oral environment limits the types of adhesives used in dentistry.

True adhesion involves chemical bonds between the materials being joined, but not all bonding to tooth structures is truly adhesive. In this text, the terms "adhesion" and "bonding" will be used interchangeably, but neither will signify chemical bonding (unless specifically stated).

Micromechanical bonding of dental materials to tooth structure is common. Micromechanical bonding also occurs in everyday life, when materials such as Superglue are used. We will define **micromechanical bonding** as bonding using surface irregularities smaller than can be seen with the naked eye or felt with a dental explorer. The result of micromechanical bonding can be difficult to distinguish from true adhesion.

Macromechanical bonding is also common in everyday life and in dentistry. With this type of bonding, surface roughness can be seen and/or felt. **Macromechanical bonding** is the mechanism by which most glues join two pieces of wood, repair broken toys, and do many other things.

The mechanisms for micromechanical and macromechanical bonding are much the same. The difference is that they occur at a different scale or physical size. The glue or cement flows into surface irregularities and fills them. The glue then sets or hardens and is locked into the surface irregularities of the objects being joined. If the glue is strong, the objects are now joined together. The main advantage of micromechanical bonding is that a greater number of small surface irregularities are used compared to macromechanical bonding. In addition, force is more evenly distributed on the joint with micromechanical bonding, making it stronger than macromechanical bonding. Screws, nails, nuts, bolts, and other fasteners are examples of macromechanical joining of objects at an even larger scale. With this type of joining, stress is greatly concentrated in the vicinity of the fastener.

In dentistry, macromechanical bonding is used for cementing or luting crowns and bridges to teeth with "nonadhesive" cements. Dental cements fill in the roughness on the surface of the tooth and on the inside of the crown. The crown is luted or glued in place in the same manner as two pieces of wood are glued together. A crown is shown in Figure 1.4.

I. Adhesive Materials in Dentistry

A. Use of Adhesion/Bonding in Dentistry

1. Retention of Restorations

Adhesion is commonly used to keep restorations in place. Undercuts (as illustrated in Fig. 1.3) and other mechanical locks are not necessary when adhesive materials are used. Sometimes, adhesion is used to bond a weak esthetic restorative material, such as a porcelain veneer, to the stronger remaining tooth structure so that the tooth supports the weak restorative material. Adhesion is also used to attach orthodontic brackets and other appliances to teeth.

2. Reduction of Microleakage

Adhesion reduces or eliminates microleakage of restorations (Fig. 4.1). It also reduces postoperative sensitivity. **Microleakage** is the seeping and leaking of fluids and bacteria between the tooth/restoration junction or **interface.** Microleakage increases the likelihood of recurrent caries and postoperative sensitivity. **Postoperative sensitivity** is caused by fluids and bacteria moving in and out of the interface between the restoration and the tooth. If the pulp is irritated by fluid movement or bacterial metabolic wastes (acids), pain results.

When teeth are heated and cooled by the ingestion of hot and cold foods, expansion and contraction occur. If the coefficient of thermal expansion for a restorative material does not match that of the tooth, they expand and contract at different rates. Repeated expansion and contraction of teeth and restorations at different rates results in fluids being sucked in and pushed out at the margins of a restoration. This phenomenon is called **percolation** and is illustrated in Figure 4.1.

Adhesion also reduces staining of the margins of esthetic materials. **Margins** are the junction of the tooth and the restoration that is clinically visible. Margins that leak frequently become dark, stained, and unesthetic. Sealing the margins of restorations reduces or eliminates microleakage and reduces postoperative sensitivity and staining.

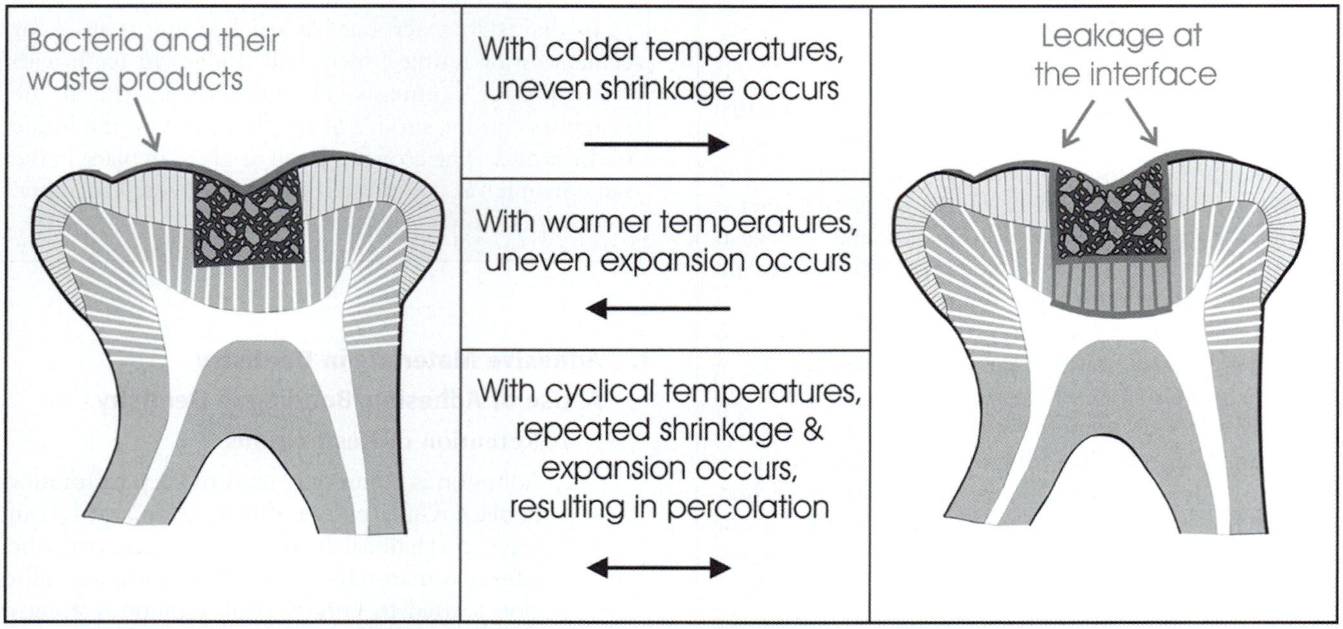

FIGURE 4.1 Illustration of the effects of temperature changes and microleakage. When the coefficient of thermal expansion of a restorative material does not match that of the tooth structure, uneven expansion and contraction occur. In turn, gaps and leakage occur at the interface of the restoration and the tooth.

3. Reduction of Recurrent Caries

The most important reason to reduce microleakage is to minimize the likelihood of recurrent caries (secondary decay). Recurrent caries is decay that occurs at the margin of a restoration. If no space exists between the restoration and the tooth, bacteria do not have a well-protected niche in which to colonize and proliferate. Smooth surfaces of teeth and sealed margins are much more resistant to decay than are pits, fissures, and gaps at the margins of restorations.

B. Development of Dental Adhesives

1. Historical Perspective

Acid etching was initially conceived by Dr. Michael Buonocore in the 1950s to seal pits and fissures. An acid is applied to enamel to etch the surface. The etched surface is rough, allowing a low-viscosity adhesive (resin system) to flow into the irregularities and then cure (or set). **Acid etching** is a micromechanical bonding technique that was first used to retain pit and fissure sealants. Later, when dental composite restorations were developed in the 1960s, acid-etching techniques were used when placing composite restorations to reduce leakage and staining of margins.

Many other uses for acid etching and composite materials were developed in the 1970s and 1980s. With composite materials and acid etching techniques, orthodontic brackets could be bonded to the labial surface of teeth rather than needing to be welded onto a metal band for every tooth. Soon, researchers learned that the enamel of the tooth and the metal of the bridge could both be etched and then bonded together. Plastic, composite, and porcelain veneers were developed that could be bonded to the labial surface of anterior teeth to hide discolored enamel, to close spaces, and to change the shape of teeth. Dentists used etched composites to bond together mobile, periodontally involved teeth; to stabilize replanted, avulsed teeth; and to stabilize segments of fractured jaws. The acid-etched composite is the "gold standard" of adhesion in dentistry, against which all other materials and techniques are compared to judge strength of bond, utility of use, and longevity.

2. Chemical Adhesion in Dentistry

Acid etching solved the problem of bonding dental materials to enamel, but bonding dental materials to dentin was more difficult. In the 1970s, Dennis Smith developed the first chemically adhesive dental cement, called polycarboxylate cement. **Polycarboxylate cements** use polyacrylic acid and zinc oxide. Later, Wilson, Crisp, and McLean developed glass ionomer cement. **Glass ionomer cements** also use polyacrylic acid, but they include glass powder instead of zinc oxide. Both materials are based on polyacrylic acid, and both chemically bond to dentin and enamel. They are discussed later in this chapter.

A number of glass ionomer materials were developed for various uses, with luting and restorative materials being the most popular. However, glass ionomer materials lack the esthetic appearance and mechanical toughness of dental composites.

3. Dentinal Bonding Agents

In the 1970s and 1980s, products were developed that supposedly bonded composite materials to dentin. By the 1990s, dentinal bonding of composites had become a clinically proven reality. Because dentinal bonding incorporates acid etching, it should be thought of as an extension of the acid etching process rather than as a replacement for it. Dentinal bonding systems continue to be developed and are now used to bond amalgam and cast restorations to dentin and enamel. In fact, nearly every restorative material can now be bonded to dentin or enamel with the use of some product and technique. However, the longevity and efficacy of some of these bonding techniques have yet to be confirmed by clinical research.

C. Surface Factors

1. Cleanliness

When applying an adhesive to an object, the surface must be clean. Otherwise, the adhesive will bond to the dirt and debris on the surface rather than to the surface itself. This would be like putting a Band-Aid on Pig-Pen of the "Peanuts" comic strip. (Pig-Pen is the character who is so dirty that a dust cloud follows him wherever he goes.) The Band-Aid would bond to the dirt rather than to Pig-Pen. Adhesives will not bond to any surface irregularities that are filled or covered by debris. If the surface and the adhesive are not somewhat chemically compatible, the adhesive will not wet the surface adequately, the adhesive will not flow into the irregularities, and the bonding will be poor. Whether the adhesive bonding is macromechanical, micromechanical, or truly adhesive (chemical), the surface must be clean to allow intimate association of the adhesive (bonding material) and the **adherend** (the surface).

2. Biofilms

In the oral cavity, it can be difficult to keep surfaces clean. A clean surface is one that is uncontaminated by oral fluids, such as saliva, blood, or crevicular fluid. Once a surface is contaminated by any oral fluid, it immediately becomes covered by a layer of biofilm. A **biofilm** is a coating that derives from organisms, both large and small. Biofilms in the mouth start as molecular coatings (the enamel pellicle) and grow into a community of microorganisms (plaque). For bonding purposes, the surface is no longer amalgam, enamel, or composite; the surface the adhesive "sees" or "feels" is biofilm. Biofilms reduce (or even prevent) bonding of many dental adhesives. To remedy this, use of a dental rubber dam is recommended when working with adhesive materials. The biofilm from saliva helps to lubricate the food bolus for swallowing, so it should not be surprising that biofilms are readily soluble in stomach acid and, therefore, do not inhibit the digestion of food. Luckily, biofilms are easily removed when acids are used to etch enamel and dentin.

D. Testing Adhesion—Optional

Much work has been done to measure the bond strength of various materials that are bonded to dentin and enamel. Usually, a small portion of material is bonded to a tooth and then pushed or pulled in an attempt to remove it. The force necessary to push or pull the bonded material off the tooth is measured in megapascals (mPa). One megapascal is equal to 145 pounds per square inch (psi). The resulting numbers are used to compare the effectiveness of the adhesive. A bond strength of 20 to 25 mPa (2,900–3,400 psi) is necessary for clinical success in high-stress areas of the mouth. Such numbers are useful only for general comparisons, however. In addition, one must know how the material broke off the tooth (where the fracture occurred). If the adhesive came off cleanly, then the break occurred at the interface. This type of break is called an **adhesive failure.** This is a test of bond strength. If the failure occurred inside the bonding material, the break is called a **cohesive failure.** This is a measure of the strength of the bonding material, not of the bond itself. If, during the testing procedure, the adhesive breaks the tooth, this is also a cohesive failure, and it signals that the strength of the bond is greater than the strength of the teeth. A bond that is stronger than tooth structure provides no advantage because the teeth, rather than the restoration, will break during failure.

II. Acid Etching

Acid etching was the first successful technique for bonding dental materials to tooth structure (Fig. 4.2). Acid creates a microscopically rough enamel surface, as shown in Figure 4.3. This roughened surface has sometimes been termed **"enamel tags"** or **"micropores."** A low-viscosity liquid polymer system is applied to the roughened surface. This liquid must wet the surface adequately so that it will flow into the micropores created by the etchant. The polymer system reacts chemically (polymerizes), changing from a liquid into a solid. The new solid is now bonded to the

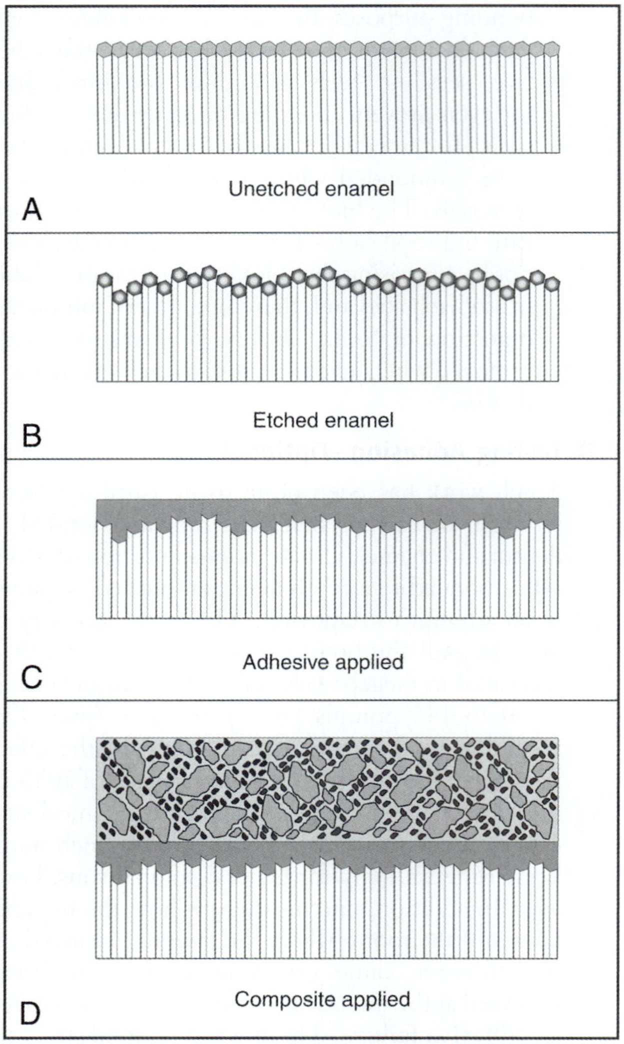

FIGURE 4.2 Schematic representation of the acid etching process for enamel. **A.** Vertical bars represent a clean surface composed of enamel rods. **B.** Etching dissolves some of the enamel rods, creating spaces between them at the surface. **C.** Adhesive flows into the spaces between the rods. The adhesive then sets and covers the surface with a layer of resin. The adhesive is micromechanically locked into the spaces between the enamel rods. **D.** The composite restorative material is applied and bonds to the underlying resin.

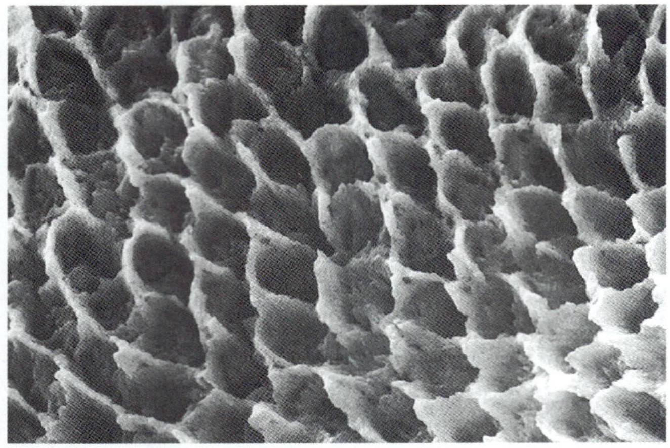

FIGURE 4.3 Scanning electron micrograph of etched enamel. (Reproduced with permission from Hormati AA, Fuller JL, Denehy GE. Effects of contamination and mechanical disturbance on the quality of acid-etched enamel. J Am Dent Assoc 1980;100(1): 34–38.)

micromechanically roughened enamel surface. A variety of acids and polymer systems are possible, but because of time restrictions and oral conditions, only a few are suitable for dental use.

A. The Acid Etching Process

First, the enamel surface is cleaned with pumice or a similar abrasive. The debris and pumice are then rinsed away with water, and the area is dried with compressed air (Fig. 4.2*A*). The acid or etchant, which is typically 37% **orthophosphoric acid,** is applied for 15 to 30 seconds. The term "etchant" is preferred in front of a patient rather than any word or words that use the term "acid." Sometimes, the etchant is called a "conditioner." However, that term can be confusing because other different dental materials are also called conditioners. The acid is rinsed away with water, and the surface is dried again with compressed air (Fig. 4.2*B*). Next, the liquid bonding resin (polymer system) is applied. The polymer system chemically reacts or "cures" (Fig. 4.2*C*). Finally, layers of restorative materials are chemically bonded to this initial layer of bonding resin (Fig. 4.2*D*).

B. Enamel

1. The acid etching technique is used to bond materials to enamel, but not to dentin. The technique is simple and micromechanical, and it has not changed appreciably over the years.
2. It is more effective to bond the polymer resin to the ends of enamel rods than to the long axis of the rods.
3. The acid etching technique has a "built-in" quality-control check. If the enamel is properly etched, it appears chalky or frosty white, as shown in Figure 4.4.
4. Years of clinical data demonstrate the advantages of using acid etching techniques for bonding to enamel. Pit and fissure sealants prevent caries, and the margins of composite restorations stain less frequently. Composites can be bonded to teeth to correct fractures, rotations, or other defects.

C. Acids

Many acids have been used to etch enamel. Orthophosphoric acid at 37% (or 3/8) concentration is the most commonly used today. Etching removes part of the enamel rod, leaving a microscopically rough surface, as shown in Figure 4.3. Etching may dissolve the periphery of enamel rods,

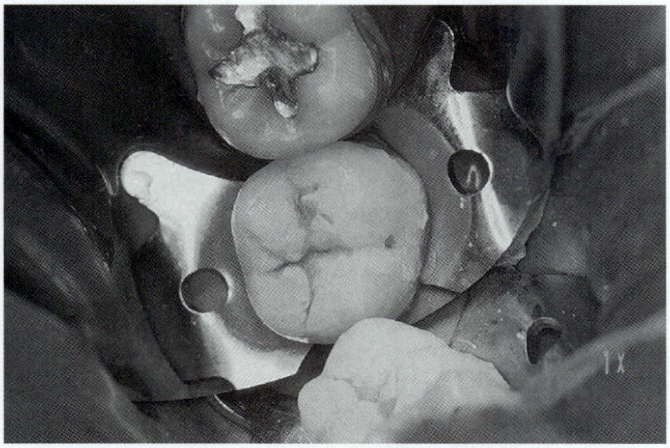

FIGURE 4.4 Photograph of etched enamel on the second molar (taken in a mirror). Note the chalky or frosty appearance of the surface, and compare this with the glossy surface of the unetched first molar. (See color images.) (Courtesy of Dr. Ronald House, Morgantown, WV.)

the core of the rods, or both in different areas. One can overetch, however, and crystals can form (precipitate) from the calcium and phosphate ions initially dissolved. Such precipitated crystals can inhibit bonding.

D. Time

The recommended time for etching enamel is typically 15 to 30 seconds. Deciduous teeth need to be etched for a longer time than permanent teeth. The enamel rods of deciduous teeth are less regularly arranged, so a longer etching time is required to obtain a surface with sufficient roughness for bonding. The results of acid etching of deciduous teeth are less reliable, however, than those of permanent teeth.

E. The Surface

Although the technique is simple, one must keep the surface clean and dry. The surface is very sensitive to contamination after etching. Reasons for a clean surface were explained previously.

F. Resin Systems (Materials Used With Acid Etching)

1. Low-Viscosity Resin

The first low-viscosity resin system to be used was polymethyl methacrylate. Resin systems, later developed for use as restorative dental composites, were used in conjunction with acid etching techniques. All resins used today wet the etched surface well and flow into the microscopic irregularities. The low-viscosity resin system is also called **enamel bonding resin** (or, simply, "the adhesive"). All resin systems used today set via addition polymerization. (Addition polymerization will be presented in Chapter 5.) Polymerization, or the setting process of the resin, can be activated (started) with light or a chemical reaction.

2. Composite Material

After the bonding resin is set, a composite restorative material is placed. The composite material sets by the same chemistry as low-viscosity resin and chemically bonds to the resin. A chemically activated acid-etched composite kit is shown in Figure 4.5.

III. Dentinal Bonding

Once acid etching was shown to be an effective clinical procedure, the focus turned to the development of techniques for bonding to dentin. The typical cavity preparation has more dentin than enamel available for bonding. A number of assorted complex chemical systems were developed. These systems were designed to chemically bond to collagen and other components of tooth structure. The intimate association of adhesive and tooth structure that is required for chemical bonding results in good wetting of the tooth surface. Chemical bonding was the intent, but micromechanical bonding was the result. Current **dentinal bonding** systems function by way of micromechanical bonding and secondary atomic bonds. It is doubtful that any of these systems bond to tooth structure principally by primary atomic bonds. In reality, dentinal bonding systems are an extension of the acid etch technique.

A. Dentinal Bonding Systems

1. Tooth Tissues

Dentinal bonding systems bond to both enamel and dentin. Because enamel is the outer layer of tissue, it is important that these systems bond to enamel. Without a strong bond to enamel,

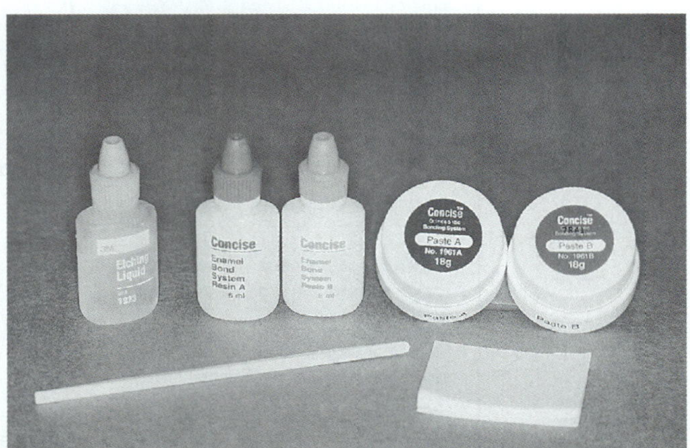

FIGURE 4.5 An enamel bonding system. The acid etchant is on the *left,* two chemically activated resin bottles are in the *center,* and two jars of the chemically activated composite restorative materials are on the *right.*

microleakage at the enamel–composite interface would increase the likelihood of recurrent caries even if a sufficient bond to dentin prevented deeper penetration of bacteria.

2. Structure of Dentin

Dentin is composed of intratubular dentin, intertubular dentin, and dentinal tubules filled with odontoblastic processes. Intratubular dentin and intertubular dentin are highly mineralized, but the odontoblastic processes are mostly water. In addition, different types of dentin exist: primary, secondary, reparative, sclerotic, and dead tracts. As one can see, dentin is much more variable and complex than enamel. Bonding to dentin has been a difficult problem for scientists to solve.

3. Smear Layer

When dentin is cut or prepared by dental instruments, a layer of debris called the **smear layer** is produced on the surface (Fig. 4.6*A*). It is similar to sawing green, sap-filled, sticky pine wood; the sawdust and sap stick to the newly cut surface. The smear layer on dentin also extends a short distance into the dentinal tubules. It is made of ground dentin that weakly adheres to the cut dentin surface. Enamel, on the other hand, cuts more cleanly because it is a more highly calcified tissue.

4. Historical Fallacies and Dentinal Bonding

The historical development of dentinal bonding systems in the United States is interesting in that several "sacred cows" had to be sacrificed before clinical use was widely accepted:

a) First, it was believed that composites irritate the pulp and so should not be placed directly on dentin.

In the 1980s, it was learned that composites, if properly cured, do not cause the problem. It is the microleakage of composites or other dental materials that causes pulpal irritation.

b) Second, it was common wisdom that one should not etch dentin.

It was believed that etching dentin would irritate pulp tissue, remove the smear layer that protects the pulp and cause postoperative problems. In the 1990s, the "Total Etch Technique" was accepted. Etching dentin and enamel at the same time was accepted.

In summary, current research supports the etching of dentin and the use of dentinal bonding systems to reduce microleakage. While some believe that any and all dentin should be etched, more conservative clinicians will, on rare occasions, place a protective material in deep cavity preparations to protect the pulp from irritation by the acid. Etching dentin close to the pulp is thought to be like

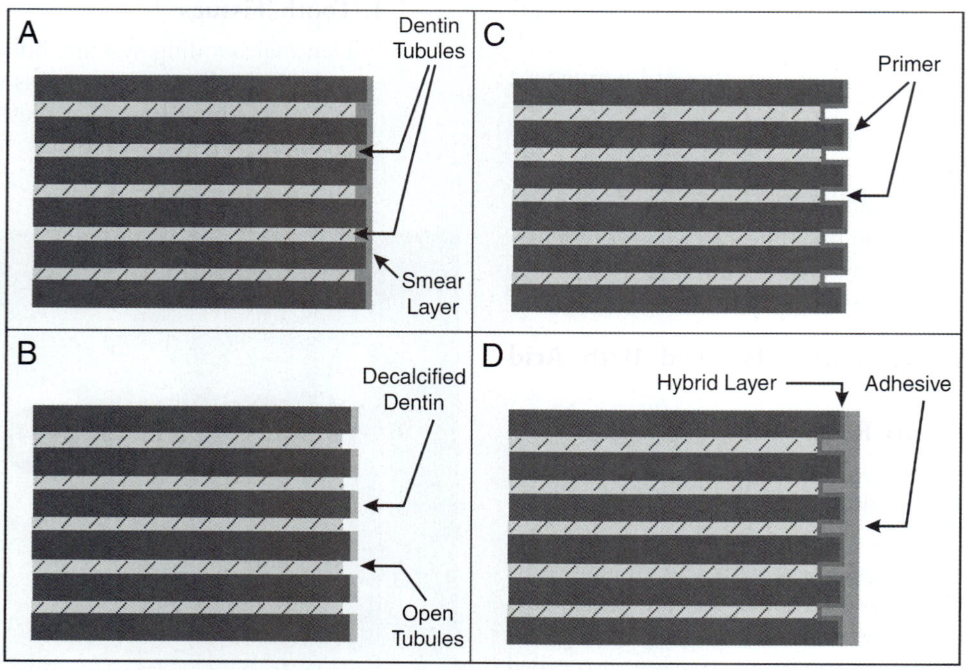

FIGURE 4.6 Schematic representation of a three-step dentinal bonding system. **A.** Prepared dentin is covered by a smear layer. **B.** When the enamel and dentin are etched, the smear layer is removed, the surface of the dentin is decalcified, and the dentinal tubules are opened. **C.** Primer flows into the open tubules and the decalcified dentin. **D.** Adhesive covers the primer and the hybrid layer.

rubbing salt in an open wound, with the deeply prepared dentin being the open wound.

5. History of Dentinal Bonding Systems

Dentinal bonding systems started out quite complex, requiring as many as six materials to be applied to the cavity preparation. Enamel and dentin were treated differently. Enamel only (not the dentin) was first etched, rinsed, and dried. Next, the dentin was "conditioned" with a weaker acid or a chelating agent. Chelating agents form molecular complexes with calcium and other ions, and they are used to remove the smear layer and to decalcify the dentin surface. Application of a dentin primer was next, and that was followed by the resin adhesive. With many products, two liquid components were mixed to obtain the primer or the adhesive materials before they were applied to the tooth. Primers were air-dried or cured or both, depending on the system. Adhesive resins were cured before the composite material was placed.

Today, a variety of relatively simple dentinal bonding systems abound, see Figure 4.7. Three-step systems, not much different than the two-step acid etching technique (etch and apply bonding resin), have demonstrated long-term clinical success. Simpler two-step systems have been become quite popular. Recently, one-step systems that use self-etching primers were introduced. In general, as the number of steps was reduced, the system may be easier to use but not always better. A generic three-step dentinal bonding system is described in detail in the following section to provide a theoretical understanding of the clinical process. Please note it is important to understand and follow the manufacturer's directions for each product used.

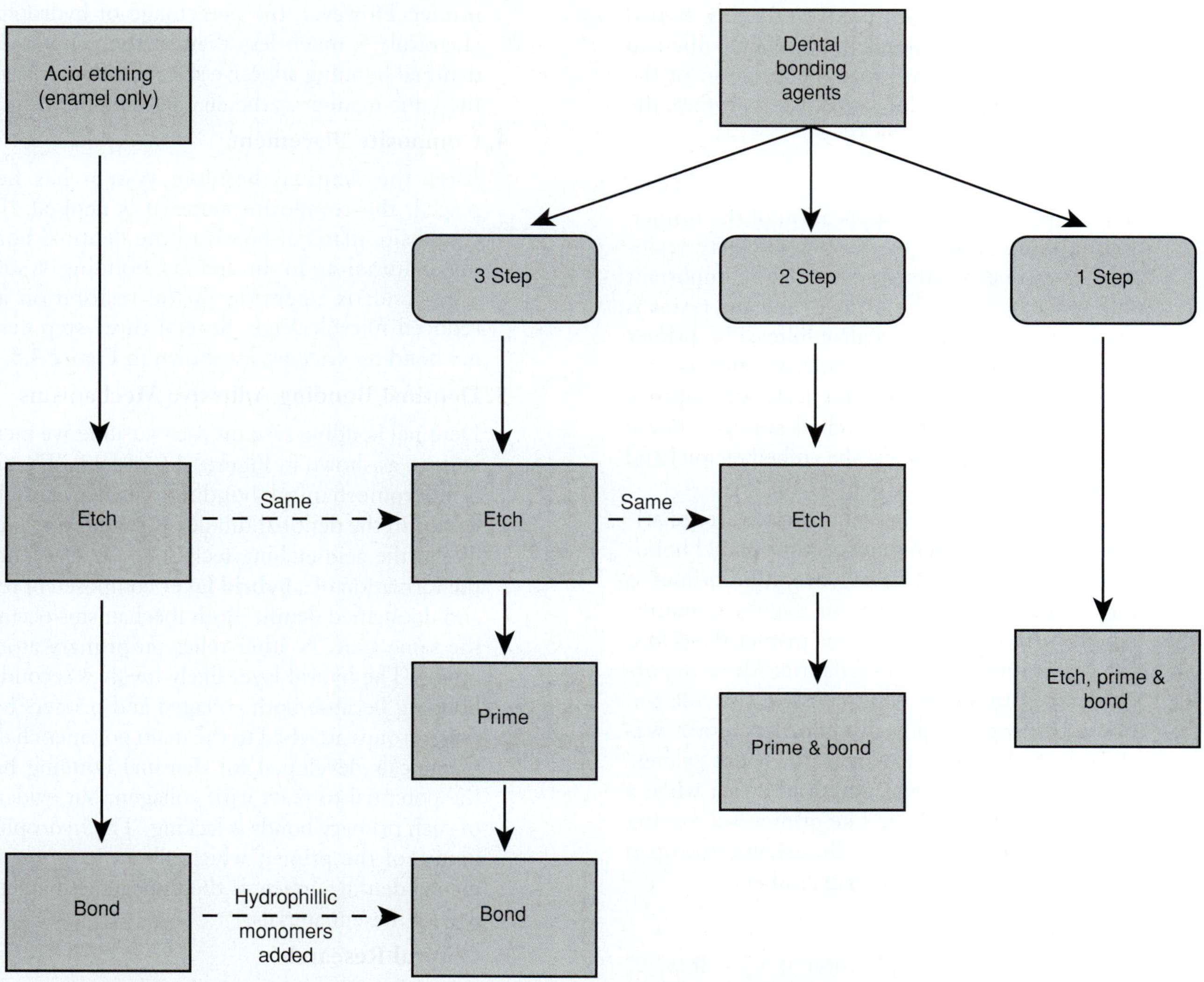

FIGURE 4.7 Diagram of the relationship of the various steps in acid etching for enamel bonding and dental bonding of enamel and dentin.

B. Three-Step Dentinal Bonding System

1. Etch Dentin and Enamel

The first step is the etching of both dentin and enamel as in the acid etch technique, as shown in Figure 4.6*B*. Typically, 37% orthophosphoric acid is used. Etching dentin removes the smear layer from the surface of the dentin as well as the plugs of material forced into the dentinal tubules during cavity preparation. Some etchants have small amounts of additives that are supposed to disinfect the tooth surface. These additives may also reduce the fluid that oozes from the cut odontoblastic processes and the opened tubules. Reducing this fluid makes the surface less wet and aids in application of the resin. Etching also decalcifies a layer of dentin several microns thick. Collagen fibers, a major organic component of dentin, are left on this decalcified surface. After etching, the surface is rinsed with water (as with acid etching), but the surface is only slightly dried (not desiccated), either with a gentle stream of air or by blotting. Overdrying etched dentin can cause the decalcified collagen fibers to "collapse" into a dense mat. Penetration of the mat by the primer is less effective, therefore, the bond to dentin is weaker.

2. Apply Primer

The second step is the application of the primer. **Primers** are similar to the low-viscosity resins used in enamel bonding systems. The important difference between the primers and the resins is that primers are more hydrophilic. The primer may also contain a volatile solvent, such as acetone, to thin the organic chemicals and improve flow and wetting of the etched surface. These hydrophilic chemicals wet the etched enamel and dentin surfaces well.

The primer flows into the surface irregularities of etched enamel, much as the enamel bonding resin did. In fact, the hydrophilic primer is more tolerant of a moist (or even a contaminated) surface. In addition, the primer flows into the open tubules of etched dentin. More importantly, the primer also flows around the collagen fibers that were exposed when the dentin was etched, as shown in Figure 4.6*C*. Most primers do not set on their own; rather, they set when a third material is applied. The primer is a wetting agent that aids flow of the adhesive into the open tubules and around the collagen fibers.

3. Apply Adhesive

The third step is the application of the "adhesive" material, as shown in Figure 4.6*D*. The adhesive material is a low-viscosity resin, much like that used in enamel bonding resin systems. The difference is that the dentinal bonding adhesive contains some hydrophilic chemicals, as in the primer. However, the percentage of hydrophilic chemicals is much less than in the primer. The dentinal bonding adhesive sets, or polymerizes, in the same manner as the enamel bonding resin.

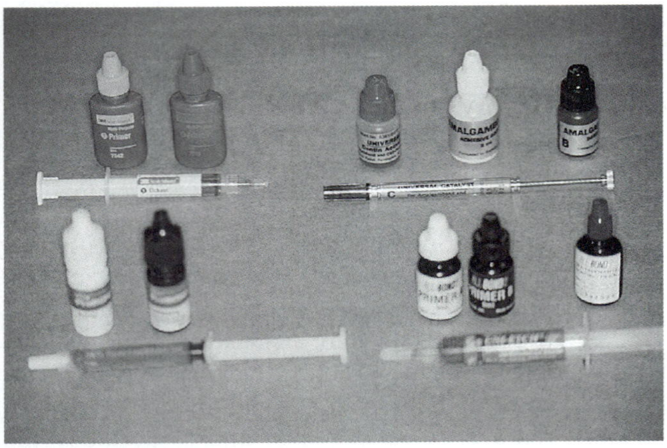

FIGURE 4.8 Photographs of four three-step dentinal bonding systems. From *top left* and then *clockwise:* Scotchbond Multi-Purpose, AmalgamBond, All-Bond 2, and Probond.

4. Composite Placement

After the dentinal bonding system has been placed, the composite material is applied. The composite material bonds to the dentinal bonding material as in an enamel bonding system. The result is retention of the restoration and reduced microleakage. Several three-step dentinal bonding systems are shown in Figure 4.8.

5. Dentinal Bonding Adhesive Mechanisms

Dentinal bonding systems use two adhesive mechanisms, as shown in Figures 4.6 and 4.9. The first is micromechanical bonding; resin material is locked in the dentinal tubules as **resin tags,** much like in the acid etching technique. The second is the formation of a **hybrid layer** composed of resin and decalcified dentin. Both mechanisms occur at the same time. Neither relies on primary atomic bonds. The hybrid layer likely involves secondary bonding because both collagen and primers have polar groups attached to the main polymer chains. Chemicals developed for dentinal bonding have the potential to react with collagen, but evidence of such primary bonds is lacking. The hydrophilic nature of the primer, which allows it to wet the etched dentin surface, is the important characteristic of these materials.

6. Clinical Research

Several products have more than 15 years of clinical data to support their effectiveness. The

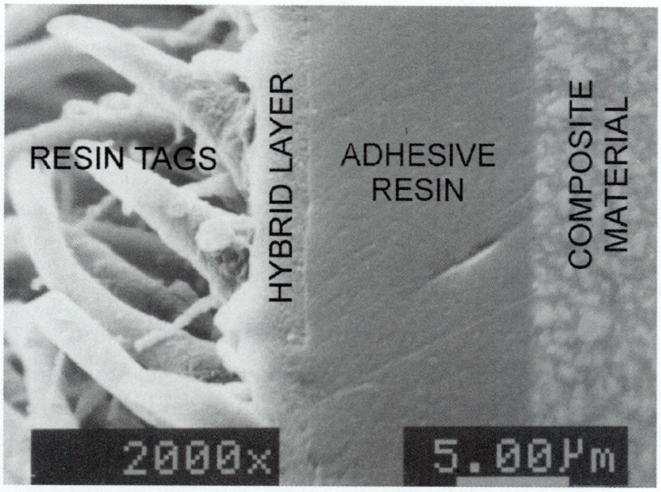

FIGURE 4.9 Scanning electron micrograph of a dentinal bonding system. A dentinal bonding system and composite were applied to the dentin. The dentin was removed by etching with an acid. The micrograph shows material that was in dentinal tubules (resin tags) and the hybrid layer. (Courtesy of BISCO, Inc.)

problem is that most dentinal bonding products on the market are "new." Dental bonding systems continuously change. Only short-term, 6- or 12-month data are available for many products. Surprisingly, the clinical performance of several "old" three-step systems is as good as or better than many of the new easier products.

C. Two-Step Dentinal Bonding Systems

Newer dentinal bonding systems have reduced the number of steps to two. Several products are shown in Figure 4.10. While they would seem to be more convenient, some two-step systems have little advantage in terms of time needed to apply materials. A few two-step products actually take longer than some three-step products. Some advocate the use of these systems when placing sealants or orthodontic brackets because the adhesive is more tolerant of contamination by saliva or other oral fluids.

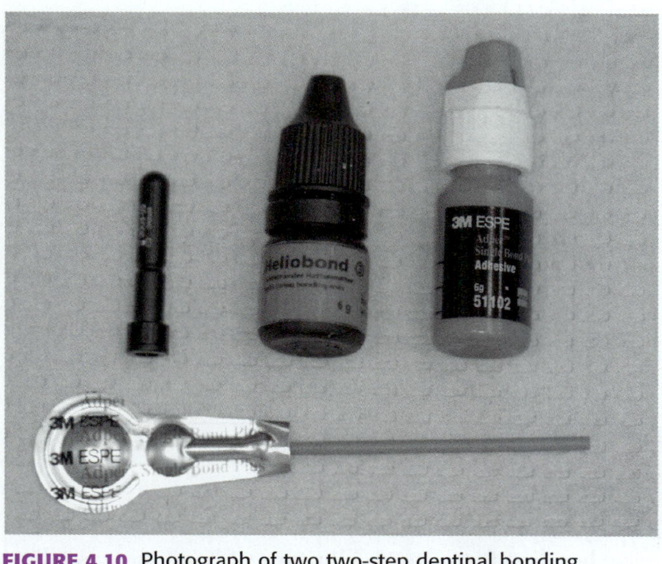

FIGURE 4.10 Photograph of two two-step dentinal bonding systems. Top left to right, Prime N Bond NT (unidose), Heliobond, Single Bond and bottom, Single Bond (unidose). Note the acid etchant utilized for two-step dentinal bonding systems is not pictured.

1. Etch

Dentin and enamel are etched the same as three-step systems using the same products. The smear layer is removed and surface dentin is decalcified. The rinse water is carefully removed by gently blowing with compressed air or blotting because desiccation of the dentin must be avoided.

2. Apply Adhesive

The adhesive of a two-step system is a combination of the primer and adhesive of the three-step system. The resin system is more hydrophilic than three-step systems. Solvents are present and aid in the wetting of the etched surface. Solvents are evaporated by gently blowing with air. For many products, two layers of the adhesive are required. The adhesive is light cured and the composite restorative material placed.

D. One Step Systems With Self-Etching Primers

One step systems that use self-etching primers seem to be the ultimate simplification of dentinal bonding. Several products are shown in Figure 4.11. The self-etching primers are very acidic organic chemicals that etch the enamel and dentin. Solvents are included to aid in surface wetting and evaporation of water. Hydrophilic resins are also included. Several problems can occur with some of these new products. Several do not etch uncut enamel well. Shelf-life may also be a problem. Complete polymerization of the resin is very important because any uncured resin components will irritate the pulp. There is one advantage of using self-etching primers. Any part of the tooth etched by the primer will be covered and protected by the adhesive.

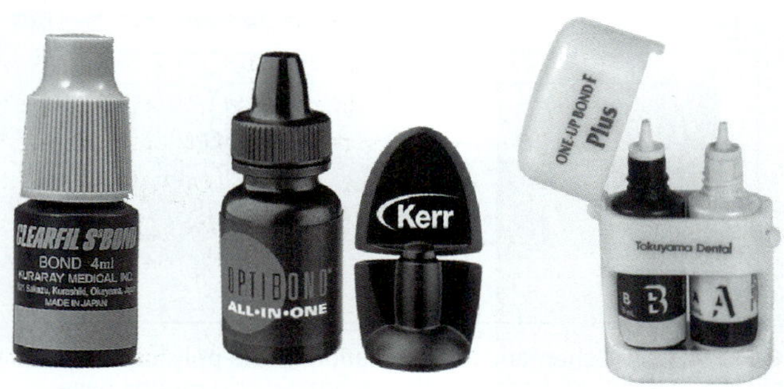

FIGURE 4.11 One-step dentinal bonding systems; left to right. Clearfil S^3 Bond, Optibond All-In-One (bulk and unidose) and One-Up Bond F Plus. Note: One-Up Bond is a two component, one-step system.

Etched enamel not covered by the adhesive of other systems has an increased susceptibility to decay. Laboratory and clinical results for these one-step systems are promising. After applying the adhesive following the manufacturer's directions, the adhesive is light cured and the composite restorative material placed.

IV. Glass Ionomers

A. Materials Based on Polyacrylic Acid

Glass ionomers are one of the two adhesive materials that are based on polyacrylic acid. The other is polycarboxylate cement, which will be covered in greater detail in Chapter 7. Glass ionomers started as a separate category of dental materials. They have evolved to become one end of a continuum of products, with dentinal bonding systems/composites at the other end. This will be discussed more in Chapter 5 and is illustrated in Figure 5.13.

B. Polycarboxylate and Glass Ionomer Cements

Polycarboxylate cement was developed by Dennis Smith in London in the 1970s. He combined the common dental cement powder, zinc oxide, with a new liquid, polyacrylic acid dissolved in water (yes, a polymer dissolved in water). Wilson and Crisp combined Smith's new liquid with the other common dental cement powder, which was finely ground or powdered glass. Their new material was named glass ionomer cement. Polyacrylic acid is a long-chain molecule with acid (carboxyl) groups hanging off the side, as shown in Figure 4.12*A*. The acid groups react with the powder when the material sets to form a solid mass. The acid groups can also react with tooth structure and chemically bond to dentin and enamel (see Figs. 4.12*B* and 4.12*C*).

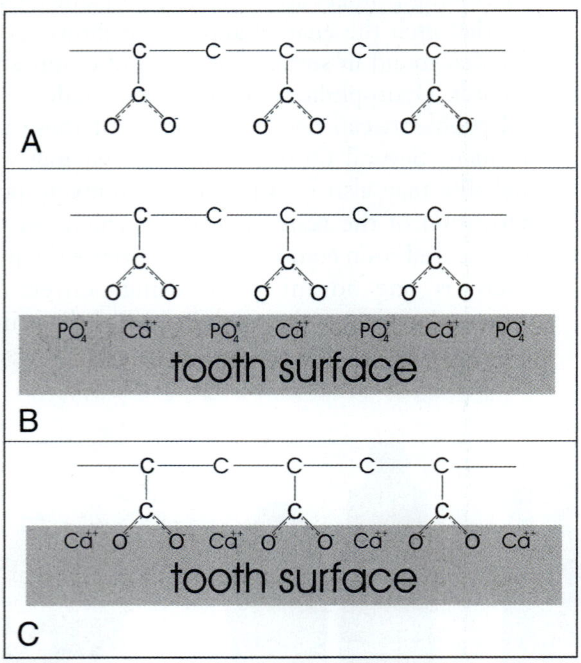

FIGURE 4.12 A. Schematic representation of the polyacrylic acid molecule in solution. Note that the carboxylic acid groups have ionized. **B.** Schematic representation of bonding between carboxylic acid groups and calcium ions in tooth structure. **C.** Schematic representation of bonding carboxylic acid groups substituting for phosphate ions in tooth structure.

C. Bonding Mechanisms of Glass Ionomers

Bonding "true" glass ionomer materials to enamel and dentin is simple compared to dentinal bonding systems and composites. No separate adhesive is placed and then followed by the restorative material. Instead, the glass ionomer material itself is the adhesive and the restorative material. In addition to chemical adhesion, micromechanical retention is possible if the surface has microscopic irregularities, such as partially open dentinal tubules. Glass ionomer materials will be covered in more detail in Chapter 7.

At first, glass ionomer materials were directly applied to dentin and enamel. Later, dentin surfaces were cleaned or "conditioned" with an aqueous solution of polyacrylic acid before placement of the glass ionomer material. The result is a cleaner surface (with the smear layer removed) and better bonding. The dentin tubules are not opened, as when dentin is acid-etched, and dentin is not decalcified to produce a hybrid layer.

V. Uses of Bonding in Dentistry

Depending on the clinical situation, the dentist will choose among a variety of adhesive materials. Acid etching of enamel is still used to place pit and fissure sealants and to bond orthodontic brackets. Dentinal bonding systems are the norm when composite restorations are placed and are used to reduce the sensitivity of exposed root surfaces of teeth. Glass ionomer materials are the materials of choice for many clinicians when a cervical lesion has margins in both enamel and dentin or the patient has a high risk for caries. All adhesive materials require proper handling and a clean surface for maximum bonding.

SUMMARY

Many materials in dentistry rely on the property of adhesive bonding for success. This type of bonding is usually considered to be micromechanical because the bonding occurs at a level too small to be seen by the naked eye. An example of macromechanical bonding in dentistry is the cementing of crowns and bridges to teeth, similar to the manner in which two pieces of wood are glued together.

Uses of adhesive materials in dentistry include retention of restorations, reduction of microleakage, and reduction of recurrent decay. Cleanliness and biofilms are important factors to consider before using adhesive materials. For bonding success, the surface must be clean to allow intimate association of the adhesive (bonding material) and adherend (the surface).

Today, the acid etching process is used to micromechanically bond dental materials to tooth structure. A microscopic rough surface is created, which allows a low-viscosity polymer resin to flow into the rough "enamel tags" or "micropores." The procedure requires that the surface be cleaned with an abrasive, etched with orthophosphoric acid, and coated with a bonding resin before the restorative material can be applied. Between these steps, the tooth surface is thoroughly rinsed and dried.

To bond to the dentin, an extension of the acid etch technique is used. Cut or prepared dentin differs from enamel in that it is covered by a "smear layer." The traditional, three-step dentinal bonding process consists of etching dentin and enamel, applying primer, and then applying adhesive, after which the tooth is ready to accept the restorative material. Dentinal bonding systems utilize two adhesive mechanisms: micromechanical bonding and the formation of a hybrid layer. The hybrid layer is composed of resin and decalcified dentin. Both mechanisms occur at the same time, and neither relies on primary atomic bonds.

Another adhesive dental material is glass ionomer cement, which is composed of polyacrylic acid and finely ground or powdered glass. No separate adhesive is placed and then followed by the restorative material because the glass ionomer itself is chemically adhesive to tooth structure. The glass ionomer can serve as both the bonding agent and the restoration.

Depending on the patient's needs, the dentist will choose among the available adhesive materials. All adhesive materials must be handled properly to ensure maximum bonding.

Learning Activities

1. Obtain several extracted teeth, and place composite material on both etched and unetched enamel. Push off the composite material with an instrument. Is there a difference in the force needed to remove the composite from the differently prepared surfaces?
2. Place a drop of adhesive from a dentinal bonding system on enamel that has been etched and on enamel that has been etched and then contaminated with saliva. Is there a difference in the contact angles formed by the adhesive on the two surfaces?
3. Make 1-mm-thick specimens of a hybrid composite (or any composite material on hand) and a glass ionomer restorative material. Compare the appearance (surface texture, color, and opacity) of these materials.

Review Questions

1. Postage stamps are now self-adhesive. The paper (actual stamp) is referred to as the ______________, and the sticky material on the back of the stamp is termed the ______________.
   a) Adherend, adhesive
   b) Adhesive, adherend
   c) Adhesive, bonding agent
   d) Adherend, biofilm
2. Kristin has orthodontic appliances, commonly known as "braces." These include metal brackets directly bonded to the facial surface with a bonding material. One bracket breaks off, and the "failure" occurs within the bonding material. This type of failure is considered to be:
   a) Adhesive
   b) Adherend
   c) Cohesive
   d) Macromechanical

3. On the lines below, use the numbers 1 through 8 to place the steps of the acid etching process and restoration placement in correct sequence.

_____ Clean surface is rinsed with water.
_____ Etched surface is rinsed with water.
_____ Bonding resin is applied.
_____ Enamel is cleaned with pumice.
_____ Cleaned surface is dried with air.
_____ Etched surface is dried with air.
_____ Restorative material is applied.
_____ Etchant is applied.

4. Orthophosphoric acid (enamel etchant) is commonly used in a ______ concentration.
a) 27%
b) 30%
c) 37%
d) 47%
e) None of the above

5. Why do primary teeth need to be etched longer than permanent teeth?
a) It compensates for potential behavioral management problems
b) The enamel is denser on primary teeth
c) The enamel rods are more regularly arranged than on permanent teeth
d) The enamel rods are less regularly arranged than on permanent teeth

6. Dentinal bonding systems function by way of:
a) Micromechanical bonding and secondary atomic bonds
b) Macromechanical bonding and secondary atomic bonds
c) Micromechanical bonding and primary atomic bonds
d) Macromechanical bonding and primary atomic bonding

7. The "dentin debris" that is created when dentin is cut or prepared by dental instruments is called:
a) Adhesive layer
b) Smear layer
c) Primer layer
d) Chelating agent

8. The use of bonding in dentistry serves all of the following functions EXCEPT:
a) Reduction of recurrent caries
b) Retention of color in the restoration
c) Reduction of microleakage
d) Retention of restorations

9. An adhesive mechanism of a dentinal bonding system is a hybrid layer. It is composed of:
a) The smear layer and resin
b) Dentin primer and decalcified enamel
c) Resin and decalcified enamel
d) Resin and decalcified dentin

10. The following are all historical fallacies about dentinal bonding except one. Which one is the EXCEPTION?
a) Composites irritate the pulp
b) Dentin should not be etched
c) The smear layer is "dentinal debris"
d) The smear layer should be left to protect the pulp

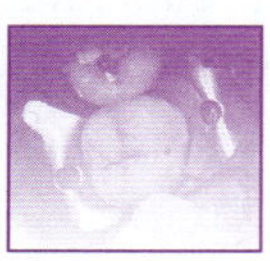

Supplemental Readings

Christensen GH. Bonding to dentin and enamel: Where does it stand in 2005? J Am Dent Assoc 2005;136(9)1299–1302.

Cox CF, Suzuki S, Suzuki SH. Biocompatibility of dental adhesives. J Calif Dent Assoc 1995;23(8):35–41.

Latta MA, Barkmeier WW. Dental adhesives in contemporary restorative dentistry. Dent Clin North Am 1998;42(4):567–577.

Soderholm KJ. Does resin based dentine bonding work? Int Dent J 1995;45(6):371–381.

Swift EJ. Bonding systems for restorative materials—a comprehensive review. Pediatr Dent 1998;20(2):80–84.

Tay FR, Pashley DH. Dental adhesives of the future. J Adhes Dent 2002;4(2):91–103.

Van Meerbeek B, Perdigao J, Lambrechts P, Vanherle G. The clinical performance of adhesives. J Dent 1998;26(1): 1–20.

5

Direct Polymeric Restorative Materials

Objectives

After studying this chapter, the student will be able to do the following:

1. Name the two types of polymerization reactions commonly seen in dental materials, and explain the meaning of "addition" in "addition polymerization."
2. Discuss the following properties of restorative resins:
   - Polymerization shrinkage
   - Coefficient of thermal expansion
   - Abrasion resistance
3. Summarize the relationship between a filler particle, the matrix, and the coupling agent of a composite restorative material.
4. Compare the advantages and disadvantages of light-cure and chemical-cure composite materials.
5. Explain the importance of proper eye protection when light-curing dental materials.
6. Relate the importance of the following procedures and/or characteristics of dental composites:
   - Depth of cure
   - Addition of material in increments
   - Inhibition by air
   - Unreacted C=C bonds
   - Shades
   - Shortcomings of the matrix
7. Summarize the importance of the following properties in relation to the fillers (particles) found in dental composites:
   - Composition
   - Size
   - Amount
   - Abrasion resistance
   - Refractive index
   - Clinical detection
8. Choose one of the three types of dental composites, and justify its use in the following dental situations:
   - Bonding orthodontic brackets to enamel
   - Class V "gingival notch" restoration
   - Small Class I or II restoration
9. Briefly explain the reason(s) for the development of flowable and condensable composites.
10. Discuss the role the dental hygienist should play in the placement and maintenance of pit and fissure sealants.
11. Discuss the use of a primer with pit and fissure sealants.
12. Briefly describe "preventive resin restoration" and "composite cements."
13. Assess the positive and negative characteristics of light-cure and chemical-cure glass ionomer cements.
14. Discuss the similarities between compomers, glass ionomers, and composites.

Key Words/Phrases

activation
addition polymerization
compomer
condensable composites
crazing
depth of cure
diluent
filler particles
flowable composites
free radical
hybrid composite
incremental addition
inhibitor
initiation
macrofilled composite
matrix
microfilled composite
monomers
oligomer
percolation
pit and fissure sealants
polymers
polymerization
preventive resin restoration
propagation
silane coupling agent
termination
thermoplastic polymers
thermoset polymers

INTRODUCTION

Polymers are materials that are made of large, long molecules formed by chemically reacting molecular building blocks called monomers. A variety of polymers exist, and they exhibit a variety of properties. The chemical reaction that links the monomers together to produce a polymer (macromolecule) is called **polymerization.** Common polymers or "plastics," such as polyethylene and Plexiglas (an acrylic resin), are made via addition polymerization and are used to make soda and milk bottles and many other everyday objects. Polyethylene materials have long, linear chains that are easily recycled because they can be remelted and reprocessed. These materials are called **thermoplastic polymers** because they can be heated (thermo) and molded or shaped (plastic) after the polymerization reaction, similar to wax.

Polymers with a cross-linked rather than a linear structure tend not to melt. Rather, they decompose. These materials are called **thermoset polymers.** They cannot be heated and molded, so their use requires them to be in the final shape when the polymerization reaction occurs. They tend to be stronger and tougher than thermoplastic materials. Most dental resins are cross-linked and are therefore thermoset.

Polymers were introduced in Chapter 2. In this chapter, we will discuss acrylic resins and dental composites used to replace and restore teeth.

I. Acrylic Resins

Acrylic resins were first used in dentistry for denture bases (see Figs 1.6 and 1.7). A denture base is the pink plastic part of a denture that simulates the gingiva and lost alveolar bone. Denture teeth are bonded to the base to form the denture. Dental acrylic resin is the same polymer used in Plexiglas, a tough plastic that serves as a glass substitute in windows. Acrylic resins are used in dentistry for a variety of devices and will be covered in greater detail in later chapters. The chemistry of acrylic resins will be presented in this chapter because it is the same chemistry as that of most direct polymeric restorative materials. Acrylic resins were once used for anterior restorations but were very susceptible to recurrent decay. When dental composites became available, direct acrylic restorative materials were made obsolete. The shortcomings of acrylic resins and the improved performance of composite materials will be discussed in this chapter.

A. Addition Polymerization—Optional

The polymerization reaction of acrylic resins, called addition polymerization, is very common in dental materials. The other common polymerization reaction, condensation polymerization, will be covered when impression materials are discussed. Acrylic resins and composite materials, such as restorative materials, cements, sealants, and adhesives, all set via addition polymerization. The common factor relating all these materials to each other is the same chemical structure of the reactive or functional group. The functional group is the part of the molecule responsible for its important chemical properties.

1. Functional Groups

Monomers are molecules with a reactive group that participates in the polymerization reaction. This reactive group is called the functional group. The functional group of acrylic resin monomers is the carbon–carbon double bond. We will denote this bond as C=C. The "double bond" has two pairs of electrons shared by the two carbon atoms, so four electrons are involved in the double bond. Although C=C is the reactive part of the monomer, other atoms and side groups (besides hydrogen) can be bonded to either or both of the carbon atoms of the C=C. The side groups become pendants (like a charm on a charm bracelet) on the polymer chain, and they determine the chemical and physical properties of the resulting polymer.

2. Free Radicals

The chemical (polymerization) reaction of acrylic resins is called free radical or addition polymerization. The first name, free radical polymerization, is used because a free radical, an unpaired electron, is involved in the reaction. The other name, **addition polymerization,** is used because one monomer at a time is added to the polymer chain as the reaction proceeds. Addition polymerization is a very common polymerization reaction used to make a variety of polymers or plastics.

B. Steps in Addition Polymerization—Optional

1. Initiation

The first step in addition polymerization reaction is called **initiation.** Actually, initiation can be thought of as two reactions. The first involves the formation of a **free radical,** which is a molecule with an unpaired electron. Several **activation** methods are used (Fig. 5.1*A*. In the second reaction, the free radical reacts with a monomer molecule to start a growing chain (Fig. 5.1*B*).

a) Formation of Free Radicals (Polymerization Activation)

An initiator molecule can become activated (changed into a free radical) by heat, light, or a chemical reaction. Several types of chemical

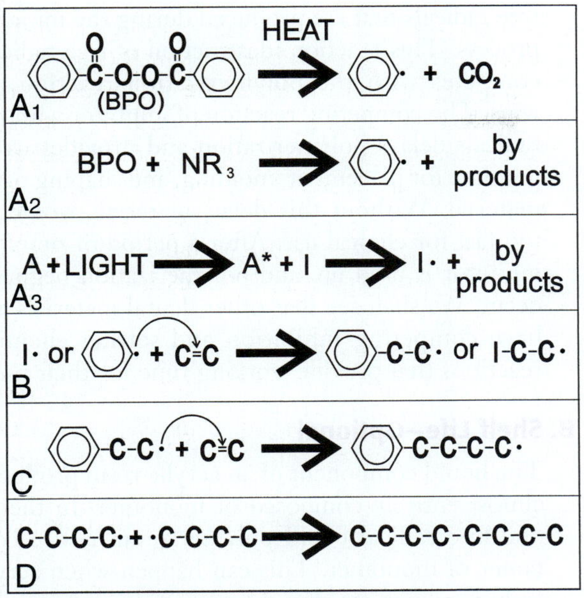

• denotes an unpaired electron, a free radical
* denotes a excited molecule

FIGURE 5.1 Initiator molecules are activated by heat (**A_1**), chemical reaction (**A_2**), and light (**A_3**) to form free radicals. Initiation of chain growth (**B**), propagation of chain growth (**C**), and one example of chain termination (**D**) are also illustrated. *A,* activator; *I,* initiator; *BPO,* benzoyl peroxide; *NR3,* tertiary amine; •, unpaired electron, a free radical; *, an excited molecule.

reactions are used in dentistry to form free radicals. One is a chemical reaction that begins when chemicals are mixed together. The other is a chemical reaction that is started by light (Fig. 5.1*A*).

As a result of the various activation methods, materials are classified as heat-activated (also known as heat-cure), chemically activated (also known as cold-cure or chemical-cure), or photoactivated (also known as photo-cure or light-cure). In this text, heat and chemical activation will be presented in detail, while light activation will be described only in general terms.

b) Reaction of Free Radical and Monomer

Regardless of the method by which the free radical is formed, the second reaction during initiation of polymerization is for the free radical to react with the C=C of the monomer. As previously mentioned, a free radical is an unpaired electron. An unpaired electron is "unhappy" (high-energy state) and wants to form an atomic bond by pairing with another electron (forming a lower-energy state). In addition polymerization, it does so by reacting with one of the electron pairs of the C=C of the monomer. A group of three electrons, however, is not the result. Rather, a single C–C bond and another free radical on the end of the growing chain are formed, as illustrated in Figure 5.1*B*. The first "link" in the growing chain has been added.

2. Propagation

Figure 5.1*C* illustrates the second step in addition polymerization, which is the growth or lengthening of the chain. This step is called **propagation.** The free radical of the "initiated chain" reacts with a monomer, and the chain is one monomer longer. The process is similar to initiation. Propagation involves adding the second, third, fourth, and later monomers to the growing chain until that chain is hundreds or even thousands of monomers long. Polymerization continues as long as monomers are available to react with the free radical at the end of the growing chain. Polymerization reactions result in a long chain of monomers. Such addition polymerization reactions are also called chain-lengthening reactions.

3. Termination

Two free radicals at the ends of two growing chains may react. If they do, they will form a carbon–carbon bond, as illustrated in Figure 5.1*D*. At this point, no free radicals are left to continue growth of the chain. **Termination** of polymerization of both chains is the result; thus, termination is the name given this step. Free radicals also react with contaminants, which may also cause termination of polymerization.

C. Activation of Addition Polymerization

1. Heat Activated

Heat-activated acrylic resins typically use benzoyl peroxide (BPO) as the initiator. Heat is the activator. When heated to 60°C, BPO breaks down into CO_2 and free radical molecules, as illustrated in Figure 5.1A_1. Heat-activated acrylic resins come from the manufacturer as a powder/liquid system. The powder and liquid are mixed to form a dough for molding into the desired shape, but the polymerization reaction does not start until the material is heated, typically in a hot water bath. Most complete and partial dentures use heat-activated acrylic resins for the denture base.

2. Chemically Activated

Chemically activated acrylic resins also commonly use BPO as the initiator. A variety of chemicals are used as the activator. Activators used in dental polymers belong to a group of chemicals called tertiary amines, which are organic molecules with a nitrogen atom bonded to three carbon-containing groups. We will use

NR_3 to denote a tertiary amine. Figure 5.1A_2 shows the reaction of the tertiary amine with BPO and the formation of free radical molecules. Chemically activated materials are typically a powder and a liquid that are mixed together to start the polymerization process. Chemically activated acrylic resins are used to make temporary crowns, custom impressions trays, orthodontic retainers, and many other dental devices.

3. Light Activated

Light-activated acrylic resins and other light-cure dental materials use several activator and initiator chemicals. The activator absorbs light and then reacts with the initiator. Figure 5.1A_3 represents the formation of free radical–containing molecules by light activation. Light-activated materials are supplied as a single paste; no mixing is required. The polymerization process does not begin until the material is exposed to a very bright light source. The "set on demand" nature of light-activated materials has made them very popular. The most common light-activated dental materials are composite restorative materials, but other light-activated acrylic products exist.

4. Dual-Cure Materials

Several dental materials have both chemical- and light-activated capabilities. These materials are called dual-cure materials. Polymerization is started with a curing light, but material that cannot be reached by the intense light sets via the chemical-cure mechanism.

D. Addition Polymerization Is an Exothermic Reaction

In chemical factories, the heat of this rapid exothermic polymerization reaction must be removed, or the rise in temperature can become dangerous. Dental acrylic resins react via addition polymerization and are also exothermic. In a later chapter, we shall see that controlling the rise in temperature is important for the proper processing of an acrylic denture.

II. Inhibitors and Competing Reactions

A. Working Time

Polymerization reactions can occur very rapidly. For a dental material to be useful, the reaction must either occur when desired (as with light-activated materials) or be delayed after mixing and occur somewhat slowly (as with chemically activated products). The reaction of chemically activated materials is initially delayed for several minutes by the presence of a chemical called an inhibitor. An **inhibitor,** typically hydroquinone, reacts with (destroys) the first free radicals that are produced during the initiation process. This reaction (destruction of free radicals) competes with the polymerization reaction and wins. The competing reaction of inhibitor with free radicals delays polymerization and provides working time for placement, molding, and shaping of the material. Without this delay, materials would set too fast for clinical use. After a period of time, the inhibitor is used up, and polymerization begins to occur. We shall see that other dental materials also have competing inhibition and setting chemical reactions that provide working time for their use.

B. Shelf Life—Optional

The liquid component of an acrylic resin product is almost entirely composed of monomer. In theory, one free radical could polymerize an entire container of monomer. This can happen when acrylic resin products are stored for several years. To prevent this and provide a reasonable shelf life for their products, manufacturers add a small amount of inhibitor to materials that contain monomer. Inhibitors are present at a much smaller concentration in light-activated and heat-activated products than they are in chemical-activated systems. Inhibitors provide shelf life for monomer-containing mixtures of materials. Without an inhibitor, what was once a liquid or a paste would become a solid chunk of polymer over time.

III. Problems With Unfilled Resins

Polymers without filler additives are not suitable for use as restorative materials. A discussion of several problems will aid our understanding of the importance of fillers.

A. Polymerization Shrinkage

Polymerization reactions make a few very large polymer molecules from many small monomer molecules. Atoms and molecules become packed much closer together when polymerized, and the resulting material is smaller in volume than the starting components. Polymerization shrinkage is an important problem with the use of polymers. In dentistry, polymeric restorative materials shrink when they set; thus, they have the potential to open gaps at the margins of these restorations. Bonding materials to tooth structure reduces the potential for these gaps and the resulting microleakage.

B. Coefficient of Thermal Expansion

Polymeric materials have high coefficients of thermal expansion compared to tooth structure. In fact, these coefficients can be from 2 to 10 times greater. Repeated expansion and contraction of polymeric

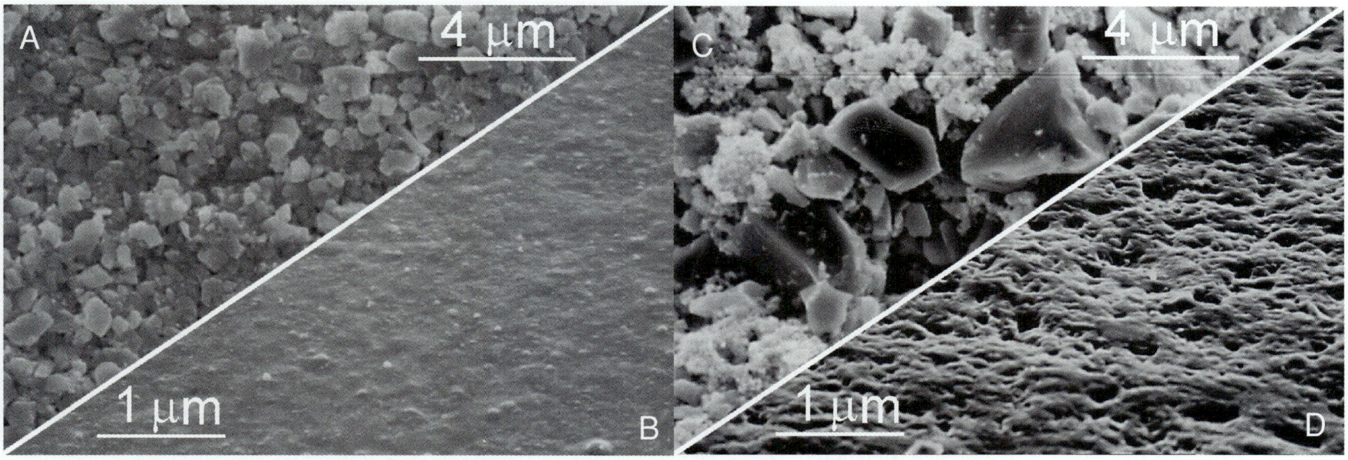

FIGURE 5.2 Scanning electron micrographs of two dental composites (**B** and **D**) and their filler particles (**A** and **C**). The smaller filler particles result in composite restorations with a smoother surface. (Courtesy of BISCO, Inc.)

restorative materials can open and close gaps at the margin of a restoration. This phenomenon is called **percolation** and is illustrated in Figure 4.1. As a result, leakage increases, and recurrent caries are much more likely.

C. Strength and Abrasion Resistance of Polymeric Materials

Even the best polymers are unable to withstand occlusal forces in the oral environment. They lack strength and abrasion resistance. Polymeric materials are useful in dentistry, however, because they can be placed into a cavity preparation as a plastic mass and then molded and shaped. Next, they are polymerized in the mouth, forming a replacement for lost tooth structure. Processing directly in the mouth is very useful, but time and temperature limit which polymers can be used.

IV. Improvements to Dental Resins

Several techniques have been used to improve dental resins. These techniques originated in nondental industries, but they have greatly improved polymeric restorative materials. The most successful and notable individual in this process was Dr. Raphael Bowen, who developed the first dental composites.

A. Fillers and Silane Coupling Agents

Industrial uses of polymers greatly expanded when strong, hard fillers were added to strengthen plastics to form composites. Fiberglass is one such material. It combines a polymer with glass fibers and is much stronger and useful compared to the polymer alone. Composite materials were introduced in Chapter 2. **Filler particles** are typically inexpensive, strong, hard ceramic materials. Many fillers are naturally occurring minerals, but others are specially prepared glass materials.

Dr. Bowen incorporated a strong ceramic filler particle into his polymer system to form a much stronger dental restorative material. Two examples of dental composites are shown in Figure 5.2. To obtain the maximum benefit from the addition of these particles, the polymer (or matrix, as it is called in a composite system) is bonded to the filler particle with a coupling agent. The coupling agent couples, or transfers, stress from the relatively weak matrix to the relatively strong filler. Dental composites use ceramic filler particles coated with silane coupling agents. Silane coupling agents work a bit like soap; they have a different chemical group at each end of the molecule. **Silane coupling agents** are long molecules that react with the polymer matrix at one end and with the ceramic filler at the other end, as illustrated in Figure 5.3. The end that reacts with the polymer matrix has a C=C that

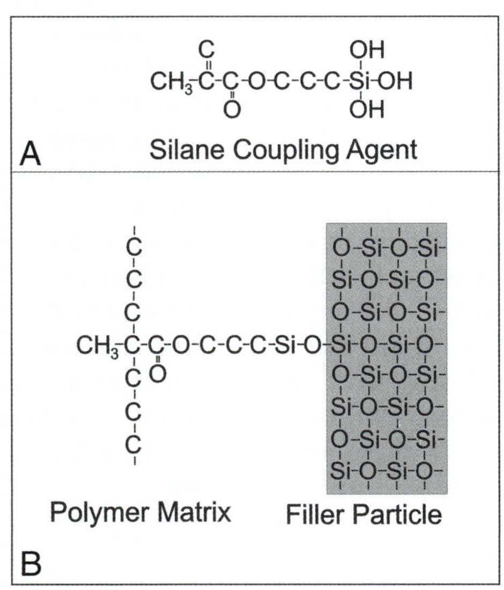

FIGURE 5.3 Example of silane coupling agent (**A**) and its reaction with the polymer matrix on the *left* and the filler particle on the *right* (**B**).

participates in the addition polymerization reaction. The other end has a silane group, hence the name silane coupling agent. The silane group has silicon and oxygen atoms that react with the silicon and oxygen on the surface of the ceramic filler particle.

Fillers are selected for their physical properties. Luckily, the strong, hard ceramic materials that are chosen also have low coefficients of thermal expansion. When mixed with polymers, the resulting dental composites have coefficients closer to that of tooth structure than the polymers on which they are based. Because a composite has less polymer in the system, polymerization shrinkage is reduced when the material sets.

Manufacturers try to maximize the filler content of their dental composites because adding more filler increases strength, decreases polymerization shrinkage, and decreases thermal expansion to nearer that of tooth structure. However, there is a limit to the amount of filler that can be added. When mixing dough for bread, excess flour results in a defective product; the same is true for filler in dental composites. If all filler particles are not properly wetted by the liquid monomers, voids and gaps between the filler particles result. As previously mentioned, voids do not resist any stress placed on a material; they also concentrate stress in the material in the vicinity of the void.

B. Bowen's Resin—Optional

In addition to adding fillers to form composites, Dr. Bowen also developed a polymer for dental composites. This molecule is actually a combination of several monomer molecules to form what is called an **oligomer.** The notable features of Dr. Bowen's oligomer are polar side groups that increase chain-to-chain hydrogen bonding and two reactive C=C groups. Because each C=C group can participate in the formation of a growing polymer chain, the oligomer is called bifunctional. Bifunctional monomers and oligomers result in cross-linking and greatly improve the strength of the resulting polymer. Dr. Bowen's oligomer is called bis-GMA and is illustrated in Figure 5.4 along with methyl methacrylate, the monomer most commonly found in dental acrylic systems, and triethylene glycol dimethacrylate. The bis-GMA is a very viscous material and needs to be diluted with other bifunctional monomers, such as triethylene glycol dimethacrylate, when dental composites are formulated. Although bis-GMA is more properly called an oligomer, we shall use the term monomer when referring to it.

V. Composite Materials

Composite materials are the combination of two materials. The result is a material that is superior to either component alone.

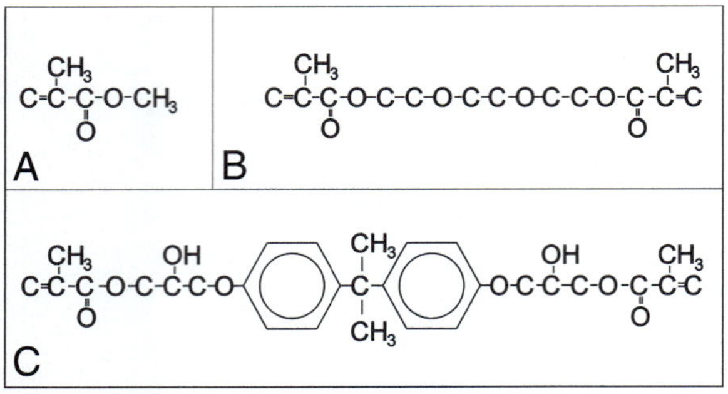

FIGURE 5.4 Structure of methyl methacrylate (**A**), triethylene glycol dimethacrylate (**B**), and bis-GMA (**C**).

A. Dental Composites

Dental composites are supplied in a variety of shades (colors) and handling characteristics. Their use continues to expand and replace other materials. Before dental composites were introduced, other esthetic materials were used, such as acrylic resins, but they lacked clinical efficacy. Acrylic resin materials had a high coefficient of thermal expansion, and polymerization shrinkage was excessive. Recurrent caries around and under acrylic resin restorations was typical. Silicate cements were also used as an esthetic material, but they dissolved too quickly and required frequent replacement. In the 1960s, when dental composites were developed, they quickly replaced acrylic resin and silicate restorative materials.

B. Components of a Dental Composite

Dental composites are composed of two phases: matrix and filler. The matrix is soft, weak, flexible, and prone to wear compared to the filler. In addition, two "molecular components" are present: a silane coupling agent and a polymerization system.

1. Matrix

The **matrix** of a dental composite is a polymer, typically bis-GMA or a similar monomer. An organic chemical called a **diluent** is added to control the viscosity of the final product. For both bis-GMA and the diluent, C=C is the functional group. The matrix of a dental composite polymerizes via chemical reaction (addition polymerization). Polymerization is activated via a chemical reaction (chemical activation) or light activation (light-cure). Light-activated materials are the most commonly used dental composites, but chemically activated materials have their uses.

The polymer matrix of dental composites is chemically similar to enamel and dentin adhesives.

Composites chemically bond to primers and adhesives of dental bonding systems because both have C=C functional groups and both set via addition polymerization, as discussed earlier. Adhesives of enamel bonding systems and dentinal bonding systems are typically bis-GMA and diluents formulated to have the proper viscosity. The currently used dentinal bonding systems, composite restorative materials, and resin cements are very compatible with each other. It is common to use a dental bonding system from one manufacturer and composite restorative material from another.

The matrix of a dental composite has several important functions. The matrix is the phase that polymerizes to form a solid mass and that bonds to the tooth structure. However, the matrix has several shortcomings. It is the weakest and the least wear-resistant phase of a dental composite material. It also absorbs water and can stain and discolor. Therefore, manufacturers minimize the matrix content of composite materials by maximizing the filler content. Stronger composite materials result.

2. Fillers

In the beginning, fillers in dental composites were naturally occurring quartz materials (sand). Quartz materials are strong, hard, and chemically stable in the oral environment. Recently, manufacturers have "engineered" glass materials for dental composites. These engineered glass materials are formulated to have the proper strength, hardness, and chemical as well as optical properties for use in dental composites. The glass is ground to have the proper-size particle coated with a silane coupling agent. The silanated filler is mixed with monomers, diluents, coloring agents, and other chemicals to form the paste that is purchased from the manufacturer.

a) Filler Size

The size of the filler in a dental composite determines the surface smoothness of the resulting restoration. Larger particles result in a rougher surface (see Fig. 5.2). Composites are most often classified by the size of their filler particles. This text will discuss three categories of dental composites: macrofill, microfill, and hybrid (blends). In reality, each category of composite has some range of particle size. It would be needlessly expensive for manufacturers to select a narrow range of particle size.

b) Evolution of Fillers

Filler particles have evolved from the strongest, most abrasion-resistant materials to somewhat softer, less abrasion-resistant materials. A softer particle is more likely to wear down rather than to be pulled out of the matrix when abrasion occurs. If a particle is pulled out, the surface is now soft resin that will wear away quickly. If the particle wears and stays partially embedded in the matrix, however, the surface has an overall greater abrasion resistance and wears at a slower rate.

c) Filler Content (Amount of Filler)

With the exception of proper handling, the percentage of filler is the most important determinant of the physical properties of dental composites. As the filler content increases, the resin content decreases. Therefore, polymerization shrinkage decreases, and the coefficient of thermal expansion becomes more like that of tooth structure. Hardness and abrasion resistance increase as well.

3. Silane Coupling Agents

Although not a true phase in a dental composite, the silane coupler is a very important component of the material. The silane coupler must be chemically compatible with both the filler and the resin phases. Manufacturers have accomplished this, and the stress placed on a restoration is thus transferred from the weaker resin phase to the stronger filler phase. Dentistry has recognized the effectiveness of silane couplers and now uses them to silanate ceramic restorations, such as a crown, in the dental lab or at chairside. The silane coupling agent enables adhesive materials to bond ceramic restorations to tooth structure.

One theory of composite wear proposes that the bond between the silane coupler and the filler particle is slightly soluble in the oral environment. As the bond is broken, the filler particles are pulled out of the resin matrix, exposing the soft resin. The resin is then worn away, exposing more filler particles to the oral environment, and the cycle continues.

4. Polymerization Systems

Two polymerization systems are used to convert the matrix–filler paste to a solid composite material. All dental composites use addition polymerization.

a) Chemically Activated Materials

Chemically activated materials are two paste systems, as shown in Figure 5.5. One paste contains the tertiary amine, and the other contains the BPO initiator. The pastes have different colors and are mixed at chairside until the two colors blend into one. The pastes are supplied in small plastic jars or screw-type syringes. When the two pastes are mixed, the

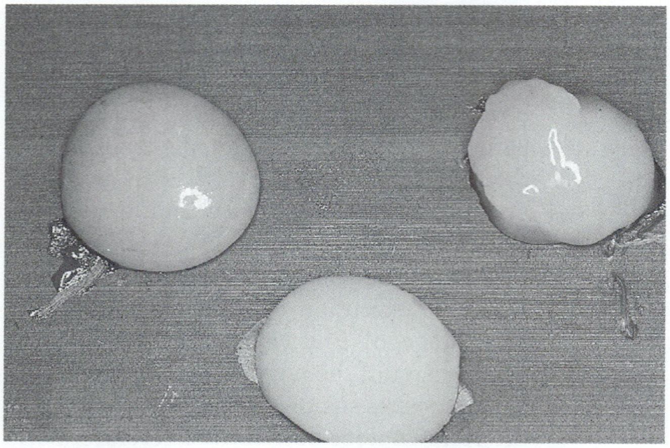

FIGURE 5.5 Photograph of the base and catalyst pastes *(top)* of the Concise system shown in Figure 4.5 and the mixed composite material *(bottom).*

inhibitor destroys the free radicals that are produced for a short period of time, as previously described. This results in a limited amount of working time to place and contour the material. When the inhibitor has reacted completely, polymerization begins. Because two pastes are mixed, air bubbles are unavoidably incorporated during mixing. Any porosity, such as these air bubbles, weakens the set material and increases staining. Care must be taken to minimize these defects in the final product.

b) Light-Activated Materials

Light-activated materials are single-paste materials that are mixed by the manufacturer, as shown in Figure 5.6. Because no chairside mixing occurs, manufacturers can make the paste thicker, with less matrix and more filler particles. In addition, voids are minimized by the manufacturing process; a stronger restoration is the result.

Light-activated materials set when exposed to a very bright light. As a result, the working time is variable and can be quite long if the operator desires. The setting time is short. The wavelength of the light source is matched to the activator chemical in the material. The intensity of the light source is greatest around 470 nm. Light absorption of the activator is also greatest at 470 nm. Light with a wavelength of 470 nm is blue light that is visible to the human eye. Because the light is very bright, direct viewing of the light source will damage the eye. Even indirect (reflected) observation of the curing light is contraindicated. Light shields have been incorporated into current curing lights to protect the operator's eyes, as shown in Figure 5.7*A*.

Light sources include halogen lights (Fig. 5.7*A*), plasma arc lights, argon lasers, and blue light-emitting diodes (Fig. 5.7*B*). Halogen lights are similar to slide projector bulbs. Plasma arc lights are similar to some high-intensity commercial outdoor lighting. Light-emitting

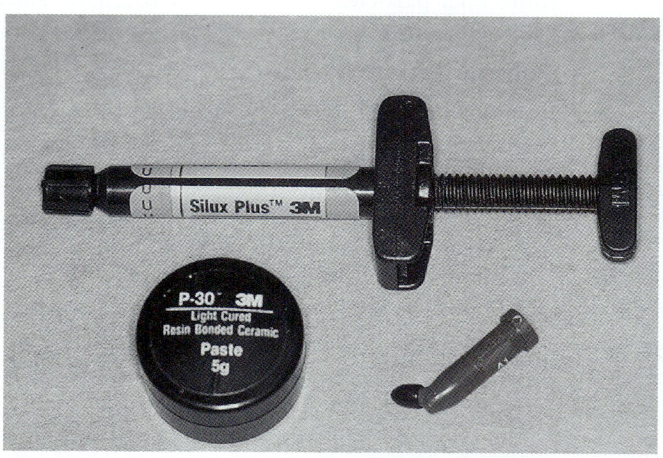

FIGURE 5.6 Light-cure composites are supplied as a jar (or tub), screw-type syringe, and compule (unit dose).

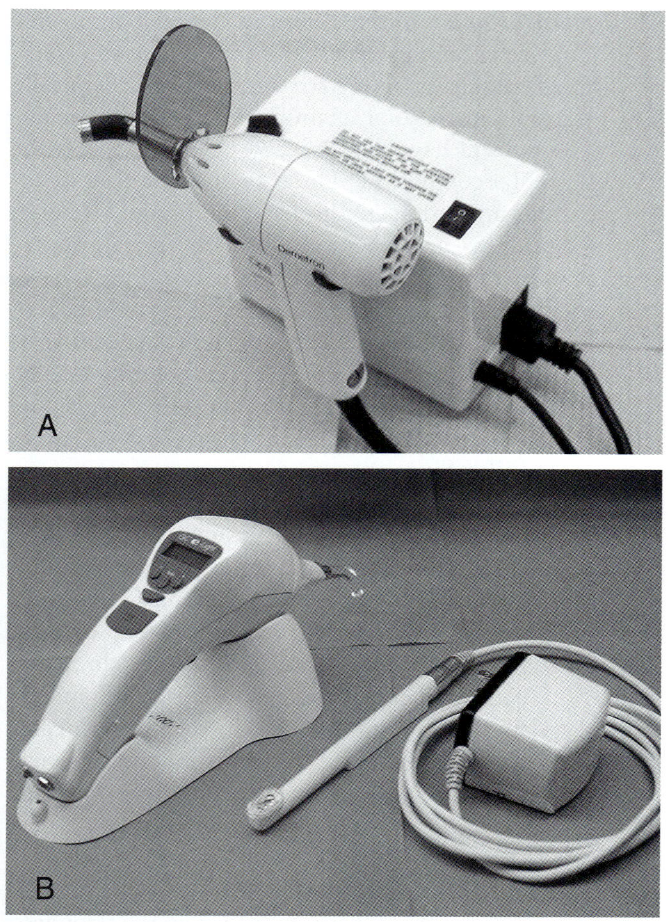

FIGURE 5.7 Photograph of dental curing lights. **A.** A conventional halogen curing light with a shield designed to protect the operator's eyes from the intense light. **B.** Two light-emitting diode curing lights.

diodes are common in automobile dashboards and traffic signal lights. Features that aid the operator in controlling curing time include: timer, on/off switches, sound effects, and other "bells and whistles." Because the working time of light-cure materials is determined by the user, they are widely popular and have replaced chemically activated materials for most uses. Chemically activated composites are used when light cannot reach the composite material, such as when cementing a metal crown with a composite cement.

C. Types and Properties of Dental Composites

1. Macrofilled Composites

The first type of dental composite to be developed in the 1960s is now called macrofilled composite. A **macrofilled composite** is illustrated in Figure 5.8*A*. The filler is a quartz material with particle sizes of 10 to 25 μm. Filler content is 70% to 80% by weight. There is a difference between filler content as measured by weight and by volume. Because the filler phase is much denser than the resin phase, the volume percentage is typically 10% to 15% lower than the weight percentage. Manufacturers like to report the weight percentage because it is higher. Physical properties are determined by the volume percentage, so it is the favorite of scientists. Either percentage can be used to evaluate materials, but it is important to know which scale (weight percentage or volume percentage) is being used.

The large size of the filler particles in macrofilled composites results in a restoration that feels rough to the dental explorer and can appear rough to the eye. The likelihood of plaque accumulation and staining is greater with macrofilled than with other types of composites. The typical macrofilled composite will turn slightly gray when rubbed with an instrument. This aids in the location of macrofilled composite restorations. Macrofills have little clinical importance at this time except that some orthodontists still use them. The rough feel and easy detection give them an advantage during the removal of bonded orthodontic brackets or appliances and the accompanying bonding material.

The strength and other physical properties, except wear resistance and surface roughness, of macrofilled composites are adequate for Class III, IV, and V restorations. Excessive wear when used for Class I and II restorations limited their posterior use. Macrofills were used before dentinal bonding systems were developed; placing them in posterior teeth resulted in postoperative sensitivity, leakage, and recurrent decay.

2. Microfilled Composites

In the late 1970s, **microfilled composites** were marketed. The particle size of microfilled composites is far smaller than in macrofill composites (0.03–0.5 μm). Microfill composites polish very smooth and lustrous (Fig. 5.8*B*), and the surface appearance is very similar to enamel. The very small filler particles are typically fused silica. The problem with microfilled composites is the low percentage filler (40–50%). The surface area of the very small filler particles requires much more resin to wet the surface of the filler particles. This high resin content results in an increased coefficient of thermal expansion and lower strength.

The polymerization shrinkage of microfilled composites is less than expected based on the total resin content. Some (or all) of the filler particles are actually "composite filler particles" (Fig. 5.8*B*). The resin of these "composite filler particles" has already been polymerized. Therefore,

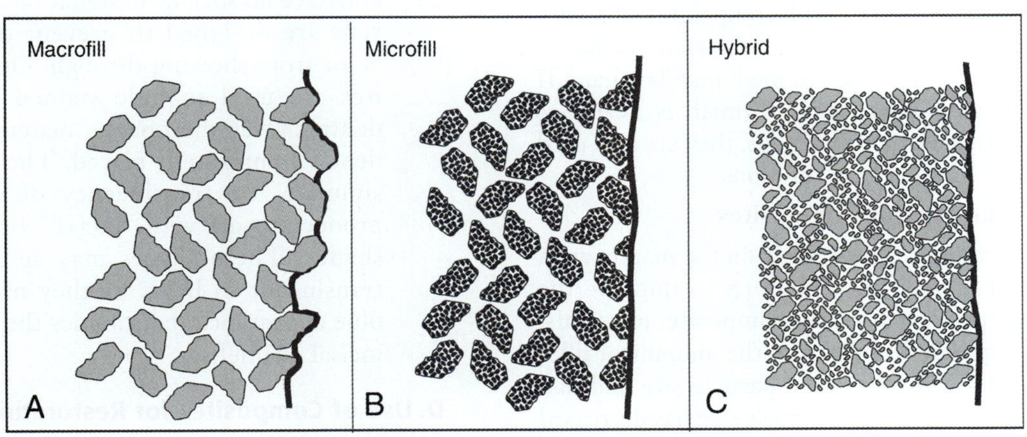

FIGURE 5.8 Schematic representation of different types of composites and their surface roughness after polishing or wear. **A.** Macrofilled composite. **B.** Microfilled composite. **C.** Hybrid composite.

this resin cannot polymerize and does not increase polymerization shrinkage. It does increase the coefficient of thermal expansion. Additional uncured matrix components are combined with the "composite filler particle" to make the microfilled composite paste.

Microfill composites were enthusiastically received by the dental profession when introduced in the mid-1970s. Smooth, lustrous composite restorations were a significant improvement over the available macrofilled composites. Microfilled materials were tried in Class I and II restorations, but the performance of most of the products was not much better than that achieved with macrofilled composites. Microfilled composites were used when esthetics are the dominant concern. Large composite restorations, such as an extensive Class IV restoration, are built in layers of several different shades and translucencies. The first layers to be placed are a hybrid composite selected for strength. The final layer, a veneer of sorts, is a microfilled composite selected for surface luster.

Microfilled composites are also used in Class V restorations at the cemento–enamel junction. Microfills have a lower modulus of elasticity and flex with the tooth better than the strongest composite materials. Clinical research has shown Class V microfill composite restorations are more likely to be retained than other composite materials.

3. Hybrid Composites

The next type of composite was developed in the late 1980s and is called a **hybrid composite.** These composites are strong and polish well. Their filler content is 75% to 80% by weight. The filler particles average 0.5 to 1 μm in size, but with a wider range of particle sizes (0.1–3 μm) (Fig. 5.8*C*). They are called hybrid (or blended) composites because they have a range of particle sizes. Hybrid composites are very popular; their strength and abrasion resistance are acceptable for small to medium Class I and II restorations. Their surface finish is nearly as good as that of microfills; thus, they are also used for Class III and IV restorations.

4. Improved Hybrid Composites

Hybrid composites currently on the market are a result of manufacturers' efforts to improve the clinical performance of composite materials. They continue to maximize the amount of filler present by controlling the particle size and distribution. The average particle size has decreased and nano-sized particles have been added. The results are slight improvements in strength and polymerization shrinkage. The most notable improvement is the smooth surface of modern well-polished composite materials.

5. Special Use Composite Materials

Two special use composite materials are available. Several manufacturers are marketing flowable composites, and others are marketing condensable composites. Because composite materials are more difficult to place in the cavity preparation than amalgam, both types are designed to make the placement of composite materials easier.

a) **Flowable composites** flow into the cavity preparation because of their lower viscosity. Manufacturers have decreased the filler content of the material to reduce the viscosity and increase the flow of these materials. A weaker, less abrasion-resistant material results. Flowable composites are typically used as the initial increment of a composite restoration and then covered with a hybrid material.

b) **Condensable composites** (or, more properly, compactible composites) are another attempt to make placement of the material into the cavity preparation easier. In general, condensable composites have a filler particle feature that inhibits the filler particles from sliding by one another. A "thicker, stiffer feel" results, and the manufacturers call these products condensable. Clinical research has shown these materials with a different "feel" are not an improvement over hybrid composite materials.

6. Shades and Opacities of Dental Composites

Dental composites and porcelains are manufactured in several shades to match the color and translucency of teeth. By layering materials with different shades and translucencies, a more natural restoration can be placed. The most commonly used composite materials match the body of the tooth in translucency and have no specific designation. Opaque materials are designed to prevent the underlying color from showing through. Opaque composites are used to hide stained or discolored dentin. Over the opaque material, the typical dental composite is placed. The last layer may simulate the translucency of enamel; some products come with "incisal" or "translucent" shades. These shades may actually be more translucent to light, or they may just have a blue appearance that mimics the appearance of incisal enamel.

D. Use of Composites for Restorations

Composite restorations are the material of choice for directly placed esthetic restorations, as shown in

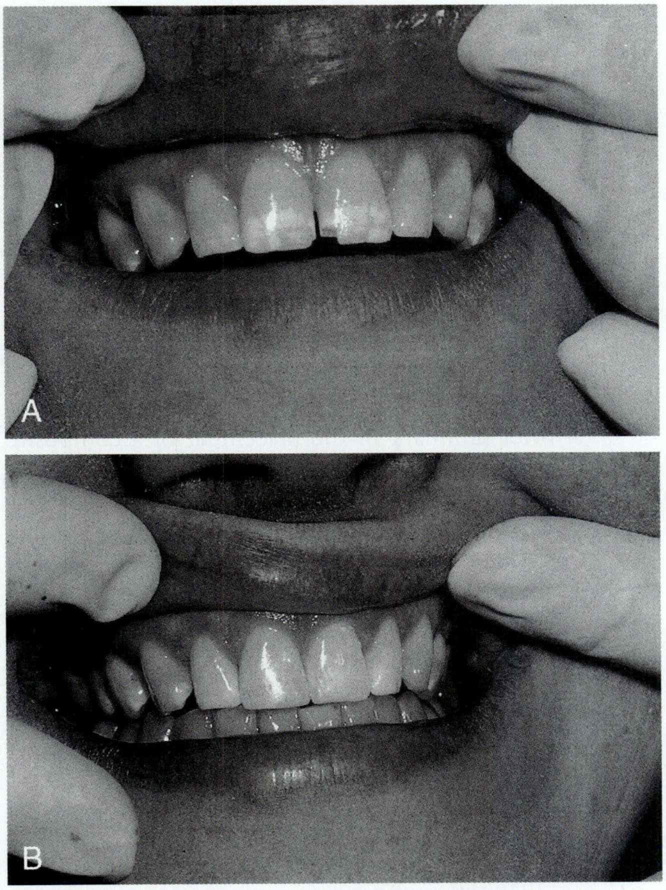

FIGURE 5.9 A. Patient with chipped mesial of a central incisor, small diastema, and enamel discoloration. **B.** Both central incisors were restored with a hybrid composite bonded to the mesial and facial surfaces, restoring the fracture, closing the diastema, and covering some of the discolored enamel. (See color images.)

Figure 5.9 and summarized in Table 5.1. Composites are one of several materials called "tooth-colored" materials. Composites have the smoothest surface and best translucency of any direct esthetic restorative material, but they are still considered to be inadequate for the characteristic of life-like appearance when compared to all ceramic restorations. However, ceramic restorations, although superior in terms of esthetics, are more costly because they are indirect restorations that require a second appointment for cementation and involve a lab fee. Ceramic restorations will be discussed in a later chapter.

Composite materials are also inadequate in the mechanical property of fracture toughness when compared to metallic restorative materials. The use of directly placed dental composites is limited to restorations that are subjected to a range of low to moderate stresses. The current practice of dentistry requires bonding the restoration to tooth structures.

Hybrid composites dominate composite materials currently in use. They function well in moderate stress restorations where esthetics are important. Their use has expanded to all surfaces of all teeth where isolation during placement is possible, see Figures 1.15, 1.16, and 5.9. As the size of the restoration increases, the stress on the restorative material increases. Composites do not have the mechanical properties for long-term success in large high-stress restorations such as cusp replacement restorations. With proper treatment planning and placement, composite restorations will succeed for many years.

E. Factors Affecting the Placement of Composites

1. Depth of Cure

Typical use of dental composites involves etching of tooth structure, priming, and application of the adhesive and composite restorative material. Unfortunately, the curing light can only penetrate through several millimeters of composite to polymerize the underlying material. The thickness of

Table 5.1 Types of Composites

Property	Microfill	Macrofill	Hybrid
Filler size (μm)	0.03–0.5	10–25	0.5–1
Filler (wt%)	40–50	70–75	75–80
Strength	Low	Fair	Good
Abrasion resistance	Good	Poor	Very good
Thermal expansion	Poor	Fair	Good
Current uses	Class III, IV, and V; veneers	Few	Class I, II, III, and IV
Polishability	Very good	Poor	Good
Examples	Durafill VS	Adaptic	Venus
	Renamel	Concise	TPH^3
	Heliomolar		Premise
			Aelite
			Filtek Z250

composite that is cured by a light source is called the **depth of cure.** The depth of cure varies depending on the time of light exposure, the composite product, the shade of that product, and the curing light. If the composite material nearest the pulp is not fully cured, pulpal irritation and postoperative sensitivity are more likely to occur. To prevent uncured material at the bottom of the preparation because of an excess thickness of material, dental composites are placed in layers or increments and are cured after each layer is placed.

2. Incremental Addition

Placing dental composites in layers, which is commonly called **incremental addition,** not only assures adequate polymerization but provides a secondary benefit as well. Composites shrink approximately 2% when they set. Polymerization shrinkage continues to be a problem with dental composites, just as it was (although to a much greater extent) with acrylic resin materials. Dentists learned to place acrylic resins in layers, allowing the first layer to set and shrink toward the tooth before adding additional layers. The same process is used with dental composites. The first layer is placed into the cavity preparation and is cured. If placed properly, the first layer shrinks toward the tooth. The second and any subsequent layers are then placed and cured until the tooth is adequately restored to form and function.

3. Air Inhibition

When composite materials are placed in increments, each increment chemically bonds to the previous one. Chemical bonding occurs because addition polymerization is inhibited by atmospheric oxygen. This inhibition of the reaction results in a thin layer of unreacted material on the surface of a newly set composite (if the surface was exposed to air when it set). The thin, air-inhibited layer does not cure, regardless of whether light-activation or chemically activated material is involved. When a second layer is added, it excludes oxygen, and the air-inhibited layer and the new material are chemically bonded together when the second layer is cured. The air-inhibited layer on a dental composite has a tacky feel. Composite surfaces adjacent to the tooth structure or a matrix band are not exposed to atmospheric oxygen, and their setting reaction is not inhibited.

4. Unreacted C=C Bonds

Not only can composite materials be placed in layers and bonded together, but also new composite will bond to old composite. Why? Not all C=C bonds react when a dental composite sets. Typically, only about 50% of the C=C bonds react. Therefore, it is possible to repair or add to a composite restoration by cleaning the surface and then properly adding new material. Some of the unreacted C=C bonds in the old material will react with the setting matrix of the new material. The strength of the bond is much lower than that of a newly placed, solid piece of material, but adding new composite material to an old composite is not uncommon.

F. Placement of a Composite Restoration

A brief summary of the placement of a composite restoration is provided:

1. Diagnose the lesion.
2. Determine the shade or shades that are needed.
3. Isolate the area to be treated, preferably with a rubber dam.
4. Cut the cavity preparation, including beveling enamel margins.
5. Determine the need for a cavity liner, and place if necessary. (The liner protects the pulp from the acid etchant when the cavity preparation is very deep.)
6. Etch, prime, place, and cure the adhesive.
7. Incrementally place and cure the composite material.
8. Finish (proper anatomical contours).
9. Check for proximal contacts.
10. Examine for voids and marginal defects with a mirror and explorer. Use dental floss to detect any overhangs.
11. Polish (lustrous surface).
12. Remove the rubber dam.
13. Check for occlusion.

G. Detecting Composite Restorations

Detecting a well-placed composite restoration can be difficult. A good shade match and excellent margins may make composite restorations nearly "invisible," but they do feel a bit softer than enamel to a sharp explorer. Composite restorations appear either radiopaque or radiolucent on radiographs, depending on the filler in the product. Composite materials have evolved from being very radiolucent to having a radiopacity somewhat like that of tooth structure. The radiopacity of composites aids in their detection and in the detection of recurrent caries. The radiopacity of composites is accomplished by making the fillers radiopaque. Barium and other heavier elements have been added to the engineered glass that is the starting material in the manufacture of fillers. Chapters 14 and 15 discuss the clinical detection and radiographic appearance of composite restorations, respectively.

H. Pit and Fissure Sealants

Pit and fissure sealants are preventive materials applied to the susceptible pits and fissures of teeth to prevent or reduce caries. Current recommendations for use of pit and fissure sealants are based on the clinical and radiographic assessment of the tooth and the caries risk of the patient. Caries risk factors include past history of caries, diet, salivary flow and buffering capacity, fluoride exposure, and oral hygiene.

1. Purpose

Fluoridation of water and toothpaste has greatly reduced smooth surface dental caries. However, pit and fissure caries continue to be common. If one examines a few patients older than 25 years of age, one commonly sees that the pits and fissures of their molars have been restored.

Pit and fissure sealants are effective in reducing caries and the need to restore teeth. The goal is to fill susceptible pits and fissures with a polymeric material, thus depriving cariogenic bacteria of a niche to colonize, as illustrated in Figure 1.11. Pit and fissure materials use the acid etch technique to bond the material to enamel. It is an acceptable responsibility of the dental hygienist to place and maintain sealants.

2. Placement of Sealants

Placement of a sealant begins with isolation of the surface, using a rubber dam or other means. Next, the surface is typically cleaned with a slurry of pumice. The tooth is then etched and rinsed with water. The sealant is placed as a final step. The sealant is allowed to set if the material is chemically activated, but currently, light-activated sealants are more commonly used. This is the same acid etching procedure that was used for composite restorations before the development of dentinal bonding agents. Isolation during the procedure is very important. Sealant products vary in filler composition and color. Some sealant materials have no filler; others have a small percentage of filler. Some products are clear; others are opaque white in appearance. The placement of pit and fissure sealants is presented in detail in Chapter 25.

3. Use of Primers With Sealants

If a rubber dam cannot be used for isolation, an alternative procedure is to etch, use a primer from a dentinal bonding system or a one-step self-etching adhesive, and then place the sealant. The primer is believed to help the sealant wet a slightly contaminated surface. Improved retention of the sealant results.

4. Maintenance of Sealants

Sealants commonly wear and chip during function as a result of occlusal forces. Periodic examination of sealants for loss, fractures, or caries is an important responsibility of the dental hygienist. Some sealants will need to be reapplied when they are lost. However, the clinical reduction of dental caries with the use of pit and fissure sealants is well established.

I. Preventive Resin Restoration

Some research has shown sealed dental caries to remain inactive, but most clinicians are not ready to routinely leave decay in developmental pits by sealing over this potential problem. A conservative approach to pit and fissure decay, called **preventive resin restoration** (PRR), was developed in the 1980s.

1. Placement of PRR

The PRR shown in Figure 5.10 is a combination of pit and fissure sealant and composite restoration. The suspicious pit is opened with a bur, and existing caries are removed. The tooth is then etched and primed, and the adhesive is placed. The prepared pit is filled with a hybrid composite material. Any pits and fissures not filled by the composite or adhesive are filled with sealant. A great deal of tooth structure is preserved by placing a PRR compared to the traditional Class I cavity preparation developed by G.V. Black in the late 1800s.

2. Air Abrasion Systems

Many clinicians are using air abrasion systems to remove debris and decay from pits and fissures and then placing sealants and preventive resins. Air abrasion systems (or dental "sandblasting" units) have been recently introduced. A high-velocity stream of air carries very hard ceramic particles (aluminum oxide) and abrades the tooth, similar to industrial sandblasters. These systems are different from the "prophy jet" that uses baking soda to remove stains from the surface of teeth. Air abrasion systems can effectively cut enamel and dentin, cut cavity preparations, and remove composite materials. Eliminating the use of pumice and prophy cup to prepare (clean) enamel surfaces is another advantage of air abrasion systems. However, a rubber dam is required to protect the patient's airway from the dust and debris that result from an air abrasion system.

3. Hard Tissue Lasers

Dental lasers that cut enamel, dentin, and composite materials are becoming common. Many patients do not require anesthesia for the use of

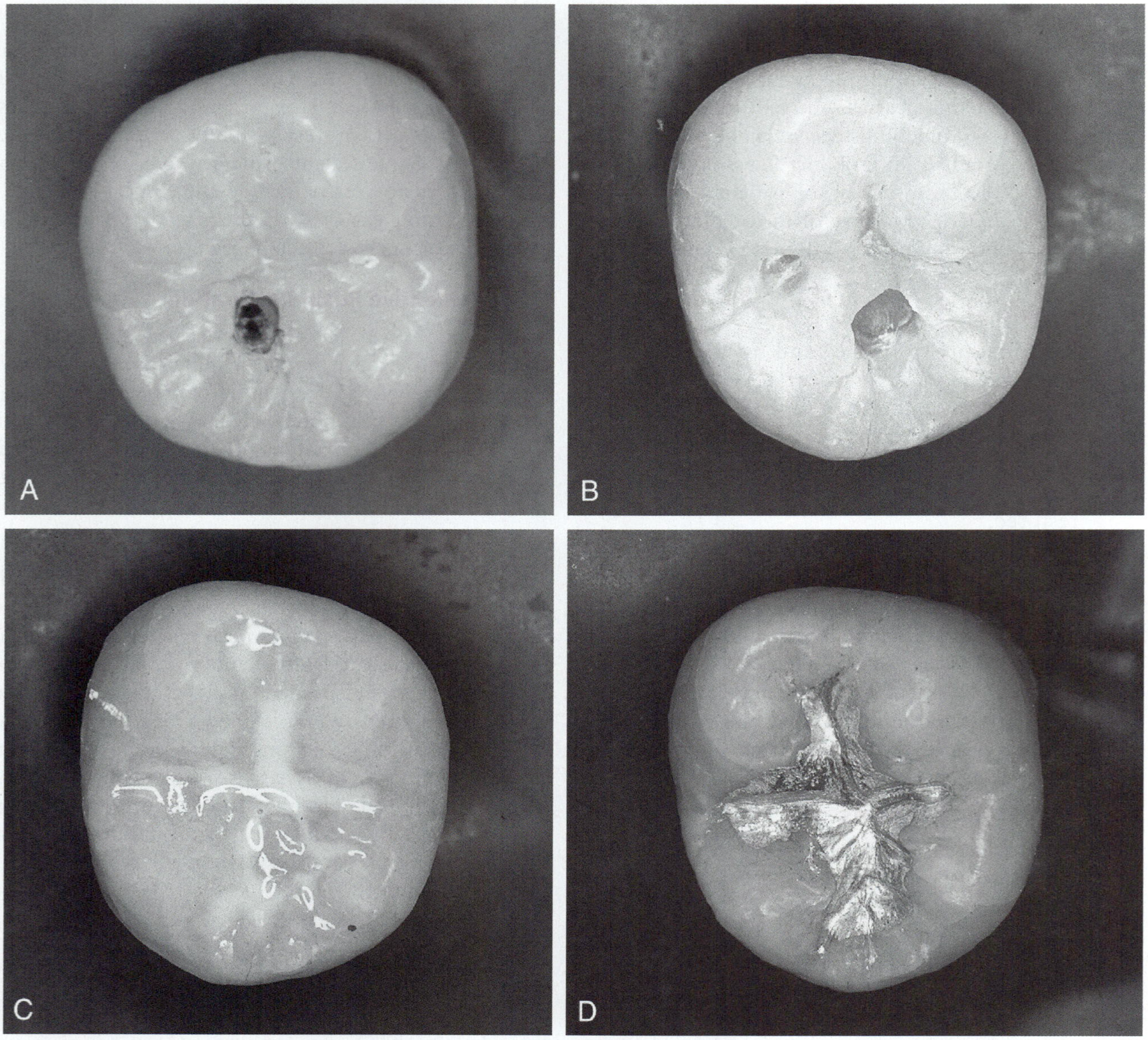

FIGURE 5.10 Photographs of molar with decay in several pits (**A**), the decay removed and the central groove opened (**B**), restored with a preventive resin restoration (**C**), and with the preventive resin restoration removed and restored with a conventional cavity preparation and amalgam (**D**). Note the amount of tooth structure conserved by the preventive resin restoration.

such lasers. Hard tissue lasers are ideal for cleaning debris from pits and fissures when placing sealants and preventive resin restorations.

J. Composite Cements

1. Composition

Composite cements or luting materials have the same structure as other dental composites. They are a resin matrix reinforced with filler. Composite cements have a greater percentage of resin to increase flow and smaller-sized particles for a lower film thickness. Composite cements will be presented in greater detail in Chapter 7.

2. Use

One advantage of composite cements is their ability to bond restorations to the tooth structure. Composite cements are the luting material of choice for ceramic restorations. They are also used when retention of a preparation is less than desired. Examples include crown preparations that are short in height or of a shape with "little holding power" (excessive taper).

K. Other Uses of Composite Materials

1. Indirect Composite Restorations

Composite restorations can be made indirectly by a dental laboratory. To improve strength, indirect composite materials can be processed at higher temperatures and pressures than the oral cavity can tolerate. Laboratory-processed composite restorations require an impression of the prepared teeth and a cast. A second appointment is needed to cement the restoration. Recently, several innovative laboratory-processed composite materials have been introduced, including CAD/CAM techniques. Fiber reinforcement is being used to increase strength to enable the construction of composite crowns and short-span bridges.

2. Composites as Alternatives to Acrylic Resins

Because composite materials are superior in strength and other properties to acrylic resin materials, they have begun to replace acrylic resin materials in a variety of uses. This replacement has been slow to occur, however, because of the increased expense of composite materials. Some of these acrylic resin replacement composites are a polyester resin cross-linked with a bis-GMA–type monomer via addition polymerization monomer. (This is how fiberglass is made.) Composite materials are now used for temporary crowns, denture teeth, custom tray materials, and other laboratory uses. One example of a crown and bridge temporary material and mixing gun are shown in Figure 5.11. The construction of temporary crowns is presented in Chapter 35. Several products are laboratory light-cure materials, and again, additional details will be presented in Chapter 11.

VI. Glass Ionomer Materials

A. Chemical-Cure Glass Ionomer Products

The original glass ionomer products set via an acid-base chemical reaction. These are sometimes called chemical-cure glass ionomers. Glass ionomer materials were the first truly adhesive restorative materials. They chemically bond to enamel and dentin as

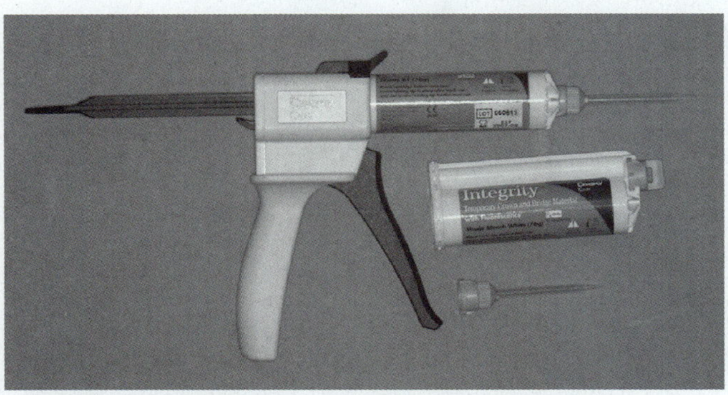

FIGURE 5.11 A crown and bridge temporary material. This paste/paste system is mixed in the baffle of the mixing tip, as is common with impression materials.

described in Chapter 4. Glass ionomer materials release fluoride over time; it is commonly thought that this fluoride inhibits recurrent decay. The chemistry of glass ionomer and other dental cements will be covered in Chapter 7. Glass ionomer restorations are "tooth colored" but opaque in appearance. Their esthetics are inferior to those of dental composites. In this chapter, the use and properties of glass ionomer restorative materials will be presented.

Glass ionomer restorative materials (acid-base reaction only) are supplied as powder/liquid systems; a variety of shades are available for most products. Proper mixing and placement are critical. The proper powder/liquid ratio is mixed, and a viscous material (much like icing for a cake) results. Many products are available in preproportioned capsules that are mixed with an amalgamator (see Fig. 7.7*A*). The freshly mixed material is placed into the cavity preparation without delay and then contoured to the proper shape. Sometimes, plastic strips are used to hold the material in the proper shape while it sets.

Placement of chemical-cure (acid-base reaction only) glass ionomer restorations is technique sensitive. If mixing is too slow or placement is delayed, the adhesive property of the material is lost. In addition, these glass ionomer materials are susceptible to dehydration during the initial setting of the material and the finishing of the restoration. If not protected from dehydration, surface crazing occurs. **Crazing** is the formation of many shallow surface cracks. After the initial finishing, a protective sealant is painted on to cover the newly placed glass ionomer material. Enamel bonding resins, as described in Chapter 4, or special varnishes are used as a protective sealant. The final polishing of these glass ionomer materials is typically delayed for 24 hours to allow the material to set completely. At a subsequent appointment, the final polish achieves optimum surface smoothness and esthetics. Chemical-cure glass ionomer materials have a high initial solubility in oral fluids, but their solubility is low after the setting reaction is complete.

The advantages of adhesion and fluoride release make chemical-cure glass ionomers useful materials, but their shortcomings have limited their clinical use. Glass ionomer products are very popular for use as luting cements and as restorative materials in low-stress areas of teeth. Chemical-cure glass ionomer restorative materials are brittle. Poor wear resistance and fracture toughness limit their use to Class I and II restorations in deciduous teeth. The fluoride release makes glass ionomer restorative materials the material of choice for Class V lesions in patients with a high risk of caries.

Table 5.2 Brand Names of Glass Ionomer and Compomer Restorative Materials

Glass Ionomer Products	Predominant Uses: Luting Cements	Liners	Restorative Material
Acid-base reaction only	Ketac-Cem Fuji I	HI	Fuji II; Fuji IX Ketac-Silver Ketac-Fil Fuji Miracle Mix
Acid-base reaction and chemically activated polymerization	GC Fuji Cem RelyX	N/A	N/A
Acid-base reaction and light-activated polymerization[a]	HI	Vitrebond GC Fuji Lining LC Vivaglass Liner	Fuji II LC Photac-fil Vitremer
Compomers (light-activated polymerization)	N/A	N/A	Compoglass F Dyract F2000

HI, mostly products of historical interest only; N/A, not applicable.
[a]Some products also include chemically activated polymerization.

B. Resin-Modified Glass Ionomer Products

Resin-modified glass ionomer products were developed in the late 1980s (Table 5.2). They are also called resin-reinforced glass ionomers. They have an acid-base setting reaction in addition to free radical polymerization, light or chemically activated. Light-activated polymerization products set when exposed to the same curing light that is used for composites. Light-activated products are popular because of their "cure on demand" setting reaction. They are still adhesive, and they release fluoride. Light-activated glass ionomer restorations are easier to place and finish, and they are not as sensitive to dehydration as their chemical cure counterparts. At the time of placement, light-activated glass ionomers are finished and polished. They are a little stronger and tougher than chemically activated glass ionomers. Light-activated glass ionomers are currently quite popular for Class III and V restorations; several Class V restorations are shown in Figure 5.12. In addition, light-activated glass ionomer liners are currently the mostly commonly used base/liner products.

C. Acid-Base Chemically Activated Resin-Modified Glass Ionomer Products

The superiority of resin-modified glass ionomer restorative materials in terms of mechanical properties resulted in a market for similar luting materials. Because light is ineffective in curing material under a metal crown, chemically activated (addition polymerization) glass ionomer materials, which also

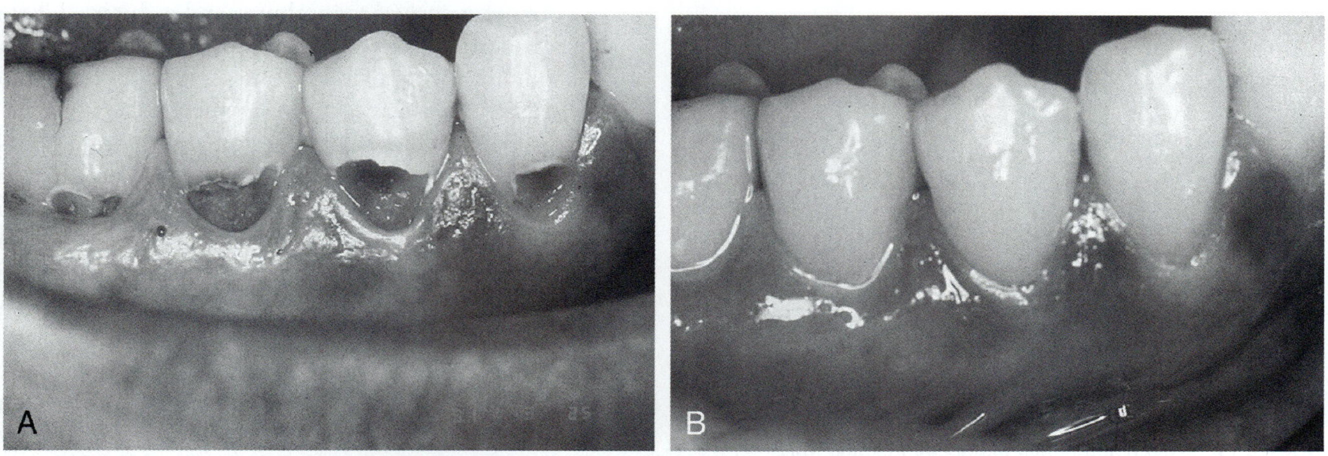

FIGURE 5.12 Several Class V carious lesions (**A**) and light-cure glass ionomer restorations (**B**). (Courtesy of GC America, Inc.)

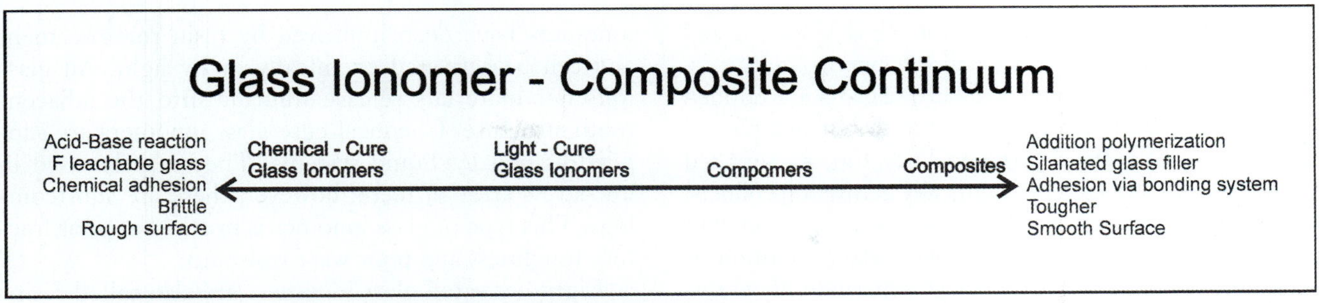

FIGURE 5.13 A comparison of direct esthetic restorative materials.

incorporate the acid-base reaction, have been developed. They are considered by many to be the "state of the art" for luting metal and porcelain-fused-to-metal crowns.

D. Recharging Fluoride in Glass Ionomer Materials

Laboratory studies have shown that glass ionomer materials release fluoride. Dentists use glass ionomer materials in hopes of preventing decay via this fluoride release. This fluoride release decreases over time. Other laboratory studies have shown that glass ionomer materials can have their fluoride "recharged" with topical fluoride treatments. The result is a significant increase in the fluoride released by "old" glass ionomer material. Acid-base glass ionomer materials, both initially and after recharging, release more fluoride than resin-modified materials.

VII. Compomers

Because of the popularity of glass ionomer materials and composite/dentinal bonding systems, a combination of the two materials has been developed and has become quite popular. The "**compomer**" label is used to describe materials that bond and set like dentinal bonding/composite systems but that initially release some fluoride like glass ionomers. Some of these products are a bit like glass ionomers, but most are very much like composites. Compomers typically use the same dentinal bonding systems as composites do. Some initially release fluoride, but clinical data showing a reduction in recurrent caries are lacking. The promise of fluoride release and good handling characteristics has resulted in the large number of compomer products now available.

VIII. Selecting Restorative Materials

The current market in adhesive polymeric restorative materials is a continuum, ranging from chemical-cure glass ionomers at one end to light-cure glass ionomers to compomers to, finally, composites at the other end, as illustrated in Figure 5.13. Many times, choosing a product for a particular restoration in an individual patient is a matter of the dentist's personal preference rather than a decision based on a material's physical properties or clinical data. The patient's desires for an esthetic material and the strength required by the location of a restoration are also significant factors in the selection of a product. Handling characteristics are an important consideration as well. Brand names of adhesive restorative materials are included in Tables 5.1 and 5.2.

SUMMARY

The first acrylic resins used in dentistry were the "pink portion" of a denture base. Later, they were also used as a tooth-colored restorative material. Since then, materials scientists have developed composite materials with greatly improved properties. Filler particles made of ceramic materials were added to improve strength. Silane coupling agents, a coating over the filler particles, transfer the stress from the unfilled matrix portion of the composite to the filler particle.

Composite restorative material may be cured two ways: chemical reaction (chemically activated) or light activation (photo-cure). Chemically activated materials are two-paste systems that blend into one color. Working time to place and contour the material is limited because of the "auto" setting reaction. It is also easy to incorporate bubbles during mixing. Light-cure materials are more commonly used and are supplied as single-paste materials. No mixing is required; therefore, voids are minimized and result in a stronger restoration. With light-cure composites, working time is essentially unlimited because they will not set until the curing light is activated.

Dental composites fall into three categories: macrofilled, microfilled, and hybrid. The categories are named for their particle size. The current practice of dentistry is dominated by hybrid composite materials. Hybrid composites are strong and result in a smooth surface. Microfills are indicated for Class V lesions and times when surface luster is a major concern.

For the most part, pit and fissure sealants are unfilled (or slightly filled) resins that flow into the enamel pit and fissures areas of occlusal surfaces. They, too, are supplied as either light-activated or chemically activated products. The acid etch process is used before sealant placement, and primers may be used to improve sealant retention. It is the responsibility of the hygienist to periodically examine sealants for loss, fracture, or caries.

Preventive resin restorations are a combination of a pit and fissure sealant with a composite restoration. The suspicious pit is opened with a bur. Caries are removed, and the pit is then etched and primed. Finally, the adhesive is placed.

Another use of composite materials is for restorations made indirectly in a dental laboratory. This type of restoration requires an impression, and the patient must return for a second appointment for the cementation. Still other uses include temporary crowns, denture teeth, and custom tray materials.

Glass ionomers are another esthetic restorative material that chemically bond to enamel and dentin. They were the first truly adhesive restorative materials. Glass ionomers have been improved by resin reinforcement and can be activated chemically or by light. All glass ionomer materials release fluoride into the adjacent tooth structure. Chemical cure glass ionomers are supplied as powder/liquid systems. They may be used in low-stress areas of teeth; however, there are shortcomings. This type of glass ionomer is brittle, has poor fracture toughness and poor wear resistance.

Light-activated glass ionomers are also called resin-modified glass ionomers. They are easier to place and finish, less sensitive to dehydration, and a little stronger and tougher. They are used for Class III and V restorations.

This chapter has presented many adhesive polymeric restorative materials from which a dentist may choose. The choice may be made based on the dentist's personal preference rather than on the material's physical properties or clinical data. The patient's desire for esthetics and the strength required of the restoration are other significant factors. Composites and glass ionomers are two of the many dental materials that the dental hygienist must be able to identify as well as assess and maintain during the patient's routine dental visits. The remaining chapters will assist the clinician in accomplishing these goals.

Learning Activities

1. Cure a 1-mm-thick (5- by 5-mm) sample of composite with one side against a Mylar strip (bottom) and the other side exposed to air (top). Feel the sticky air-inhibited layer on the top, and compare this surface with the bottom.
2. Place additional composite material on the top surface of the above sample. Cure and attempt to push the second increment off the first. Describe the force required.
3. Make composite samples of several types of composites listed in Table 5.1. Feel the surface with an explorer. Compare the surfaces for roughness and surface luster.
4. Make Rice Krispies® treats with different marshmallow/cereal ratios. How do the different mixtures feel when eaten? Crunchy? Chewy? What happens if too much cereal is added? Give the leftovers from the bad batches to your least favorite teacher. Send the good stuff to our troops overseas.

Review Questions

1. One problem with polymers is their high coefficients of thermal expansion. These coefficients can be ________ to ________ times greater than that of tooth structure.
   a) 1 to 3
   b) 3 to 5
   c) 2 to 5
   d) 2 to 10
2. Which of the following components of restorative resins acts as a "coating" and serves to transfer stress from a weak component to a stronger one?
   a) Matrix
   b) Filler particle
   c) Silane coupling agent
   d) Polymers
   e) Adhesives

3. What advantage do microfill composites have compared to macrofilled composites?
a) Low coefficient of thermal expansion
b) Smooth and lustrous polished surface
c) Greater overall strength
d) Higher percentage of filler

4. Which of the following characteristics best describes chemical-cure composite restorative materials?
a) Unlimited working time
b) Supplied as single paste materials
c) May incorporate air bubbles during mixing
d) Contains less matrix and more filler particles

5. A specific amount of composite (thickness) that is cured by a light source is termed:
a) Depth of cure
b) Incremental addition
c) Depth of addition
d) Incremental polymerization

6. The size of the filler particles in a dental composite determines the:
a) Polymerization reaction
b) Technique for incremental additions
c) Etching time before the primer and adhesive are placed
d) Surface smoothness of the resulting restoration

7. The __________ composite restorative materials are those with a lower viscosity (decreased filler) to aid in placement.
a) Preventive resin
b) Hybrid
c) Flowable
d) Condensable

8. Hybrid composites are recommended for:
a) Surface luster
b) Areas needing strength
c) Low-stress areas
d) Class V restorations

9. A combination of a pit and fissure sealant and a composite restoration is termed:
a) Flowable composite
b) Condensable composite
c) Compomer
d) Preventive resin restoration

10. Abrasion resistance for hybrid composite restorative material is said to be:
a) Poor
b) Fair
c) Good
d) Very good

11. Thermal expansion for microfill composite restorative material is considered to be:
a) Poor
b) Fair
c) Good
d) Very good.

12. Which composite material has the largest percentage of filler by weight?
a) Microfill
b) Hybrid
c) Macrofill
d) Flowable

13. Composite materials that polymerize using light activation are:
a) Initiated by mixing
b) Not as popular as chemically activated resins
c) Supplied as a single paste
d) Lack the "set on demand" characteristic

14. A restorative material that initially releases some fluoride like glass ionomers but bonds and sets like composites is called:
a) Flowable composites
b) Condensable composite
c) Compomer
d) Preventive resin restoration

15. Which of the following best describes microfill composite materials?
a) Abrasion resistance is poor; filler size is 10–25 microns
b) Abrasion resistance is poor; strength is high
c) Polishability is poor; strength is high
d) Polishability is very good; strength is low

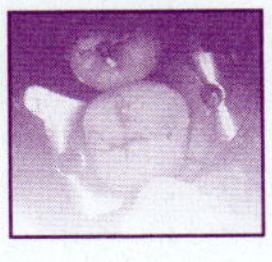

Supplemental Readings

Berg JH. The continuum of restorative materials in pediatric dentistry—a review for the clinician. Pediatr Dent 1998; 20(2):93–100.
Beun S, et al. Characterization of nanofilled compared to universal and microfilled composites. Dent Mat 2007;23(1):51–59.
Feigal RJ. Sealants and preventive restorations: review of effectiveness and clinical changes for improvement. Pediatr Dent 1998;20(2):85–92.
Ferracane JL. Current trends in dental composites. Crit Rev Oral Biol Med 1995;6(4):302–318.
Fissure caries. Operative Dent 2001;26:324–327.
Visible light curing. J Am Dent Assoc 2002;133(10): 1430–1431.

6

Amalgam and Direct Gold

Key Words/Phrases

admixed alloy
amalgam
amalgam alloy
amalgamation
amalgamator
annealing gold foil
blended alloy
cohesive gold
copal varnish
creep
delayed expansion
dental amalgam
direct gold
gold foil
lathe-cut alloys
precipitation
spherical alloys
trituration
triturator
working time

Objectives

After studying this chapter, the student will be able to do the following:

1. Differentiate between an amalgam alloy and a dental amalgam.
2. Describe the composition of conventional and high-copper dental amalgams.
3. Describe the function (effects) of the major elements of dental amalgams.
4. Describe the self-sealing property of amalgam.
5. Describe the following shapes of amalgam alloy particles:
   - Lathe cut
   - Spherical
   - Blend or admix
6. Describe the effect of moisture contamination on amalgam.
7. Describe acceptable mercury hygiene practices.
8. Describe the use and advantages of direct gold restorations.

OPTIONAL

9. Explain the trituration and setting processes.
10. Describe the reactions involved in both conventional and high-copper amalgams.
11. Describe the composition, relative strength, and relative corrosion resistance of the four most common amalgam phases.

INTRODUCTION

Dental amalgam is a very old, but still widely used, restorative material. The present forms of amalgam evolved from the "silver paste" that was developed in the 1800s. The popularity of dental amalgam results from its cost-effectiveness and ease of use. During the 1970s and 1980s, more than a million amalgam restorations were placed each year. Probably more than half of the single-tooth restorations currently in posterior teeth are amalgam restorations. Dental amalgam is used in all surfaces of posterior teeth and, occasionally, in the lingual pits of anterior teeth. Use of dental amalgam is decreasing as caries prevention becomes more and more successful. Composites are also widely used as an alternative material.

I. What Is Dental Amalgam?

A. Amalgam is a metal alloy of which one of the elements is mercury (Hg).

B. Dental amalgam is made by mixing approximately equal parts (by weight) of a powdered metal alloy with liquid mercury. These components are illustrated in Figure 6.1. The powdered metal is called an amalgam alloy and is predominantly silver (Ag) and tin (Sn). The mixing process of the alloy with the liquid mercury is called **amalgamation** or **trituration.** A mechanical device called an **amalgamator** or **triturator,** as shown in Figure 6.2, "shakes" the capsule containing the alloy powder and mercury at high speed, mixing the two components into a plastic mass, as shown in Figure 6.3. The triturated material is reacting or setting while it is forced, or condensed, into the cavity preparation.

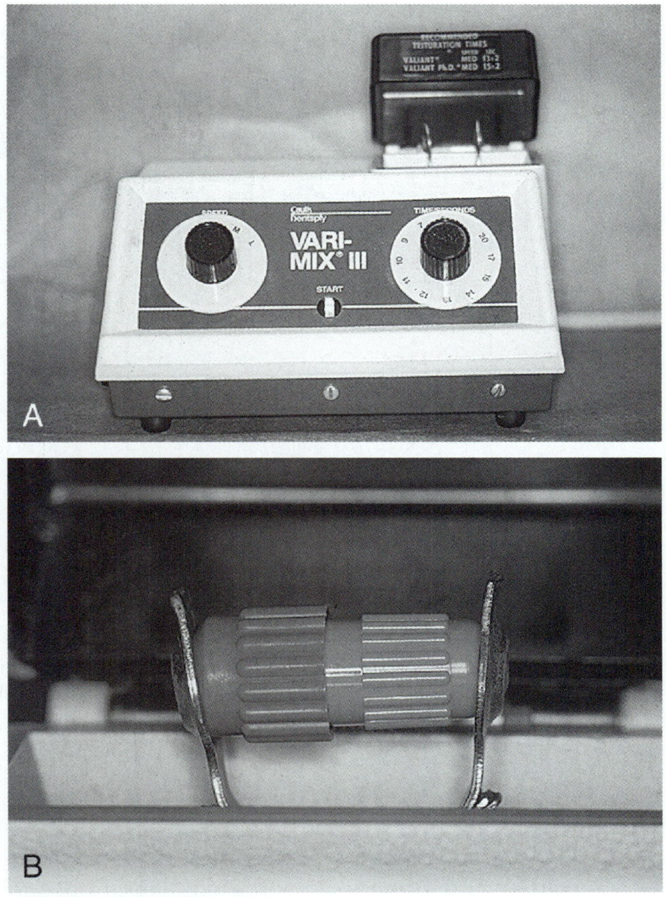

FIGURE 6.2 Photographs of a triturator **(A)** and an amalgam capsule in place, ready to be triturated **(B)**.

The cavity preparation is always overfilled with amalgam. The excess is then removed (carved) to restore the original anatomy of the tooth. The condensation and carving procedures are illustrated in Figure 6.4.

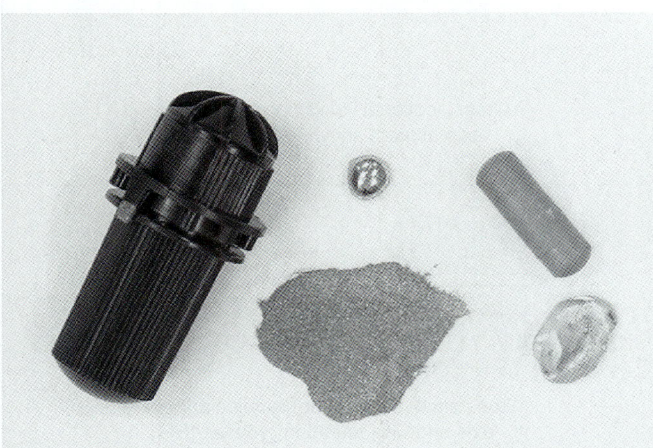

FIGURE 6.1 Starting at the *left* and moving *clockwise:* capsule, liquid mercury, pestle, freshly mixed amalgam, and powdered amalgam alloy.

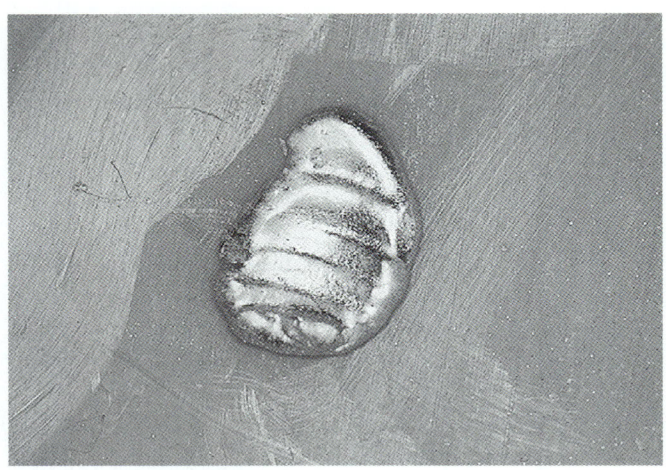

FIGURE 6.3 Photograph of properly triturated dental amalgam.

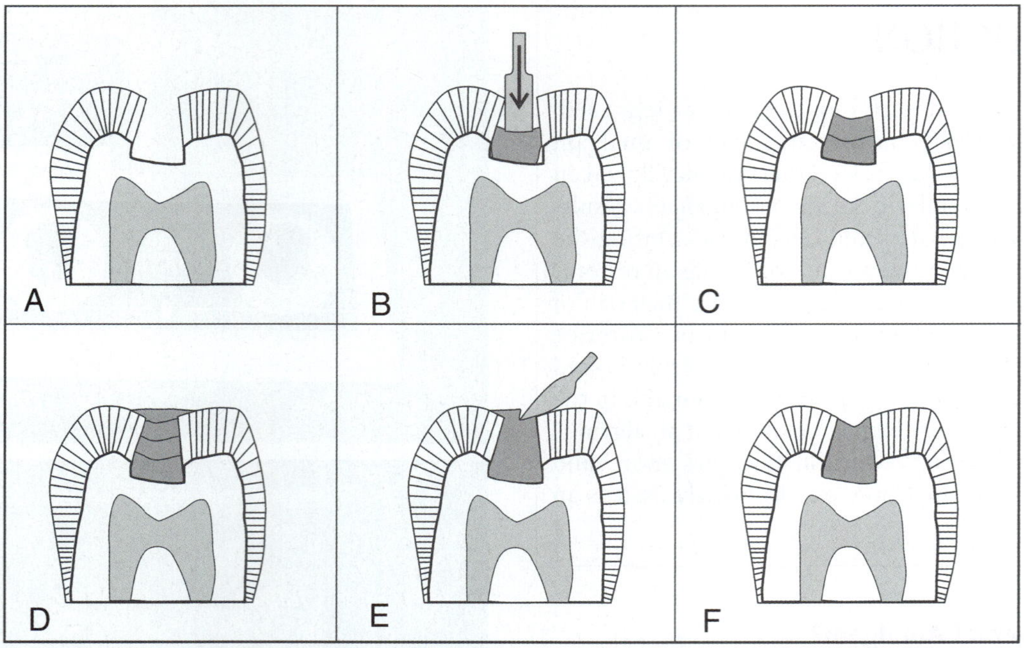

FIGURE 6.4 Illustration of condensing and carving procedures. **A.** The cavity is prepared. **B.** The first increment of amalgam is placed in the preparation and condensed to eliminate voids. **C** and **D.** The second and succeeding increments are placed until the preparation is overfilled. **E** and **F.** While still "soft," the material is carved to reproduce the proper anatomical contours.

C. The setting reaction of amalgam starts during trituration and progresses while condensation and carving take place. The **working time** of amalgam (the time that is needed to condense and carve) is not directly controlled by the dentist, as it is with light-activated composites.

D. Amalgam is a direct restorative material that is held in place by mechanical retention. Examples of mechanical retention include undercuts and grooves that are placed by the dentist in the cavity preparation with a handpiece and bur. Examples of convergent undercuts and retentive grooves are shown in Figure 6.5.

E. The particles of the amalgam alloy may be formed by two methods.

1. The first method used to produce dental amalgam particles is grinding an ingot of metal to produce filings. Such amalgam alloys are called **lathe-cut alloys,** and an example is shown in Figure 6.6*A*.
2. The second method used to produce dental amalgam particles is to spray molten metal into an inert atmosphere. The droplets cool as they fall, producing **spherical alloys,** as shown in Figure 6.6*B*.
3. Some products are a mixture of both lathe-cut and spherical particles, as shown in Figure 6.6*C*. These products are called **admixed or blended alloys.**

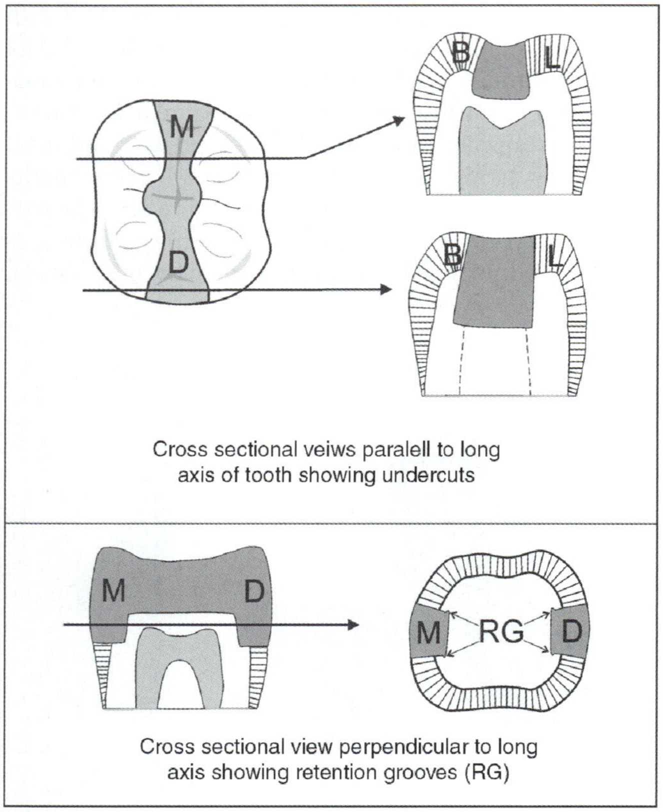

FIGURE 6.5 Illustration of the retentive features of an amalgam restoration. Buccal (*B*), distal (*D*), lingual (*L*), and mesial (*M*) surfaces are labeled for orientation.

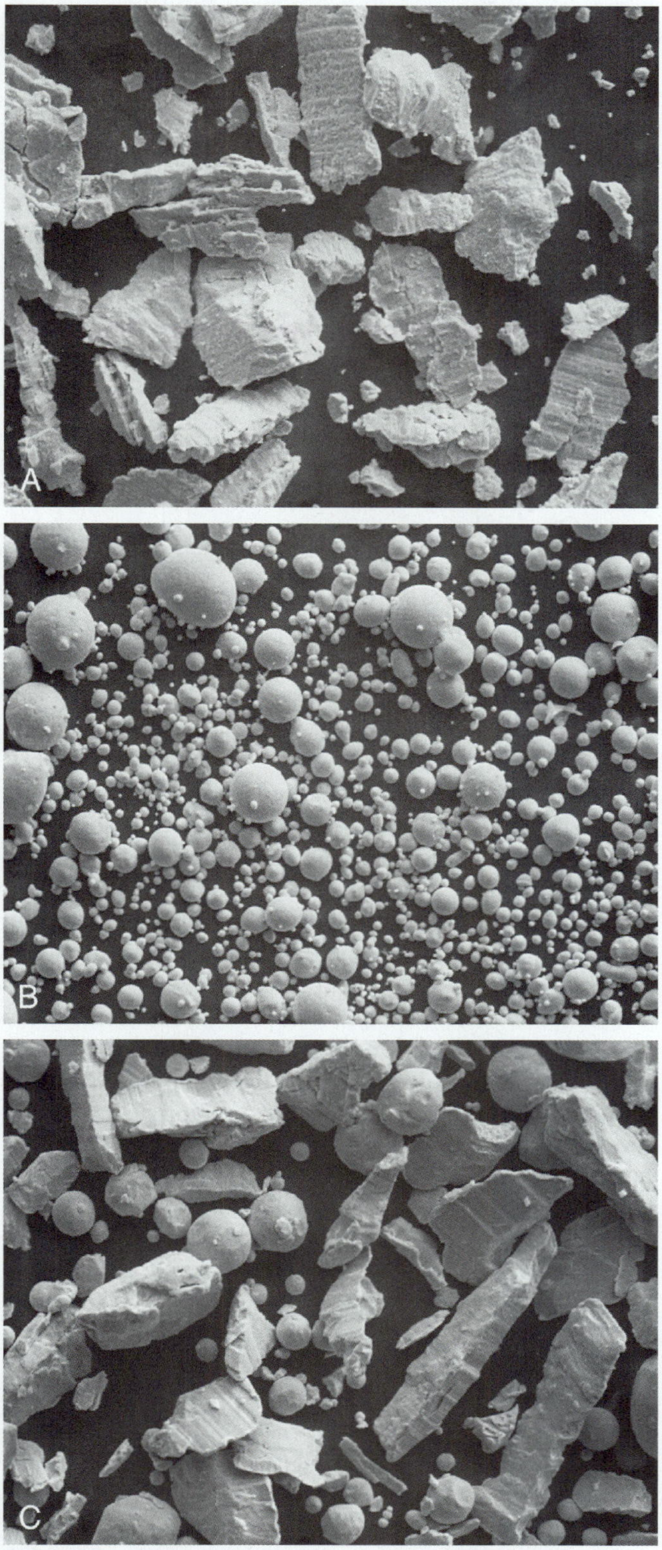

FIGURE 6.6 Scanning electron micrograph of amalgam particles. **A.** Lathe-cut amalgam alloy. **B.** Spherical amalgam alloy. **C.** Admixed amalgam alloy. (Courtesy of Special Metals Corporation, Ann Arbor, MI.)

4. Regardless of the production method used, the particles are mixed and react with liquid mercury. The result is dental amalgam.

F. It is important to note that the term "amalgam alloy" does not mean the same thing as "dental amalgam." **Amalgam alloy** is the Ag-Sn powdered metal before it is mixed with mercury. Dental amalgam is the result of mixing the powdered metal with mercury and is used to restore teeth. Many times, including in this text, the terms "amalgam" and "amalgam alloy" are used. Most of the time, little confusion results. Occasionally, however, it is important (usually for test questions) to understand which material is being discussed: amalgam alloy, the resulting dental amalgam, or both.

II. Advantages of Using Dental Amalgam

Because of its toughness and wear resistance, amalgam is a long-lasting, cost-effective restorative material. In addition, amalgam has the ability to seal its margins during service. As the margins corrode, the tooth/restoration interface fills with corrosion products so that microleakage is reduced. Often, margins of a dental amalgam may look broken down but are actually well sealed just below the surface. Clinical research has shown that marginal integrity of dental amalgams is a poor predictor of recurrent decay.

Amalgam is the least technique-sensitive permanent restorative material that is available to the dentist. In addition, it is the only material that might work when placed in a wet, contaminated environment.

The life expectancy of an amalgam restoration, like that of any other direct restorative material, is indirectly related to the size of the restoration. As the restoration increases in size, the stress within the restoration also increases, and the life expectancy of the restoration decreases. Based on clinical research, the life expectancy for a conservative Class I amalgam is 15 to 18 years. A Class II amalgam should last 12 to 15 years. It is important to remember that the patient has a great deal of influence on the longevity of restorations. The patient's diet and oral hygiene practices are very important and can contribute to a longer life expectancy of their restorations.

III. History of Dental Amalgam

A. Initial Development

Dental amalgam was developed in France in the 1800s. It was introduced to the United States in 1833, and the mercury toxicity controversy started immediately. This controversy divided U.S. dentists into pro-amalgam and anti-amalgam groups. At that time, the only alternatives for direct restorative materials were direct gold and dental cements. Casting techniques could not produce satisfactory restorations. The composition of dental amalgam was improved greatly by the work of Flagg and Black. A "balanced" formulation resulted, in which the expansion effects of the silver in the alloy offset the contraction effects of the tin.

B. Specification 1

In the 1920s, the National Bureau of Standards (now the National Institute of Standards and Technology) was asked by the U.S. government to develop a set of standard tests for dental amalgam. The standard was enthusiastically received by the field of dentistry and became Specification #1 of the American Dental Association (ADA). Specifications are discussed in Chapter 1. In the first half of the twentieth century, most amalgam alloys followed the formula of G.V. Black because his composition was included in the specification.

C. Introduction of High-Copper Amalgam

Around 1960, an amalgam alloy with a higher copper (Cu) content was developed. Increasing the copper content reduced the percentage of the weakest phase of the resulting dental amalgam. Clinical performance improved markedly. Today, numerous high-copper dental amalgams are on the market, and a variety of particle shapes and compositions are available. The copper content ranges from 10% to 30%.

IV. Low-Copper Dental Amalgam

Low-copper amalgams are included in this text for historical perspective. In addition, they are a good starting point because of their simple composition and chemistry. Today, high-copper amalgams are the state of the art and dominate the market.

A. Composition

The composition of a low-copper, "traditional" or "conventional" amalgam alloy is based on Black's composition: approximately 65% silver, 25% tin, less than 6% copper, and sometimes, 1% zinc.

B. Function of Components

1. Silver causes setting expansion and increases strength and corrosion resistance.
2. Tin causes setting contraction and decreases strength and corrosion resistance.
3. In low-copper amalgams, copper functions much the same as silver.
4. If the zinc content is greater than 0.01%, the amalgam is called a zinc-containing amalgam. If the content is less, the amalgam is called a nonzinc amalgam. During manufacture, zinc reduces oxidation of the other metals in the alloy. For many years, the clinical effect of zinc was debated. Recently, clinical research has shown that zinc-containing dental amalgams have a longer clinical life expectancy than nonzinc amalgams.
5. Many other elements, mostly metals, have been added to dental amalgam alloys in the range of a few percent. These metals include gold, palladium, indium, and even mercury.

C. Setting Reaction of Low-Copper Amalgam—Optional

$$\text{excess } Ag_3Sn\ (\gamma) + Hg \rightarrow$$
$$\text{unreacted } Ag_3Sn\ (\gamma) +$$
$$Ag_2Hg_3\ (\gamma_1) + Sn_8Hg\ (\gamma_2)$$

Or, simply,

$$\gamma + Hg \rightarrow \gamma + \gamma + \gamma_2$$

1. γ is the Greek letter gamma and is used to designate the Ag-Sn alloy, or gamma phase.
2. γ_1, or gamma-one, is used to designate the Ag-Hg phase.
3. γ_2, or gamma-two, is used to designate the Sn-Hg phase.
4. When the liquid mercury is mixed with the amalgam alloy, the mercury is both absorbed by the alloy particles and dissolves the surface of the particles.
5. Silver and tin continue to dissolve in the liquid mercury, which becomes saturated with silver and tin. New γ_1 and γ_2 phases begin to precipitate. These are new compounds, the result of the setting reaction. **Precipitation** is a process in which a solid is formed from material dissolved in a liquid. Examples of precipitation include freezing water (ice is the precipitate), sugar that forms in old honey, and the curdling of milk (milk protein is the precipitate).
6. Precipitation of the γ_1 and γ_2 phases continues until the mercury is consumed and a solid mass results. The setting reaction may take as long as 24 hours to complete, when strength reaches a maximum.

D. Mercury/Alloy Ratio

The composition of the set dental amalgam depends on several factors. The mercury/alloy ratio is the amount of mercury that is mixed with the amalgam alloy. Using more mercury increases the mercury-containing reaction products. Using less mercury decreases the mercury-containing reaction products. Proper trituration and condensation techniques can also reduce the mercury content of the set amalgam. Because the mercury-containing reaction products are weaker than the Ag-Sn starting material, minimizing mercury results in an improved restoration.

The strength of the amalgam is increased, and marginal breakdown is reduced. Remember, as with other dental materials, the liquid mercury must wet all alloy particles and form a cohesive mass without voids. An inadequate mercury/alloy ratio results in voids and poor restorations.

E. Development of Other Shapes

The early amalgam alloys of the 1800s were large, rough particles by today's standards. In the 1940s and 1950s, manufacturers changed the shape of the particles to increase early strength and produce "smoother carving" amalgams. Lathe-cut alloys became "micro-lathe cut alloys," which were smaller-sized lathe-cut particles. Next, spherical particles were introduced. Spherical alloys pack together better and require less mercury for an acceptable mix. However, major improvements in the clinical performance of amalgam restorations did not result.

F. Microstructure of Low-Copper Amalgams—Optional

Dental amalgams are a mixture of elements and phases.

1. The γ (Ag-Sn) phase is typically the strongest and most corrosion-resistant phase. It is approximately one-quarter of the volume of a dental amalgam.
2. The γ_1 (Ag-Hg) phase is somewhat strong and corrosion resistant, but it is also brittle. The γ_1 phase makes up approximately half of the amalgam and is the matrix phase that holds this multiphase material together.
3. The γ_2 (Sn-Hg) phase is the weakest and most corrosion prone. It makes up approximately one-tenth of the material, but is the "weak link" in the structure.
4. It is important to realize that the chemical formulas for amalgam phases do not include minor components, which affect the properties of each phase and of the resulting amalgam. The γ_1 (Ag-Hg) phase usually contains some copper, tin, zinc, and other amalgam alloying elements.

V. High-Copper Dental Amalgams

Starting in the 1960s, a variety of high-copper dental amalgams were developed. The clinical performance of many, but not all, of these amalgams is superior to that of the best low-copper amalgams. The significant factor that determined improved performance is elimination of the weak γ_2 phase. Strength is increased, and corrosion and marginal breakdown are reduced. Currently, high-copper amalgams dominate the dental market. These high-copper amalgams can be categorized into several groups.

A. Admix High-Copper Amalgam

"Blended," "admix," or "dispersion" alloys are a mixture of two kinds of particles, as shown in Figure 6.6*C*.

1. These high-copper amalgams contain lathe-cut particles with the same composition as those of the low-copper amalgam alloys, silver and tin. The other particles are spherical and contain 28% copper and 72% silver. This composition is called the Ag-Cu eutectic.
2. The first high-copper amalgam was "Dispersalloy," developed by Innes and Yondelis in Canada in 1963. It was originally sold to Johnson & Johnson, but the patent and trademark have since been sold several times to other dental materials companies. Several admix amalgams are available, but Disperalloy maintains a significant market share.

B. Spherical High-Copper Amalgams

Single-composition, high-copper, spherical dental amalgams have only one shape of particle, as shown in Figure 6.6*B*. The particles are a combination of silver, tin, copper, and other elements.

The first single-composition spherical dental amalgam, "Tytin," was developed by Kamal Asgar. Again, the trademark has been sold. Many spherical single-composition alloys are available, but Tytin remains very popular and has a significant market share. Dispersalloy and Tytin are good examples of dentists' brand loyalty.

C. Setting Reactions of High-Copper Amalgams

The setting reaction of high-copper amalgams is a little more complex than in low-copper amalgams. The following is a simplified reaction; its notable feature is the lack of a γ_2 (Sn-Hg) product:

$$\text{excess AgSnCu (the alloy)} + \text{Hg} \rightarrow$$
$$\text{unreacted alloy} + Ag_2Hg_3\ (\gamma_1) + Cu_6Sn_5$$

1. The alloy contains 10% to 30% copper.
2. Silver reacts in the same manner as a low-copper amalgam, forming a γ_1 (Ag-Hg) reaction product.
3. Tin reacts with copper to form several Cu-Sn reaction products. No Sn-Hg reaction product is formed as occurs in the low-copper amalgam reaction. The microstructure of an admixed amalgam is shown in Figure 6.7.

D. Why So Many Different Amalgam Products?—Optional

Why do so many kinds of amalgam exist? The answer is that each has different handling characteristics.

1. Shape of the Alloy Particle

The shape of the alloy particle affects the handling characteristics of the material. Lathe-cut

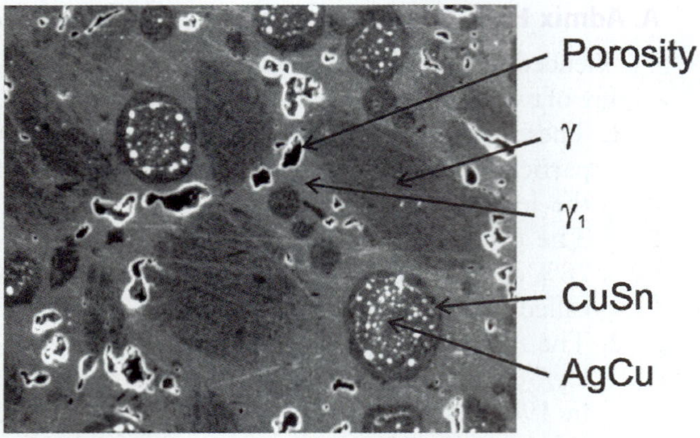

FIGURE 6.7 Scanning electron micrograph showing the microstructure of a high-copper admixed dental amalgam. (Courtesy of Drs. Bill and Sally Marshall, San Francisco, CA.)

particles are rough and do not slide past each other easily. Therefore, the resulting freshly triturated lathe-cut amalgam requires more force during condensation than is required with spherical particles. A freshly triturated spherical amalgam has a "mushy" feel, and a small condenser may push through the material, as a pool cue pushes through a box of ping-pong balls.

a) It is easier to restore proximal contacts (Class II restorations) with a lathe-cut or admix amalgam than with a spherical amalgam. Restoring proximal contacts of teeth with a direct restorative material requires use of a matrix band to obtain the proper anatomical shape. The matrix band is positioned around the tooth. Along with the remaining tooth structure, it functions as a temporary wall to form the mold into which the restorative material is placed. When the freshly mixed amalgam is condensed against the matrix band, the band can be deformed if needed and pushed against the adjacent tooth. This creates the necessary contact point. The matrix band may rebound to its original position, however, unless the amalgam holds it in the deformed position. Lathe-cut and admix amalgams maintain this position against the adjacent tooth better than spherical amalgams.

b) Particle shape greatly affects the amount of liquid mercury that is needed to wet the surface of the particle. Of all solids, a sphere has the lowest ratio of surface area to volume. Therefore, spherical particles need less mercury to wet the particles, and less mercury means that the reaction is finished sooner, with a faster-setting amalgam as the result.

c) With less mercury used or a lower mercury/alloy ratio, the relative percentage of mercury-containing reaction products is reduced. Because mercury-containing phases are the weaker phases, reducing the amount of mercury increases the strength and other properties of the dental amalgam.

d) Proper mixing and handling also affect the composition of the resulting dental amalgam. Proper mixing and condensation will keep porosity to a minimum. In addition, mercury can be "squeezed out" of the freshly triturated, nonspherical amalgams by using a proper condensation technique. The particles are forced together by condensation pressure, and the excess mercury is forced to the surface. Personal preference for the "feel" of amalgam when condensing and carving is a very important factor when selecting products for purchase.

2. Silver Content of the Alloy

The silver content of an amalgam alloy affects the cost. Several alloys have as much as 30% copper. As the copper content increases, the silver content decreases, and so does the cost of the product. The cost of amalgam itself is a minor factor in the overall cost of an amalgam restoration. On the other hand, recycling amalgam scrap is both environmentally and economically beneficial.

VI. Factors Affecting Handling and Performance

Both the manufacturer and the dentist control factors that affect the handling and performance of dental amalgam.

A. Manufacturer

The manufacturer controls:

- Alloy composition
- Alloy particle shape
- Particle size
- Particle size distribution.

The manufacturer also controls the rate of the setting reaction by heat treating the particles and by washing the surface of the particles with acid to remove surface oxides.

Manufacturers supply amalgam alloy in several forms, as shown in Figure 6.8. Amalgam alloy can be purchased as a powder, as a powder pressed into tablets (looking much like a silver aspirin), and as preproportioned disposable capsules containing both the alloy powder and mercury. With current concerns for mercury hygiene and clinical infection control, preproportioned disposable capsules are considered the standard form in most practice settings.

B. Dentist

Mixing and handling by the dentist and the auxiliary personnel also affect the properties of the set amalgam.

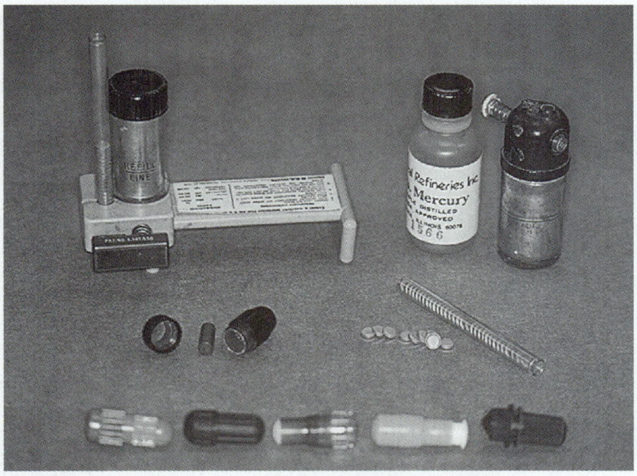

FIGURE 6.8 Several forms of amalgam alloy as supplied by their manufacturers. **Top row** (moving *left* to *right*). Alloy pellet and mercury dispenser, bulk mercury in a plastic bottle, mercury dispenser. **Center row.** Reusable capsule and amalgam alloy pellets. **Bottom row.** Several precapsulated amalgam products.

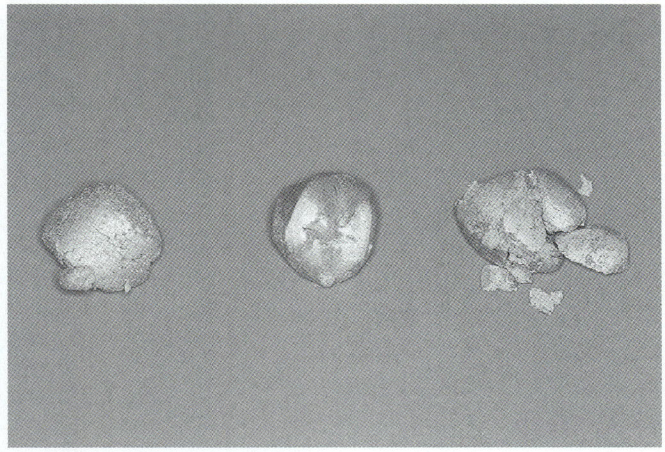

FIGURE 6.9 From *left* to *right,* undertriturated, properly triturated, and overtriturated amalgam.

1. The manufacturer controls the mercury content when preproportioned capsules are used, but other forms of alloy require the assistant to precisely control the amount of mercury that is mixed with the alloy. Excess mercury increases the mercury-containing reaction products, which tend to be the weaker phases.
2. Proper trituration technique is required. Both the speed and time of trituration are set to obtain the proper consistency of the mix. Overtrituration and undertrituration also affect the working time and strength of the material.
   a) Overtriturated amalgam tends to crumble and is difficult to condense. It exhibits a shortened working time. In addition, voids will likely result in the restoration.
   b) Properly triturated amalgam is a cohesive mass that might be slightly warm to the touch. The surface is smooth, and the mass has a plastic feel. Such a mix is easily condensed and exhibits the proper working time.
   c) Undertriturated amalgam has a mushy-grainy feel because not all of the particles are broken up. The mass is difficult to properly condense.
   d) Examples of overtriturated, properly triturated, and undertriturated amalgam are shown in Figure 6.9.
3. Proper condensation techniques reduce or eliminate voids, which are the worst component of the amalgam. Although amalgam is probably the only material that might work in a wet environment, it should be condensed in a clean, dry cavity preparation. Contamination with saliva increases leakage of the restoration. Zinc-containing amalgams expand excessively if contaminated by moisture when they are condensed.
4. The dentist controls the anatomical form and finishing techniques. Open interproximal contacts, overhanging margins, and other improper contours increase the likelihood of periodontal problems. Poor condensation with defects at the margins increases the likelihood of recurrent decay. Finally, undercarved occlusal surfaces cause trauma to the supporting tissues.

VII. Amalgam Properties

Several physical properties of amalgam hold particular interest for the clinician. Proper handling of the material is required for optimum results.

A. Dimensional Change

Minimal change in dimension after condensation is important. Excessive contraction leads to leakage and postoperative sensitivity. Excessive expansion can also cause postoperative sensitivity. Dimensional change is affected by many factors, such as the mercury/alloy ratio as well as trituration and condensation techniques. The best results are obtained by following the manufacturer's recommendations.

B. Strength

Amalgam restorations must resist the biting forces of occlusion. At one time, it was thought that the 1-hour compressive strength of amalgam was an important property, and this strength was incorporated into the specification. The 1-hour strength of spherical alloys is much greater than that of lathe-cut or admix amalgams. Strength at 24 hours is greater for all types of amalgams, and strength differences between the types of amalgams are much less after 24 hours. Again, the strength of the amalgam depends on the phases that are present. Having more of the stronger phases results in a stronger material.

Dental amalgam has a high compressive strength, but the tensile and shear strengths are comparatively low. Therefore, amalgam should be supported by tooth structure for clinical success in the long term, which is approximately 10 to 20 years. Also, amalgam needs sufficient bulk. A thickness of 1.5 mm or more is needed to withstand occlusal forces.

C. Creep

Creep was discussed previously in Chapter 3. **Creep** is a slow change in shape caused by compression. Creep of dental amalgam specimens is a common test and is included in the amalgam specification. It was once thought that creep provided a good indicator of clinical performance. Supposedly, amalgam could be pushed by adjacent and opposing teeth to cause open, chipped, and overhanging margins. Recurrent decay would then result. However, when high-copper amalgams were developed, creep became less of a predictor of clinical success. Remember, because the γ_2 phase has been eliminated in high-copper amalgams, the phase that is most susceptible to creep is no longer present.

D. Corrosion of Dental Amalgam

Amalgam galvanically corrodes in much the same way that iron rusts. Galvanic corrosion occurs when two dissimilar metals exist in a wet environment. An electrical current flows between the two metals, and corrosion (oxidation) of one of the metals occurs. The likelihood of galvanic corrosion increases if two metallic phases are present in a metal. Dental amalgams always have more than two phases, and they also exist in a corrosive environment, the oral cavity. Therefore, amalgams corrode and, eventually, fail.

Corrosion occurs both on the surface and in the interior of the restoration. Surface corrosion discolors an amalgam restoration and may even lead to pitting. Surface corrosion also fills the tooth/amalgam interface with corrosion products, reducing microleakage. Internal corrosion (in the interior of the restoration) is hidden from the clinician. Such corrosion will lead to marginal breakdown and, occasionally, fracture. Assessing the status of an amalgam restoration for marginal breakdown and internal corrosion is beyond the current clinical diagnostic techniques. Instead, alleged recurrent decay is the dominant reason for replacing amalgam restorations. Although the restoration may look unesthetic and the margins may appear to be "ragged," the amalgam is still sealed at the interface and serves the patient well.

An acidic environment promotes galvanic corrosion. Poor oral hygiene and a cariogenic diet will expose both teeth and restorative materials to a destructive environment. The same factors that promote caries will accelerate corrosion. Therefore, patient behavior can affect the longevity of amalgam and other restorations.

E. Working and Setting Times

The working and setting times of dental amalgams are not well-standardized properties. Fast-set and slow-set versions of many brands are sold. The fast-set version of a given product will set faster than the regular-set version of that product. However, that same fast-set version may not be faster than the regular-set version of a different product. Personal preference for working and setting times is a very important factor when selecting products for purchase.

VIII. Use of Dental Amalgam

Amalgam is used to restore many different types of carious lesions and tooth fractures, as shown in Figure 6.10. Again, amalgam is a very cost-effective restorative material and is used to restore Class I, II, V, and VI carious lesions. At times, amalgam is used for small cingulum pits in the lingual of anterior teeth. Amalgam is also used as a foundation for a crown to restore a severely decayed tooth, as shown in Figure 6.11. The foundation is called an "amalgam buildup" or "amalgam core." An amalgam buildup that has been prepared for a crown is shown in Figure 8.1*A*. Such a large amalgam restoration may function adequately for 5 to 6 years, but not

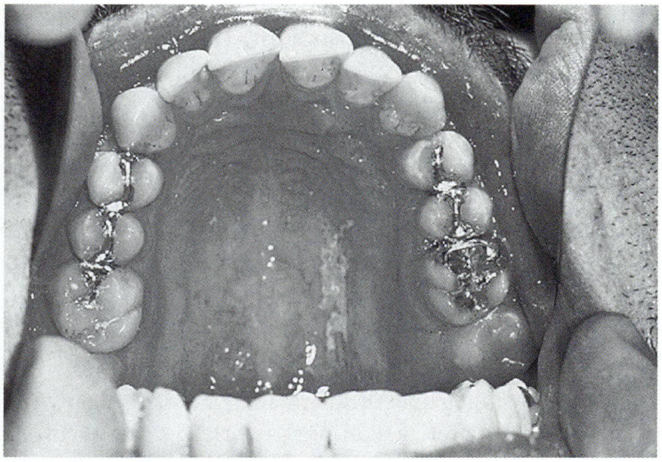

FIGURE 6.10 Photograph of a maxillary arch with several amalgam restorations. (See color images.) (Courtesy of Dr. Ted Stevens, Morgantown, WV.)

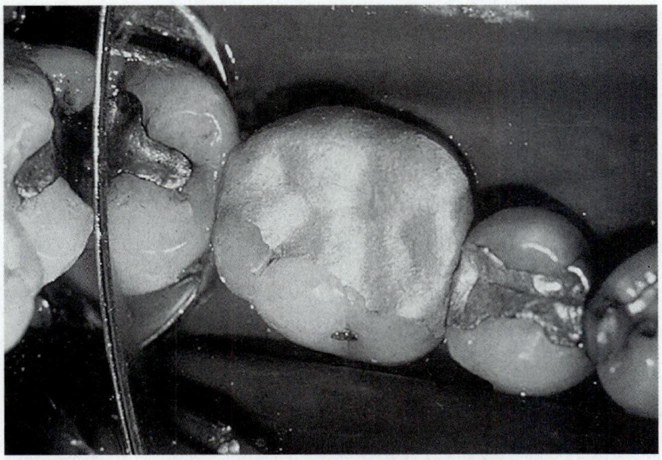

FIGURE 6.11 Photograph of a large amalgam restoring the mesial, distal, occlusal, and lingual surfaces of a mandibular first molar. This could function as a permanent restoration or be prepared and serve as a core for a crown, as shown in Figure 8.1*A*. (See color images.) (Courtesy of Dr. Ted Stevens, Morgantown, WV.)

nearly as long as it may function when covered by a crown (15–20 years) (see Fig. 1.4).

A. Use With a Cavity Varnish

For many years, amalgam has been used with a cavity varnish. The most common is copal varnish. **Copal varnish** is a resin dissolved in a solvent. Varnish is painted on the cavity preparation, much like varnish is painted on woodwork in a house. The amalgam is then condensed and carved. The intent is to reduce initial leakage by sealing the margins before corrosion products form. Postoperative sensitivity is supposedly reduced, along with the amalgam's tendency to discolor adjacent tooth structure. Today, cavity varnish is being replaced by a variety of materials. Dental bonding systems have been developed to bond amalgam to tooth structure. At this time, however, the reduction of postoperative sensitivity or increased clinical life expectancy of "bonded" amalgam restorations has not been demonstrated by clinical research.

B. Selection of the Amalgam Alloy

It is recommended that dentists use only ADA-accepted, high-copper alloys. If not using a precapsulated product, use only ADA-accepted mercury. Many outstanding products are on the market. These products have differences in particle shape, rate of set, and other factors that affect the "feel" of these materials. One must choose an alloy based on personal preference, but the product should have independent clinical research data available that details its clinical life expectancy. Some products are definitely better than others.

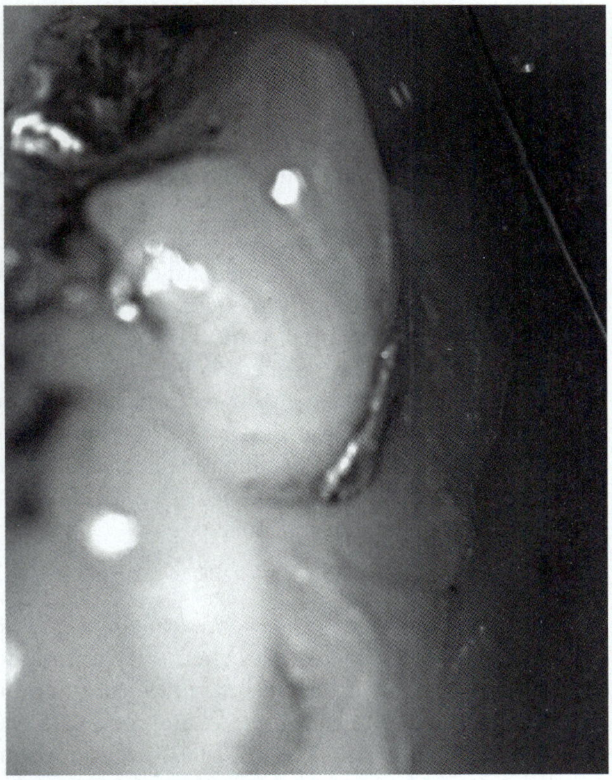

FIGURE 6.12 Amalgam condensed in a contaminated cavity preparation that has expanded.

C. Effect of Moisture

As with any dental material, the quality of an amalgam restoration is reduced if it is placed in a wet or contaminated preparation. Zinc-containing amalgams are more affected than nonzinc materials by moisture. Zinc reacts with water to produce hydrogen gas. The hydrogen gas causes the amalgam restoration to expand, seeming to push out of the preparation. **Delayed expansion** is illustrated in Figure 6.12. Increased corrosion and reduced clinical longevity result. Amalgam should not be handled with bare hands because even the moisture from one's skin can cause problems. Current standard precautions, however, make this a moot point.

D. Finishing and Polishing

The relative value of polishing amalgam restorations is debatable. It is not uncommon for the first few amalgams placed by a dental student or auxiliary to need finishing and polishing at a second appointment. In addition, an amalgam (placed by another dentist) may need to be recontoured or smoothed on occasion. It is important for the dentist to recontour any amalgam needing such care regardless of when or where it was placed. Providing such treatment is considered to be quality patient care.

The goal of finishing an amalgam restoration is to produce margins that are continuous with adjoining tooth structure and to produce proper contours. Polishing produces a smooth and lustrous surface that reduces both the likelihood of corrosion and the ability of plaque to adhere to the surface. Polishing lathe-cut and admix amalgams should be delayed for 24 hours to allow the amalgam to set and become hard enough to withstand the polishing procedure. Spherical amalgams set much faster; some can be polished 20 minutes after being placed. Appropriate finishing and polishing of amalgam restorations improve their appearance, as illustrated in Figure 6.10. The finishing and polishing of amalgams are presented in Chapter 26 and are a typical responsibility of the dental hygienist.

E. Mercury Toxicity

Mercury toxicity is a concern in dentistry because mercury and its chemical compounds are toxic to the kidneys and the central nervous system. Proper handling of mercury will prevent harm to office staff. The most significant danger is from mercury vapor. Mercury has a high vapor pressure and evaporates at room temperature. The lungs absorb most of the mercury vapor in air when inhaled. Poor mercury hygiene will subject office staff to unnecessary risk. It is important that the ADA recommendations for mercury hygiene are followed. These recommendations include proper handling and storage along with prompt cleaning of all mercury spills. Safety in the dental office is addressed in Chapter 20.

Mercury toxicity is not a problem for patients. Numerous government and nongovernment scientific panels have rebuffed claims of mercury toxicity in patients. The only exception is patients who are truly allergic to mercury. Very few cases (<0.1% of patients) of mercury allergy have been reported in the scientific literature. Dentists who urge patients to replace amalgam restorations to cure medical problems are not practicing ethical dentistry. Several such dentists have lost their licenses.

Mercury in the environment is an important problem. The role that dentistry plays in mercury contamination is under investigation. Significant mercury contamination problems are from industrial sources, however, and not from dentistry.

IX. Direct Gold Restorations

Pure gold will cold-weld to itself at room temperature. In dentistry, pure or nearly pure gold is used to place small restorations, as shown in Figure 6.13. **Gold foil** is also called **direct gold** or **cohesive gold.** Gold foil restorations require extreme attention to detail and considerable skill.

When using direct gold restorations, the operatory field must be clean because contamination will prevent cohesion of the gold. Gold foil comes from the manufacturer covered with a thin layer of chemical protectant. This protectant is burned off with a 100% ethyl alcohol flame. This heating operation is called **annealing gold foil.** This use of the term “annealing,” however, is a misnomer. Annealing has a very different meaning in the field of metallurgy. Gold foil is condensed or compacted using hand pressure or other mechanical means.

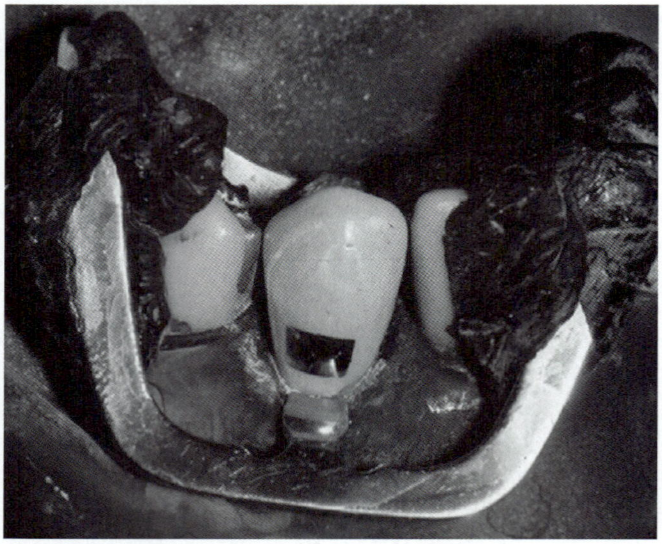

FIGURE 6.13 A gold foil restoration. (Courtesy of Dr. Birgitta Brown, Morgantown, WV.)

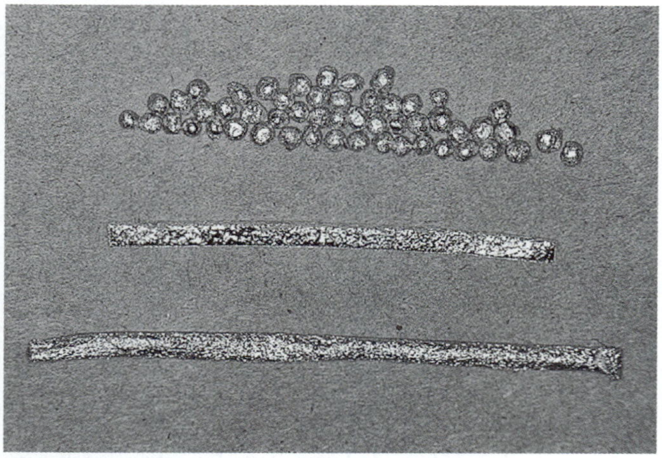

FIGURE 6.14 Several forms of cohesive gold: gold powder wrapped in gold foil called Easygold **(top)**, rope gold **(middle)**, and mat gold **(bottom)**.

Although gold foil can be carved with special knives, it is typically shaped with rotary instruments and then polished. Because the labor costs (not the cost of the material) are high, other materials have significant economic advantages. Gold foil comes in a variety of forms (mat gold, rope gold, and other commercial products), as shown in Figure 6.14. If properly placed, gold foil restorations are very long lasting. Use of gold foil is limited to small Class I, II, III, and V restorations because it lacks strength compared to other metallic restorations. Direct gold is also used to repair defects in gold crowns.

SUMMARY

Dental amalgam is a direct restorative material that is used in all surfaces of the posterior teeth and, sometimes, in the lingual pits of anterior teeth. Dental amalgam is made by mixing approximately equal parts of a powdered metal alloy with mercury. It is held in the cavity preparation by mechanical retention. The particle shape of the alloy is manufactured in two forms: spherical and lathe-cut (filings). A combination of both comprises admixed (also called blended or dispersion) alloys. Use of dental amalgam has several advantages. It is long lasting, cost-effective, and able to seal its margins over time. The development of high-copper amalgams has significantly improved the clinical performance of amalgam as a restorative material. The restorations are stronger and have less marginal breakdown.

The manufacturer and the dentist both control the handling and performance characteristics of dental amalgam. The manufacturer controls the alloy composition, particle shape, particle size, and particle size distribution. The manufacturer also controls the rate of the setting reaction and the form in which it may be purchased. The dentist controls the trituration technique, the method of condensation, and the anatomical form and finishing techniques.

Dental amalgam reaches its maximum stress after 24 hours. The compressive strength is high, but the tensile and shear strengths are comparatively low. It is used for Class I, II, V, and VI carious lesions. It can also be used as a foundation for a crown when the tooth is severely decayed. This is called an "amalgam buildup" or an "amalgam core."

Finishing and polishing of dental amalgam will extend the lifetime of the restoration. The goal of finishing is to produce a continuous margin with the adjoining tooth structure. Polishing produces a smooth and lustrous surface that reduces corrosion and plaque adherence. It is a well-accepted responsibility of the hygienist to finish and polish amalgams.

Mercury toxicity has been a concern in dentistry for decades. If not handled properly, mercury can be harmful to both patients and office staff. The recommendations by the ADA as well as mandates from Occupational Safety and Health Administration that address proper handling, storage, and cleaning greatly minimize the risk of using this material. As of this writing, no scientific evidence shows that dental amalgam is harmful to the patient or to dental personnel.

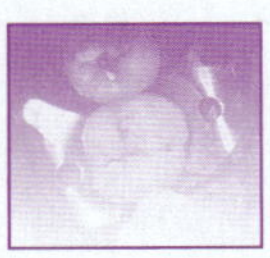

Learning Activities

1. Condense a spherical amalgam and an admix amalgam into a simple simulated cavity preparation, such as a washer from a hardware store. Note any difference in the handling or "feel" between the two materials.
2. Overtriturate (by increasing the speed and time settings on the triturator) an amalgam mix, and note the difference in handling characteristics compared to those mixed in learning activity 1.
3. Observe the amalgam restorations in the mouth of a classmate or the restorations charted for several patients. Which surfaces of their teeth are restored with amalgam? Discuss the advantages of amalgam compared to alternative materials, such as a composite resin.

Review Questions

1. Which of the following elements is used in the highest amount in an amalgam restoration?
a) Tin
b) Copper
c) Silver
d) Mercury
e) Aluminum

2. Amalgam is strongest in __________ strength after it has set.
a) Shear
b) Tensile
c) Compressive
d) Bending

3. The elements composing the gamma-two (γ_2) phase (the weakest and most corrosion-prone phase) of the amalgam reaction are:
a) Silver and tin
b) Silver and mercury
c) Tin and mercury
d) Tin and tin

4. The function of silver in the amalgam reaction is to:
a) Reduce strength and corrosion resistance
b) Increase strength and corrosion resistance
c) Minimize oxidation
d) Maximize oxidation

5. Control of the mercury content during mixing and condensing of amalgam must be carefully considered because:
a) The higher the mercury content, the higher the strength and the lower the marginal breakdown
b) The lower the mercury content, the higher the strength and the lower the marginal breakdown
c) The higher the mercury content, the higher the strength and the greater the marginal breakdown
d) The lower the mercury content, the higher the strength and the greater the marginal breakdown

6. The single most important feature that accounts for the clinical success of amalgam restorations is:
a) Finish and polish
b) Marginal seal
c) Economy
d) Ease of manipulation

7. The manufacturers of dental amalgam control all of the following except:
a) Alloy composition
b) Rate of setting reaction
c) Proper trituration technique
d) Particle size

8. An amalgam restoration that has been finished and polished:
a) Reduces the ability of plaque to adhere
b) Resists tarnish and corrosion
c) Will not have any voids
d) Is more likely to have continuous margins with tooth structure
e) All of the above
f) a, b, and d
g) a, c, and d

9. In the low-copper or traditional amalgam reaction, tin reacts with mercury. In the high-copper amalgam reaction, tin reacts with:
a) Silver
b) Copper
c) Zinc
d) Mercury

10. The life expectancy of an amalgam restoration is indirectly related to the size of the restoration. As the restoration increases in size, internal stresses decrease, as does the life expectancy.
a) The first statement is true; the second statement is false.
b) The first statement is false; the second statement is true.
c) Both statements are true.
d) Both statements are false.

11. Ashley was condensing an amalgam during lab and she noticed that the triturated amalgam had a softer, "mushy" feel. She most likely used what type of alloy in the mixed amalgam?
a) Spherical
b) Lathe-cut
c) Admixed
d) Blended

12. Just after Jennifer triturated her amalgam, the appearance of it was "crumbly" and dry. It already looked set. The amalgam was most likely:
a) Mixed with an increased mercury/alloy ratio
b) Over-triturated
c) Properly triturated
d) Under-triturated

13. Amalgam may be used for a variety of restorative procedures. ALL of the following pertain to the use of amalgam EXCEPT:
a) Good service to patients at a reasonable cost
b) For cingulum pit areas on the lingual of anterior teeth
c) Amalgam cores
d) Restoring Class I, II, IV, and V caries

14. It has been reported in the scientific literature that ______% of dental patients have a TRUE mercury allergy.

a) 0.01
b) 0.05
c) 0.1
d) 1.0

15. The use of gold foil is limited to small restorations because of its:

a) Short-term longevity
b) Low strength compared to other restorative materials
c) High cost of gold foil compared to other materials
d) Unique handling characteristics

Supplemental Readings

ADA Council on Scientific Affairs. Dental mercury hygiene recommendations. J Am Dent Assoc 2003;134:1498–1499.

Anusavice KJ. Phillips' Science of Dental Materials. 11th ed. Philadelphia: Saunders, 2003, Chapter 17.

Greener EH. Amalgam—yesterday, today, and tomorrow. Operative Dent 1979;4:24–35.

Letzel H, van't Hoff MA, Vrijhoef MMA, Marshall SJ, Marshall GW Jr. A controlled study of amalgam restorations: survival, failures and causes of failure. Dent Mat 1989;5:115–121.

Marshall SJ, Marshall GW Jr. Dental amalgam: the materials. Adv Dent Res 1992;6(Sept):94–99.

Powers JM, Sakaguchi RL, eds. Craig's Restorative Dental Materials. 12th ed. St. Louis: Mosby, 2006, Chapter 11.

7

Dental Cements

Key Words/Phrases

base
composite cements
eugenol
glass ionomer cement
liner
luting agent
obtundent
polycarboxylate cement
resin cements
silicate cement
temporary cements
varnish
zinc oxide–eugenol (ZOE) cement
zinc phosphate cement

Objectives

After studying this chapter, the student will be able to do the following:

1. Describe the use of dental cements as a:
   - Luting agent
   - Base
   - Filling material
   - Temporary restoration
   - Intermediate restoration
   - Periodontal pack
   - Temporary cement
2. Explain the importance of adhesion and microleakage to the clinical use of a dental cement.
3. Differentiate between a base and a liner.
4. Describe the use of a cavity varnish or cavity sealer.
5. Describe the relative properties of the component liquids and powders of dental cements.
6. Explain the setting reaction of a typical dental cement.
7. Based on the properties of the liquid and the powder, discuss the properties of:
   - Zinc oxide–eugenol (ZOE) cement
   - Zinc phosphate cement
   - Polycarboxylate cement
   - Glass ionomer cement
   - Composite cement
   - Calcium hydroxide base
8. Summarize the mixing process for the first four cements in objective #7 and how it relates to the setting reaction.
9. Describe the use and advantages of a composite cement.

I. Use of Dental Cements

Dental cements are used to lute inlays, crowns, bridges, and other restorations and appliances in place, as shown in Figure 7.1. In addition, dental cements are used for a variety of other dental procedures depending on the material. Chapter 23, which presents the laboratory and clinical application of five of the materials, may be used to supplement this chapter.

A. Luting Agent

The term "cement" implies that the material will be used to lute or glue things together. Although other uses are common, use as a **luting agent** has given this group of materials their name, cements. Dental cements hold appliances and restorations in place with micromechanical and macromechanical retention. Some dental cements are adhesive via chemical bonds, but most are not. Adhesion was discussed in Chapter 4.

When a crown is luted to the preparation, the cement is mixed and then painted (or even filled) inside the crown, as shown in Figure 7.1*A*. The crown is seated in place on the preparation, causing the excess cement to ooze out at the margins, as shown in Figure 7.1*B*. The cement is allowed to set either partially or completely, and the excess is removed, much like scaling calculus from teeth. It is critical that all the excess cement is removed because any excess cement left behind will cause gingival irritation.

Luting cements have the most demanding requirements of any dental material. They must set in the mouth, changing from a fluid liquid to a rock-hard solid in a matter of minutes. The resulting material must be biocompatible and insoluble in oral fluids. Because cements are much more soluble than the overlying restorative material, accurate fit of the restoration to be luted is critical. Crown margins should precisely fit the preparation to minimize the amount of cement that is exposed to the oral environment. Poorly fitting margins increase the solubility of the cement and the likelihood of recurrent decay.

A patient's oral hygiene and diet can also affect the longevity of a luted restoration. As bacteria ferment sugars, the pH in the mouth drops. Dental cements are much more soluble in an acidic environment. As the cement dissolves, a gap is created between the tooth and the restoration. The tooth structure at the gap will have a high risk for caries. Plaque control and proper diet will reduce the probability of recurrent decay for a variety of reasons, including maintenance of a less destructive environment for dental cements and other materials.

B. Pulp Protection

Dental cements are also used as an intermediate base or liner when the remaining dentin is believed to be less than 2 mm thick. A base or liner is placed on the dentin between the pulp and the restorative material. A base and a liner are illustrated in Figure 7.2*E* and 7.2*F*. Because the solubility of dental cements is much greater than that of the overlying restorative material, bases and liners must not be applied on margins.

1. Liners

A **liner** is used to protect the pulp from chemical irritation, as illustrated in Figure 7.2*F*. A liner may stimulate secondary dentin formation or release fluoride. Liners are too thin (<0.5 mm) to provide thermal insulation, and they may be too weak to support the restorative material or to resist amalgam condensation forces.

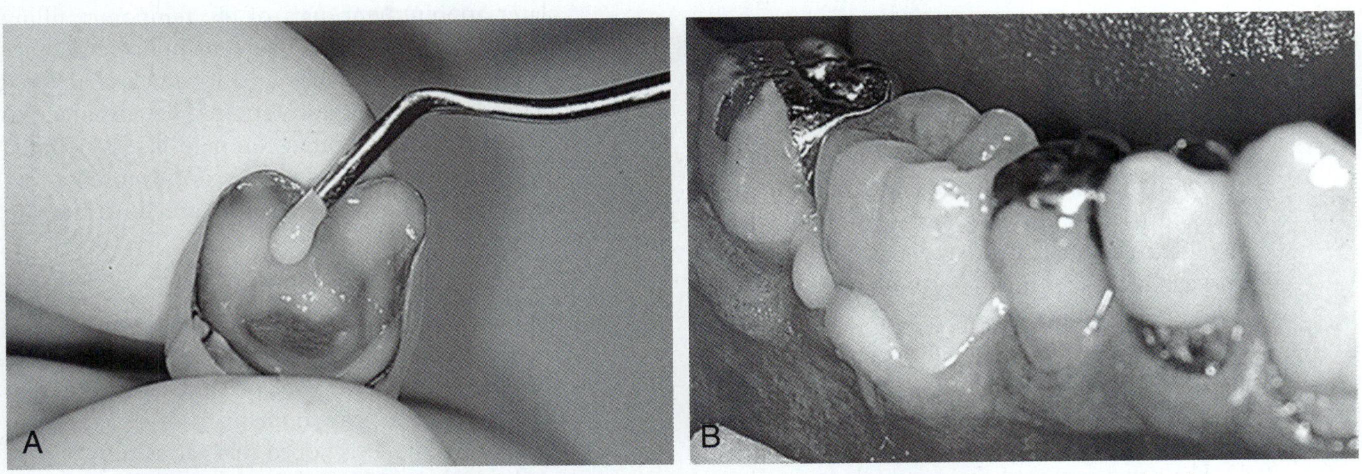

FIGURE 7.1 **A.** When luting a crown, the inside of the crown is painted with cement. **B.** The crown is seated on the prepared tooth, and the excess cement is forced out at the margins. (Courtesy of GC America, Inc., Alsip, IL.)

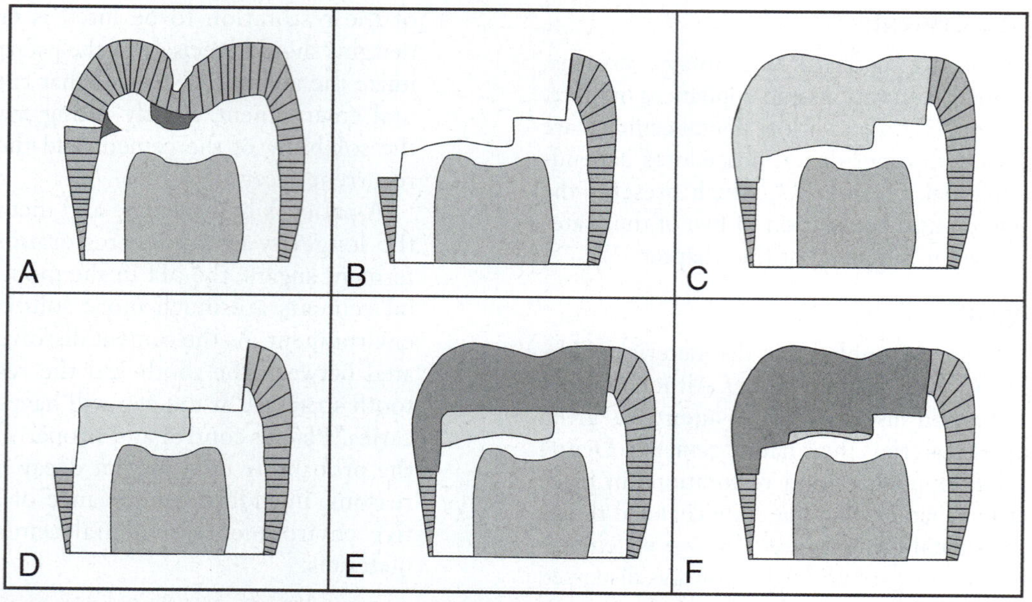

FIGURE 7.2 Several uses of dental cements for pulpal protection. **A.** Carious lesions are present. **B.** The tooth is prepared. **C.** A temporary filling is placed. **D.** At a later appointment, the temporary filling is cut back, leaving a cement base. **E.** The base is covered with a permanent restoration. **F.** A liner is much thinner than a base.

Several lining materials were originally used as a paint-on barrier composed of a solvent and calcium hydroxide or zinc oxide. Methylcellulose was commonly added to increase viscosity and improve handling. Liners were used to prevent chemical irritation. Originally, they were very weak and soluble, and they were frequently covered with a stronger base material, such as zinc phosphate cement. Liners were also used under composites, when it was believed that the composites themselves were irritating. Dentistry has learned that composites are not irritating and the use of liners has dramatically decreased.

2. Bases

A **base** is stronger and thicker than a liner, as illustrated in Figure 7.2*E*. A base provides thermal insulation. Some support the restorative material and may release fluoride, and some are irritating to the pulp before the setting reaction has completed. Such a base may be used in conjunction with a liner. Previously, the distinction between bases and liners was clear. Today, liner materials are much stronger, and the distinction between bases and liners is quite blurred.

C. Temporary Restoration

Some of the same dental cements that are used to lute crowns and that serve as a base may also be used as a temporary restorative material (Fig. 7.2, *A–C*). For some cements, the material is mixed to a thicker consistency than is used for luting. Other cements have formulations that are designed for use as temporary and permanent restorations.

1. Temporary Restorative Materials

Many dental cements are used as a temporary restorative material. The specific cement is chosen based on the particular clinical requirements of the situation. A temporary restoration (filling) may be placed as an emergency procedure when time restraints prevent a more complex treatment. Also, when pulpal pain and other symptoms do not result in a definitive diagnosis, such as reversible versus irreversible pulpitis, a temporary restoration might be placed.

2. Temporary Material as a Base

At times, a temporary filling is placed, and at a later appointment, part of the temporary filling material is removed. The remaining temporary material then becomes a base, which is covered with a permanent restoration. The advantage to such procedures is that the pulp is less irritated when the overlying dentin is not exposed a second time. These procedures are illustrated in Figure 7.2, *A–E*.

3. Caries Control

When patients have a high number of carious lesions (>10), caries control procedures may be implemented. The goal of caries control is to change the oral environment from cariogenic to noncariogenic. It is hoped that caries control procedures change the oral flora from acid-producing and -loving bacteria to other nonpathogenic species. Caries control includes quick, efficient removal of as much decay as possible in the shortest time possible, placement of temporary restorations, diet improvement, and fluoride supplements. Two dental cements that are frequently used for caries control are zinc oxide–eugenol (ZOE) and glass ionomer cement. If all the decay is removed from a lesion, the temporary restoration can later function as a base, as previously described. Light-cure glass ionomer materials will bond to composite materials to a certain extent. Light-cure glass ionomers may be used for caries control and then veneered with composite material to improve esthetics and surface roughness. The ZOE materials are snow white in appearance and, for many patients, are not suitable for use in the anterior teeth.

D. Other Formulations of Dental Cements

Formulations of dental cements are also used as endodontic sealers and surgical/periodontal packs; these formulations are discussed later in this and in other chapters.

Still other cement formulations include impression materials and bite-registration materials. These formulations are discussed in the following chapter.

E. Cavity Sealers

Cavity sealers will be discussed in this chapter because both these and dental cements are used to protect the pulp.

1. Varnish

In dentistry, copal varnish and other varnish formulations are used much like varnishes are used to protect wood. **Varnish** is composed of resins dissolved in a solvent. Figure 7.3 shows an example of a cavity varnish. The varnish is painted onto the entire cavity preparation, including the margins. The solvent then evaporates and leaves behind a very thin layer of resin. Varnish is frequently used under amalgam restorations. It can also function as a chemical barrier, protecting the pulp from an irritating base or a luting cement. It decreases the initial microleakage of the amalgam restoration until corrosion products form at the interface. Varnish is not thick enough to affect thermal sensitivity, and it is not used with composite materials because it would interfere with adhesion.

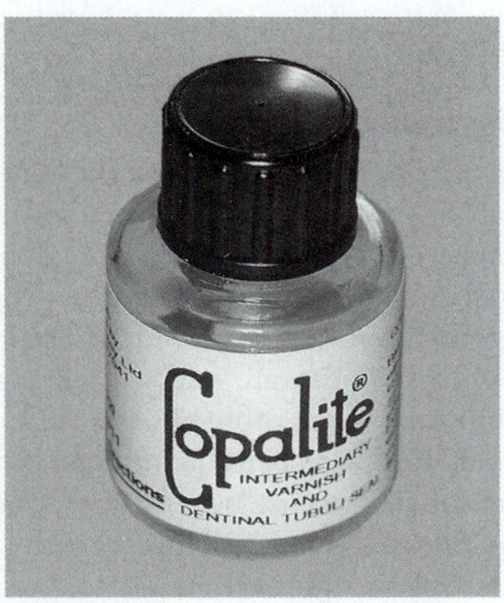

FIGURE 7.3 Cavity varnish.

2. Dentinal Bonding Agents

Some dentists are substituting dentinal bonding agents for varnish. Several of these products will bond the amalgam to the tooth structure. Clinical studies of postoperative sensitivity, however, do not support the routine use of dentinal bonding systems with all amalgam restorations. Some dentists are using Gluma primer as a substitute for varnish. Gluma is a brand name for one of the original dentinal bonding systems. The original Gluma system has been completely reformulated, but the original primer is still available and becoming more popular with time.

3. Order of Placement

If more than one base, liner, varnish, or dentinal bonding system is used, the properties of the materials determine their order of placement. Adhesive materials are placed first. Irritating materials are placed last. For example, when a calcium hydroxide liner is used, it is first covered with the varnish, and then the amalgam is condensed.

II. Chemistry of Dental Cements

With the exception of composite cements, dental cements are brittle, ceramic materials. Their chemistry is a simple acid-base reaction. The resulting product is insoluble in water and oral fluids.

A. Formulation

1. Dental cements are typically a powder/liquid system.
2. The liquid is an acid.
3. The powder is a base. The powder must be insoluble in oral fluids but reactive with the acid.
4. If one understands the properties of the components of a dental cement, then one will be able to predict the properties of the resulting set material.

B. The Reaction

1. The reaction is

acid + excess base → residual base + insoluble salt

2. In terms of the components of the dental cement, the reaction is

liquid + excess powder → residual powder + matrix

3. The residual powder and the matrix must be insoluble in oral fluids.
4. The end result is a "cored structure," much like that in set amalgam.

C. Composite Cements

The chemistry of composite cements is the same as that of acrylics and composites. This chemistry was presented in Chapter 5.

III. Powders Used in Dental Cements

Two materials are used to make powders for dental cements: zinc oxide and glass. The manufacturing process grinds and sieves the powders to obtain the proper particle size. The size of the particles determines the film thickness of the resulting mixed cements. Film thickness determines how well a casting or other restoration can be seated on a preparation. Excessively large particles result in high film thickness, open margins, and recurrent decay.

A. Zinc Oxide

1. Zinc oxide is the only insoluble, nontoxic, reactive oxide or hydroxide that is available to react with an acid. Common additives to the zinc oxide powder are aluminum oxide (alumina) and other oxides that control the setting rate, such as magnesium oxide. Aluminum oxide is very strong and, chemically, very inert. It mechanically reinforces the resulting cement.
2. Zinc oxide has some antibacterial effects and is included in diaper rash, sunscreen, and foot powder products.

B. Powdered Glass

1. Silicon oxide, the chemical formula of glass, is very unreactive. However, if oxides of sodium, calcium, and potassium are added in sufficient quantity, the glass will react with a strong acid. As expected, the powder is white because it is made of small, translucent glass particles.
2. The glass formulation also contains fluoride. Fluoride is a common glass additive because it reduces the melting temperature and improves the flow of the molten glass. Fluoride in the glass powder gives the resulting dental cement the ability to release fluoride and inhibit recurrent caries.

C. Reactivity of Powders

The reactivity of the powder components is controlled by the manufacturer and is matched to the reactivity of the liquid component.

IV. Liquids Used in Dental Cements

The composition or strength of the acid determines the reactivity of the cement liquid. The manufacturer controls this.

A. Eugenol

Eugenol is an organic liquid that is also a weak acid. Eugenol is a major component of oil of cloves. As a result, eugenol has the distinctive smell and taste (of cloves).

1. Eugenol is a phenol derivative that is antibacterial and also obtundent to the pulp. **Obtundent** means that it reduces irritation.
2. Eugenol inhibits free radical polymerization. This limits the use of eugenol-containing cements because they will inhibit the set of composite restorative materials.
3. Other organic liquids have been added to eugenol to formulate dental cements. The most notable of these added organic liquids is ethoxybenzoic acid.

B. Phosphoric Acid

The phosphoric acid used in dental cements is approximately two-thirds phosphoric acid and one-third water by weight. This formulation is very acidic and can be quite irritating to biologic tissues in or out of the oral cavity. The amount of water present affects the reactivity of the liquid by changing the ionization of phosphoric acid. Therefore, it is important not to dispense the liquid until one is ready to mix the cement. High or low humidity will affect the water content and, therefore, the pH, reactivity, and properties of the resulting cement. If the liquid appears cloudy, it has outlived its shelf-life and should be discarded.

C. Polyacrylic Acid

Several dental cements use an aqueous solution of polyacrylic acid. These solutions are 30% to 50% polyacrylic acid by weight and are very viscous liquids.

1. Dispensing

Dispensing these liquids requires more attention than dispensing other cement liquids. If one is not careful, the viscous liquid does not form independent drops. Instead, the drops can "run together," and the amount of liquid dispensed will not be accurate and will vary greatly with each mix. Like phosphoric acid, the liquid should not be dispensed until one is ready to mix the cement because water can evaporate, changing the reactivity and the cement properties. These cement liquids should not be stored in the refrigerator because some will gel and become unusable.

2. Bonding

The carboxyl groups of polyacrylic acid bond to calcium in tooth structure. This bond is believed to be relatively stable in a wet environment. Adhesion of glass ionomer materials was presented in Chapter 4.

3. Water Hardening Cements

"Water hardening" or "water setting" cements use anhydrous, freeze-dried polyacrylic acid. The manufacturer mixes zinc oxide or glass powder with the powdered anhydrous polyacrylic acid. This combined powder is mixed with a companion liquid that is predominately water. When mixed, the polyacrylic acid first dissolves in the water and then reacts with the zinc oxide or powdered glass.

V. Powder/Liquid Ratios and Systems of Dental Cements

Dental cements combine these three liquids and two powders, as shown in Table 7.1. The properties of the resulting cements are based on the properties of the components involved. The manufacturer adjusts the reactivity of both the liquid and powder components to obtain proper setting characteristics and other properties. Do not mix powders and liquids of different cements or different products of the same type.

A. Components Dictate Handling and Mixing

1. The ZOE cement and zinc phosphate cement are mixed with a powder/liquid ratio that depends on the intended use. A base or temporary restoration mix is thicker than a luting mix. The higher the powder/liquid ratio, the greater the strength, the lower the solubility, and in general, the better the cement. On the other hand, working time decreases, and viscosity increases. If a luting mix becomes too thick, the restoration may not seat adequately. In this case, the marginal gap is increased, as is the likelihood of caries. In addition, micromechanical retention is reduced.
2. The powder/liquid ratio is limited in that the liquid must wet all the powder for the cement to function adequately.
3. Glass ionomer and polycarboxylate cements have powder/liquid ratios that are determined by the manufacturer; it is important to follow the manufacturer's directions. Mixing time is also important. If the mixing procedure is too slow, two problems can occur. The first involves the resulting mix becoming too thick. In this case, the restoration may not adequately seat when luted, which increases the marginal gap. The second involves adhesion. The mixed cement must be fluid enough to wet the tooth for both micromechanical and chemical adhesion. If the mixing process is too slow, the carboxylic acid groups react with the powder and are not available to react with the tooth structure. Chemical adhesion is then reduced or even eliminated.
4. Paper pads are available for mixing many dental cements and other dental materials. One must be careful, however, if a paper-mixing pad is used for mixing a dental cement. Cement liquids may weaken the paper surface, causing it to become abraded. The abraded paper particles are then incorporated into and weaken the resulting cement. Some mixing pads use paper that has been coated with a thin layer of plastic. This type of pad is commonly used with glass ionomer and polycarboxylate cements. A thick glass slab is favored for mixing zinc phosphate cement; typically, the slab is cooled to improve the resulting mix.

B. Systems

Most cements come as powder/liquid systems, but some are paste/paste systems. Paste/paste systems are dispensed by equal lengths, as are other paste/paste dental materials.

Each dental cement has its own advantages and disadvantages. Use and mixing of dental cements are summarized in Table 7.2. The remainder of this chapter will focus on the following dental cements:

1. ZOE
2. Zinc phosphate
3. Glass ionomer
4. Polycarboxylate
5. Composite
6. Others

Table 7.1 Components and the Resulting Cements

Components	Zinc Oxide Powder	Glass Powder
Eugenol	Zinc oxide–eugenol (ZOE) cement	No reaction
Phosphoric acid	Zinc phosphate cement	Silicate cement
Polyacrylic acid	Polycarboxylate cement	Glass ionomer cement

Table 7.2 Reference Guide for Liners, Bases, and Cements

Cement	Use	Mixing Technique	Mixing Time[a]	Characteristics of a Proper Mix	Setting Time[a]
Calcium hydroxide	Cavity liner	Mix quickly in a small area of paper pad	10 seconds	Uniform color	2–3 minutes
Zinc phosphate	Luting agent	Add divided increments in specified time, using large slab area	1–1.5 minutes	Mix will stretch 1 inch between slab and spatula	5.5 minutes
	Base	Same as luting agent (above)	1–1.5 minutes	Thick, putty-like (nonsticking) consistency	5.5 minutes
Glass ionomer	Luting agent	Add powder to liquid in one portion	30–45 seconds	Use while glossy	7 minutes
	Base	Same as luting agent (above)	30–45 seconds	Use while glossy	7 minutes
Zinc oxide–eugenol (ZOE)	Base and temporary restoration	Add half-scoop increments, using small mixing area	1.5 minutes	Thick, putty-like (almost crumbly) consistency	2.5–3.5 minutes
Polycarboxylate	Luting agent and intermediate base	Add powder to liquid in one portion	30 seconds	Use while glossy	10 minutes
Temporary	Temporary luting agent	Equal lengths; mix all at once	30 seconds	Uniform color	5 minutes
Composite	Luting agent	Mix equal amounts of pastes	30–45 seconds	Uniform color	5 minutes

[a]These are approximate time periods. Check the manufacturer's instructions for specific mixing times, measurements, and setting times.

VI. ZOE Cement

When zinc oxide is mixed with eugenol, **zinc oxide–eugenol (ZOE) cement** is the result.

A. Products

1. Unreinforced ZOE products are still on the market, but they should only be used when strength and solubility are not critical. Such ZOE formulations for temporary cements are popular and perform adequately.
2. Reinforced ZOE products are stronger and less soluble than unreinforced products. Reinforced ZOE products are used for temporary restorations and intermediate bases. Additives include alumina, rosin, and polymethyl methacrylate resin.

B. Properties

1. Formulations of ZOE have been developed for nearly every use of dental cements. This cement works very well for some uses, but not for all. Unfortunately, ZOE products including reinforced ZOE do not have adequate strength and are too soluble for use as a permanent cement.
2. The ZOE cement is obtundent and, therefore, very useful when pulpal protection is desired or a sedative filling is needed.

C. Mixing

1. Paste/Paste Products

The two pastes are dispensed in equal lengths on a paper-mixing pad. The pastes have different colors. Mixing with a cement spatula swirls the two pastes together. Mixing continues until a homogeneous color is obtained.

2. Powder/Liquid Products

The powder is measured and dispensed with a scoop, as shown in Figure 7.4. The liquid is dispensed as drops. A glass slab is commonly used for mixing powder/liquid ZOE products. The powder is forced into the liquid with a cement spatula. The mixing process first incorporates large increments of powder, followed by smaller increments, as adding powder becomes more difficult. The mixing process requires time to incorporate enough powder to obtain acceptable properties.

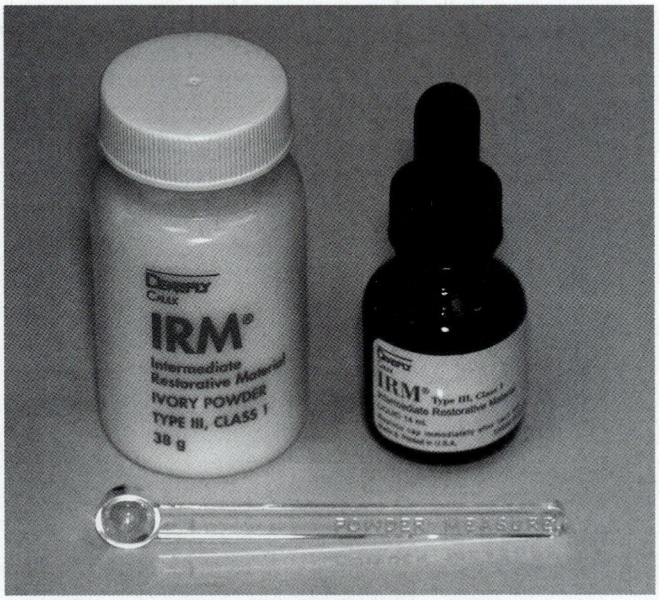

FIGURE 7.4 Zinc oxide and eugenol cement.

3. Cement Consistencies

When a luting mix is desired with a powder/liquid product, mixing is continued until a consistency is obtained such that a "1-inch string" of material occurs when the flat surface of the cement spatula is pulled from the mixed material. When a base consistency is desired, mixing is continued until the material has the consistency of pie dough (can be rolled into a ball with fingers covered with cement powder but has a bit of a crumbly nature). If too little powder is used, the mixed mass will be sticky and difficult to handle. A proper base mix will not stick to instruments and can be pushed or condensed into place and even carved.

4. Clean-up

As with all dental cements, the set material is nearly insoluble in water. Therefore, it is important that the cement spatula and glass slab are washed with water before the material sets. Soap assists with clean-up because eugenol is an organic liquid that is only slightly soluble in water. If one delays clean-up, the set material is difficult to remove from the instruments used. Set ZOE materials can be dissolved with a variety of organic solvents, such as alcohol, orange solvent, and others.

5. Setting Reaction

Water accelerates the ZOE setting reaction. Therefore, ZOE materials set faster in the mouth than they do when out of the mouth, making them quite useful and popular.

6. Removal of Excess ZOE

Removing excess ZOE luting material is very easy if the material is allowed to set and become a brittle mass, after which it cleanly breaks off at the margins. With an instrument such as a scaler or an explorer, it usually breaks off in large chunks. If one is impatient, the soft material breaks into little pieces, making removal more difficult.

D. Uses

1. ZOE cement is a very old and yet still useful material. Its obtundent property makes it very useful for sedative and temporary fillings. Its use as a base has declined greatly. Other cements that release fluoride have replaced ZOE.
2. A reinforced ZOE base can withstand amalgam condensation forces and support the overlying amalgam restoration.
3. Biocompatibility is very good because ZOE seals very well. However, eugenol causes hypersensitivity reactions in some patients. In addition, eugenol can irritate the skin of dental personnel.

VII. Zinc Phosphate Cement

Zinc phosphate cement is formed when zinc oxide powder is mixed with phosphoric acid. Zinc phosphate cement has been used in dentistry for centuries. At one time, it was the strongest and least soluble cement that was available. This is no longer true, but zinc phosphate cement remains an option for several uses.

A. Products

1. Zinc phosphate cement is supplied by manufacturers as a powder and liquid, as shown in Figures 7.5 and 7.6*A*. The powder and liquid are mixed to a thick or thin consistency depending on the clinical use.

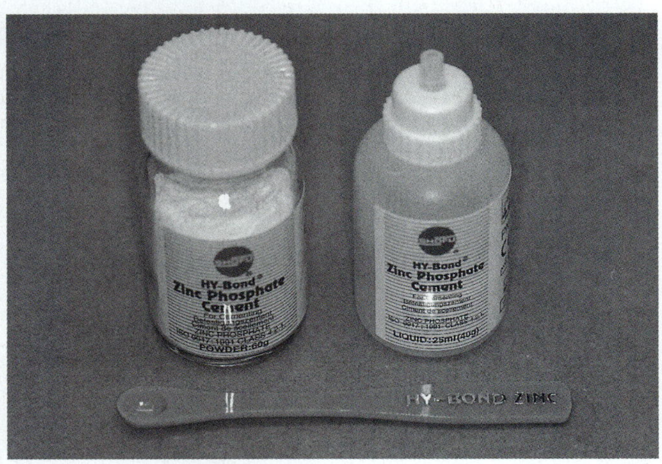

FIGURE 7.5 Zinc phosphate cement.

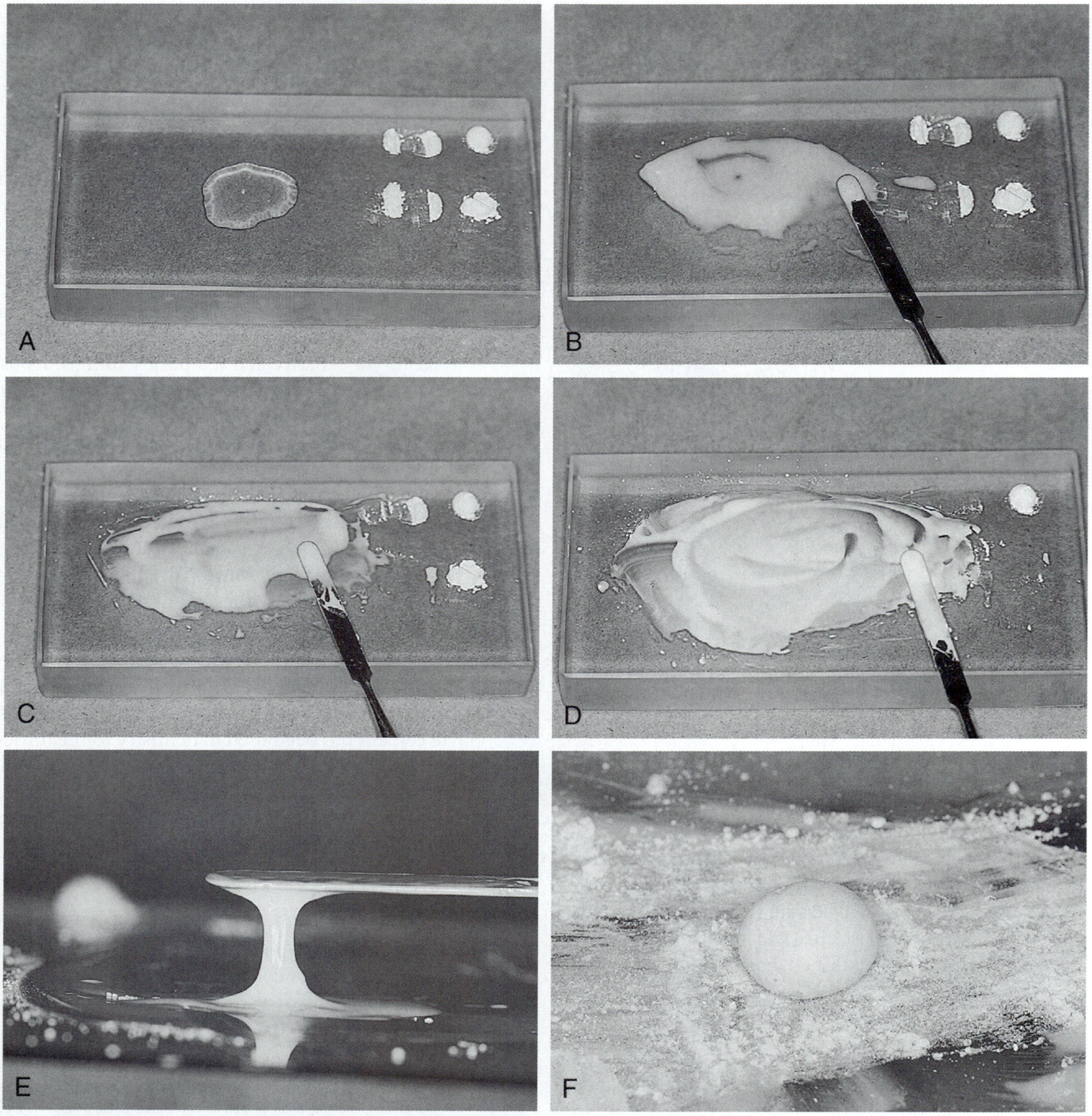

FIGURE 7.6 The mixing process for zinc phosphate cement. **A.** Powder and liquid are dispensed on a chilled glass slab. The powder is divided into increments. **B.** The first increment is mixed into the liquid. **C** and **D.** Increments are added to the mix, using the entire surface of the glass slab. **E.** When mixed for luting, the cement will "string" 1 inch. **F.** A mix for a base can be rolled into a ball.

2. Zinc phosphate cement powder comes in shades. The color of a cement can affect the esthetics of a translucent restorative material. When a translucent ceramic crown, such as an all-porcelain crown, is cemented, the shade of the cement is chosen to maximize the esthetics of the restoration. Zinc phosphate cement powder is mixed with water for trial cementing of the restoration. If the shade is acceptable, the cement is then mixed with cement liquid, and the crown is luted in place.

B. Properties

1. As mentioned, zinc phosphate cement is strong and has a low solubility compared to other cements.

2. Because the mixed cement has a low pH until it has set, zinc phosphate cement is irritating to the pulp. When zinc phosphate cement is used as a base, often a liner is placed or a varnish is applied to the preparation first.
3. Zinc phosphate cement sets to a hard, brittle material. It can withstand amalgam condensation forces and support the overlying amalgam restoration. Removing excess luting material is very easy if the material is allowed to set and become a brittle mass, after which it breaks off cleanly in large chunks. If one is impatient, the soft material breaks into little pieces, making removal more difficult.

C. Mixing

1. Zinc phosphate cement is dispensed as scoops of powder and drops of liquid. A cement spatula and glass slab are used to mix the material. The mixing process is shown in Figure 7.6.
2. Zinc phosphate cement is mixed to the proper consistency, which depends on the intended clinical use. The mix is thinner (lower powder/liquid ratio) when used as a luting agent and thicker (higher powder/liquid ratio) when used as a base. Proper mixing is critical. When improperly mixed, zinc phosphate cement is difficult to handle and has inferior properties.
3. The setting reaction is very exothermic. The heat of the reaction accelerates the setting rate. It is important to dissipate this heat. Zinc phosphate cement is mixed slowly and over a large area of a chilled glass slab to dissipate the heat of the setting reaction. Each increment of Figure 7.6 is mixed for 10 to 15 seconds (for a total of 90 seconds) to facilitate the transfer of heat to the glass slab. The chilled glass slab absorbs the heat given off and slows the setting reaction, enabling more powder to be incorporated into the liquid. Using the entire surface of the slab facilitates heat removal, as shown in Figure 7.6*D*. The powder is incorporated into the liquid with force, as with ZOE cement. The significant difference is that the powder for zinc phosphate is added first in small increments and then in larger ones. The heat of the reaction of the first, small increments is dissipated into the glass slab if mixing is slow enough.
4. When a luting mix is desired, mixing is continued until a "1-inch string" occurs when tested with the cement spatula, as shown in Figure 7.6*E*. When a base consistency is desired, a higher powder/liquid ratio is used. In this case, mixing is continued until the material has the consistency of putty and can be rolled into a ball with fingers covered with cement powder, as shown in Figure 7.6*F*. If too little powder is used, the mixed mass will be sticky and difficult to handle. A proper base mix will not stick to powder-covered instruments and can be pushed or condensed into place.
5. As with all dental cements, the set material is nearly insoluble in water. Therefore, it is important that the cement spatula and glass slab are washed with tap water before the material sets. If one delays clean-up, the set material becomes very difficult to remove from the slab and the instruments. If the mix is allowed to set on the spatula or slab, clean-up is much easier if the instruments are soaked in a baking soda-water solution.

D. Uses

1. Zinc phosphate cement is used for luting inlays, crowns, bridges, orthodontic bands, and other appliances. Zinc phosphate cement has a long working time compared to those of other luting cements.
2. Zinc phosphate cement is also used as a base material. It is acidic, however, and the pulp may need to be protected with a liner or a varnish.
3. Years of clinical use have demonstrated the longevity of zinc phosphate cement.

VIII. Glass Ionomer Cements

Glass ionomer cements are formed when a glass powder is mixed with an aqueous solution of polyacrylic acid. Glass ionomer cements have become quite popular because of their physical and mechanical properties and their clinical performance. A multitude of products are on the market. The first glass ionomer cements set via an acid-base reaction, like most other dental cements. We will call them A/B (acid-base) cements. "Resin-modified" or "resin-reinforced" products have become more popular. They set via two reactions: acid-base and addition polymerization. Glass ionomer products were discussed in Chapter 5 and are summarized in Table 5.2.

A. Products and Uses

1. Luting Materials

Glass ionomer cement is one of the most popular luting materials. Both A/B and resin-reinforced products exist. Resin-modified glass ionomer cement has been called the material of choice for luting all-metal and ceramometal crowns. These glass ionomer products are stronger and tougher than those products that set via an acid-base reaction only.

Light-activated, resin-reinforced glass ionomer luting materials appeared on the market only recently, but problems with their use were soon noted. They were intended for use with translucent ceramic crowns. Unfortunately, light-cure glass ionomer luting materials absorb water in the mouth and swell excessively. This causes an unacceptable number of crowns to fracture after weeks or months of use. These products generally are no longer marketed.

2. Restorative Materials

Glass ionomer restorative materials were discussed in Chapter 5. The restorative materials have the same setting reactions as luting materials but are thicker, stronger materials with a much higher film thickness.

3. Base/Liner Materials

A number of base and lining A/B materials have been developed. With the introduction of light-activated, resin-reinforced glass ionomer liners, however, use of A/B products has greatly diminished. Light-activated glass ionomer liners have adequate strength for use as a base and are quite popular. At times, dentists will use a glass ionomer restorative material for a temporary restoration or a large base.

4. Glass Ionomer Cements

Glass ionomer cements are available in three forms, as shown in Figure 7.7. One form is supplied as a powder and a liquid. The powder is measured with a scoop and is mixed with a specific number of liquid drops from a bottle. It is important that the cement is mixed quickly and the working time is not exceeded.

The second form is a premeasured, single-dose capsule (much like amalgam). These unidose capsules are mixed with an amalgamator. The capsule has a "spout" where the mixed material is expressed from the capsule with a "gun or dispenser." Capsules are easy to use and very popular, but they are also more expensive.

The third system is a paste/paste system common for many dental materials. The pastes are dispensed and mixed until they become one homogenous color. Many resin reinforced glass ionomer luting materials are paste/paste products supplied in a double barrel dispensing device, see Figure 7.7C. These dispensing devices assure proper proportioning of the two pastes.

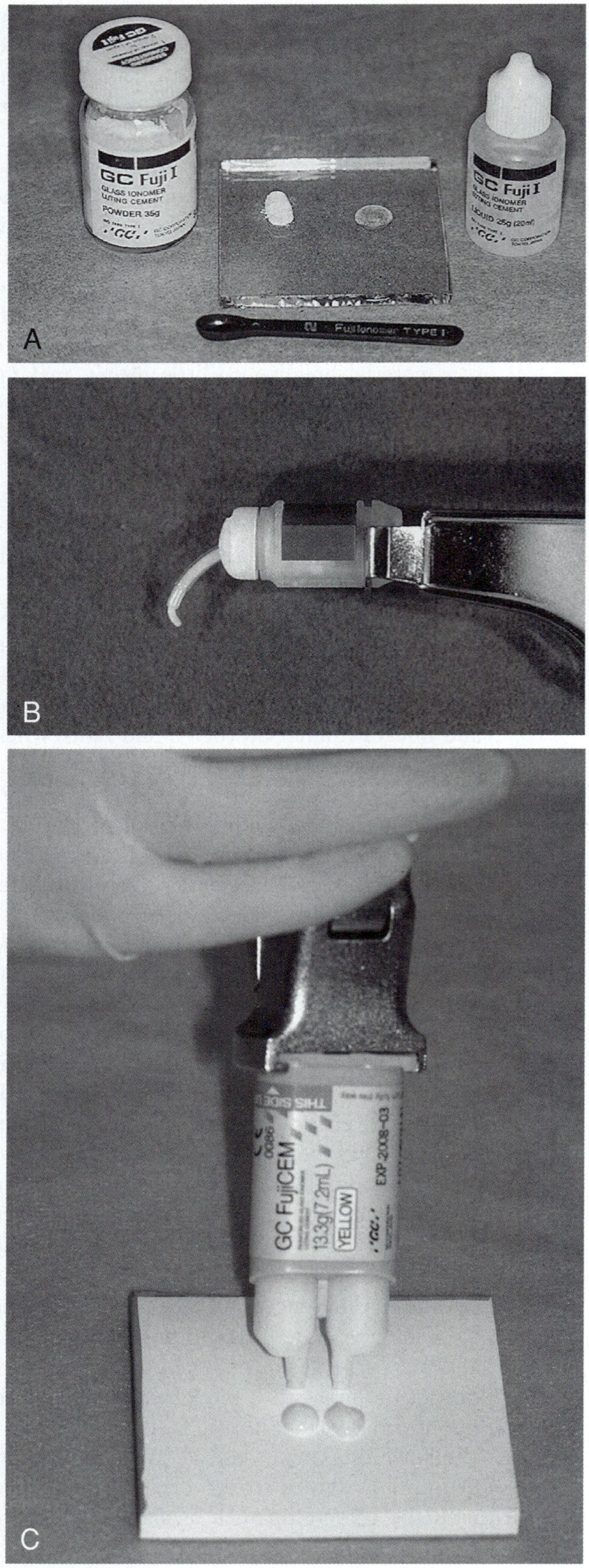

FIGURE 7.7 Glass ionomer products. **A.** Powder and liquid. **B.** Premeasured capsule. Note the cement being expressed from the capsule tip. **C.** Paste/paste dispenser.

B. Properties

1. Glass ionomer materials are the strongest and least soluble dental luting cements (with the

exception of composite cements). They are also adhesive and release fluoride, and they have good biocompatibility. This combination of properties makes them quite popular.

2. Glass ionomer materials bond to tooth structure. In addition, they bond to stainless steel and alloys for ceramometal crowns.

C. Mixing

1. It is critical that glass ionomer cement is properly mixed and handled. If it is not, a nonadhesive material results. The powder is dispensed with a scoop, and the liquid is dispensed as drops. A cement spatula and paper pad are typically used. The cement manufacturer supplies special mixing pads that consist of sheets of plastic-coated paper. The plastic coating protects the paper from abrasion and prevents the liquid from being absorbed by the paper. It is important that the drops form and fall separately. Glass ionomer cement is not mixed to a desired consistency, as ZOE and zinc phosphate cements are. The manufacturer's recommended powder/liquid ratio should be followed. The mixing process is much quicker than that for ZOE or zinc phosphate cement. Mixing should be completed in 30 seconds or less, and the restoration should be seated within 2 minutes from the start of mixing. Typically, the powder is mixed into the liquid in two increments. The mixed material must be placed while the cement surface appears glossy; beyond that time, adhesion is reduced or lost.

2. Clean-up with water is easy and should be done as soon as possible. Remember that the set material will bond chemically to the stainless-steel cement spatula.

IX. Polycarboxylate Cement

A. Properties and Use

Polycarboxylate cement is formed when zinc oxide powder is mixed with an aqueous solution of polyacrylic acid (Fig. 7.8). Polycarboxylate cement was the first adhesive material developed for use in dentistry. Polycarboxylate cement bonds to tooth structure, and this results in very little leakage. It is not as acidic as zinc phosphate cement, is very biocompatible, and is used as a luting cement and an intermediate base. Unfortunately, polycarboxylate cement is not very strong and has a moderate solubility. Glass ionomer cements have the same adhesive properties along with better strength, solubility resistance, and fluoride release. Glass ionomer and zinc phosphate cements have a much greater market share than polycarboxylate cement.

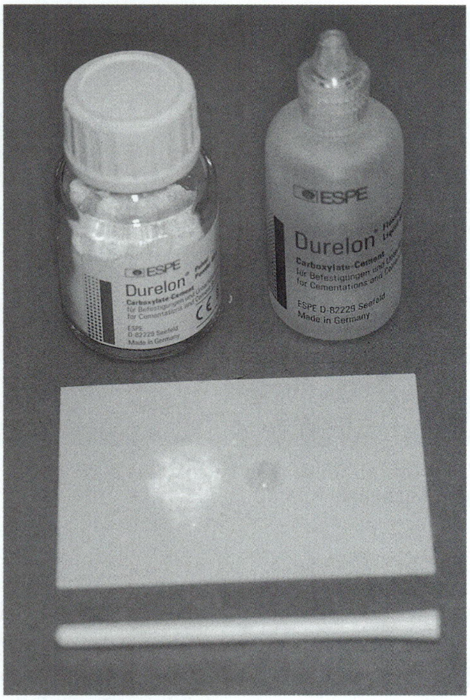

FIGURE 7.8 Polycarboxylate cement.

B. Mixing

Polycarboxylate cement is mixed in the same manner as glass ionomer cements. The powder and liquid are dispensed and mixed on a paper pad with a cement spatula. The mixing time is similar to that of glass ionomer cements because adhesion depends on unreacted carboxylic acid groups. The mixed material must be placed inside the crown and the crown seated while the cement is still glossy.

X. Composite Cements

Composite cements are composite materials (see Chapter 5) with a higher percentage of resin and smaller particle sizes to reduce viscosity. They are sometimes referred to as **resin cements.** Originally they had a very high film thickness. Before the development of dentinal bonding systems, leakage of composite cements was common and caused postoperative sensitivity. Modern composite cements have an improved film thickness (thinner). With the use of a dentinal bonding system (Fig. 7.9), composite cements are the favorite luting material of many clinicians. They are the material of choice for luting all ceramic restorations. If the ceramic material is properly etched and silanated, composite cement will bond the restoration to the underlying tooth structure. Composite cements are also useful for recementing poorly fitting

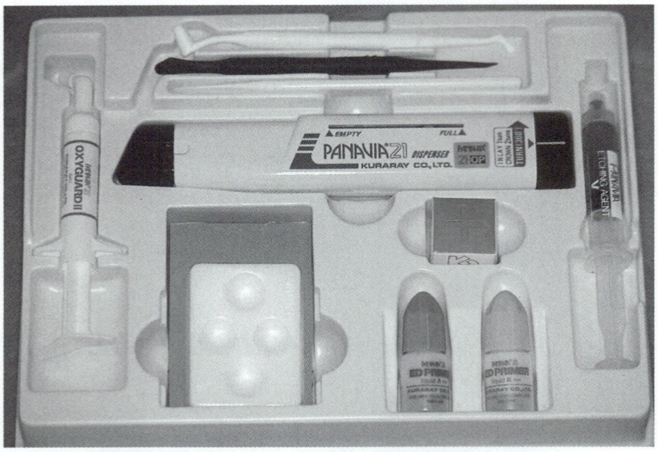

FIGURE 7.9 A composite cement kit containing the cement and a dentinal bonding agent.

crowns when the patient does not wish to have the inadequate crown remade.

Many types of composite cement systems are available. They come as chemically activated, light activated and dual-cure systems. Their use can be quite complex and requires attention to detail. Many times the dentinal bonding system must be altered to change the light activated bonding system to a dual-cure bonding system. The self-etching primers of most dentinal bonding systems are not compatible with chemically activated composite cements. Regardless of product used, the tooth must not be contaminated by oral fluids during the application of the dentinal bonding agent and cement, and the seating of the crown. While one assistant may be adequate, for some products, use of a second assistant is wise.

Composite cements come as a single paste if light activated. Single paste light activated materials are used to bond veneers and orthodontic brackets. Dual-cure and chemically activated products are supplied as two pastes and are mixed on a paper pad with a plastic spatula. As composite cements are used with esthetic restorations such as veneers, composite cements come in a variety of shades. The color of the cement can change the appearance of an esthetic restoration. Some products include try-in pastes to allow evaluation of the restoration with a specific shade.

XI. Other Dental Cements and Cement Uses

A. Silicate Cement

Silicate cement is formed when a glass powder is mixed with phosphoric acid. Silicate cement is an old material and is not used today; however, a short discussion is included for historical perspective. At one time, silicate cement was the only available esthetic anterior restorative material. Silicate cement is very acidic, very irritating to the pulp, and highly soluble. It also leaks excessively. As a result, silicate cements were used with liners. Silicate cement restorations needed to be replaced often; however, recurrent decay was rare. It was discovered that the infrequent occurrence of recurrent decay was caused by fluoride release. Fluoride was present in the glass powder. Thus, fluoride release became a desirable property for many dental materials.

B. Calcium Hydroxide Liners and Bases

At one time, calcium hydroxide liners and bases were very popular materials and were placed under most composite restorations. Calcium hydroxide products promote the formation of secondary dentin. They are still recommended when a cavity preparation leaves little dentin covering the pulp or when a "micro pulp exposure" is suspected. At this time, they are the recommended materials for direct pulp-capping procedures. A direct pulp cap is a material that is placed on vital pulp tissue when the overlying dentin is removed and the pulp is exposed. The tooth is then restored without root canal therapy. Success of a direct pulp cap is not guaranteed, and root canal therapy or extraction may be required.

Calcium hydroxide materials are paste/paste systems, as shown in Figure 7.10. One paste contains calcium hydroxide; the other contains salicylate. Salicylate is a weak acid that is chemically similar to eugenol and reacts with the calcium hydroxide. Titanium oxide is added as a filler. The oldest calcium hydroxide products were weak and used as liners. Improvements have strengthened the material, however, and now some products are strong enough to be used as a base. With the development of dentinal bonding systems and our current understanding of the biocompatibility of

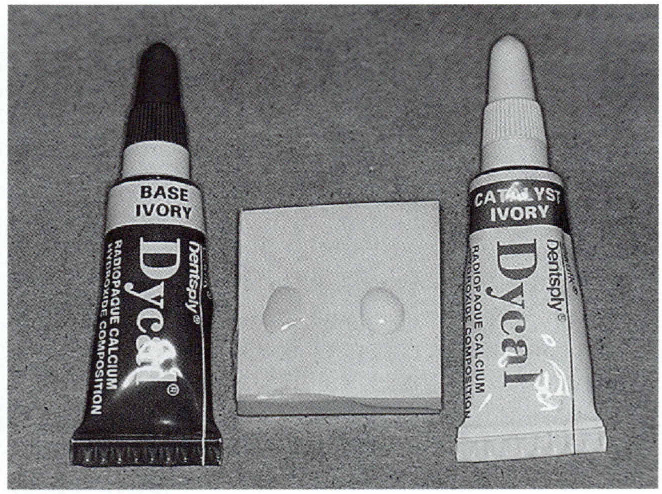

FIGURE 7.10 A calcium hydroxide product.

composite materials, use of calcium hydroxide products has greatly diminished.

The setting reaction of calcium hydroxide materials is accelerated by water. The moisture in dentin is sufficient to cause the material to set within seconds of its application onto the dentin surface. This feature makes calcium hydroxide very easy to use.

C. Temporary Cements

Temporary cements are used to retain a temporary restoration while the permanent restoration is being fabricated. Temporary cements are typically paste/paste systems, as shown in Figure 7.11. They are a unique group of materials in that both a maximum and a minimum strength are required (remember Goldilocks). If the temporary cement is too weak, the temporary restoration will be lost prematurely. If the temporary cement is too strong, the dentist may have trouble removing the temporary crown, and damage to tissues may occur.

Many temporary cements are paste/paste ZOE formulations. The composition of one paste is zinc oxide and vegetable oil. The other paste contains eugenol. The ZOE temporary cements mix easily and set quickly in the humidity of the mouth. The set material is brittle, and the excess cement is easily removed. The obtundent property may even settle down an irritated pulp after it has been insulted by tooth preparation, impression procedures, and construction of a temporary crown. This describes a nearly ideal material—so what's the problem?

With the development and use of resin cements, many dentists believe that using ZOE temporary cement will inhibit the set of resin cement. Remember that eugenol inhibits free radical polymerization. As a result, temporary cements were developed that do not contain eugenol; instead, fatty acids and other chemicals are used to react with zinc oxide. These products have similar properties, but they do not handle as well. Many are not brittle. Rather, they are "gummy," and the excess cement can be difficult to remove.

At times, a temporary crown or bridge refuses to stay in place. It keeps coming off, frustrating both the dentist and the patient. When a stronger temporary cement is needed, a powder/liquid formulation of ZOE cement can be used but should be mixed with a lower-than-recommended powder/liquid ratio to reduce the strength.

D. Surgical/Periodontal Packs

Surgical periodontal packs are paste/paste systems. They mix and handle much like ZOE impression materials, which are discussed in the next chapter. The composition is similar to ZOE temporary cements. These products are placed over surgical sites to protect the underlying tissues. They are temporarily held in place by using the undercuts and embrasures of teeth. Surgical packs are weak materials, so they are easily removed. Because ZOE products have an unpleasant taste and smell, noneugenol products have become popular. These products are formulated in the same manner as noneugenol temporary cements, and their use is presented with those of other periodontal materials in Chapter 13. Mixing periodontal packs is presented in Chapter 33.

E. Endodontic Sealers

Many endodontic sealers are zinc oxide and eugenol preparations with added rosin and barium sulfate. Their use is presented with those of other endodontic materials in Chapter 13.

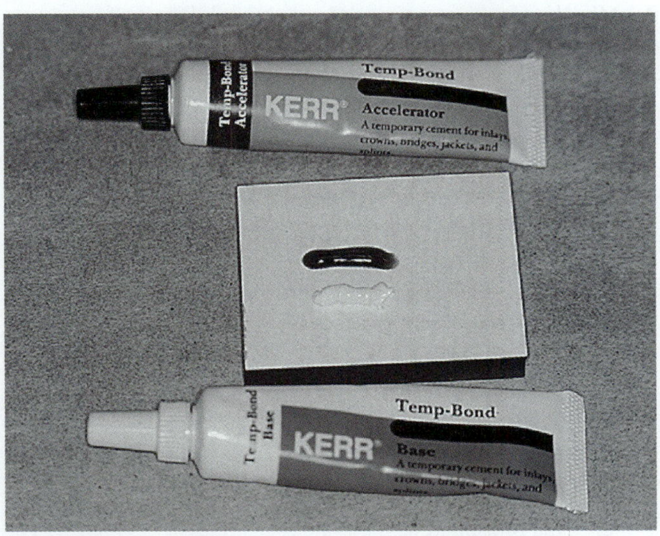

FIGURE 7.11 An example of a paste/paste temporary cement.

SUMMARY

Dental cements are used to lute restorations and appliances into place. They are also used for a variety of other dental procedures. Luting cements have the most demanding requirements of any dental material. They must be insoluble, set in a wet environment, and be biocompatible.

Dental cements are also used as an intermediate base or liner when the thickness of dentin after cavity preparation is thin. The base or liner is placed between the pulp and the restorative material. In the past, liners were thin, soluble, and weak. Today, liners are stronger, and the distinction between liners and bases has become blurred. In the current practice of dentistry, use of liners has dramatically decreased. Bases are stronger and may release fluoride.

Temporary restorations are usually cements that have been mixed thicker than when used for luting. Sometimes, part of that temporary restoration is saved and then serves as a base material under the permanent restoration.

Dental cements are a powder/liquid system, with the liquid being an acid and the powder comprising the base. The powder must be insoluble in the oral cavity yet react with the acid. The powders in dental cements are zinc oxide and powdered glass. The liquids are eugenol, polyacrylic acid, and phosphoric acid. Eugenol is a major component of oil of cloves and has an obtundent effect on the pulp.

Zinc oxide-eugenol (ZOE) cement is usually too weak and soluble to serve as a permanent cement. Because of its sedative effect, however, it is useful for protecting pulp or for soothing an irritated pulp.

Zinc phosphate is a combination of zinc oxide powder and phosphoric acid. It is the oldest cement still in use today. This cement is strong, has low solubility, and involves a very exothermic setting reaction. The heat of the setting reaction accelerates the setting rate. Therefore, it is important to mix this cement over a large area of a chilled glass slab. This allows more powder to be added to the mix for the desired strength. This cement can be used as a base as well as a permanent cement for crowns, bridges, orthodontic bands, and other appliances.

Glass ionomer cement is composed of glass powder and polyacrylic acid. It has been called the material of choice for luting metal and ceramometal crowns. Both chemically activated and light-activated materials exist. Glass ionomer materials are available in powder/liquid and paste/paste forms. Some products are supplied in pre-measured single dose capsules. Glass ionomer products are the strongest and least soluble dental cements, with the exception of composite cements. They also release fluoride, are biocompatible, and are truly adhesive to tooth structure.

Polycarboxylate cement consists of zinc oxide powder and polyacrylic acid. It, too, will bond directly to tooth structure. This cement is very biocompatible but not very strong. Its solubility resistance is rated as only moderate.

Composite cements are also called resin cements. They contain a higher percentage of the resin matrix material to reduce viscosity and are the materials of choice for luting all ceramic restorations.

Temporary cements are usually paste/paste systems and are used to retain a temporary restoration while the permanent restoration is being fabricated. They are unique in that both a minimum and a maximum strength are required. If the cement is too weak, the temporary restoration will be lost prematurely. If the cement is too strong, the dentist may have difficulty removing the temporary restoration and may damage tissue and tooth structure.

Dental cements are a broad category of materials with a broad range of uses. Proper mixing and handling typically have a greater effect on the resulting cements than on other categories of dental materials.

Learning Activities

1. Mix zinc phosphate cement on both chilled and room-temperature glass slabs. Note the amount of powder incorporated into each mix.
2. Mix ZOE cement with and without a drop of water. Use a consistent powder/liquid ratio. Note the setting time for each mix.
3. Mix glass ionomer cement. Apply it to a clean surface on an extracted tooth and to a surface contaminated with saliva. Allow the cement to set, and then scrape on the cement with an instrument. Was there any difference between the two applications in the amount of adhesion?

Review Questions

1. Which of the following cements are available in a single-dose capsule, much like that of silver amalgam filling material?
   a) Polycarboxylate
   b) Silicate
   c) ZOE
   d) Glass ionomer
   e) Zinc phosphate

2. Two dental cements that are used for caries control are:
a) ZOE and zinc phosphate
b) ZOE and polycarboxylate
c) Zinc phosphate and glass ionomer
d) Glass ionomer and polycarboxylate
e) Glass ionomer and ZOE

3. All of the following are true for ZOE EXCEPT:
a) It releases fluoride.
b) It lacks strength.
c) It is an obtundent material.
d) It protects the pulp.

4. Which of the following cements is most soluble?
a) Glass ionomer
b) Zinc phosphate
c) ZOE
d) Polycarboxylate

5. When glass ionomer is mixed too slowly, the resulting mix is:
a) Thin
b) Thick
c) Lumpy
d) Granular

6. Cements are ____________ soluble than the overlying restoration.
a) More
b) Less
c) Equally
d) None of the above

7. During mixing, which of the following cements should use as much of the area on the slab as possible to reduce the exothermic reaction?
a) Polycarboxylate
b) Glass ionomer
c) ZOE
d) Zinc phosphate

8. Which of the following dental materials promotes the formation of secondary dentin?
a) Composite cements
b) Silicate cement
c) Calcium hydroxide
d) Temporary cements

9. Which of the following is a common additive to glass powder, reduces melting temperature, and improves the flow of molten glass?
a) Quartz
b) Fluoride
c) Silicate
d) Oxides

10. The cement of choice for luting ceramic restorations to tooth structure is
a) ZOE
b) Zinc phosphate
c) Polycarboxylate
d) Composite

11. The disadvantage, or drawback, of using polycarboxylate cement is:
a) Lack of strength
b) Ability to bond to tooth structure
c) Biocompatibility
d) Lack of sufficient clinical data for long term use

12. ZOE may be used for the following:
a) Temporary restorations
b) Intermediate bases
c) Permanent restorations
d) Luting temporary crowns
e) Luting permanent crowns
f) a, b, and c
g) a, b, and d
h) a and d only

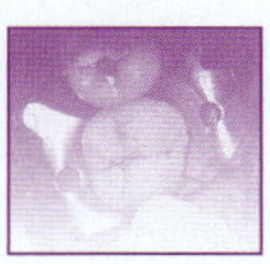

Supplemental Readings

Anusavice KJ. Phillips' Science of Dental Materials. 11th ed. Philadelphia: Saunders, 2003, Chapter 16.
Burke FM, Ray NJ, McConnell RJ. Fluoride-containing restorative materials. Int Dent J. 2006;56:33–43.
Hilton TJ. Cavity sealers, liners and bases: current philosophies and indications for use. Operative Dent 1996;21:134–146.
Leinfelder KF. Changing restorative traditions: the use of bases and liners. J Am Dent Assoc 1994;125:65–67.
Powers JM & Sakaguchi RL, eds. Craig's Restorative Dental Materials. 12th ed. St. Louis: Mosby, 2006, Chapter 20.

8 Impression Materials

Key Words/Phrases

automix
bite registration tray
casts
custom trays
die
gel
hydrocolloid conditioner
hysteresis
imbibition
impression materials
- addition silicones
- alginate
- condensation silicone
- impression compound
- irreversible hydrocolloid
- polyether
- polysulfide
- reversible hydrocolloid
- zinc oxide–eugenol (ZOE)

impression tray
retraction cord
sol
stock trays
study model
surfactants
syneresis
triple tray
viscosity

Objectives

After studying this chapter, the student will be able to do the following:

1. Describe the use of impression materials during indirect restorative procedures.
2. List the oral structures from which impressions are made.
3. Differentiate between a model, a cast, and a die.
4. Describe the various types of impression trays.
5. List the desirable qualities of an impression material.
6. Differentiate between:
    - Elastic and inelastic impression materials
    - Reversible and irreversible impression materials
7. Describe the composition and setting mechanism of:
    - Wax and impression compound
    - Zinc oxide–eugenol (ZOE)
    - Agar or reversible hydrocolloid
    - Alginate
    - Polysulfides
    - Condensation silicones
    - Polyethers
    - Addition silicones
8. Compare the properties, use, and cost of the above impression materials.
9. Describe the effect of water temperature on the setting rate of alginate.
10. Describe the effect of water and heat on the setting rate of polysulfides.

I. Impression Materials

A. General Comments

Impression materials are used to make replicas (models or casts) of teeth and other oral tissues. In dentistry, we take impressions of teeth and their supporting structures. These supporting structures include gingiva, alveolar bone or residual ridge, hard and soft palate, and frenums, which are muscle attachments. The replicas are used to construct restorations and other appliances. The impression is a negative reproduction, whereas the replica (model or cast) is a positive reproduction, as illustrated in Figure 8.1. The impression must be an accurate duplication of the hard and soft tissues of interest and be stable enough to allow disinfection and production of a model.

Not all impression materials are compatible with all model materials. Because impression materials are used for many purposes, a wide variety of products are available to make impressions of oral tissues. Some uses are simply to produce a physical model of the oral tissues for study, called a **study model.** Study models are used in diagnosis and treatment planning. Other uses require very exact (within 0.1%) replication of the size and shape of a preparation for the construction of a restoration or appliance. These replicas are called **casts.** A replica of a single tooth is called a **die.**

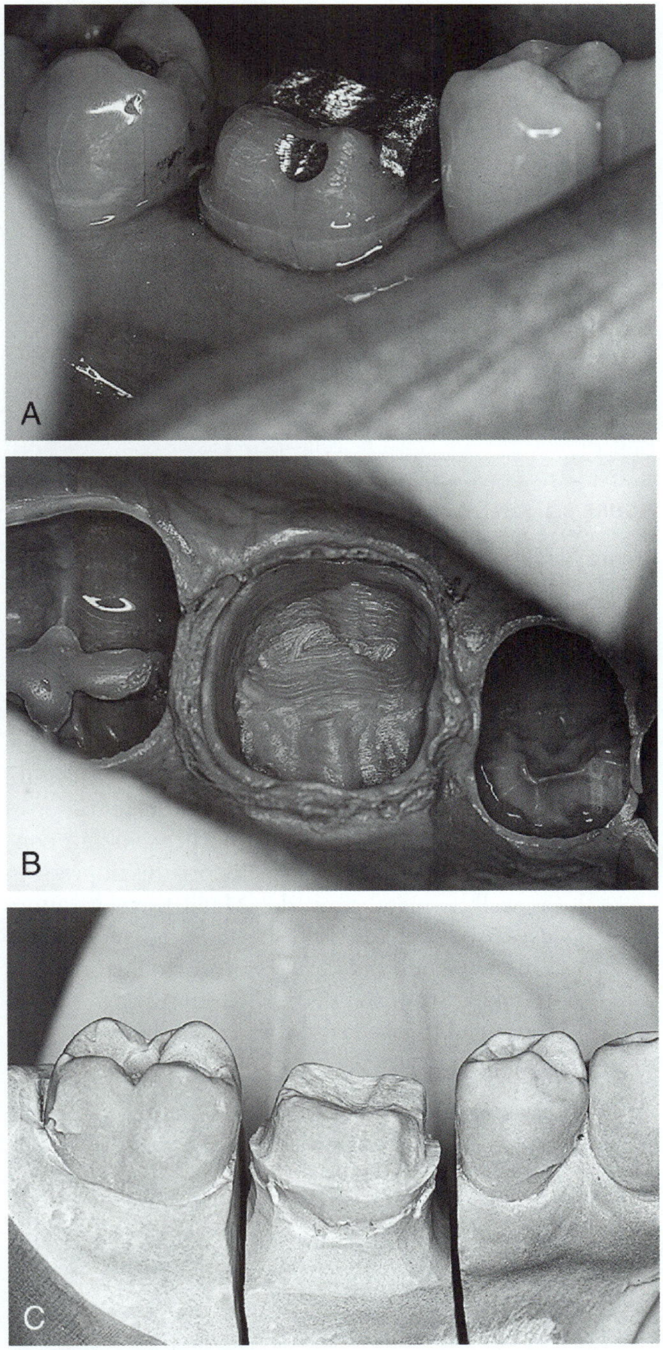

FIGURE 8.1 Photograph of a crown preparation (**A**), an impression (**B**), and a cast (**C**).

B. Impression Material Systems

Impression materials are supplied in a variety of forms. Some are powders that are mixed with water; others are paste/paste systems. Several materials are softened or melted by heating. Regardless of their form, impression materials are mixed (or heated) to make a thick paste or liquid. They are then loaded into an impression tray, placed in the mouth, and seated onto the tissues of interest. The tray functions as a carrier and can stabilize the set impression material. Several impression trays are shown in Figure 8.2. It is interesting to note that dental impression materials are also used to make impressions for medical prostheses, such as artificial eyes.

Paste/paste impression materials (and many other dental materials) come in tubes, much like toothpaste tubes. The orifice of each tube is sized to provide the proper ratio of the two pastes when equal lengths are dispensed. Thus, if the size of the two orifices is the same, one should dispense equal lengths. If the orifice of one tube is larger than that of the other tube, then again, one should dispense equal lengths. Examples are shown in Figure 8.3.

C. Cost

The cost of impression materials varies greatly, from pennies per impression to as much as several dollars. An accurate cost analysis needs to include the percentage of first impressions that are acceptable and the number of restorations that need to be remade. Unacceptable restorations made on casts from cheap impression materials can make dentistry a nonprofit enterprise.

D. Impression Trays

1. Use of Impression Trays

Impression trays are used to carry the impression material into the mouth, and the handle of the tray is used to remove the impression. The

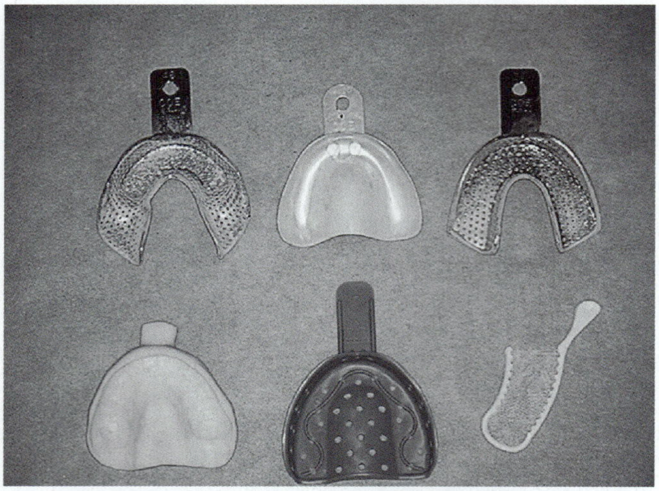

FIGURE 8.2 Several impression trays (from *upper left* moving *clockwise*): a metal perforated tray for partially edentulous impressions, a solid metal tray for edentulous impressions, a metal tray for dentulous impressions, a bite registration tray, a plastic tray for dentulous impressions, and a custom tray.

tray can also support a weak material impression and improve accuracy. Trays are supplied in a variety of shapes and sizes, and they are made from several materials. Plastic disposable trays are very popular and work well with current asepsis practices. Plastic trays are inexpensive and convenient, but they do not support the impression as well as metal trays do. Metal trays are more expensive but reusable. In addition, metal trays are stiffer and, thus, are less likely to distort when removed from the mouth. Cleaning and sterilizing metal trays adds to the cost of their use.

2. Stock Trays

Stock trays are "off-the-shelf" items that come in a variety of materials, shapes, and sizes. The different-shaped trays are designed to take impressions of different oral conditions: edentulous mouths, partially edentulous mouths, and mouths with a full complement of teeth. Such trays are illustrated in Figure 8.2. Stock trays also come in a range of sizes, from very small trays for pediatric patients to very large trays for large adult mouths.

3. Custom Trays

The most accurate impressions are made with custom trays. **Custom trays** are made on a model of the patient's arch with acrylic or other resin. Therefore, two impressions are taken when a custom tray is used. A preliminary impression is taken with a stock tray and an inexpensive material. A gypsum product is poured into the impression, and the resulting model is used to construct the custom tray. The custom tray is then used to take a final impression.

Custom trays are used to take final impressions for full dentures, inlays, crowns, bridges, and some removable partial dentures. Custom trays use less impression material than stock trays because they fit around the teeth better than a stock tray. Some say that custom trays are cost-effective because they use less material. Others say that custom trays are cost-effective because they make the impressions easier to take and accurate impressions result more frequently than with stock trays. Two techniques for the fabrication of custom trays for crown and bridge impressions are presented in detail in Chapter 29. It is important to note that proper mixing and handling of the impression material are the factors most critical for success.

4. Special Use Trays

A variety of special use trays have been developed. **Bite registration trays,** as shown in Figure 8.2, record the occlusal surfaces of both arches. Bite registrations are used to relate the upper and lower casts in the dental laboratory in precisely the same manner as they come together in the patient's mouth. Use of a bite registration without a tray is shown in Figure 8.4.

Another popular impression tray is the **triple tray,** which is used with the dual-arch or closed-mouth impression technique. The triple tray is a quadrant tray with a "J" shape that curls around the posterior of the most distal molars (Fig. 8.5, *A* and *B*). With the dual-arch technique, the loaded tray (on both sides) is seated on the arch with the prepared tooth. The patient then closes to their normal bite, and the technique records an impression of the prepared tooth, an impression of the opposing teeth, and a bite registration, all at the same time (Fig. 8.5*C* and *8.5D*).

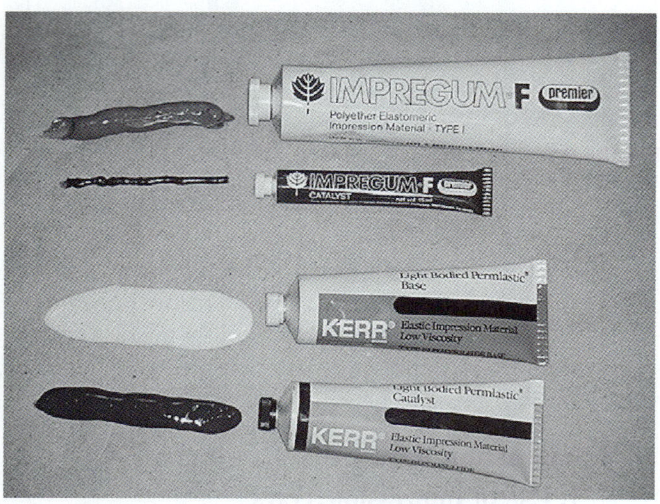

FIGURE 8.3 Polysulfide (*lower*) and polyether (*upper*) impression materials. Note that the lengths dispensed, but not the volumes, are equal.

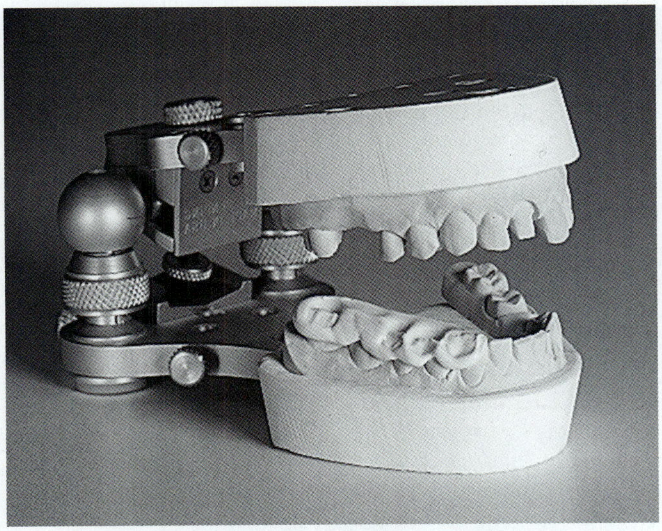

FIGURE 8.4 A bite registration and models mounted on a simple articulator. (Courtesy of GC America, Inc., Alsip, IL.)

E. Classification of Impression Materials

1. Chemical Reaction or Physical Change

Impression materials set either by a chemical reaction or by a physical change. Some set by chemical reactions to form elastic rubber materials; these impression materials are called thermoset. The chemical reaction involves chain lengthening, cross-linking, or both. Other impression materials set by a physical change when they cool, either by solidification or by gelation. Solidification occurs when molten wax cools and goes from a liquid to a solid. Gelation is the process by which gelatin, such as Jell-O, changes from a liquid to a semisolid state when it cools. Impression materials that undergo a physical change when cooled are called thermoplastic. In general, thermoplastic materials are not as stable as thermoset materials.

2. Use

a) Elastic/Inelastic

Because impression materials are used for a variety of purposes, the requirements of a particular procedure determine which impression materials can be used. Impressions of dentulous mouths use trays and materials different from those for edentulous patients. Teeth typically have nooks and crannies that require an elastic material to be used. Edentulous impressions may use elastic or inelastic impression material. Inelastic impression materials set hard and rigid compared to elastic impression materials and would "lock" around teeth if used in a dentulous patient.

b) Accuracy

The accuracy required by the restoration or prosthesis determines which impression materials can be used. Not all impression materials have sufficient accuracy for crown and bridge impressions. Study models are not considered to be highly accurate reproductions of oral tissues. Therefore, alginate is an acceptable impression material for study models, but it is an unacceptable impression material for the fabrication of bridges, crowns, and inlays. Nearly all impression materials are acceptable for full denture impressions.

c) Flow and Detail Reproduction

Many kinds of impression materials come in a variety of viscosities. **Viscosity** is a measure of a liquid's ability to flow. There are (from thinnest to thickest consistency) light body, medium body, monophase, heavy body, and putty materials. Light body materials are typically used with an impression syringe and are injected around preparations. They are the most "runny" of the impression materials, and they best record the details of tooth preparations (small grooves, edges, and margins).

Many times, a **retraction cord** is placed in the gingival sulcus to facilitate crown and bridge impressions. In most instances, the patient will have had local anesthesia to ensure their comfort. The retraction cord pushes the gingiva away from the tooth, as shown in Figure 8.6. Frequently, the cord will contain a hemostatic or astringent medicament to control bleeding. After the cord has been in place for several minutes, it is usually removed, just before the impression is taken. There are exceptions, however, as the cord may be kept in place during the impression. Use of a retraction cord allows the low-viscosity material to flow to and, thus, to reproduce areas of a preparation that are difficult to reach. The cord moves the gingival tissue slightly away from the tooth and also controls the moisture in the area.

Putty materials are the thickest impression materials, but they can still record the details of a fingerprint. Heavy body and putty materials are placed in the impression tray, and their high viscosity reduces running and dripping of the impression material out of the tray and onto the operator or patient. They are typically used with a light body material. The light body material records the preparation and its margins while the thicker material becomes the bulk of the impression. The impression tray, which is filled with high-viscosity material, is

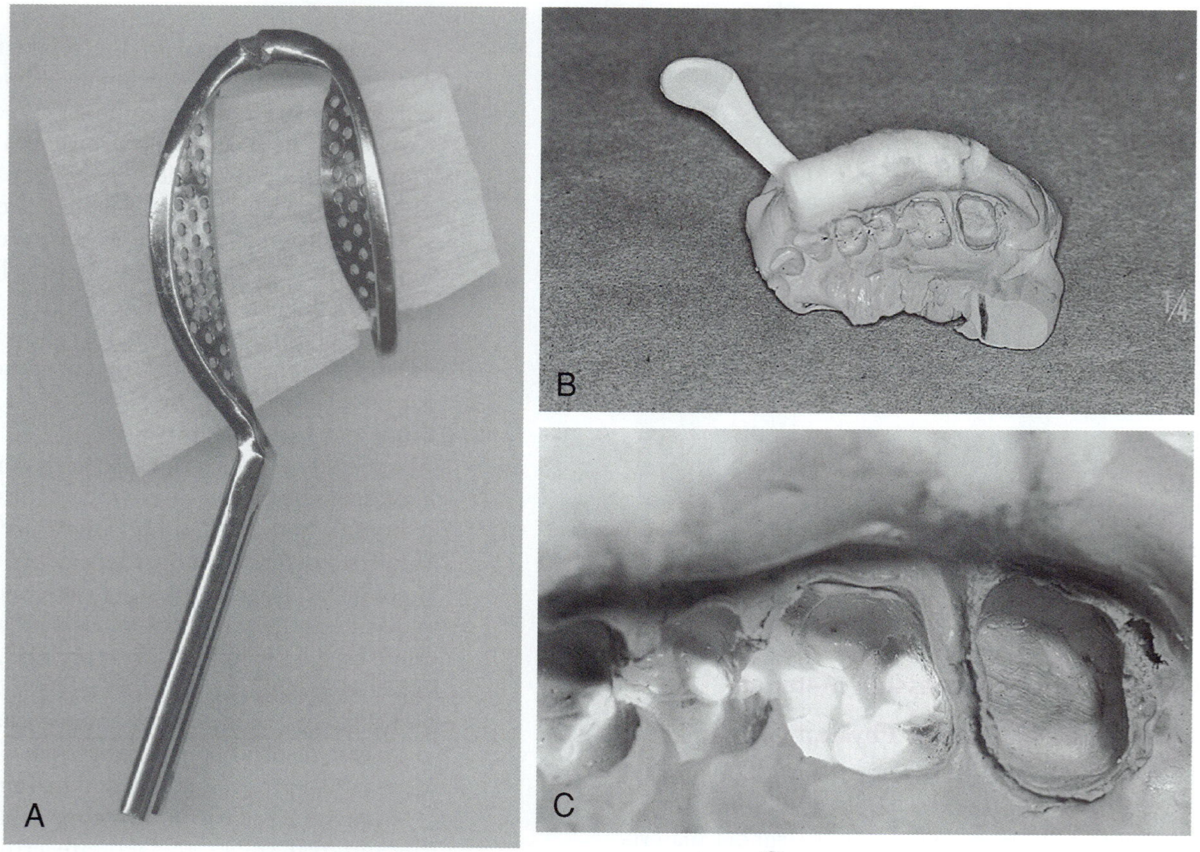

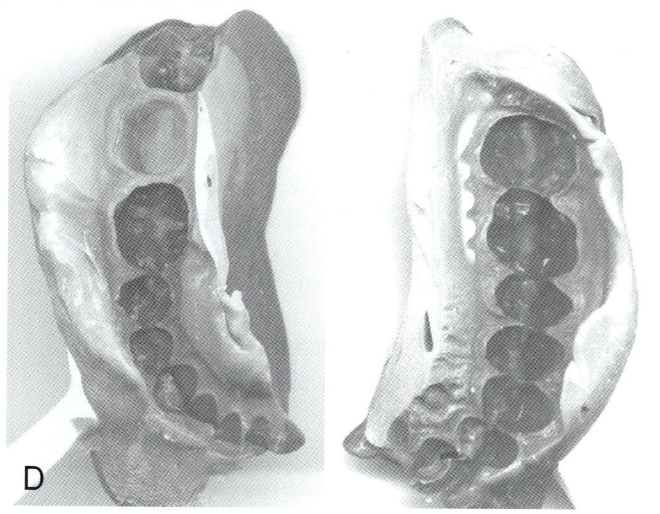

FIGURE 8.5 **A.** A metal triple tray. **B.** Impression taken with a plastic disposable triple tray. **C.** A close-up of the impression. The material is very thin, and light shines through where the teeth occlude (*left* and *middle*). Also, the impression is thicker in the area of the preparation (*right*). **D.** A close-up of both sides of another impression using a triple tray. Note the impression of the prepared second molar (*top*) and the opposing teeth (*bottom*).

immediately seated over the light body material. The materials then set together into one mass and are removed as one impression.

Medium body impression materials may be injected or used in the tray depending on the dentist's preferences. Monophase materials are designed to be used for both injection and in the tray. Therefore, only one mix of monophase material is needed.

3. Types of Impression Materials

Each impression material has its own advantages and disadvantages for use in dentistry. The following sections will focus on each type of impression material and its use (Table 8.1).

a) Inelastic Impression Materials
  1) Plaster
  2) Wax and impression compound
  3) Zinc oxide–eugenol (ZOE)

b) Aqueous Elastomeric Impression Materials
  1) Alginate (irreversible hydrocolloid)
  2) Agar (reversible hydrocolloid)

c) Nonaqueous Elastomeric Impression Materials
  1) Polysulfides

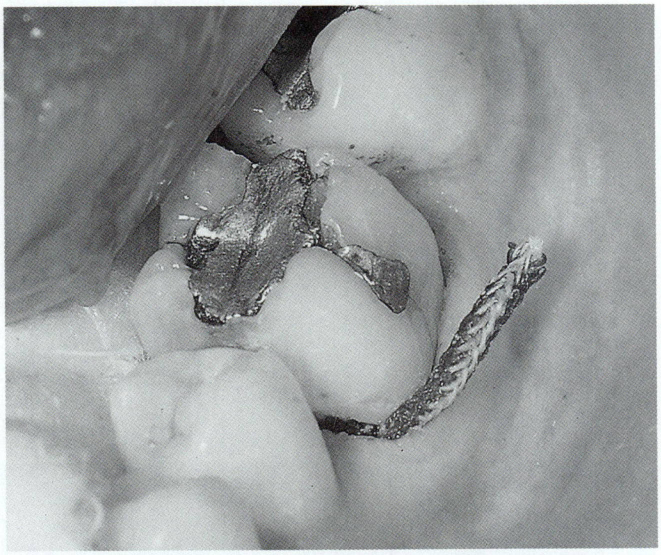

FIGURE 8.6 Retraction cord being placed in the sulcus during crown preparation. (Courtesy of Ultradent, Inc.)

2) Condensation silicones
3) Polyethers
4) Addition silicones

II. Plaster

Plaster would seem to be an unlikely impression material. However, impression plaster is still sold. It has the same setting reaction and properties as the gypsum products that are used for models and casts. Gypsum products will be discussed in Chapter 9. The major difference is that impression plaster has flavors added, and these plasters set more quickly to minimize the time the material is in the mouth. When impression plaster sets, it is hard and brittle. Its major use is for an impression of an edentulous ridge in the fabrication of a denture. Impression plaster is inexpensive compared to other materials, but its unpleasant taste makes it a seldom-used option.

III. Wax and Impression Compound

A. Wax

Wax was probably the first impression material used in dentistry. It is cheap, clean, and easy to use. A multitude of waxes are used in dentistry. Some are hard, much like paraffin wax that is used in canning jellies and jams. Others are soft and moldable at room temperature, similar to Play-Doh. Wax used for taking impressions is solid at mouth temperature but is moldable at a temperature that is tolerated by oral tissues. Wax comes in many forms (sticks, strips, tubes, etc.). Wax can be thought of as a low-molecular-weight polymer. It is a thermoplastic material. It is also very weak, and the technique of the procedure must compensate for its poor mechanical properties. Wax is used by some dentists to take impressions for full dentures.

More commonly, a variety of waxes are used as adjunctive materials in the dental laboratory for the

Table 8.1 Classification and Use of Impression Materials

Type of Impression Material	Elastic vs. Inelastic	Setting Process	Used for the Construction of: Full Denture	Partial Denture[a]	Inlay, Crown, or Bridge	Study Models
Plaster	Inelastic	Chemical	Preliminary	No	No	No
Wax or impression compound	Inelastic	Physical	Preliminary	No	No	No
ZOE	Inelastic	Chemical	Final[b]	No	No	No
Reversible hydrocolloid (agar)	Elastic	Physical	Not used[c]	Yes	Yes	No
Irreversible hydrocolloid (alginate)	Elastic	Chemical	Preliminary	Yes	No	Yes
Polysulfide	Elastic	Chemical	Final[b]	Yes	Yes[b]	No[d]
Condensation silicone	Elastic	Chemical	Final[b]	Yes	Yes	No[d]
Addition silicone	Elastic	Chemical	Final[b]	Yes	Yes	No[d]
Polyether	Elastic	Chemical	Final[b]	Yes	Yes	No[d]

[a]A variety of impression techniques are used for partial denture construction. This table does not address all possible techniques.

[b]Use of a custom tray is recommended.

[c]Edentulous trays for hydrocolloid use are not common.

[d]These materials could be used, but their use is not economical.

fabrication of crowns, bridges, and other restorations. Wax is softened or melted and then formed into the desired shape. The wax piece is surrounded by a mold material. The wax is melted away, and the mold is filled with a restorative material, such as gold. These processes will be described in more detail in later chapters.

B. Impression Compound

Impression compound is wax with added filler to improve handling and stability. It is stronger and more brittle and, when softened, flows much less compared to wax. Impression compound is supplied as sticks or cakes of material, as shown in Figure 8.7*A*. It is softened in a warm water bath, as shown in Figure 8.7*B*. Because the thermal conductivity of impression compound is low, time and patience are required to soften the material properly. The heated, softened, and moldable material is placed in an impression tray, resoftened, and then seated in the mouth. When the material has cooled to mouth temperature, it returns to a rigid state and is removed. Impression compound is a stiff, thermoplastic material and is used by many dentists to make preliminary impressions for complete dentures, as shown in Figure 8.7*C*. Other impression materials that record fine details are better suited for final impressions.

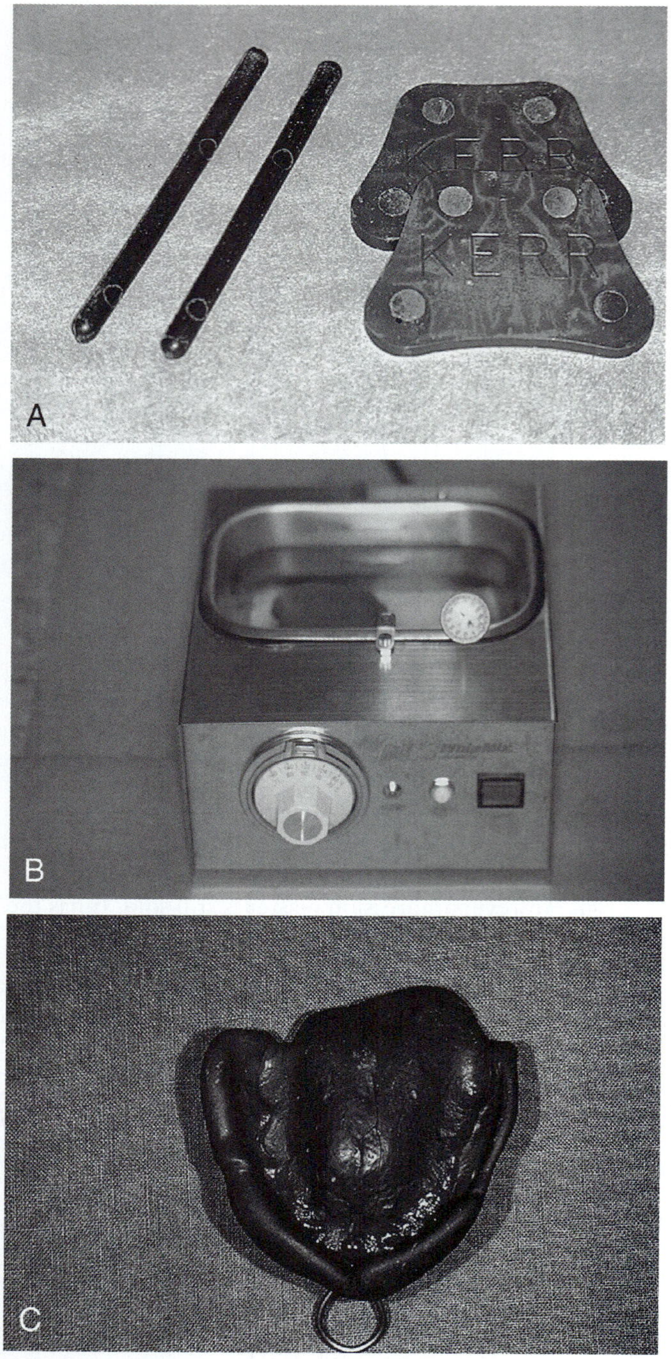

FIGURE 8.7 A. Impression compound sticks and cakes. **B.** Tray with impression compound in a water bath. **C.** Preliminary impression for a complete denture. (Courtesy of Dr. James Overberger, Morgantown, WV.)

IV. Zinc Oxide–Eugenol (ZOE)

Zinc oxide–eugenol (ZOE) has been formulated for a wide variety of uses in dentistry, including as an impression material. The chemistry of ZOE materials is covered in Chapter 7.

A. Form of the Material

The ZOE materials come as two pastes. One paste contains eugenol and inert fillers; the other is formed by using zinc oxide powder mixed with vegetable oil. Eugenol is a major component in oil of cloves. Therefore, ZOE materials smell and taste of cloves. For some patients, this is unpleasant. The two pastes come in tubes much like toothpaste, as shown in Figure 8.8. Equal lengths of material from each tube are dispensed. Typically, the two pastes of ZOE (and other materials that come in tubes) are different colors. The pastes are swirled, stropped, and scraped together during mixing until one homogeneous color is obtained.

B. Use

The ZOE impression materials set to a hard and brittle mass, which limits their use to impressions of edentulous ridges for removable dentures. They are inexpensive and easy to use and were once very popular. They are commonly used in a custom tray for the final impression for a complete denture. Today, however, ZOE materials have been replaced by newer materials, such as addition silicones. The newer materials have little advantage in terms of performance and are much more expensive. The simple advantage of stocking one less impression material in the dental office is likely the reason for declining use of ZOE impression materials.

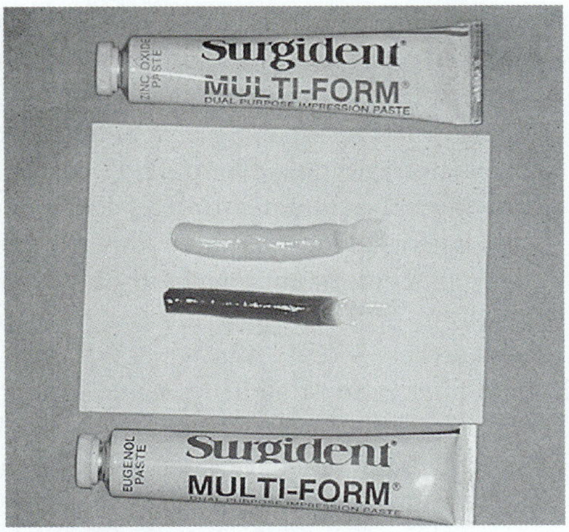

FIGURE 8.8 ZOE impression paste.

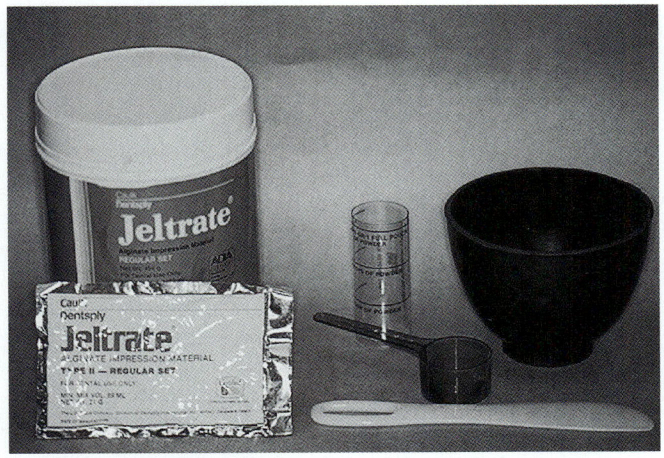

FIGURE 8.9 Alginate impression materials in a bulk container, premeasured envelope, scoop for bulk powder, water measure, mixing bowl, and spatula.

V. General Aspects of Hydrocolloid Impression Materials

Two impression materials are considered to be hydrocolloid materials because the major component is water. Both materials change from a viscous liquid, called the sol, to a semisolid, rubbery material, called the gel. The **sol** state is a solution of one material dissolved in another. In the **gel** state, two phases exist, much like a foam of soap bubbles. The first phase is a solid carbohydrate polymer network, like the soap of the foam. The second phase is water trapped in very small pockets, like the air in the foam. Colloids were discussed in Chapter 2.

The hydrocolloid that sets via a chemical reaction is called **irreversible hydrocolloid.** It is commonly called **alginate.** If we were to heat alginate that was set, we would get warm alginate; it would not reverse back to the sol (fluid) state. The other hydrocolloid that gels by a physical change (cooling) is called **reversible hydrocolloid.** This impression material would actually reverse back to a sol state when heated, then change again to a gel when cooled, hence the name reversible hydrocolloid. Reversible hydrocolloid is also called agar or agar-agar (or sometimes simply hydrocolloid).

VI. Alginate (Irreversible Hydrocolloid) Impression Materials

A. Properties

Alginate materials are termed irreversible impression materials because they will not reverse to a sol once they react and become a gel. They have advantages and disadvantages similar to those of reversible hydrocolloid materials because both types of materials are predominantly water. Alginate materials are not as accurate as reversible hydrocolloid materials, but they are much easier to use. Alginate materials are supplied as powders that are mixed with water, as shown in Figure 8.9.

B. Composition

1. The powder contains potassium alginate. It is a carbohydrate polymer that dissolves in water, forming the sol. Carboxylate groups (-COOH) react with calcium ions and cross-link the material to form a gel. The reaction is similar to that of polycarboxylate and glass ionomer cements. Potassium alginate is derived from algae.
2. Another main component of the powder is an inert filler, such as diatomaceous earth (silica). The filler gives the mixed material "body" that allows acceptable handling. Without filler, the mixed material would be too runny for use.
3. Several other chemicals are present in the powder: the reactor for the cross-linking reaction (calcium sulfate), the retarder for working time (sodium phosphate), colorants, and flavors.
4. Some alginate products have antimicrobial agents added to the powder. The purpose is to reduce the microbial content of the powder as provided by the manufacturer more than to disinfect the impression after it has been taken.
5. Both reversible and irreversible hydrocolloid materials are predominantly water. Thus, several advantages and disadvantages result when their use is compared to that of other impression materials.
   a) **Advantages**
   Reversible and irreversible hydrocolloid will wet a tooth surface that is contaminated by oral fluids. Fewer air bubbles are trapped between the tooth and the impression material. Hydrocolloid materials will even absorb a limited amount of oral fluids. These two effects occur because water-based liquids mix

together easily, like a mix of soda pop and fruit juice used to make punch.

The second advantage of being composed predominantly of water is that pouring the impression with gypsum products is easier than with elastomeric impression materials. Again, the gypsum product, when mixed with water, easily wets the surface of the impression material, which is predominantly water. Hydrocolloid impression materials are quite hydrophilic, but the same cannot be said for all impression materials.

b) Disadvantages

The disadvantage of the material being predominantly water is that water evaporates from the surface of the impression if it is left exposed to air. When the water evaporates, the impression shrinks and is no longer accurate. To prevent evaporation of water from hydrocolloid (alginate and reversible hydrocolloid), impressions should be poured as soon as possible after disinfecting.

Hydrocolloid materials contract slightly after setting and exude water. This process is called **syneresis.** Syneresis occurs very slowly, but it is a second reason to pour hydrocolloid impressions as soon as possible.

When disinfecting a hydrocolloid impression, however, it is important to limit the time that the impression is exposed to an aqueous disinfecting solution. The hydrocolloid will absorb water, swell, and distort. This is called **imbibition.**

C. Setting Reaction—Optional

Alginate materials set by a chemical reaction that cross-links a carbohydrate polymer.

1. Working time is provided by a competing reaction that initially delays cross-linking. When the powder is mixed with water, the alginate powder dissolves, as does the calcium sulfate and sodium phosphate.
2. Initially, the calcium ions react with the phosphate ions and precipitate out of solution. The calcium ions do not react with the dissolved alginate until all the phosphate ions have reacted.
3. After the retarder (the phosphate ions) has reacted, the setting reaction becomes the dominant reaction. The calcium ions react with the alginate, cross-linking the polymer chains, and gelation occurs. The set material is a hydrogel that is composed mainly of water.

D. Use and Handling

1. Alginate is supplied in preweighed envelopes or bulk containers. With bulk containers, dispensing is achieved with a scoop that is supplied by the manufacturer. The alginate powder tends to settle in bulk containers during shipment and storage. Before opening a new bulk container, the material should be "fluffed" by shaking or turning the container upside down and right side up for about a minute. This will remix the heavier components with the lighter ones, resulting in the proper amount of material in each scoop.
2. The filler in most alginate materials is a silicate material. Silicate dust causes lung problems in miners. Additives have been included in some alginate products to reduce the dust that occurs when alginate is used; these products are called dustless alginates. Regardless, it is not healthy to breathe any dust. A mask, as commonly worn when treating patients, will reduce exposure to alginate dust.
3. Water is dispensed with a calibrated water measure that is also supplied by the manufacturer. If one is unhappy with the consistency of the mixed material, the solution to this problem is to change brands. Do not alter the water/powder ratio to make the mix thicker or thinner.
4. The temperature of the water controls the rate of the setting reaction. Warmer water increases the setting rate, and cooler water slows the setting reaction. Alginate is supplied by most manufacturers in regular-set and fast-set varieties. Regular-set materials gel in 3 to 4 minutes, whereas fast-set materials gel in 1 to 2 minutes.
5. Mixing the alginate material is an aggressive aerobic activity. First, the powder and water are gently stirred together. Once all the powder has been wetted by the water, the effort should be greatly increased. The paste is pushed against the side of the rubber mixing bowl to force the water and powder together. For better spatulation, the mixing spatula should have a curved side that follows the curve of the mixing bowl. Aggressive spatulation continues until a smooth creamy mix is obtained. The typical mixing time is 1 minute. The mixed alginate material is scooped from the mixing bowl with the spatula, placed in the tray, and seated in the patient's mouth. Taking alginate impressions is presented in Chapter 27.
6. Regardless of the setting time of the alginate material, removal of the impression is delayed for 2 to 3 minutes after gelation. Strength and elasticity improve during this additional setting time. The impression is removed with a quick motion. Alginate tends to be stronger when it is stressed quickly. Slowly removing impressions

can increase distortion and tearing whether the material is a hydrocolloid or an elastomer.

7. As with irreversible hydrocolloid materials, alginate impressions must be disinfected and poured with care. Gain or loss of water (evaporation, syneresis, or imbibition) will affect the accuracy of the resulting cast. If an alginate impression cannot be poured immediately, it should be sprayed with disinfectant, sealed in a plastic bag, and poured as soon as possible. No satisfactory method exists to store hydrocolloid materials for more than 30 minutes.
8. Alginate impression material is used for a variety of purposes. It is inexpensive and easy to use but lacks the accuracy for precisely fitting restorations. Proper mixing and handling will result in acceptable study models and casts on which to fabricate mouthguards and bleaching and fluoride trays.

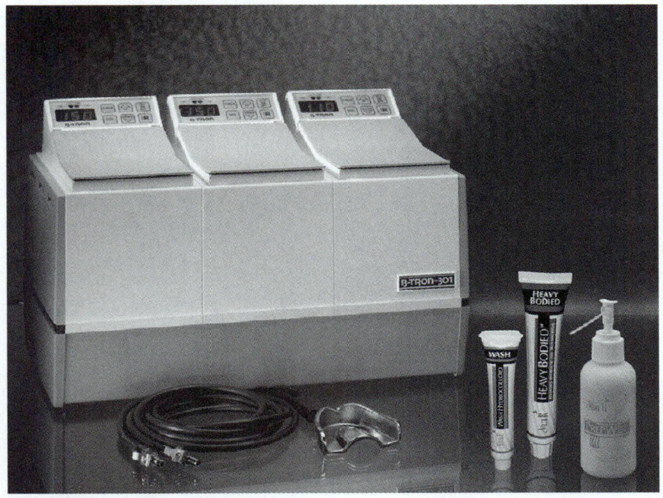

FIGURE 8.10 Hydrocolloid impression material (in tubes) and equipment for its use. The water bath (*top*) has three compartments with three different temperatures. (Courtesy of Van R Dental.)

VII. Agar (Reversible Hydrocolloid)

A. Form of the Material

Reversible hydrocolloid is premixed by the manufacturer and supplied as a semisolid material in tubes and sticks. The sticks look and feel like a long, thin pencil eraser, except they feel wet because of their high water content. Reversible hydrocolloid is made of predominantly water with added agar. Agar is a carbohydrate polymer. It is also the same material used in microbiology as a growth medium. Other components of reversible hydrocolloid include colorants, flavors, mold inhibitors, and a sulfate compound. The sulfate compound improves the hardness of the gypsum model that is poured into the impression.

B. Use

1. Equipment

Reversible hydrocolloid requires special equipment to heat, store, and temper the materials, as shown in Figure 8.10. In addition, special impression trays that circulate cooling water are needed. The special equipment that is required to use reversible hydrocolloid limits the popularity of this excellent material. Reversible hydrocolloid itself is very inexpensive and results in a very accurate impression.

2. Preparation of Material

Reversible hydrocolloid must be prepared for use before taking the impression. This can be done at the beginning of the day or the week. Special equipment is required. This equipment is called a hydrocolloid conditioner (Fig. 8.10) and has three compartments.

a) In the first compartment, the reversible hydrocolloid is boiled to change the rubbery material (the gel) into a viscous liquid (the sol).

b) In the second compartment, the material is stored in a 150°F (65°C) water bath until needed. Material can be stored for as long as several days.

c) Several minutes before it is to be used for an impression, the reversible hydrocolloid is placed in a 110°F (45°C) water bath. This step is called tempering. Tempering lowers the temperature to a point at which the oral tissues are able to tolerate the impression material. At mouth temperature, the material gels and returns to its elastic state. Circulating cold water through tubing and a special tray facilitates cooling. A hydrocolloid impression is shown in Figure 8.11.

3. Hysteresis

Hysteresis is unlike the common phase changes of water, which melts and freezes (or boils and condenses) at the same temperature. It is important to note that reversible hydrocolloid does not melt at the same temperature at which it gels. It melts at a much higher temperature than boiling water. On the other hand, it gels at a much cooler temperature, mouth temperature. The characteristic of melting and gelling at different temperatures is called **hysteresis**.

4. Advantages and Disadvantages of Reversible Hydrocolloid

Reversible hydrocolloid works well in a wet environment. Therefore, reversible hydrocolloids

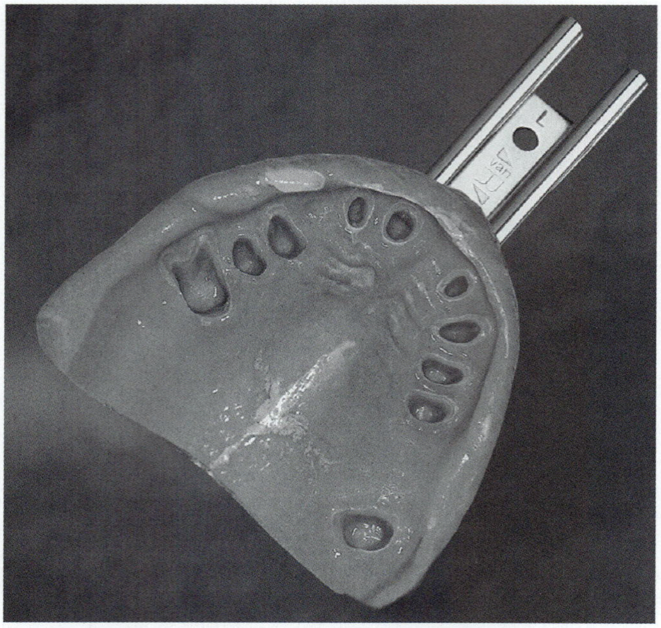

FIGURE 8.11 A hydrocolloid impression. (Courtesy of Van R Dental.)

are very useful for taking impressions when the margins of a crown preparation are subgingival or not easily kept dry. In fact, some dentists wet the teeth with water just before taking the impression. On the other hand, these materials require special equipment for heating, cooling, and use. Another shortcoming of these materials is their poor tear strength compared to nonaqueous elastomeric impression materials.

5. Popularity of Reversible Hydrocolloid

With the various advantages and disadvantages of reversible hydrocolloid material, one would expect dentistry to have a love/hate relationship with this material. Few dentists use reversible hydrocolloid, but those who do love it. They work around the weaknesses of the material and are able to produce excellent results.

VIII. General Aspects of Nonaqueous Elastomeric (Rubber) Impression Materials

A variety of rubber-like impression materials have been developed for dentistry. A variety of names are used to describe this group of materials: nonaqueous elastomeric impression materials, rubber base materials, elastomers, and others. These materials set via polymerization reactions and are more stable than hydrocolloid materials, but they are also more expensive. They are named based on their polymerization chemistry: polysulfide, condensation silicone, polyether, and addition silicone.

IX. Polysulfides

Polysulfide impression material was the first nonaqueous elastomeric "rubber" impression material developed for dentistry. Often, polysulfide materials are called "rubber" or "rubber base" materials, even though polyether and silicone materials are also rubber materials. Polysulfide, polyether, and silicone materials are also called nonaqueous elastomeric impression materials. They all undergo cross-linking and chain-lengthening polymerization reactions. They have similar, but not identical, mixing and handling properties. One very important difference between types of elastomeric impression materials is the adhesive that is used to bond the impression material to a nonperforated tray. Each impression material has its own adhesive, which will not work with other types of material.

A. Condensation Polymerization

Polysulfide materials set via a condensation polymerization reaction. This is the same chemical reaction that joins together the building blocks of biologic polymers. Biologic polymers (proteins) are important components of the tissues of the body. In a typical condensation reaction, a hydrogen atom and a hydroxyl group (OH) are taken from the monomers and are combined to form water (H_2O). The functional groups of the monomers can be carboxylic acid and amine groups that produce proteins (or nylon). The functional groups of polysulfide impression material are mercaptan groups (sulfur and hydrogen atoms) and oxygen from lead oxide, as shown in Figure 8.12. Reaction by-products other than water are produced by other condensation polymerization reactions, but water is the most common by-product. The name "condensation" polymerization is based on the production of water.

B. Composition of Polysulfide Impression Materials

Polysulfide impression materials are supplied as two pastes in tubes. Typically, one paste is dark brown,

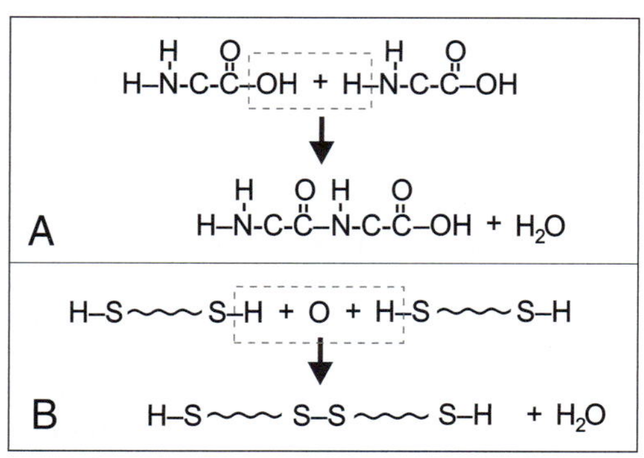

FIGURE 8.12 Condensation polymerization reactions that produce proteins (**A**) and polysulfide impression material (**B**).

and the other paste is white. The white "base" paste contains a low-molecular-weight polysulfide polymer mixed with an inorganic filler, such as titanium oxide. The brown "accelerator" paste contains lead oxide and an "oily" organic chemical that does not react. A few percent sulfur is also included in the brown paste because it promotes the polymerization reaction.

C. Mixing Polysulfide Impression Materials

The two pastes are dispensed in equal lengths on a paper mixing pad. An impression material spatula is used to mix the two pastes. The impression material spatula has a long (~4 inches), straight-sided blade. The pastes are swirled and stropped together until a homogeneous paste is obtained. Mixing may take from 30 to 90 seconds depending on the amount and viscosity of material. The side of the spatula blade is used to scrape unmixed material off the paper pad and then to mix it into the rest of the material. The mixed material is loaded into the tray and placed in the mouth as a viscous paste. The same procedure is used to mix other nonaqueous elastomeric impression materials, such as polyether and silicones. The mixing process for polysulfide impression material is shown in Figure 8.13.

D. Polymerization Reaction of Polysulfide Impression Materials—Optional

The polymerization reaction starts when mixing begins and proceeds slowly. The low-molecular-weight polysulfide polymer has mercaptan groups (-SH) on the end of the short polymer chains and as pendant groups hanging off the middle of the chains. Two hydrogen atoms from two different short polymer chains react with oxygen (from the lead oxide) to form water. The sulfur acts as a catalyst and helps to link the two sulfur atoms together, joining the two polymer chains together. The same reaction lengthens the polymer chains and cross-links the chains.

E. Properties of Polysulfide Impression Materials

Polysulfide impression materials are much more accurate than alginate. With proper handling, polysulfide impression materials can be used for inlays, crowns, and bridges. However, they are not as accurate as other nonaqueous elastomeric materials. A polysulfide impression should be poured within several hours after mixing. Custom trays are recommended for optimum results. Polysulfide impression materials have a disagreeable smell and taste. They stain clothing and are generally

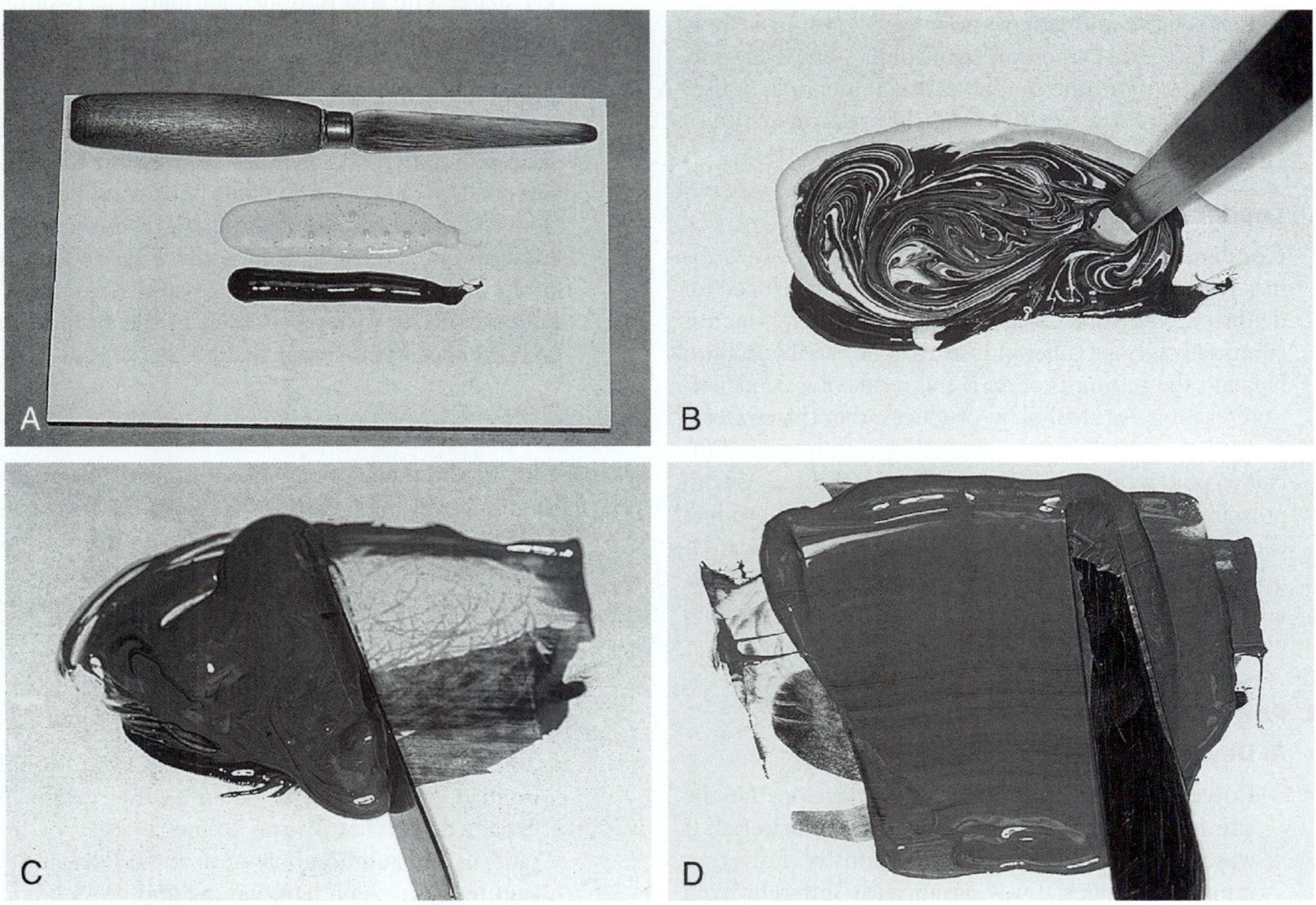

FIGURE 8.13 Mixing process for paste/paste impression materials.

regarded as unpleasant materials. Polysulfide impression materials do have one advantage: They have the longest working time of any elastomeric material (4–6 minutes). As a result, they are useful for impressions of multiple preparations. Along with the long working time comes the longest setting times. Impressions need to be held in place in the mouth for as long as 15 minutes.

The water by-product of the setting reaction can be lost through evaporation; distortion is the result. The working and setting times of polysulfide impression materials are significantly accelerated by heat and humidity. The setting time on hot, humid summer days will differ from that on cool, dry days. One technique using polysulfide impression material for a full denture impression actually mixes a drop of water with the material to accelerate the set.

F. Use of Polysulfide Impression Materials

Polysulfide impression material is often used with custom trays to increase the accuracy of the impression. For impressions of crowns and bridges, light body material is injected around the preparation, and heavy body material is used in the tray. Light body and medium body materials are used for complete denture impressions.

Polysulfide impression materials are relatively inexpensive and easy to pour with gypsum materials. They are somewhat hydrophilic; however, only a single pour (one model) is recommended. Subsequent pours using the same impression may not have the required accuracy.

X. Condensation Silicones

Condensation silicone impression materials were the next elastomeric impression material to be developed for dentistry. They are based on silicone rubber, which is commonly used in other industries. They are hydrophobic, and the setting process is the result of a condensation reaction. An alcohol by-product rather than water is formed. They are cleaner materials to use, but it is difficult to pour a model without voids and bubbles. As with polysulfide materials, loss of the reaction by-product through evaporation can result in distortion. Condensation silicone impressions must be poured without delay. These materials are not popular at present because newer materials provide better results.

XI. Polyethers

A. Development

Polyether impression material was developed in the late 1960s for use as a dental impression material. It was not borrowed from another industry. Polyether impression material was significantly different from the other materials available at that time.

B. Chemistry—Optional

These materials have an ether group in the molecular structure. An ether group is an oxygen atom that is bonded to two carbon atoms. Polyether impression materials set via a unique, ring-opening polymerization reaction that is thought to offset some polymerization shrinkage. The polymerization reaction is called cationic polymerization. Cationic polymerization is very similar to addition polymerization, except that instead of a free radical, a cation (positive ion) is the reactive molecule. No reaction by-product is produced.

C. Properties and Use

The working and setting times are shorter than those for polysulfide materials; they are more like those of addition silicone materials. Polyether impression materials are very stiff compared to other materials, and they set quickly. Polyether impression materials come in a single viscosity, much like the medium viscosity of other types of materials. They are clean materials to use but have an unpleasant taste. Polyether impression materials are very accurate and easy to pour with gypsum products. These properties and ease of use make polyethers very popular materials with a large market share. The cost of polyether materials is similar to that of addition silicone materials. They are very stiff, which makes them well suited for use with a disposable triple tray, as shown in Figure 8.5.

Impregum is the most popular polyether product. The popularity of polyether impression materials has resulted in addition silicone "Impregum clones." The additional silicone clones have the same viscosity, stiffness, and even purple color. These clones are often called monophase impression materials. A single-viscosity material is used in the syringe and the tray (just as polyether materials are used).

XII. Addition Silicones

Addition silicones are the most popular type of elastomeric impression material, especially for crown and bridge impressions. They are clean and do not have an unpleasant taste or smell. They are the most accurate, stable, and expensive impression materials. Addition silicone impression materials are also called vinyl polysiloxanes and polyvinylsiloxanes.

A. Polymerization Reaction

The reactive group is a carbon–carbon double bond (C=C), which is called a vinyl group. As expected, polymerization occurs by way of free radicals and addition polymerization. Polymerization involves chain lengthening and cross-linking to a stable rubber material. No evaporation of a

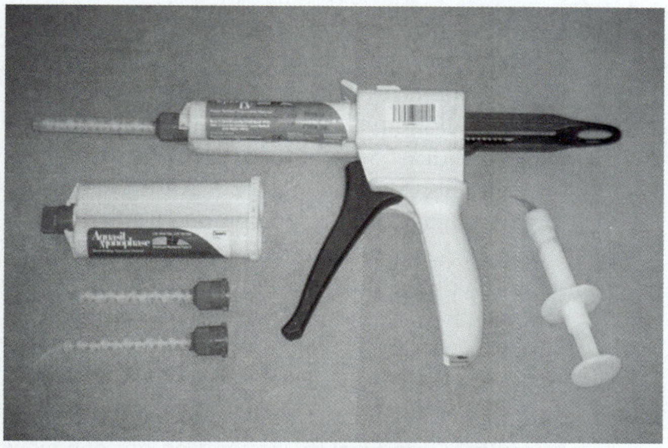

FIGURE 8.14 Automixing gun, cartridge, tips, and impression syringe.

reaction by-product occurs because no by-product is formed.

B. Viscosities and Mixing

The material supplied by the manufacturer is composed of short silicone rubber molecules with several reactive groups on each molecule. Fillers are added (to obtain the proper viscosity) along with a "catalyst," which functions as an activator. Manufacturers produce addition silicone materials in as many as five viscosities: light body, medium body, heavy body, monophase, and putty. Each viscosity comes in the form of two different-colored pastes. The pastes (except for putty) are mixed in the same manner as polysulfide materials. Addition silicones are also supplied in double-barreled cartridges for use in an "**automix** gun," as shown in Figure 8.14. The automix system forces the two pastes through a tip, which contains a spiral-shaped "baffle." In the tip, the baffle causes the material to swirl around and flow in a turbulent manner that mixes the two pastes together. A second, smaller tip may be added to the main tip; this second tip is designed to dispense the impression material intraorally. The automix system is very popular and has been adapted for other types of dental materials, such as acrylic resins for temporary crowns and bridges.

C. Use of Putty

1. Purpose

Putty is used in combination with a low-viscosity material. Putty fills the majority of the tray. It is covered by a low-viscosity material in the tray, or the low-viscosity material is injected around the teeth of interest. Putty's high viscosity forces the lower viscosity materials around the teeth of interest.

2. Mixing, Working, and Setting Times

Kneading the two colored materials together with the fingers mixes impression putty. The palms of the hands should not be used because the material will be slightly heated by the clinician's body (hand) temperature. Polymerization is then accelerated, and working time is decreased. Also, latex gloves must not be worn when mixing addition silicone putties. Sulfur in the latex material inhibits the polymerization reaction; therefore, the material may not set. Instead, vinyl gloves should be worn over hands that have been washed with soap and water.

Impression putty typically sets faster than light, medium, and heavy body materials. Working with two materials that set at different rates may be difficult. A variety of errors can occur when the two materials set at different times. It is very important to follow a standard impression procedure that uses a clock to time mixing, placement, and set of materials; these are called the mixing, working, and setting times, respectively. Timing the mixing, placement, and set of all chemically activated materials is recommended regardless of the material. Such procedures should follow the manufacturer's directions.

D. Additives to the Material

1. Surfactants

Current addition silicone impression materials have surfactants added to make pouring the model easier. **Surfactants** reduce the contact angle of the mixed gypsum product on the surface of the impression. Wetting is increased, and the likelihood of bubbles is decreased. Many manufacturers claim the surfactants also make taking an impression of wet teeth easier; however, such claims are without basis.

2. Hydrogen Absorbers

Another problem can occur with some addition silicone materials: If the components are not formulated in the proper ratio or with the proper purity, hydrogen gas is produced by a secondary reaction. If such a material is poured too quickly, very tiny bubbles of hydrogen form at the interface of the impression material and the model material. Small bubbles on the gypsum cast are the result. Several products have hydrogen absorbers added to the formulation to prevent this problem.

Because disinfecting an impression takes from 10 to 30 minutes, hydrogen gas bubbles are less of a problem after such a delay. Also, addition silicone materials are very accurate and stable, so addition silicone impressions are often sent to a commercial dental laboratory and poured there—even if the impression is shipped to a dental laboratory across the country. When the impression gets to the lab, sufficient time has passed for the hydrogen gas to have dissipated.

XIII. Miscellaneous Comments

A. Other Uses of Impression Materials

1. Bite Registration Materials

Most elastomeric impression materials can be used as a bite registration material. As shown in Figure 8.4, the mixed material is placed on the occlusal surfaces of the mandibular arch. The patient bites into the material. The impression material sets, recording the relationship of the maxillary arch to the mandibular arch. The bite registration is then removed and used in the dental laboratory to relate an upper cast to a lower cast in the same manner as the patient's natural bite.

2. Mold for Temporary Crowns

Putty can be used to make a "mold" for the fabrication of temporary crowns. Before the tooth is prepared for a crown, the mixed putty is placed over the tooth of interest. The putty sets and is removed, and the tooth is then prepared. The area of the prepared tooth of the putty impression is filled with a plastic temporary material. The most common temporary material is chemically activated acrylic resin. After the putty impression is filled with the acrylic resin, it is reseated in the patient's mouth. The prepared tooth forms the inside of the temporary crown, and the putty impression forms the outside of the mold of the temporary crown. The acrylic resin sets, is removed from the mouth, and is trimmed, polished, and then temporarily cemented. Construction of temporary crowns is presented in greater detail in Chapter 35.

B. Compatibility of Impression Materials With Die Materials

Not all impression materials are compatible with all model materials. All impression materials can be poured with gypsum products, but not all impression materials can be electroplated to form dies. Hydrocolloid materials are not compatible with epoxy die materials. Impression material/model material compatibility will be discussed in greater detail when model materials are presented in Chapter 9.

C. Optical Impressions

Dentistry has embraced digital technology when it is economically advantageous. One example is digital radiography, which has been adopted by many practices. Several CAD/CAM systems have been developed for dentistry. CAD/CAM stands for computer-aided design/computer-aided manufacture. CAD/CAM requires a computer model of the tooth preparation. Several techniques are used. One involves the usual dental impression with an impression material. The resulting cast is digitized at the dental laboratory. The restoration is then designed using interactive software and machined by milling (grinding) the restoration out of a piece of solid material. The dental laboratory assumes the financial burden of the cost of the equipment. The cost is spread among many dental practices.

The second technique uses an "optical" impression integrated with a CAD/CAM milling machine. The optical impression is taken with an intraoral infrared camera. The "optical" impression is stored digitally in a computer. The restoration is designed and milled in the dental office. The cost of the equipment is born by the individual dental office. In-office CAD/CAM systems are quite expensive but are increasing in popularity. In the future, optical impressions may be more common when just the camera is purchased and the resulting data file is sent to a dental lab for construction of the restoration. The common crown and bridge impression may become a memory as has the eight-track audio tape.

D. Performance of Impression Materials

Impression materials are the best performing of all dental materials. The use of impression materials has fewer restrictions than are found with most other dental materials. Impression materials only need to function for a short time (several hours to a few days). In addition, simulating clinical use of impression materials is quite simple compared to restorative materials, such as amalgam and composite. Research, product development, and quality control are greatly facilitated when clinical use can be easily simulated in the laboratory.

E. Biocompatibility of Impression Materials

Some assistants have had a skin rash on their hands that has been attributed to the manipulation of impression material. With the current practice of wearing gloves when treating patients, skin problems are first blamed on latex gloves. However, one must not forget that other dental materials can cause skin irritation, even though this is rare. Polymeric dental materials are much more likely to be irritating before they are mixed; the cured or set polymer is typically much less of a problem.

Because impression materials are used in the mouth only for several minutes, biocompatibility is usually not a significant concern. However, if residual pieces of impression material remain subgingivally or between teeth, significant irritation will occur. The clinician should inspect the oral cavity for residual material on removal.

SUMMARY

Impression materials are used to make replicas of teeth and other oral tissues. The replicas are then used to fabricate restorations and other appliances. Impression materials are supplied in a variety of forms. Some are powders mixed with water; others are paste/paste systems. They can be classified by use, type, or how they set.

The inelastic impression materials include plaster, ZOE, wax, and impression compound. Agar and alginate are aqueous elastomers. The nonaqueous elastomeric materials include polysulfide, addition silicones, condensation silicones, and polyethers.

Alginates are used frequently for diagnosis and treatment planning. They are also used to make fluoride and bleaching trays, mouthguards, and other appliances. The advantage of hydrocolloids is that while they are being poured, the gypsum easily wets the surface of the hydrocolloid because it is composed of water. The disadvantage of hydrocolloids is that they are susceptible to syneresis and imbibition, which can affect accuracy.

Addition silicones are the most popular impression material used in the construction of bridges, crowns, and other precision restorations. They are easy to use, record detail well, and have excellent properties. Their advantages include cleanliness, ease of use, lack of odor, accuracy, and stability. Their disadvantage is cost.

Each kind of impression material varies in cost, ease of use, accuracy, purpose, and mixing and setting times. Overall, impression materials are the best performing of all dental materials. They have few restrictions, and only need to function for a short time.

Learning Activities

1. Mix two different-colored toothpastes (or cake frostings). Dispense equal lengths, and mix with a cement spatula until a homogeneous color is obtained. Note the time that is required. The same can be done with two different-colored modeling clays to simulate the mixing of putty.
2. Obtain light bodied, medium bodied, and heavy bodied impression material (of the same brand). Mix and place approximately equal volumes of each material in a mound on a mixing pad. Note the "slump" of each material and the area that each covers.
3. With the materials in learning activity #2, mix and make samples of equal thickness. Bend the samples, and note the stiffness of each material.
4. With alginate and one nonaqueous elastomeric material, take an impression of a dentoform (or of several fingers) under water (in a bucket of water). Note the details recorded in the two materials.
5. Visit the Dux Dental website at http://www.duxdental.com for more information on the use of alginate and reversible hydrocolloid.

Review Questions

1. Alginate impression material is:
   a) Expensive compared to other impression materials
   b) Easy to use
   c) Not affected by gain or loss of water
   d) Well known for its long-term stability
2. Impression materials that have mechanical properties permitting considerable elastic deformation but that return to their original form are classified as:
   a) Thermoplastic
   b) Elastomeric
   c) Inelastic
   d) Resins
3. Dr. Jones requested that you mix alginate and take an impression. While measuring the water, you got involved in conversation and did not notice how warm it was. This oversight will:
   a) Make the mix unusable
   b) Lengthen the gelation time
   c) Not affect gelation time
   d) Shorten the gelation time

4. Which of the following dental materials is an example of an aqueous elastomeric?
a) Impression compound
b) ZOE impression paste
c) Polysulfide
d) Irreversible hydrocolloid
e) Addition silicone

5. The brown paste used in rubber base is called the:
a) Polymer
b) Accelerator
c) Base
d) Filler

6. Dental impression compound is known as a/an ________________.
a) Chemoplastic material
b) Irreversible material
c) Hydroelastic material
d) Thermoplastic material

7. Which of the following is an example of an inelastic impression material?
a) Polysulfide
b) ZOE impression paste
c) Alginate
d) Addition silicone

8. The term used for the setting of hydrocolloid impression materials is:
a) Crystallization
b) Polymerization
c) Curing
d) Gelation

9. The popularity of agar impression material is limited by the:
a) High cost
b) Need for special equipment
c) Poor reproduction of detail
d) Difficulty in pouring the impression

10. When an agar impression slightly contracts and exudes water, it is termed:
a) Imbibition
b) Gelation
c) Syneresis
d) Hysteresis

11. Addition silicones are the most popular type of rubber impression materials. The reason for this is cost.
a) The first statement is true; the second statement is false.
b) The first statement is false; the second statement is true.
c) Both statements are true.
d) Both statements are false.

12. Custom impression trays are made on a model of the patient's arch. Therefore, to make a custom tray, an alginate impression is also needed.
a) The first statement is true; the second statement is false.
b) The first statement is false; the second statement is true.
c) Both statements are true.
d) Both statements are false.

13. Mrs. Smith has not been to the dentist for several years. It was found that she needed extensive restorative treatment to which she agreed. You were asked to take impressions as the first step of her care. The impression material of choice would be:
a) Agar
b) Alginate
c) Dental impression compound
d) Addition silicone

14. The impression tray that is used to record the prepared tooth, a bite registration, and an impression of the opposing teeth is a:
a) Stock tray
b) Custom tray
c) Triple tray
d) Bite registration tray

15. Which of the following impression materials set by physical means?
a) Agar
b) ZOE
c) Alginate
d) Addition silicone

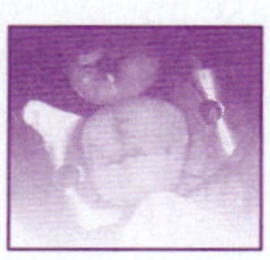

Supplemental Readings

Anusavice KJ. Phillips' Science of Dental Materials. 11th ed. Philadelphia: Saunders, 2003, Chapter 9.

Christensen GJ. What category of impression material is best for your practice? J Am Dent Assoc 1997;128: 1026–1028.

Chu CS, Smales RJ, Wei SHY. Requirements of an impression material for fixed prostheses. Gen Dent 1997;45: 548–555.

Larson TD, Nielsen MA, Brackett WW. The accuracy of dual-arch impressions: a pilot study. J Prosthet Dent 2002;87: 625–627.

Powers JM & Sakaguchi RL, eds. Craig's Restorative Dental Materials. 12th ed. St. Louis: Mosby, 2006, Chapter 12.

Thongthammachat S, Moore BK, Barco MT, Hovijitra S, Brown DT, Andres CJ. Dimensional accuracy of dental casts: influence of tray material, impression material, and time. J Prosthodont 2002;11:98–108.

9

Gypsum Materials

James Overberger, D.D.S., M.S.

Objectives

After studying this chapter, the student will be able to do the following:

1. Define the following terms: study model, cast, and die.
2. Discuss the major differences between dental plaster, stone, and improved stone.
3. Explain the meaning of initial and final setting times.
4. Give three examples of how to increase and decrease the setting times of gypsum products.
5. Discuss wet and dry strength as it relates to gypsum products.
6. Summarize the recommended technique for use of gypsum products for measuring, mixing, and filling the impression. Include hand and vacuum mixing.

Key Words/Phrases

accelerator
articulator
calcination
cast
die
dry strength
final setting time
gypsum products
high-strength stone
improved stone
initial setting time
plaster
retarder
stone
study model
water/powder ratio
wet strength
working time

INTRODUCTION

Gypsum products are supplied as fine powders that are mixed with water to form a fluid mass that can be poured and shaped and that subsequently hardens into a rigid, stable mass. An example of this powder is illustrated in Figure 9.1. Gypsum products are used mainly for positive reproductions or replicas of oral structures. These replicas are called casts, dies, or models, and they are obtained from negative reproductions, such as alginate impressions. Each replica has a specific purpose:

1. A **study model** is used to plan treatment and to observe treatment progress (Fig. 9.2*A*).
2. A **cast** is a replica on which a restoration or appliance is fabricated. A cast is more accurate than a study model and is a replica of more than one tooth, such as a quadrant or a full arch. It may be partially or completely edentulous. Examples of dental casts are shown in Figure 9.2*B*.
3. A **die** is a working replica of a single tooth, as shown in Figure 9.3. Typically, it is a removable part of a cast.

Because indirect dental restorations are fabricated on these cast or die replicas, it is essential that the particular gypsum product be carefully manipulated to ensure an accurate restoration.

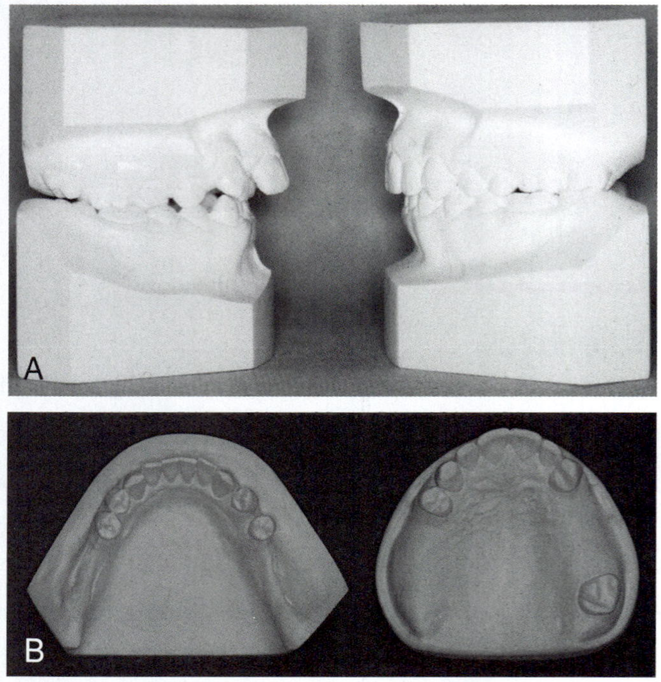

FIGURE 9.2 A. Preoperative and postoperative orthodontic study models. **B.** Dental casts made of stone for partial denture construction. (Part **B** reprinted with permission from Richardson RE, Barton RE. The Dental Assistant. 5th ed. New York: McGraw-Hill, 1978.)

I. Desirable Properties

Several properties are required of a material to be used for making casts, models, or dies. These properties are:

1. Accuracy
2. Dimensional stability
3. Ability to reproduce fine detail
4. Strength and resistance to abrasion
5. Compatibility with the impression material
6. Color
7. Biological safety
8. Ease of use
9. Cost

Not all gypsum products display all of these desirable properties equally.

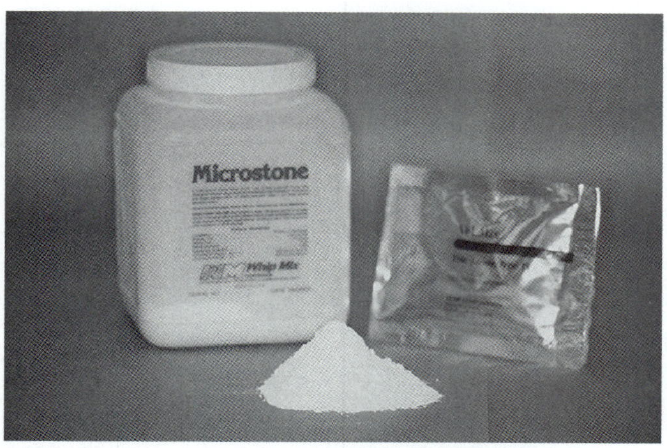

FIGURE 9.1 Gypsum powder, bulk package, and premeasured envelope.

II. Types of Gypsum Products

Gypsum products are made from gypsum rock, which is a mineral found in various parts of the world. Gypsum rock is mined, ground into a fine powder, and then processed by heating to form a variety of products. Chemically, gypsum rock is calcium sulfate dihydrate ($CaSO_4{\cdot}2H_2O$). Calcium sulfate dihydrate can also be produced synthetically. Pure gypsum is white, but in most deposits, it is discolored by impurities. Gypsum products are used in dentistry, medicine, homes, and industry. In homes, gypsum plaster is used to make walls; in industry, it is used to make molds.

In this chapter, three types of gypsum products will be discussed: plaster, stone, and high-strength or improved stone. Chemically, all three are calcium sulfate hemihydrate. They are produced as a result of heating gypsum and driving off part of the water of crystallization. This process is called **calcination** and is shown in the following equation:

$$CaSO_4{\cdot}2H_2O + \text{heat} \rightarrow (CaSO_4)_2{\cdot}H_2O$$
$$(\text{or } CaSO_4{\cdot}\tfrac{1}{2}H_2O) + 1\tfrac{1}{2}H_2O$$

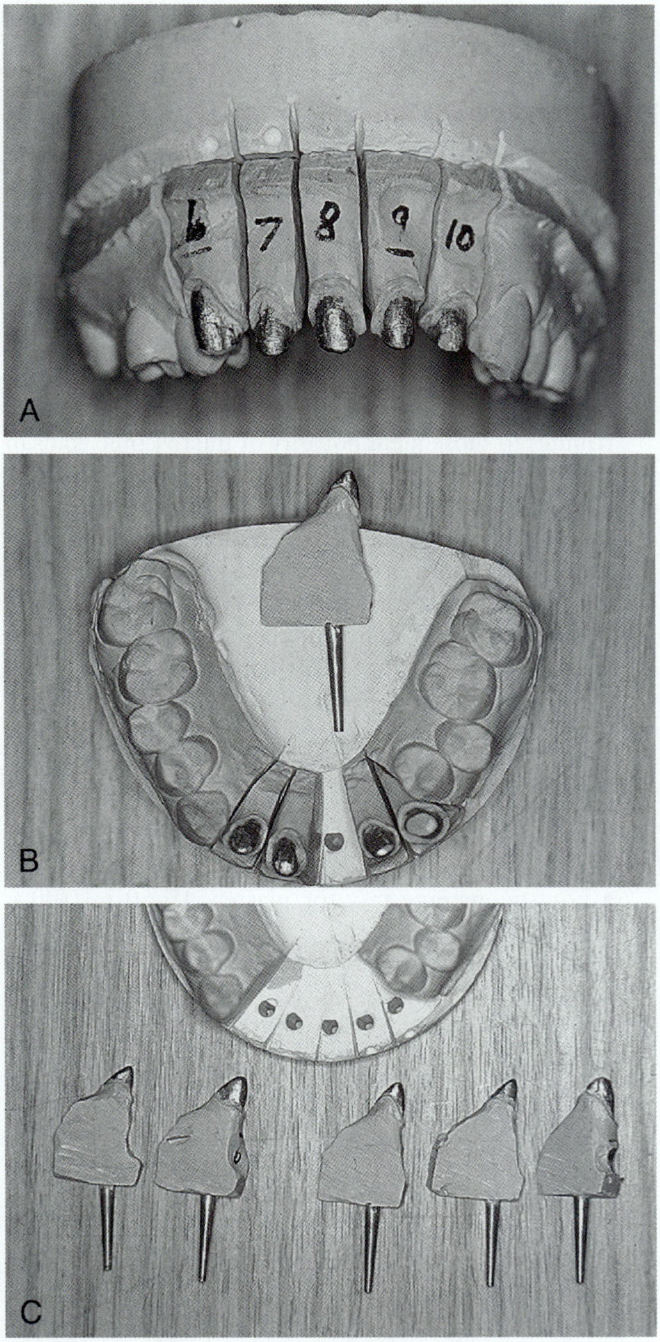

FIGURE 9.3 Cast with mounted dies. **A.** Five dies in cast. **B.** One die removed. **C.** All dies removed.

Plaster, stone, and improved stone differ in the physical characteristics of their powder particles as a result of differing calcination methods. These differences in powder particles are responsible for their different properties, which make them suitable for various uses. The manufacturers add other chemicals to improve handling and various properties.

A. Plaster

Plaster was the first gypsum product available for dentistry. It is manufactured by grinding the gypsum rock into a fine powder and then heating that powder in an open container. This direct and rapid heating in open air drives part of the water of crystallization from the crystal and shatters the crystal. The resulting powder consists of porous, irregular particles (Fig. 9.4*A*) . Plaster is the weakest and least expensive of the three gypsum products. It is used mainly when strength is not a critical requirement, such as preliminary casts for complete dentures and attaching casts to a mechanical device called an **articulator.** This device simulates the patient's occlusion and mastication process and is shown in Figures 1.8*B* and 11.6*F;* these photographs illustrate the use of plaster to secure the cast to the articulator.

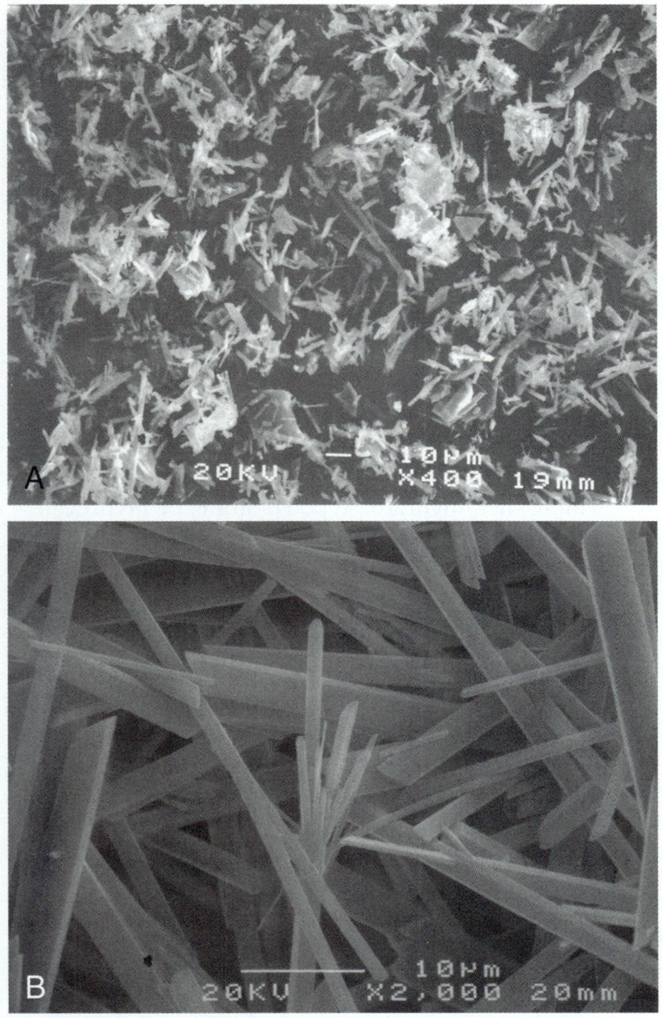

FIGURE 9.4 Scanning electron micrographs of dental plaster powder particles (**A**) and dental stone powder particles (**B**). (Courtesy of Diane Schwegler-Berry, NIOSH, Morgantown, WV.)

Plaster is usually white in color and sometimes is referred to as beta-hemihydrate or Type II. In the past, plaster was modified for use as an impression material by the addition of chemicals and was called impression plaster (see Chapter 8).

B. Stone

Stone is made from gypsum by carefully controlled calcination under steam pressure in a closed container. This method of calcination slowly releases the water of crystallization from the crystal so that the resultant powder particle (Fig. 9.4*B*) is more regular, more uniform in shape, and less porous compared to that of plaster. Stone is stronger and more expensive than plaster. It is used mainly in making casts for diagnostic purposes and casts for complete and partial denture construction, which require greater strength and surface hardness than that of plaster.

The stone is usually yellow, but it can be obtained in other colors. It is often referred to as alpha-hemihydrate, Type III stone, or Hydrocal.

C. High-Strength or Improved Stone

High-strength stone, or **improved stone,** is also made from gypsum by calcining the gypsum in a calcium chloride solution. This method of calcination results in a powder particle that is very dense, is cuboidal in shape, and has a reduced surface area. High-strength stone is the strongest and most expensive of the three gypsum products, and it is used mainly for making casts or dies for crown, bridge, and inlay fabrication. Figure 9.3 shows an example of an improved stone cast and several dies for the fabrication of crowns. This material is used because high strength and surface hardness are required during the fabrication process; the fabrication of crowns is described in the next chapter. High-strength stone is often referred to as Type IV stone, die stone, densite, and modified alpha-hemihydrate. A newly developed high-strength stone with a higher compressive strength than that of Type IV stone is also available. It displays higher setting expansion and is referred to as Type V stone.

D. Other Types of Gypsum

Other types of gypsum products are produced for special uses, such as fast set, mounting of casts on articulators, and impressions. Investments are presented in Chapter 10.

III. Setting Reaction

When any of the three types of calcium sulfate hemihydrate is mixed with water, the hemihydrate is changed back to dihydrate by the process of hydration. Heat is liberated, as shown by the following reaction:

$$CaSO_4 \cdot \frac{1}{2}H_2O + 1 \cdot H_2O \rightarrow CaSO_4 \cdot 2H_2O + \text{heat}$$

The calcium sulfate hemihydrate dissolves in the mixing water to form the dihydrate, which is less soluble than the hemihydrate. The calcium sulfate dihydrate precipitates out of solution as interlocking crystals, which form a hard mass.

IV. Water/Powder Ratio

The proportion of water to powder used to make a workable mix of a particular gypsum product is called the **water/powder ratio.** For dental use, an excess amount of measured water above the theoretically correct amount required for hydration is always necessary. This excess amount is needed to make a workable mix or slurry that can be poured and shaped. The excess water is distributed as free water in the set mass without taking part in the chemical reaction, and it contributes to subsequent porosity or microscopic voids in the set product. The proper water/powder ratio for each product depends on the physical characteristics of the powder particles. Plaster requires more gauging water (measured water) to wet the powder surfaces, fill the pores, and float the irregular porous particles. The dense particles of stone require less gauging water to float them, and their regular shape allows them to roll over one another more easily. High-strength stone, because of its very dense and cuboidal type of particle as well as modifications made by the manufacturer, requires even less gauging water than stone. For dental use, the proper water/powder ratios (quotients) are as follows:

- For the average mix for plaster, 45–50 ml/100 g (0.45–0.50)
- For the average mix for stone, 28–30 ml/100 g (0.28–0.30)
- For the average mix for improved stone, 19–24 ml/100 g (0.19–0.24)

This difference in the amount of measured water that is required to make a workable mix results in different consistencies for the products when first mixed at the proper water/powder ratio. Plaster is usually thin in consistency, like a 'smoothie,' whereas improved stone is like thick cake batter. Dental stone has an intermediate consistency. The water/powder ratio has a direct effect on the properties of each gypsum product and must be controlled for optimum results.

V. Setting Time

A. Definitions

Knowledge of the setting characteristics of a gypsum product is important for proper manipulation. The clinician should be aware of two time intervals in the setting process.

1. Working Time or Initial Setting Time

Working time or **initial setting time** is the length of time from the start of the mix until the setting mass reaches a semihard stage. It represents the available time for manipulating the

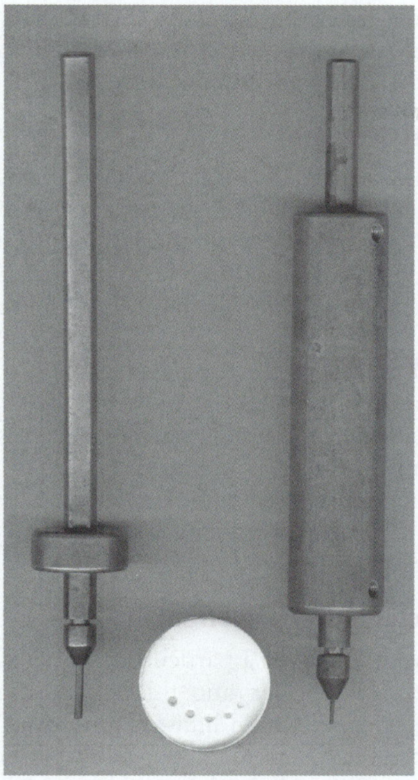

FIGURE 9.5 The 1-lb (*left*) and ¼-lb (*right*) Gillmore needles with a sample of a gypsum product.

product, and it indicates partial progress of the setting reaction.

2. Final Setting Time

Final setting time represents the length of time from the start of the mix until the setting mass becomes rigid and can be separated from the impression. The final setting time indicates the major completion of the hydration reaction.

B. Measurement

Setting times are usually measured with a surface penetration test. Gillmore needles are commonly used for this measurement and are shown in Figure 9.5. When the surface of the setting product has developed sufficient strength to support the weight of the ¼-lb needle and of the 1-lb needle, the initial setting time and the final setting time, respectively, have occurred. In other words, each designated setting time is reached when its respective needle no longer makes an indentation in the gypsum specimen. This method is somewhat arbitrary, and it is difficult to correlate directly with the setting reaction. In addition, the resulting values are mainly used for comparisons of different products. For practical purposes, loss of surface gloss can be used as a determination of the initial setting or working time; it is typically 5 to 7 minutes. The failure of penetration by a fingernail or dull knife would indicate relative rigidity and hardness and could be used as an indication of final set. Usually, a time of 30 to 45 minutes is used as a subjective criterion for the time of final set.

C. Variation in Setting Times

The setting time of a gypsum product is controlled by the manufacturer's particular formulation. Hence, several gypsum products are available with varying setting characteristics. Either a fast-setting or a slow-setting product can be purchased. Sometimes, it may be necessary to modify the setting time of a gypsum product in the dental office. Increased and decreased setting times may be obtained in the following ways:

1. Increased Setting Time (A Slower-Setting Product)

a) Decreased mixing.
b) Higher water/powder ratio (creates a thinner mix).
c) Addition of certain chemicals called retarders. A commonly used **retarder** is borax.

2. Decreased Setting Time (A Faster-Setting Product)

a) Increased mixing (the longer the mixing time, the shorter the setting time).
b) Lower water/powder ratio (creates a thicker mix).
c) Addition of certain chemicals called accelerators. A commonly used **accelerator** is potassium sulfate. Other chemicals can be used, but their effect on the setting time depends on concentration and other factors.

Improper storage and use of gypsum products can also change the setting characteristics. Because water is essential for the setting reaction, any moisture that inadvertently comes in contact with the product can change the setting time. Thus, gypsum products should be stored in airtight containers to prevent any uptake of water resulting from high relative humidity. As a result, preweighed packages have become popular for some gypsum products. The first indication of moisture contamination is faster setting of the product. If the contamination continues, slower setting occurs.

VI. Setting Expansion

All gypsum products expand externally on setting. Plaster expands the most, at 0.2% to 0.3%. Stone expands 0.08% to 0.10%. High-strength stone expands the least, at 0.05% to 0.07%. Theoretically, a contraction on setting can be calculated; however, the growing crystals of the gypsum push against each other and cause an outward crystal thrust. In turn, this thrust causes an external expansion with resulting internal porosity in the set mass. A minimal setting expansion is desirable to achieve accurate dimensional reproduction for most casts and dies. Manufacturers modify most gypsum products that are used for casts and dies to provide for minimal expansion. They do this by the addition of chemicals, which also control the setting characteristics. Thus, a particular gypsum product has both the setting time and expansion characteristics controlled by the manufacturer. The setting expansion can be controlled by manipulating variables. A thicker mix and increased spatulation will cause an increase in the amount of setting expansion; a thinner mix and decreased spatulation will cause a decrease in the amount of setting expansion. In most dental offices, however, there is little need to change the expansion characteristics of gypsum products.

If gypsum materials are immersed in or come in contact with water during the setting process, the setting expansion increases. This is called hygroscopic expansion, and it can be used to increase the setting expansion of casting investments. Casting investments are discussed in the next chapter. Although small, hygroscopic expansion is approximately twice as great as the normal setting expansion. Therefore, to prevent an inadvertent increase in size, routine casts should not be immersed in water during setting.

VII. Strength

The strength of the gypsum product is usually measured in terms of crushing or compressive strength. As expected from the setting reaction, strength develops rapidly during the first 30 to 45 minutes as hydration is completed. The strength depends on the porosity of the set material, and the porosity relates to the water/powder ratio necessary to make a workable mix. Plaster, which requires the most gauging water to make a fluid mix, is the weakest in strength, with improved stone being the strongest and stone being intermediate between the two. The 1-hour strengths of gypsum products are listed in Table 9.1.

The presence or absence of excess free water also affects strength. Two types of strength are recognized: wet strength and dry strength.

A. Wet Strength

The **wet strength** is the strength that is measured when the sample contains some or all of the water in excess of the theoretical amount required for hydration. This is the typical condition after setting. The material feels wet to the touch for many hours.

B. Dry Strength

The **dry strength** is the strength that is measured when the excess water is not present in the sample. The dry strength may be two or more times the wet strength. Usually, the cast must sit in a dry environment overnight to approach these values.

C. Factors Affecting Strength

The strength of a particular product depends on the water/powder ratio; thicker mixes will increase the strength within limits, and thinner mixes will decrease the strength. However, extremely thick mixes, particularly those of stone and improved stone, are heavy in consistency and can cause distortion of the impression as well as entrapment of air voids. Extremely thin mixes will cause a decrease in strength. Therefore, it is a good practice to follow the manufacturer's recommended water/powder ratio for optimum strength and consistency properties.

VIII. Surface Hardness

The surface hardness is related to the compressive strength, but reaches its maximum value more rapidly because the surface is the first to dry. The greatest surface hardness occurs when the product reaches its dry strength, which many times is not realized under practical conditions. Casts and dies should be allowed to set for 1 to 2 hours, or preferably

Table 9.1 One-Hour Compressive Strengths and Water/Powder Ratios of Gypsum Products

Gypsum	Minimum 1-Hour Compressive Strength (lb/in² [Mpa])[a]	Water/Powder Ratio[b]
Plaster (Type II)	1,300 (9)	45–50 ml/100 g (0.45–0.50)
Dental stone (Type III)	3,000 (21)	28–30 ml/100 g (0.28–0.30)
Dental stone, high-strength (Type IV)	5,000 (34)	19–24 ml/100 g (0.19–0.24)

[a]Adapted from Revised ANSI-ADA specification no. 25.
[b]Quotients are in parentheses.

overnight or longer, before beginning subsequent laboratory procedures. The surface hardness of set gypsum is not as high as desired. Use of a commercial hardening solution in place of water may increase the hardness and improve the abrasion resistance.

IX. Dimensional Stability

The dimensions of a hardened or set gypsum cast are relatively constant under ordinary conditions of room temperature and humidity; however, gypsum is slightly soluble in water. Occasionally, it is necessary to soak a cast in water for a laboratory procedure. If the cast is soaked in water for prolonged periods of time, the surface may be dissolved away. If the cast must be soaked in water, the water should be saturated with gypsum to prevent erosion of the surface. The safest way to soak a cast is to place it in a water bath containing particles of gypsum to provide a saturated solution of calcium sulfate at all times.

X. Technique of Use

The technical use of gypsum products is relatively simple, requiring only a mixing bowl, mixing spatula, room-temperature water, and the appropriate gypsum product. As mentioned earlier, the water and powder must be proportioned accurately for optimum properties to be obtained. The measuring and mixing technique can be summarized as follows.

A. Measuring the Water

The water is usually dispensed by volume in a graduated cylinder because 1 g of water has a volume of very close to 1 ml.

B. Measuring the Powder

The powder can be weighed in grams with a simple balance or scale. Use of a dietetic scale is a convenient method for weighing the powder. First, the water is added to the mixing bowl. Second, the scale is tared (reading is set to zero). Finally, the powder is placed into the bowl with a suitable scoop until the desired weight of powder has been added.

A measuring scale, bowl, and graduated cylinder are shown in Figure 9.6. Volume dispensers may also be used. Volume dispensing of the powder is not as accurate, however, because of the varying packing effect on the powder. Weighing with the scale is a simple and convenient method to ensure accurate proportions. Preweighed envelopes are now available that control the weight of the powder to provide accuracy and reduce both wasted powder and time required.

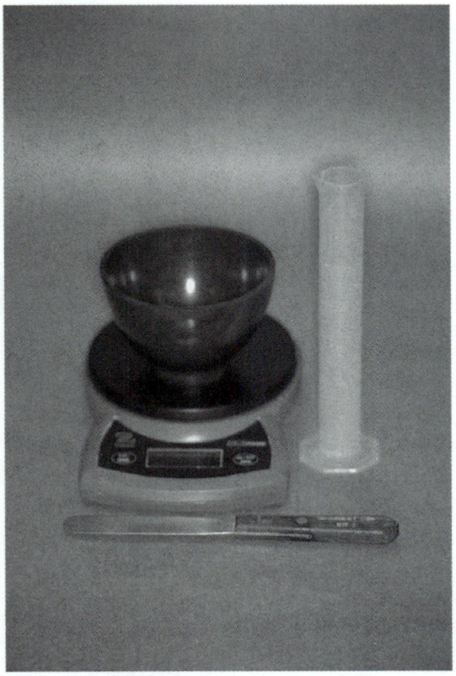

FIGURE 9.6 Equipment for mixing gypsum products: scale, rubber mixing bowl, graduated cylinder, and plaster spatula.

C. Adding Powder and Water

The preferred method of mixing is to add the measured water into the mixing bowl first, followed by gradual addition of the preweighed powder. The guesswork of repeatedly adding water and powder to achieve the proper consistency is to be avoided. It causes an uneven set in the cast, resulting in low strength and distortion.

D. Mixing

1. Hand Mixing

Hand mixing is usually done in a flexible plastic or rubber bowl with a stiff-bladed spatula to combine the powder and water. The mix should be smooth, homogeneous, workable, and free of air bubbles. A minimum of air inclusion in the mixed product is desirable to prevent surface bubbles and internal defects. Mixing is usually accomplished with a wiping motion against the sides of the bowl (to eliminate lumps and air bubbles). Use of a dental vibrator will reduce bubbles in the mix. A smooth, homogeneous mix should be obtained in approximately 1 minute. A whipping motion should be avoided.

2. Vacuum Mixing

Often, mixing is done mechanically with a vacuum mixing and investing machine. An example of this device is shown in Figure 9.7. This provides a gypsum mix that is free of air bubbles and is homogeneous in consistency. Many devices are available

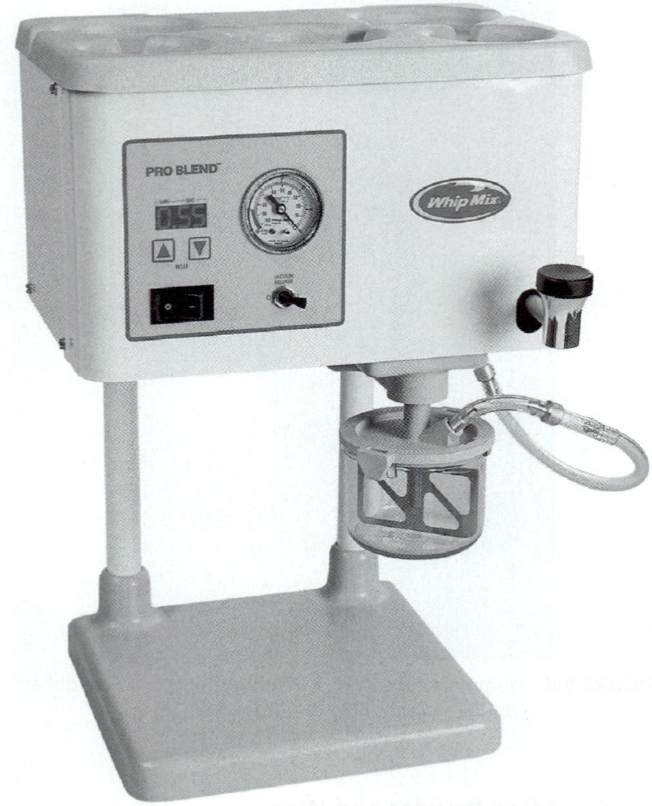

FIGURE 9.7 A vacuum mixing and investing machine. (Courtesy of Whip Mix Corp., Louisville, KY.)

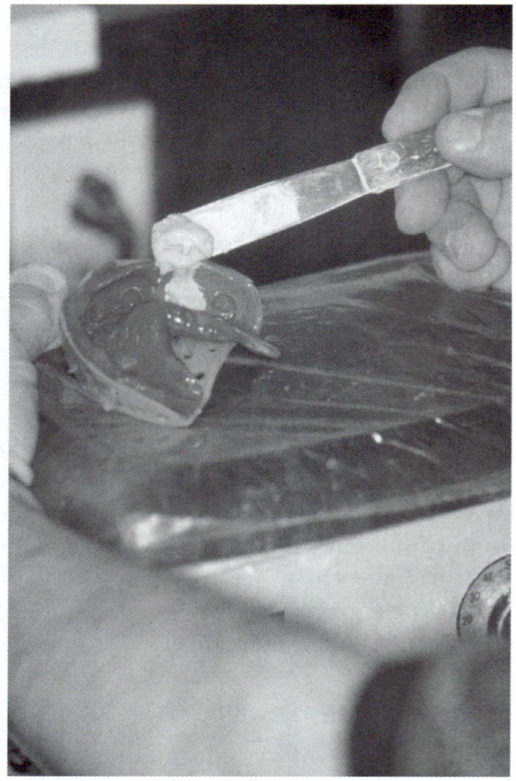

FIGURE 9.8 An impression sits on a dental vibrator as it is poured with stone.

that will mix gypsum products mechanically with or without vacuum. They are used when the elimination of voids and surface bubbles is critical.

E. Filling the Impression

When filling the impression, the gypsum mixture needs to flow slowly "ahead of itself" to prevent the entrapment of air. This is usually accomplished with a dental vibrator, as shown in Figure 9.8. This is particularly important when filling elastomeric impressions, which in many instances are water repellent. Vibrating the mix after mixing can also be used to bring air bubbles to the surface. Although relatively simple, manipulation of gypsum products requires careful attention to detail for accurate results.

SUMMARY

Gypsum products are used for making positive reproductions or replicas of oral structures. These replicas are called casts, dies, or models. Gypsum products are available in three basic types: plaster, stone, and improved stone.

The water/powder ratios vary for each type of gypsum. For plaster, the ratio is 45–50 ml/100 g. For stone, the ratio is 28–30 ml/100 g. For improved stone, the ratio is 19–24 ml/100 g. The plaster mix will be thin in consistency, whereas the improved stone mix will be like thick cake batter.

The working or initial setting time is the length of time from the start of the mix until the mass reaches a semihard stage. At this stage, the ¼-lb Gillmore needle would no longer leave an indentation. Practically speaking, the "loss of gloss" could be used as a determinant for the working or initial setting time. Final setting time is the length of time from the start of the mix until the mass becomes rigid and can be separated from the impression. At this stage, the 1-lb Gillmore needle would no longer leave an impression. Failure of a fingernail or a knife to penetrate the gypsum would indicate the final set.

Gypsum products expand externally on setting. Plaster expands the most, at 0.2% to 0.3%. Improved stone expands the least, at 0.05% to 0.07%. The strength of gypsum products is measured in terms of compressive strength. Strength develops within 30 to 45 minutes and depends on the porosity of the material. Plaster is the weakest of the three products, and improved stone is the strongest. Wet strength is the measured strength "just after it sets," and dry strength is the strength measured when excess water is not present. Casts should be protected from contact with water because gypsum is slightly soluble in water.

When mixing, the powder is added to the water. Gypsum may be mixed by hand or by vacuum. When filling the impression, the gypsum should "flow ahead of itself" so that air does not become entrapped. Use of gypsum products is relatively simple, but attention to detail ensures more accurate results.

Learning Activities

1. Place 40 g of plaster in a 50-ml graduated cylinder. Calculate the density. Now do the same for stone. Why is there a difference?
2. Mix plaster with several water/powder ratios in the range of 0.4 to 0.6. How is the setting time affected?
3. Mix plaster, using various spatulation times: 1, 2, and 3 minutes. How is the setting time affected?

Review Questions

1. The desirable strength of gypsum materials is ______________ related to the amount of water used.
   a) Directly
   b) Indirectly
   c) Not
   d) Partially
2. For gypsum products, a suitable accelerator and retarder, respectively, would be:
   a) Ethyl alcohol and oleic acid
   b) Oleic acid and glycerin
   c) Borax and potassium sulfate
   d) Potassium sulfate and borax
3. The gypsum material known as "high-strength stone" may also be referred to as:
   a) Plaster
   b) Dental stone
   c) Type III stone
   d) Improved stone
4. The final setting time for gypsum products typically is:
   a) 15 to 30 minutes
   b) 30 to 45 minutes
   c) 45 to 90 minutes
   d) 90 to 120 minutes
5. To make a correct mix for dental stone when using 50 g of powder, the amount of water would be approximately:
   a) 10 to 12 ml
   b) 14 to 15 ml
   c) 28 to 30 ml
   d) 45 to 50 ml
6. Cathy and her parents will meet with an orthodontist to discuss an orthodontic treatment plan. At a previous appointment, the orthodontist took impressions of Cathy's maxillary and mandibular arches. The replicas made from each impression to discuss the treatment plan are termed:
   a) Casts
   b) Dies
   c) Study models
   d) Molds
7. Decreasing the setting time of a dental material results in a product that:
   a) Takes less time to set
   b) Takes more time to set
   c) Does not affect the setting time
   d) Enhances the properties

8. The weakest gypsum product is:
a) Improved stone
b) Dental stone
c) Plaster
d) Die stone

9. When excess water is not present in a gypsum product, it is known as the:
a) Wet strength
b) Dry strength
c) Initial setting time
d) Surface strength

10. The best way to mix gypsum products is to:
a) "Eyeball" the amount of powder added to water
b) Add water to the powder
c) Add powder to the water
d) Add powder and water to bowl simultaneously

11. Initial and final setting times of gypsum can be determined with the use of Gilmore Needles. A practical, easy method to determine final setting time in a dental office would be to:
a) Set a timer for 20 minutes
b) Observe the change from wet to dry strength
c) Watch for the loss of gloss
d) Attempt to penetrate the material with the metal spatula

12. When the setting time of a dental material is increased, which of the following is true?
a) The material sets slower
b) The material sets faster
c) The setting reaction does not change
d) The setting reaction is increased

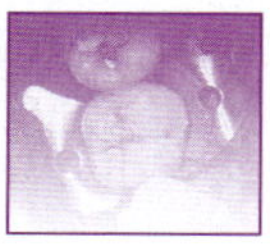

Supplemental Readings

Bird DL, Robinson DS. Torres and Ehrlich: Modern Dental Assisting. 7th ed. Philadelphia: Saunders, 2002, Chapter 47.

Duke P, Moore BK, Haug SP, Andres CJ. Study of the physical properties of type IV gypsum, resin-containing, and epoxy die materials. J Prosthet Dent 2000;83:466–473.

Powers JM, Sakaguchi RL, eds. Craig's Restorative Dental Materials. 12th ed. St. Louis: Mosby, 2006, Chapter 13.

Ragain JC, Grosko ML, Raj M, Ryan TN, Johnston WM. Detail reproduction, contact angles, and die hardness of elastomeric impression and gypsum die material combinations. Int J Prosthodont 2000;13:214–220.

10

Materials for Fixed Indirect Restorations and Prostheses

Objectives

After studying this chapter, the student will be able to do the following:

1. Discuss the factors that affect treatment planning for a fixed indirect restoration.
2. Explain the lost-wax casting process used in dentistry to make metal restorations.
3. Describe the types of alloys used to make all-metal crowns, ceramometal crowns, and partial denture frameworks.
4. Recall the types of porcelain used to simulate the color of teeth.
5. List the advantages and disadvantages of all-metal, ceramometal, and all-ceramic restorations.

Key Words/Phrases

abutment
alloys
bridge
buildups
burnishing
ceramometal restorations
coping
cores
crowns
crucible
divested
elongation
fixed restorations
gypsum-bonded investments
indirect restorations
ingate
inlays
onlays
pontics
provisional restoration
retainer
sprue
sintered
temporary restoration
veneer
wax pattern

I. Types of Fixed Indirect Restorations

There are many types of fixed indirect restorations. **Indirect restorations** are those restorations that are constructed outside the mouth. **Fixed restorations** cannot be removed from the oral cavity; they are luted (cemented) in place. Fixed indirect restorations can be classified in two ways: by the amount of tooth structure they restore or by the material from which they are made.

II. Classification by Amount of Tooth Structure Restored

A. Inlays

Inlays are intracoronal (inside the crown) restorations that replace small to medium amounts of tooth structure, as shown in Figure 1.3. They are most commonly used to restore pits, fissures, and grooves (Class I) as well as proximal surfaces (Class II) of posterior teeth. They do not restore the cusps. They are retained by luting cements.

B. Onlays

Onlays (or overlays) involve replacing more tooth structure than inlays replace. In addition to the pits, fissures, and proximal surfaces of an inlay, onlays restore one or more cusps and, at times, the entire occlusal surface of a tooth. Onlays are used when the likelihood of cusp fracture is high. The onlay protects the cusps from occlusal forces. Onlays, like inlays, are retained with intracoronal retention and luting cements. An onlay is shown in Figure 10.1.

C. Veneers

A **veneer** is a thin layer of material that covers another material (like the shell of a hard-boiled egg). In dentistry, veneers are restorations that are placed on the facial surface of anterior teeth to treat an esthetic problem, such as discolorations, rotations, or spaces (diastemata) (Fig. 10.2). Veneers are often used in conjunction with orthodontic or periodontal treatment. Two types of veneers are used.

1. Direct veneers use bonded composites, as shown in Figure 5.9. Direct veneers may not involve the removal of significant tooth structure. If tooth structure is not removed, such veneers are considered to be a reversible treatment.
2. Indirect veneers use a ceramic material, such as porcelain. The facial surface is prepared to provide space for the veneering material. Therefore, indirect veneers are not a reversible procedure. Indirect veneers involve an impression, a second appointment, and a laboratory fee, so they cost more overall than direct veneers. At one time, composite materials were also used, but discoloration was a problem. Today, porcelain is popular because a single veneer can utilize a variety of porcelain shades and translucencies. Indirect veneers are supported by, and are bonded to, the underlying tooth structure.

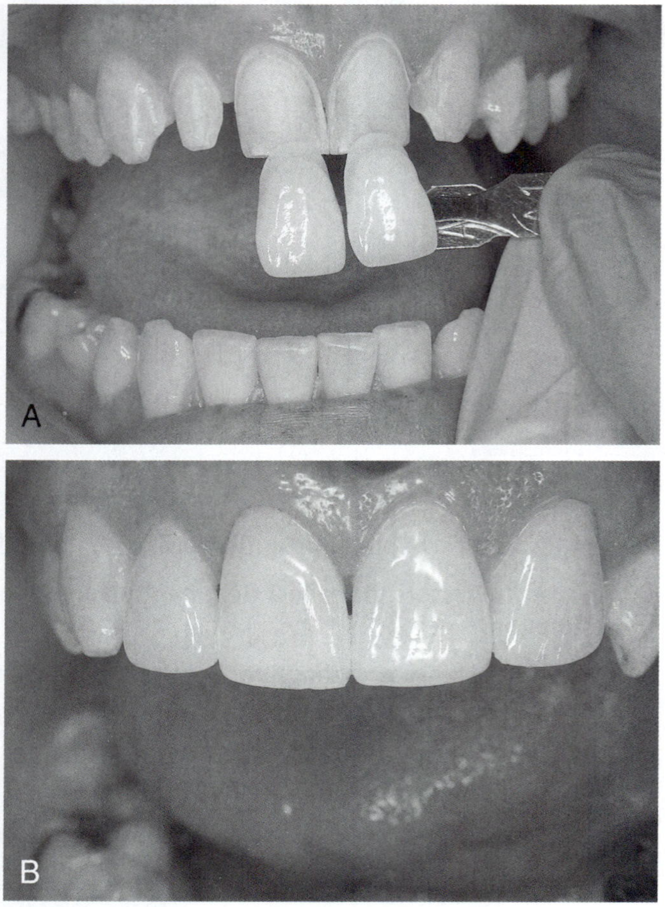

FIGURE 10.2 Photographs of teeth prepared for indirect veneers **(A)** and the veneers cemented in place **(B).** (See color images.) (Courtesy of Ultradent Products, Inc.)

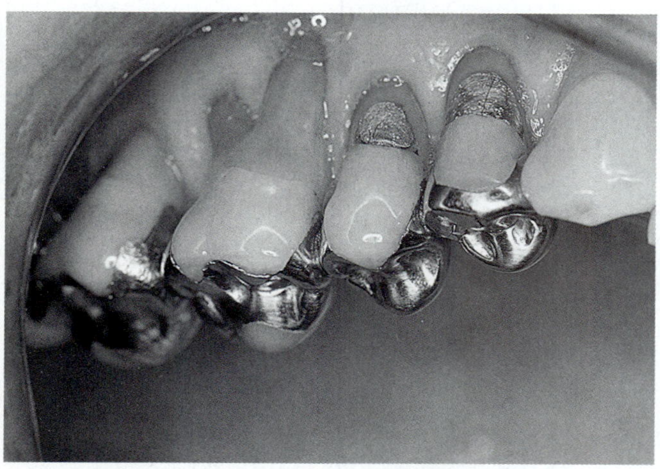

FIGURE 10.1 Photograph of several teeth restored with 30-year-old cast gold restorations. Tooth #3 is restored with an inlay. Tooth #4 is restored with an inlay/onlay combination. Tooth #5 is restored with an onlay.

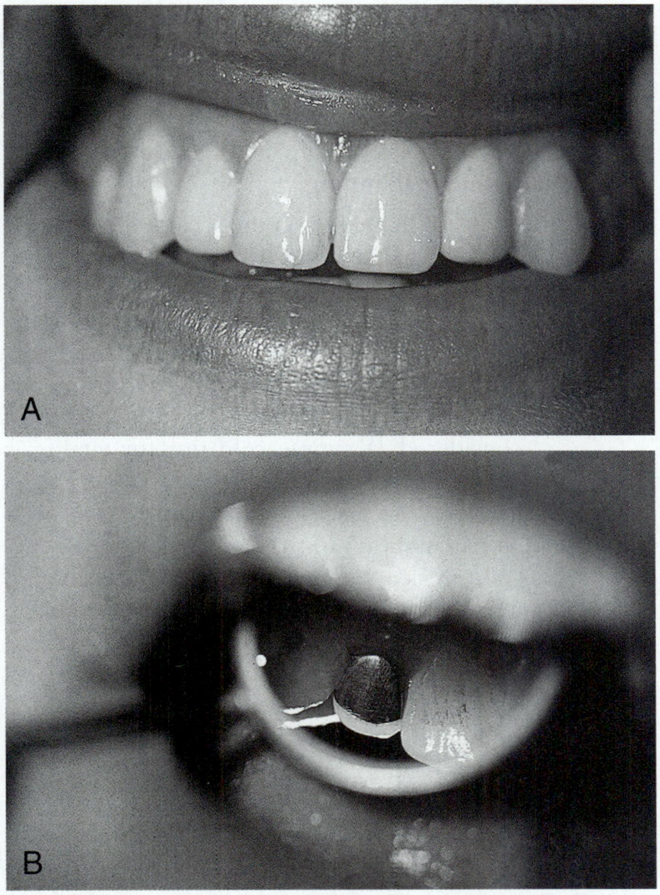

FIGURE 10.3 Photographs of porcelain-fused-to-metal crowns restoring teeth #7 and #10. **A.** Labial view of both teeth. **B.** Lingual view of tooth #10.

D. Crowns

Crowns are used to restore teeth that have lost a significant amount of tooth structure. They are used when intracoronal retention is unavailable or when the tooth needs to be surrounded and held together by the restoration. A full gold crown is shown in Figure 1.4. A porcelain crown is shown in Figure 1.10*E*. Ceramometal crowns are shown in Figure 10.3.

E. Complex Restorations

Complex restorations combine the features of inlay, onlay, and crown restorations, as shown in tooth #4 of Figure 10.1. A complex restoration is designed by the dentist after the tooth destruction has been assessed.

F. Dental Bridge

A **bridge** replaces missing teeth. Typically, a bridge has a crown, called a **retainer,** at each end. The retainers are supported by teeth called **abutments.** The replacement teeth are called **pontics.** A bridge may replace one tooth or several teeth, as shown in Figure 1.5.

III. Classification by Material

A. Metals

A variety of metals are used to restore teeth, as shown in Figures 10.1, 10.4, and 1.5. Most metallic indirect restorations are made by a casting procedure. Casting involves melting the metal and then pouring or forcing the liquid metal into a mold. The casting process allows custom, complex shapes to be easily produced. Metals are very tough and work well in high-stress situations, but their esthetics are poor.

B. Ceramic Materials

Ceramic materials are used when esthetics are important, as shown in Figure 1.10. Ceramic materials can simulate the natural colors and translucency of teeth. Porcelain is the ceramic material most commonly used in dentistry. A variety of materials and processing techniques are

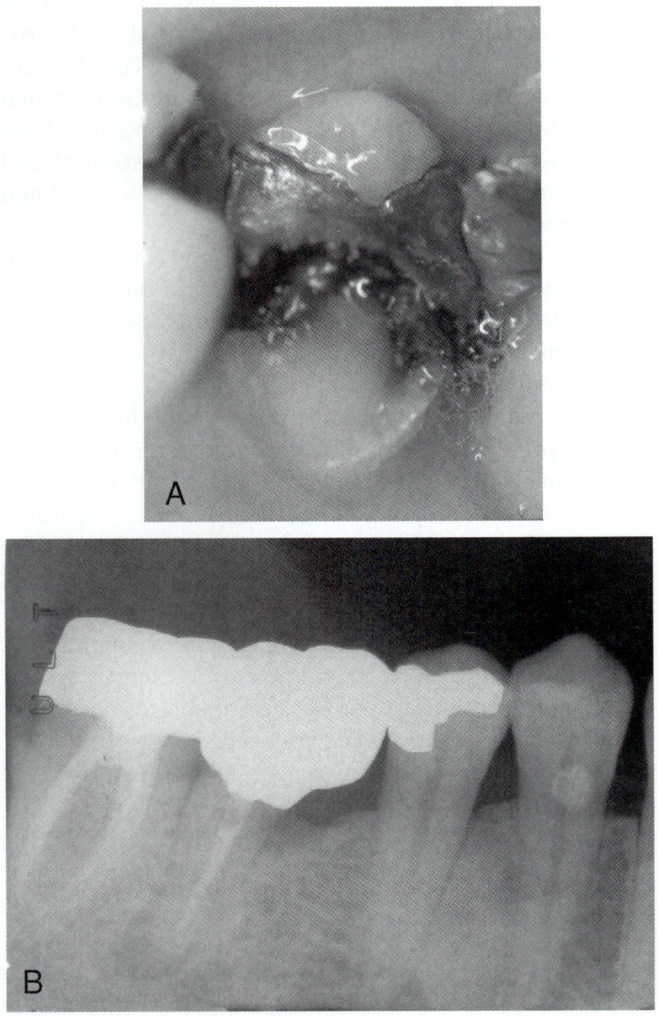

FIGURE 10.4 Two examples of the need for an indirect restoration. **A.** A fractured lingual cusp. **B.** A tooth that has had a multitude of dental treatment, including root canal therapy, root amputation, and a crown. This tooth was deemed to be hopeless and extracted because of pain, mobility, and a periapical radiolucency.

employed. Ceramic materials lack the toughness and fracture resistance required by bridges, but their esthetics can be excellent.

C. Ceramometals

A metal–ceramic combination was developed for dentistry in the 1950s. This material is made by using the same process to bake enamel (porcelain) on metal as that used to make old-fashioned pots and pans or sinks and bathtubs. The tough, strong metal supports the weak but esthetic ceramic material. The restorations are called **ceramometal restorations** (or porcelain-bonded-to-metal or porcelain-fused-to-metal restorations) and are considered to be an important "workhorse" in modern restorative dentistry. Ceramometal restorations are shown in Figure 10.3.

D. Composite Materials

Particle-reinforced composite materials (very similar to those discussed in Chapter 5) have been adapted for use as fixed indirect restorations. These materials are reinforced by irregularly shaped particles, as shown in Figure 5.8. They are cured at elevated temperatures, pressures, or both in the dental laboratory. Particle-reinforced composites have seen only limited success because their strength and toughness do not meet those required by crown and bridge materials.

Recently, fiber-reinforced composites have been developed for dentistry. These composites are similar to materials that have been developed for many other industries in which glass fibers are used to reinforce polymeric materials. Imagine a bowl of frozen, leftover spaghetti with sauce. The spaghetti represents the glass fibers; the frozen sauce represents the polymer matrix. The long fibers transfer stresses over a larger area than particles do. Automotive, aerospace, and sports equipment companies use fiber-reinforced composites to manufacture strong, lightweight products. Fiber-reinforced composites are much tougher and stronger than particle-reinforced composites. Clinical results seem promising, but because they are new, more long-term clinical data are needed.

IV. Procedures for Constructing an Indirect Restoration

A. Diagnosis, Treatment Planning, and Designing the Restoration

1. Diagnosis

Lost tooth structure and missing teeth result from a variety of causes. Caries and periodontal disease are the most common. An extreme case involving caries and periodontal disease is shown in Chapter 11. Trauma or fracture (Fig. 10.4*A*), esthetic concerns (Fig. 1.10), and congenital deficiencies (Fig. 10.2*A*) are other reasons to restore or replace teeth. Often, teeth are lost as the result of restoration and re-restoration and multiple dental treatments (Fig. 10.4*B*).

2. Treatment Planning

A variety of factors affect the success of a restoration. These factors must be assessed during treatment planning.

a) The periodontal status of the patient is critical. Without a stable foundation, the long-term success of any restoration is unlikely.

b) The endodontic status of the tooth must be considered. A simple cold test for vitality is commonly used. A periapical radiograph is important to assess the periodontal and periapical condition of the tooth.

c) Caries risk assessment and testing is becoming more common. If a crown or bridge will likely fail in several years because of recurrent caries, efforts to reduce the risk of caries should precede extensive and expensive restorations.

d) Enough tooth structure must remain to retain the restoration. Badly broken-down teeth may require **buildups** (also called **cores**) to provide retention of the final restoration, as shown in Figure 6.11.

3. Restoration Design

Many factors influence the design of a restoration.

a) The most common factor is the patient's desire for an esthetic restoration. Esthetic requirements include the shade and translucency of the restoration and influence the selection of the restorative material to be used.

b) The attrition (wear) rate of the restoration should be considered.

c) Biocompatibility of the material must be considered.

d) Location of the margins of a restoration may be placed above the gingiva or in the gingival sulcus. Margin location affects esthetics, retention, periodontal response to the restoration, and likelihood of recurrent caries.

B. Preparation

The tooth or teeth are prepared with specific restorative materials in mind. Different materials require different amounts of tooth reduction and shapes of the margins. Amalgam and inlay preparations are shown in Figure 1.3. Crown preparations are shown in Figures 1.10*B* and 8.1*A*.

C. Impressions

After the preparation is complete, an impression of the preparation, adjacent teeth, and opposing teeth

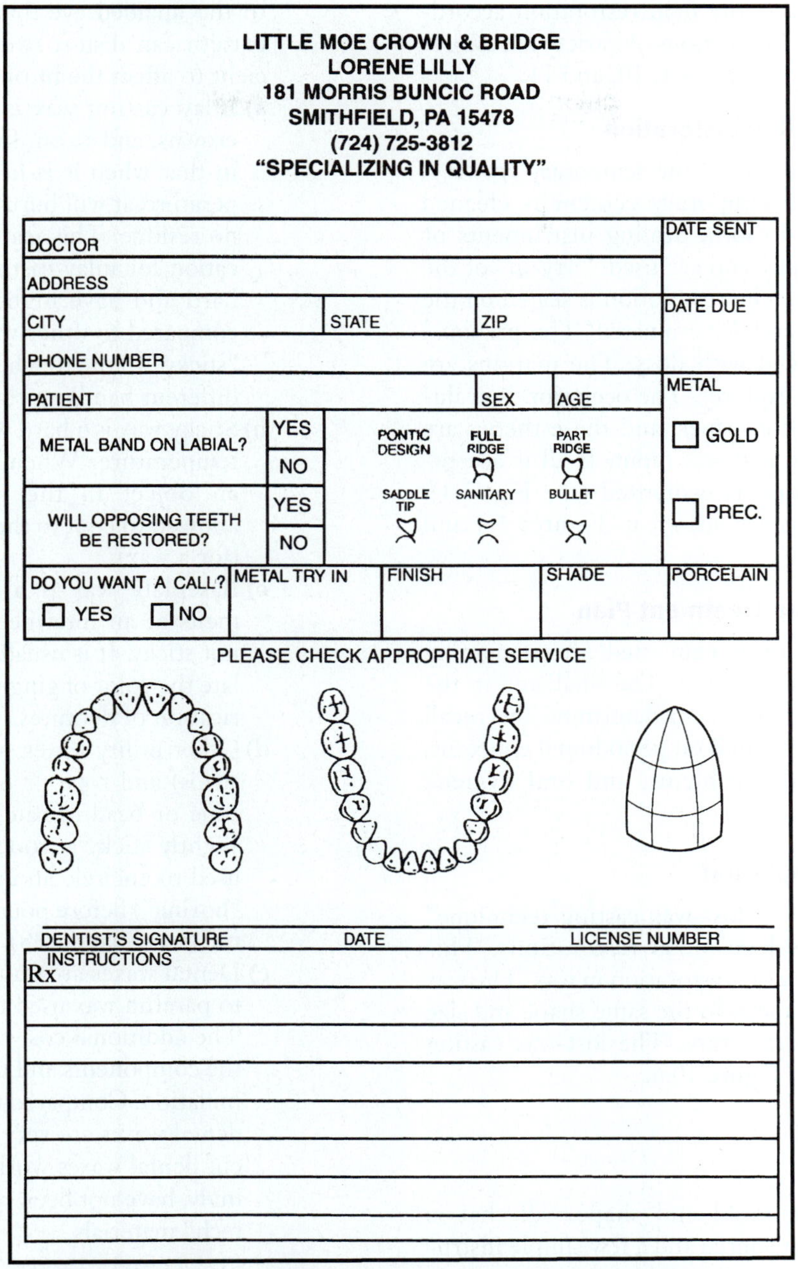
LITTLE MOE CROWN & BRIDGE
LORENE LILLY
181 MORRIS BUNCIC ROAD
SMITHFIELD, PA 15478
(724) 725-3812
"SPECIALIZING IN QUALITY"

DOCTOR
ADDRESS
CITY | STATE | ZIP
PHONE NUMBER
PATIENT | SEX | AGE
DATE SENT
DATE DUE
METAL
☐ GOLD
☐ PREC.
METAL BAND ON LABIAL? YES / NO
WILL OPPOSING TEETH BE RESTORED? YES / NO
PONTIC DESIGN
FULL RIDGE
PART RIDGE
SADDLE TIP
SANITARY
BULLET
DO YOU WANT A CALL? ☐ YES ☐ NO
METAL TRY IN
FINISH
SHADE
PORCELAIN
PLEASE CHECK APPROPRIATE SERVICE
DENTIST'S SIGNATURE
DATE
LICENSE NUMBER
INSTRUCTIONS
Rx

FIGURE 10.5 A laboratory prescription. (Courtesy of Lorene Lilly, Smithfield, PA.)

is taken. Full arch impressions result in more accurate articulation of models and less adjustment of the restoration before cementation. Several impressions were shown in Figure 1.8*A* and in Chapter 8.

D. Fabrication of a Temporary Restoration

The patient will not like the appearance and feel of the prepared tooth. In addition, exposed dentin can be very sensitive to heat, cold, and air. A **temporary restoration** (also called a **provisional restoration**) is constructed and cemented at the time of preparation, as shown in Figure 1.10*C*. The temporary restoration is left in place until the final restoration is received from the lab and permanently cemented. Chapter 35 presents techniques for the fabrication of a temporary crown.

E. Laboratory Procedures

The description and design of the restoration is written on a laboratory prescription (Fig. 10.5). This prescription becomes a part of the patient record. Impressions are disinfected, then poured in the dental office or a commercial laboratory. The laboratory constructs the final restoration according to the dentist's instructions. A variety of restorations are shown in Chapters 1, 10, and 11.

F. Cementation of the Restoration

At a second appointment, the temporary crown is removed, and the temporary cement is cleaned from the prepared tooth. Scaling instruments or pumice and a prophy cup are used. "Try-in" of the restoration is next. The restoration is seated on the preparation and carefully evaluated. The proximal contacts are checked with floss. The margins are examined with an explorer. The occlusion is evaluated with articulation paper; and the esthetics are examined with the patient's input. If all is acceptable, the restoration is cemented (see Fig. 7.1). Completed crowns are shown in Figures 1.4 and 1.10*E*.

G. Completion of the Treatment Plan

After the restoration is cemented, the remaining treatment plan is completed. The final step in the treatment plan should be to determine the recall status of the patient based on periodontal concerns, caries risk, chronic problems, and oral hygiene home care practices.

V. Casting Process—Optional

Dentistry has used the "lost-wax casting technique" for a century to produce metal restorations. This process first constructs the restoration in wax. The wax is then replaced with metal in the same shape and size as the original tooth structure. The lost-wax casting technique is shown in Figure 10.6.

A. Wax and Waxing

1. Waxing

Wax is easy to mold and shape. All that is required is a heat source and a few simple instruments. Creating the shape of the restoration in wax (**wax pattern**) requires skill and involves both the art and the science of dentistry, as shown in Figure 10.6*A*. The art is creating a reproduction of the shape of the lost tooth structure. The science is the requirement for the shape to function as the original tooth structure did (or should).

2. Dental Waxes

Dentistry uses a variety of waxes with different melting, working, and handling properties. Several are shown in Figure 10.7. The composition of a wax product is usually proprietary and is typically a combination of natural and synthetic waxes. Wax is very soft compared to other dental materials. Distortion of wax is not typically visible to the unaided eye, but wax is unstable. A wax pattern can distort over time to a degree sufficient to affect the fit of restorations.

a) Inlay casting wax is used for casting inlays, crowns, and so on. Inlay casting wax is unique in that when it is heated to a sufficient temperature, it will burn away completely, leaving no residue. This feature is part of the specification for inlay casting wax. These waxes are hard and have higher melting temperatures compared to other waxes. Inlay waxes are not "sticky" to the touch. Other dental waxes have different handling characteristics.

b) Sticky wax is a hard wax that melts at a higher temperature. When sticky wax is applied to an object in the molten state and then allowed to cool to the solid state, it sticks well (for a wax).

c) Baseplate wax is a medium-hard wax that melts at an intermediate temperature and is not sticky. It is usually pink in color (to simulate the color of gingiva) and is used in the fabrication of dentures.

d) Other utility waxes, such as boxing wax (wide strips) and rope or beading wax (like a small rope or bead of caulk), are soft, flexible, and slightly sticky at room temperature. They are used to encircle an impression (also known as "boxing") before pouring with a gypsum material (see Chapter 28).

e) Dental waxes are quite costly when compared to paraffin wax used to preserve jelly and jam. The additional cost results from the purity of the components and the complexity of the formulation. Compared to other dental materials, dental waxes are very inexpensive. The different dental waxes work quite well and, surprisingly, have not been replaced by newer, "high-tech" materials.

B. Investing and Investments

1. Investing Procedures

The casting process requires a mold space into which the molten metal flows. Embedding the wax pattern in a mold material, as shown in Figure 10.6 *D* and 10.6*E*, makes the mold space. The wax pattern is the exact size and shape that the resulting casting will be. A **sprue** is a plastic or metal tube that will create an opening (or **ingate**) for the mold. It is attached to the wax pattern, as shown in Figure 10.6*A*. With the sprue used for support, the wax pattern is attached to the sprue base, as shown in Figure 10.6*B*. The casting ring, as shown in Figure 10.6*C*, is placed over the sprued wax pattern and then filled with investment material. A casting

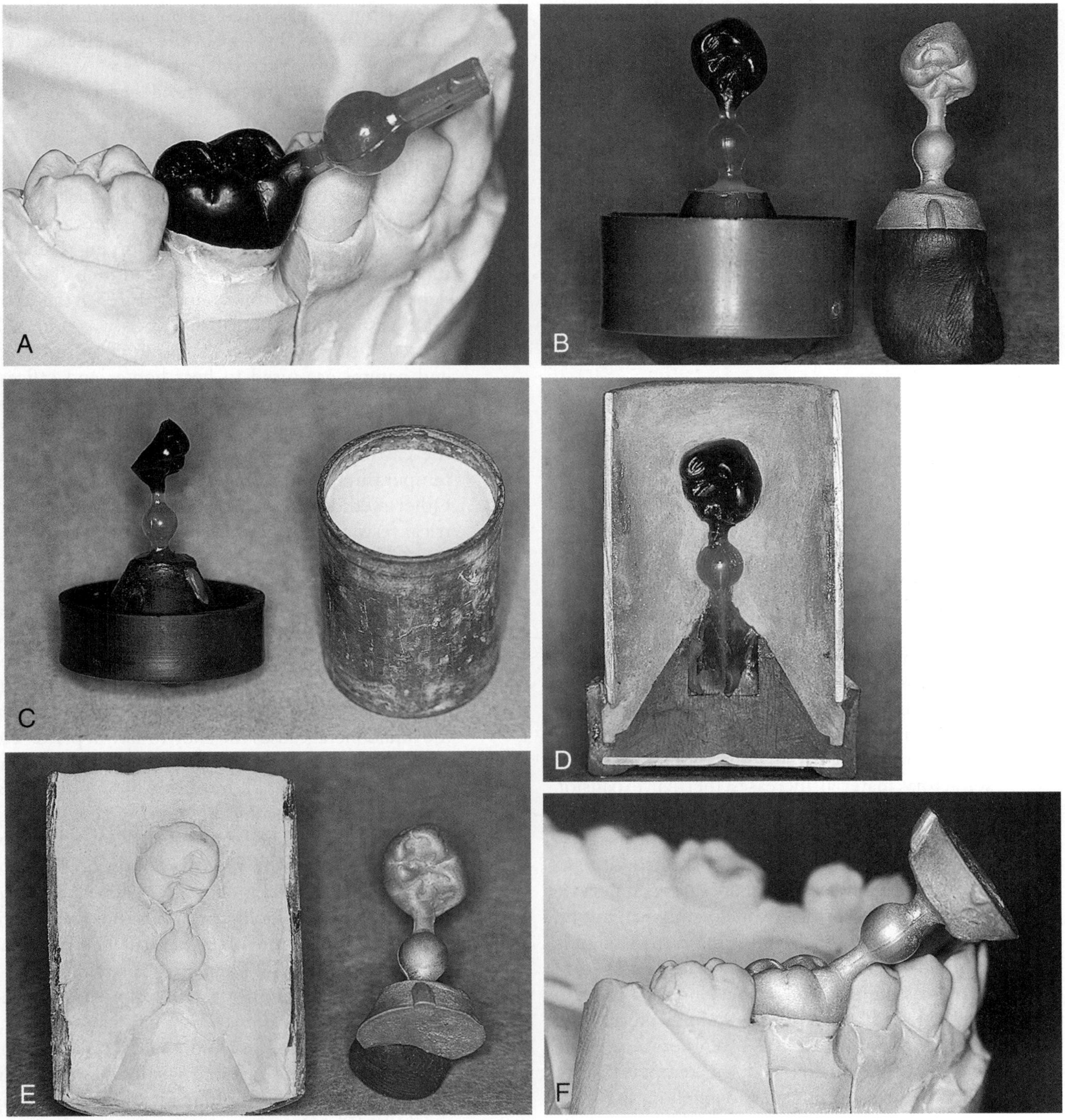

FIGURE 10.6 Photographs showing the fabrication of a full gold crown (the same crown as shown in Figures 1.4 and 8.1). **A.** Wax pattern with the sprue attached. **B.** Wax pattern attached to the sprue base (also called crucible former) and the casting. Note the reproduction of shape and size. **C.** Wax pattern and casting ring with a paper liner. The casting ring slips over the wax pattern and fits into the sprue base. **D.** Sprued and invested wax pattern inside a sectioned casting ring. **E.** Cross section through a casting ring after burnout and a completed casting. **F.** Completed casting on the die.

ring is used to form the outside of the mold, as shown in Figure 10.6*D*. The sprue and sprue base are removed, and the mold space is actually formed by the investment material. The invested pattern is heated, and the wax is melted and flows out of the mold. As the temperature rises, any residual wax is burned away. This heating procedure is called "wax burnout." Burnout results in a mold space into which the metal is cast, as shown in Figure 10.6*E*.

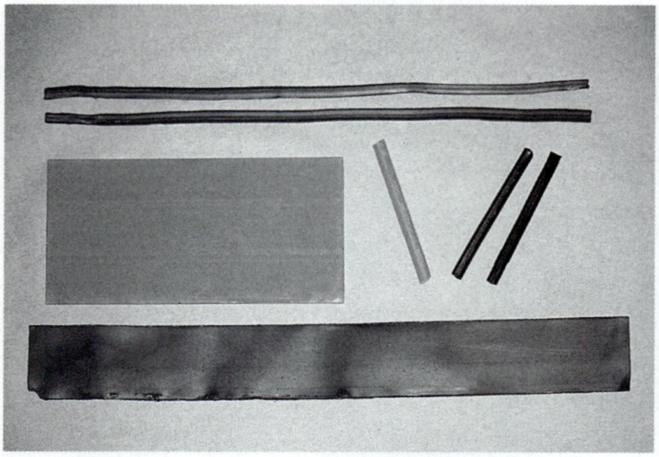

FIGURE 10.7 Photograph of several dental waxes: rope wax (*top*), baseplate wax (*middle left*), sticky wax (*middle center*), inlay wax (*middle right*), and boxing wax (*bottom*).

2. Investment Materials

The most common investment materials are gypsum-based products. The same handling characteristics discussed in Chapter 9 for gypsum products apply to gypsum-bonded investments. A silica material is added to dental stone to produce **gypsum-bonded investments.** The silica material improves the investment's resistance to heat and is called a refractory material. A second (and equally important) function is that the refractory material increases thermal expansion of the mold. The mold must be expanded to compensate exactly for the thermal shrinkage of the solid metal casting as it cools to room temperature. If mold expansion does not compensate for the thermal shrinkage, the casting will not fit. Metals typically shrink much more than ceramic materials. Luckily, the silica materials used in dental casting investments have unusual thermal properties. They exhibit a sudden increase in expansion at an elevated temperature. The amount of expansion and the temperature at which the expansion occurs depend on the silica material used in the investment. Different investment materials expand by different amounts at various temperatures.

C. Burnout

A temperature-controlled oven is used to burn out the wax pattern invested in the casting ring. The proper burnout temperature will result in proper mold expansion and a well-fitting casting. The casting ring is placed in the oven, and the mold is heated to 500 to 600°C (900–1,100°F). The wax melts and is volatilized, leaving a clean mold space. The casting ring is left in the oven after reaching the desired temperature for approximately 30 minutes to 1 hour to "heat soak" the ring. Heat soaking the ring assures that the entire wax pattern has burned out and that the mold has reached the desired temperature.

D. Casting

Several types of equipment are used to make dental castings (Fig. 10.8). The casting process involves melting the casting alloy and then forcing it into the mold space. The technique used to melt the alloy depends on the melting temperature of the alloy. Gold casting alloys for all-metal crowns are easily melted with a "blow torch" using compressed air and natural gas (used to heat homes and offices). The alloy is melted while sitting in a refractory ceramic device, called a **crucible,** which is part of the casting machine. Alloys with higher melting temperatures require oxygen or acetylene gas. Other methods to melt casting alloys include electrical resistance heating (as in a toaster) and induction melting.

The most common casting machine used to force molten alloy into the mold is called a centrifugal casting machine. It rapidly spins the mold, crucible, and molten alloy in a circle. Casting occurs when spinning suddenly starts. While the crucible, molten alloy, and mold are rapidly accelerated, the inertia of the liquid metal causes the alloy to stay in place. The alloy seems to flow out of the spinning crucible and into the spinning mold. In reality, the molten metal stays in place; the casting ring spins and collides with the molten alloy. The liquid metal is forced to flow into the ingate of the ring previously occupied by the sprue. The molten alloy flows down the sprue space and into the mold, and it fills the space previously occupied by the wax pattern. When the metal cools, it solidifies, and the casting is complete.

The most common casting machine has a coiled spring that is wound up. The energy stored in the wound spring is used to rapidly spin (accelerate) the rotating arm of the casting machine. The mold is accelerated into the molten metal as the spring unwinds. The rotating arm is composed of two parts connected by a pivot point; thus, this device is called a "broken-arm" casting machine. The pivoting of the arm keeps it at the proper angle to allow the molten alloy to flow into the mold.

Other types of casting machines use a vacuum or compressed air to force the molten metal into the mold. The crucible and casting ring are stationary; only the molten metal moves. Details of spruing, investing, and casting are beyond the scope of this textbook; interested readers are referred to the excellent dental materials texts in the suggested readings section of this chapter.

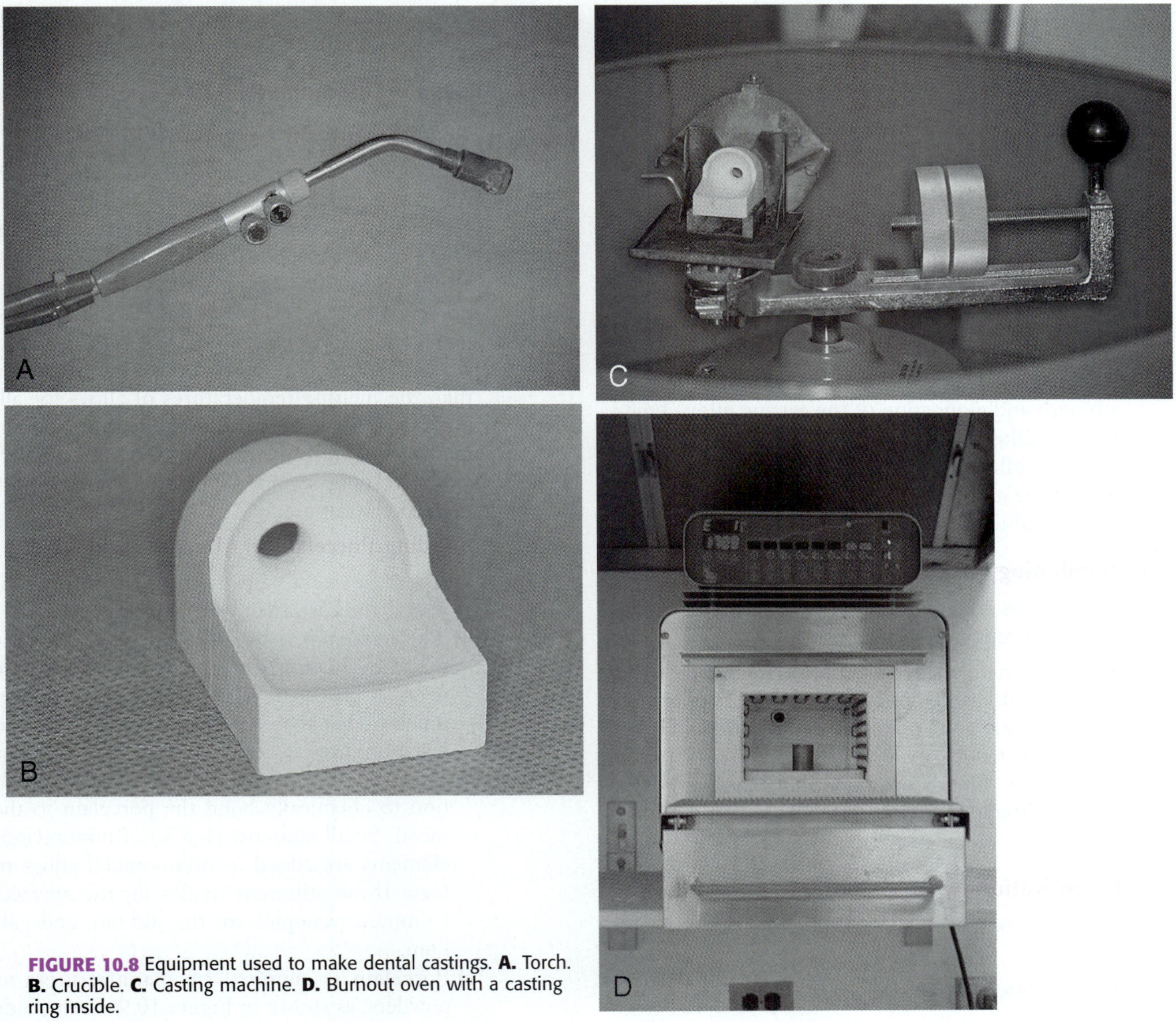

FIGURE 10.8 Equipment used to make dental castings. **A.** Torch. **B.** Crucible. **C.** Casting machine. **D.** Burnout oven with a casting ring inside.

E. Divesting, Finishing, and Polishing

After cooling, the casting is retrieved (or **"divested"**) from the ring by carving away the investment and exposing the casting. The casting is cleaned, as shown in Figure 10.6*F*. The metal that represents the sprue and casting button (excess metal) is cut off and can be reused. The casting is finished and polished, as shown in Figure 1.4. This is done by using a variety of abrasives and is described in Chapter 16.

VI. Alloys for All-Metal Cast Restorations

Cast metal restorations use alloys rather than pure metals. **Alloys** are metals that are a combination of several elements. Traditionally, casting alloys for all-metal restorations have been gold alloys, thus the name full gold crown or gold inlay. Pure gold is not used because it is too soft. Gold (~75% by weight) is combined with copper (~5%), silver (~10%), palladium (~2%), zinc (~1%), and other elements to form high-noble dental alloys. Percentages of elements vary depending on the type of casting alloy and the manufacturer. Gold alloys are easily cast with gypsum-bonded investments and relatively simple equipment.

The properties of dental casting alloys are described in the American Dental Association (ADA) specification. The specification has no composition requirements but does have performance criteria for strength, elongation, tarnish, and biocompatibility. **Elongation** is a measure of the ability of a material to be stretched before it breaks. Elongation is used to predict the ability of an alloy to be burnished. **Burnishing** margins of soft, malleable gold restoration pushes the metal against the tooth to close any gap between the tooth and the casting. Therefore, a margin or gap between the restoration and the tooth becomes smaller when it is burnished. Less cement is needed to fill in the space. Because dental cements are much more soluble than casting alloys, the likelihood of recurrent caries during clinical service is decreased when margins are burnished.

A. ADA Classification of Casting Alloys for All-Metal Restorations—Optional

Four types of casting alloys are described in the ADA specification: Types I, II, III, and IV. The differences between them are predominantly the strength and elongation of the casting alloy. Type I is the weakest, has the greatest elongation, and is used for inlays. Type IV is the strongest, has the least elongation, and is used for high-stress bridges and partial denture frameworks.

B. Terminology Used to Describe Metals

Many terms are used to describe metals. Some have precise meaning; others do not.

1. Metals are classified as noble elements based on their lack of chemical reactivity. The noble metals include gold, platinum, palladium, and other inert metals.
2. Precious metals are classified based on their cost. Precious metals are the noble metals and silver.

C. Classification by Gold Content

The gold content of alloys can be described several ways.

1. Percentage is parts per 100.
2. Carat is parts per 24.
3. Fineness is parts per 1,000.

Therefore:

$$75\% = 18 \text{ carat} = 750 \text{ fine}$$

D. Classification by Composition—Optional

Dental alloys for all-metal restorations can be classified by their composition.

1. High-gold or high-noble alloys contain 60% or more gold and other noble elements. They are usually yellow metals.
2. Low-gold or low-noble alloys contain at least 25% noble metals, with gold typically being replaced by increased silver content. Low-gold alloys are yellow or white metals.
3. A third group is the silver–palladium alloys, with approximately 70% silver and 25% palladium. These alloys are white (silver) in color.
4. Alloys with less than 25% noble elements are called predominantly base metals.
5. The term "nonprecious" is used to describe alloys without any noble elements.

E. Alloys for Ceramometal Restorations

1. Requirements for Ceramometal Alloys

Casting alloys for ceramometal restorations have the same mechanical and biocompatibility requirements as alloys for all-metal restorations. One exception is elongation because it is not usually considered to be important when bonding porcelain to metal. The ceramometal alloy must withstand the very high porcelain firing temperatures. These temperatures are much higher than the melting temperatures of alloys for all-metal cast restorations. It is important that the metal not melt or distort because the ceramometal alloy supports the porcelain during firing and clinical use.

2. Bonding Porcelain to Metal—Optional

a) After the metal substructure (or **coping**) is waxed and cast, the metal surface is cleaned.

b) The next step is to oxide the surface of the metal by heating the casting in a porcelain oven. A porcelain oven reaches temperatures much higher than a typical burnout oven and has more precise temperature control. Adherent oxides form on the metal surface and function to chemically bond the porcelain to the metal. Small amounts (1–5%) of nonprecious elements are added to ceramometal alloys to form these adherent oxides on the surface. Common examples are tin, indium, and gallium.

c) Porcelain is supplied by manufacturers as powders, as shown in Figure 10.9. Each shade has its own powder. Porcelain powders are applied (or stacked) in layers. Each layer has esthetic properties to simulate the appearance of the layers of teeth, dentin, and enamel, as shown in Figure 10.10.

d) The first porcelain layer that is applied hides the color of the metal. It is called the opaque layer and covers the gray, oxidized surface of the metal. The opaque layer is fired before adding subsequent layers of porcelain.

e) The second porcelain layer is the dentin or body porcelain shade or shades. These porcelains make up the bulk of the restoration. More than one shade of body porcelain may be used because a single tooth may vary in shade between different locations on the same tooth.

f) After the body layer, the enamel or translucent layer is applied. This is the most translucent of the porcelain materials and gives the restoration a more natural appearance.

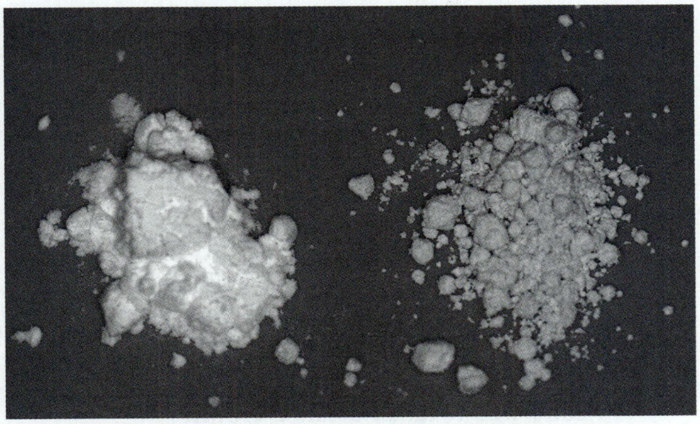

FIGURE 10.9 Two shades of opaque porcelain powder.

g) Each layer may be fired separately or in combination with another layer. Dental porcelains are fired at very high temperatures, such as 850 to 1,100°C (1,550–2,000°F). Constructing a ceramometal restoration typically involves three to five firings.

h) The procedures for bonding porcelain to metal can be found at the Vident website, http://www.vident.com/assets/downloads_cloak/VMK_95(905e).pdf.

3. Sintering Porcelain

Firing porcelain causes the powders to become **"sintered."** Sintering changes the porcelain from a powder to a solid. The powder is not melted, so the general shape is maintained. The process of sintering is similar to that of making a snowball. The snow is not melted; instead, the snow is compacted together. Sintering porcelain is the same process that is used to fire clay pots, china, and ceramic tiles. Reducing the porosity of the resulting product is very important. The less porous (more dense) the product is, the greater the strength of the final product will be.

After sintering, the final shape of the restoration is refined by grinding. Stains and glazes can be applied and fired to produce the shade detailed in the laboratory prescription.

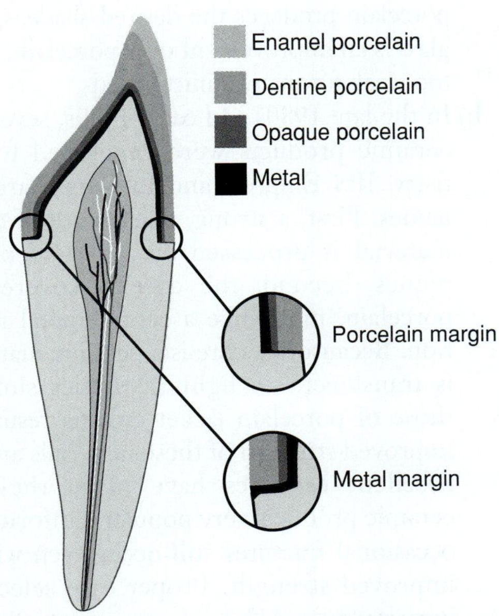

FIGURE 10.10 Illustration of porcelain layers used in construction of a ceramometal crown. A metal margin is shown on the lingual and a porcelain margin on the facial.

4. Types of Ceramometal Alloys

Ceramometal alloys can be classified in many ways. The following is one example.

a) Noble Alloys

The high-noble alloys for all-metal restorations were modified for porcelain bonding. Gold (~88%)–platinum (~4%)–palladium (~6%) alloys were developed first. No (or very little) silver and no copper are used. These alloys are yellow in color (like gold alloys for all-metal restorations) but have a higher melting temperature to withstand porcelain application firings.

Gold (~50%)–palladium (~40%) alloys are white in color. They possess better mechanical properties than gold platinum–palladium alloys. Today, these are the noble alloys of choice for ceramometal restorations.

Palladium (~60%)–silver (~30%) alloys are less costly and are white metals.

High-palladium (~80%) alloys are also white in color. They are less costly than the gold-containing ceramometal alloys but more expensive than the palladium–silver alloys.

b) Nonprecious Alloys

Nickel (~80%)–chromium (~10%) alloys are white in color and have higher melting temperatures than the noble ceramometal alloys. They tend to be stronger and harder than the noble ceramometal alloys and are much less expensive.

Chromium (~65%)–cobalt (~25%) alloys are also white and inexpensive. They have the highest melting temperatures and are the most difficult to cast. Their mechanical properties are similar to those of the strongest nickel–chromium alloys.

VII. Titanium

Titanium is the most biocompatible metal. As a result, a great deal of effort has been devoted to developing materials and methods that would allow crowns, bridges, and partial denture frameworks to be made from titanium. Current titanium use is limited. It will most likely increase in the future as titanium restorations become easier to produce. Titanium has been used as the material of choice for dental implants for decades. If handled properly, titanium can osseointegrate with bone. Osseointegration is a type of biologic bonding of bone to a material. Implants are discussed in Chapter 12.

VIII. Partial Denture Frameworks

A. Alloys

At one time, the frameworks of partial dentures were made with gold alloys. The large amount of metal required to construct a framework makes using gold alloys quite expensive. As a result, less expensive alloys from the aerospace industries, such as nickel–chromium and cobalt-chromium alloys, were adapted for removable partial denture frameworks. When the price of gold increased greatly again in the 1980s, these nonprecious alloys were modified for use as crown and bridge alloys. The high melting temperatures of these alloys require slightly different casting techniques and investment materials.

B. Silicate- and Phosphate-Bonded Investments

Silicate- and phosphate-bonded investments are used to cast high-melting partial denture framework alloys and ceramometal alloys. They can withstand much higher burnout temperatures and are more difficult to use than gypsum-bonded investments.

IX. Ceramic Restorative Materials

Dentistry has been in love with porcelain ceramic materials for more than a century. The shades and translucency of porcelain materials are unmatched in their ability to simulate the appearance of teeth.

A. Porcelain

Porcelain jacket crowns were the first all-ceramic restoration used in dentistry. The entire crown is made of porcelain, as shown in Figures 1.10*E* and 1.10*F*. Unfortunately, the mechanical properties of this brittle material are inadequate for restoring most areas of the mouth. However, the outstanding esthetics of porcelain have maintained an interest in ceramic materials.

Porcelain jacket crowns are made by applying porcelain powders in layers onto a thin layer of platinum foil that is adapted to the die. Platinum is an element with a very high melting temperature. The foil supports the porcelain powder during firing and is removed from the inside of the completed crown. No metal remains. A very translucent and natural appearing restoration results.

B. Techniques to Strengthen Porcelain Materials

1. Ceramometal

To strengthen the porcelain, it is bonded to metal. The advantages of metal include tough mechanical properties and the ability to obtain a precise fit of the crown to the preparation. The disadvantage is that metals are opaque to light, even when used in very thin layers. Light is not transmitted through the restoration as it is through tooth structure. Therefore, a ceramometal restoration is not as natural or life-like in appearance compared to an all-ceramic crown.

2. Aluminous Porcelain

Alumina (alumina oxide) was added to porcelain to increase strength. Alumina is a very strong ceramic material, and its addition slightly increases strength and clinical performance without affecting esthetics. Unfortunately, this marginal improvement was not sufficient enough.

3. Improvements in All-Ceramic Restorations—Optional

The search for stronger ceramic materials resulted in significant improvements in all-ceramic restorations. Several types of materials resulted.

a) First, castable glass materials were developed. The glass is cast much like metals are cast and is then given a strengthening heat treatment. This dental material is similar to the material used to make CorningWare® baking dishes and is called Dicor. It was developed by Corning and is marketed by Dentsply. Only one white, translucent shade of castable glass is produced. Veneering the cast glass with a thin layer of proper-shade porcelain produces the desired shade. Castable glass is an improvement over porcelain, but it is too weak for many clinical needs.

b) In the late 1980s and early 1990s, several new ceramic products were developed for dentistry. IPS Empress and In-Ceram are brand names. First, a strong, dense core of ceramic material is processed by a variety of techniques. Second, the core is covered with porcelain, much like a ceramometal restoration. Because the core is a ceramic material, it is translucent to light. Esthetics similar to those of porcelain jacket crowns result. The improved strength of these materials and their excellent esthetics have made these new ceramic products very popular. Unfortunately, occasional fractures still occur even with this improved strength. Proper case selection is important.

c) Computer-aided design/computer-aided manufacture (CAD/CAM) has been developed for dentistry. An "optical" impression, rather than a physical impression, of the preparation is made, and the restoration is machined out of a solid, single-shade piece of ceramic material via computer control. This technology is still being developed and may become an important technique for the manufacture of ceramic restorations in the future. This technology has been adapted for use with other materials, such as metals and composites.

X. Advantages and Disadvantages of All-Metal/ Ceramometal/Ceramic Restorations

A. Fracture

An all-metal restoration is least likely to fracture compared to ceramometal and ceramic restorations. Metals are tough, and fractures of metallic restorations are quite rare. On the other hand, all-ceramic restorations do fail and are only recommended for certain teeth. Restorations for teeth that do not experience high occlusal forces, such as a maxillary lateral incisor, have high success rates. Restorations for teeth that do experience high occlusal forces, such as first molars, have much lower success rates. Materials for all-ceramic restorations have improved greatly in recent years, and their use in moderate-stress areas of the mouth, such as anterior teeth and premolars, has been successful.

Ceramometal restorations are used in all areas of the mouth. Fracture of the porcelain is not common, but this is the most frequent mechanical failure. Mechanical failure of the metal substructure almost never occurs. Depending on the complexity of the restoration and the location of the porcelain fracture, this may be a nuisance or a disaster.

B. Esthetics

All-metal restorations may have acceptable or unacceptable esthetics depending on the location of the restoration and the patient's preferences. Ceramometal restorations adequately simulate the natural dentition in most situations. All-ceramic restorations reproduce the translucency of the natural dentition better than ceramometal restorations. All-ceramic restorations have the most life-like appearance of all restorative materials.

C. Wear

Unfortunately, the ceramic materials that are used for ceramometal and all-ceramic restorations are very hard. They wear the opposing enamel much more than enamel or gold alloys. The softer gold alloys wear opposing enamel much like enamel does.

D. Margins

Casting techniques for metals result in more accurate margins than those for all-ceramic restorations. An excessive gap at the margin of an all-ceramic restoration increases the risk of recurrent caries. Luckily, modern dentistry has composite cements to fill the marginal gap of ceramic restorations.

E. Selecting Materials

Advantages and disadvantages exist for each restorative material and must be assessed on a case-by-case basis. The patient should be made aware of the "pros" and "cons" of each type of material and be included in the decision. It must be emphasized that proper handling of all dental materials by all dental personnel is important to the success of any procedure.

SUMMARY

Fixed indirect restorations may be classified in two ways: by the amount of tooth structure restored or by the material from which they are made. Inlays, onlays, veneers, crowns, and dental bridges comprise the classifications based on the amount of tooth structure restored. Metals, ceramics, ceramometal, and composites comprise the classifications based on the material.

This chapter also discusses the procedures for constructing an indirect restoration, from diagnosis and treatment planning to casting and final cementation of the restoration. Classifications of alloys for all metal restorations include the ADA classification and others.

Ceramometal restorations involve many steps because the porcelain must be bonded to the metal. Ceramometal alloys include the noble and nonprecious alloys.

Porcelain crowns are an all-ceramic restoration that is unmatched regarding ability to simulate the natural appearance of teeth. However, the mechanical properties of porcelain crowns limit their use mostly to anterior teeth. Other ceramic materials have been developed that have good esthetic properties and better mechanical properties.

Composite indirect materials include particle-reinforced and fiber-reinforced composites. These materials are processed in dental laboratories by using pressure and heat to improve their polymerization and usefulness in dentistry.

Each of the all the metal, ceramometal, and ceramic restorations has both advantages and disadvantages. Areas of concern include fracture, esthetics, effects of wear, margins, and area of use.

Learning Activities

1. Assume that a member of the class needs to have a tooth restored with a crown. Discuss the advantages and disadvantages of the possible options for a maxillary lateral incisor, maxillary premolar, and mandibular molar.
2. Describe the clinical procedures necessary to construct an all-metal or a ceramometal crown.

Review Questions

1. If a mold that is created for investing and casting does not ____________ to compensate for the action of the metal alloy, the casting will not fit.
   a) Contract
   b) Equate
   c) Expand
   d) None of the above.
2. The most obvious purpose of the investment is to:
   a) Enlarge the mold by hygroscopic expansion
   b) Enlarge the mold by thermal expansion
   c) Form the mold for the casting
   d) Provide compensation for contraction
3. Porcelain is "best suited" for which of the following?
   a) Full coverage posterior crowns
   b) MODFL onlays
   c) Veneers on anterior teeth
   d) MOD inlays
4. The crown(s) portion of a dental bridge is called the:
   a) Pontic
   b) Retainer
   c) Abutment
   d) Fixed partial denture
5. Which of the following waxes is hard, leaves no burnout residue, and has a higher melting temperature?
   a) Boxing
   b) Rope
   c) Sticky
   d) Baseplate
   e) Inlay
6. During the casting procedure, a wax pattern is heated, and the wax melts and flows out of the mold. As the temperature continues to rise, any residual wax is burned away. This heating procedure is called:
   a) Shrinkage compensation
   b) Investing
   c) Burnout
   d) Crucible heating
7. Identify the correct sequence in the centrifugal casting process.
   a) Add sprue to pattern, place in crucible former, invest, and then cast
   b) Add sprue to pattern, invest, place in crucible former, and then cast
   c) Place sprue in crucible former, add pattern to sprue, invest, and then cast
   d) Place sprue in crucible former, invest, add pattern to sprue, and then cast
8. A 33% gold alloy may also be expressed as:
   a) 10 carat
   b) 16 carat
   c) 333 fine
   d) 33 fine
9. The term used to define the process of firing porcelain powder to become a solid is:
   a) Liquidating
   b) Sintering
   c) Burnishing
   d) Investing
10. One type of an all-ceramic restoration is castable glass. All-ceramic restorations are superior to ceramometal restorations in all respects.
    a) The first statement is true; the second statement is false.
    b) The first statement is false; the second statement is true.
    c) Both statements are true.
    d) Both statements are false.
11. Which of the following is considered to be a fixed indirect restoration?
    a) Amalgam
    b) Direct gold (gold foil)
    c) Onlay
    d) Composite

12. A restorative material that is placed on the facial surface of anterior teeth to "cover" or hide an esthetic problem is called a (an):
a) Coping
b) Veneer
c) Buildup (core)
d) Pontic

13. Another name for a provisional restoration is a ________________ restoration.
a) Conditional
b) Non-permanent
c) Buildup
d) Temporary

14. Silver is classified as a ______________ metal.
a) Non-precious
b) High-noble
c) Precious
d) Noble

15. An advantage of bonding porcelain to metal is:
a) A precise fit of the metal
b) The resulting opacity
c) The resulting translucency
d) Ease in plaque removal

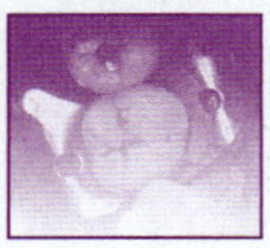

Supplemental Readings

Anusavice KJ. Phillips' Science of Dental Materials. 11th ed. Philadelphia: Saunders, 2003, Chapters 20–23 and 26.
Christensen G. Longevity Vs esthetics in restorative dentistry. J Am Dent Assoc 1998;129:1023–1024.
Farah JW, Powers JM, eds. 20 years of all-ceramic restorations: 1982–2002. Dent Advisor 2002;19(8):1–6.
Powers JM & Sakaguchi RL, eds. Craig's Restorative Dental Materials. 12th ed. St. Louis: Mosby, 2006, Chapter 14–19.
Wataha JC. Biocompatibility of dental casting alloys: a review. J Prosthet Dent 2000;83:223–234.

11

Removable Prostheses and Acrylic Resins

Key Words/Phrases

acrylic resins
chemically activated
cold-cure
complete denture
denture base
denture setup
flask
full denture
heat-activated
immediate denture
monomer
relining
removable partial denture
vertical dimension
wax try-in

Objectives

After studying this chapter, the student will be able to do the following:

1. List the uses of acrylic resins in dentistry.
2. Explain the physical and chemical stages of polymerization of acrylic resins.
3. Describe the function of the components of heat-cure and cold-cure acrylic resin systems.
4. Describe the steps involved in construction of a denture.
5. Summarize the procedures used to reline a denture.
6. Explain a dental hygienist's role in maintenance of an acrylic prosthesis.

INTRODUCTION

As with a fixed bridge, a removable denture is a prosthesis; it replaces missing teeth. This chapter will present materials and procedures that are used to construct removable prostheses: partial and complete dentures. Alloys used for partial denture frameworks are very similar to those presented in Chapter 10. This chapter will focus on acrylic materials and their use.

I. Acrylic Resins

A. What Is an Acrylic Resin?

Acrylic resins are hard, brittle, glassy polymers. The commercial plastic called Plexiglas is an acrylic resin product. Acrylic resin is clear and colorless, making it an excellent replacement material for glass in storm doors. Acrylic resins are easily colored. Technically, acrylic resins are classified as thermoplastic materials, and many commercial products are made by injection molding acrylic materials. In dentistry, however, acrylic resins are handled more like a thermoset material; after it sets, it is not heated and molded.

The most common acrylic monomer is methyl methacrylate, as shown in Figure 5.4*A*. Note the C=C bond in this illustration. Acrylic resins are long chains of such monomers. The chains have side groups that inhibit chain slippage and result in mechanical properties that provide more strength than polymer chains without side groups. Polyethylene (the same material used in "plastic" sandwich bags) is an example of a polymer without side groups.

B. Acrylic Resins as Biomaterials

Acrylic resins were developed in the 1930s and were first used in dentistry in the 1940s. They quickly replaced those materials previously used in the construction of dentures, shown in Figure 1.6. They were also used (without success) as a direct restorative material. They have been adapted for many other uses in dentistry. Their handling characteristics and mechanical properties are quite satisfactory for a variety of applications. These uses include temporary crowns, as shown in Figure 1.10*C*; custom trays, as shown in Figure 8.2; and baseplates for denture construction, to be presented later in this chapter.

It is interesting to note that a dental biomaterials scientist (Dennis Smith) suggested to an orthopedic surgeon (John Charnley) that acrylic resin would be a good material to cement artificial joints in place. In the 1960s, acrylic resin was introduced as the first bone cement and was used in hip replacements. Today, acrylic resin is still commonly used to cement hip prostheses and other orthopedic devices to bone.

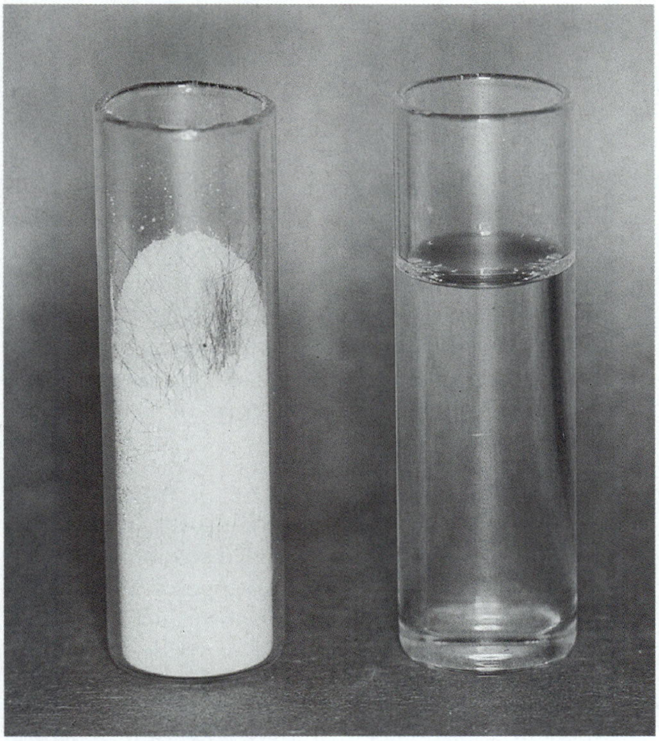

FIGURE 11.1 Photograph of an acrylic resin system, powder, and liquid.

II. Acrylic Resin Systems Used in Dentistry

Acrylic resin systems set by addition polymerization in the same manner as dental composites, which were discussed in Chapter 5. The same terms and classifications are used. They are based on the method used to initiate polymerization.

A. Cold-Cure or Chemically Activated Acrylic Resins

Cold-cure or **chemically activated** acrylic resin systems are supplied as a powder and a liquid, as shown in Figure 11.1. These are the same materials used for the "brush-bead" buildup technique for artificial nails. The typical components are listed in Table 11.1.

Table 11.1 Components of an Acrylic Resin System

	Cold (Chemical)-Cure	Heat-Cure
Liquid	Methyl methacrylate	Methyl methacrylate
	Hydroquinone	Hydroquinone
	Ethylene glycol	Ethylene glycol
	Tertiary amine	
Powder	Acrylic resin powder	Acrylic resin powder
	Benzoyl peroxide	Benzoyl peroxide
	Fibers and colorants	Fibers and colorants

1. Liquid

The liquid is mostly **monomer,** methyl methacrylate. A cross-linking agent, such as glycol dimethacrylate, is added. An inhibitor is always added to methyl methacrylate to prevent premature polymerization; hydroquinone is most commonly used. Methyl methacrylate is a powerful solvent. It can dissolve permanent marker (used for labeling things) and even some polymers. The ability of methyl methacrylate to dissolve acrylic resin, polymethyl methacrylate resin, is an important property that has a significant effect on the handling properties of acrylic resin systems.

2. Powder

The powder is predominantly polymethyl methacrylate resin with added colorants and benzoyl peroxide. It is usually composed of very small beads of acrylic resin, as shown in Figure 11.2. When activated, benzoyl peroxide forms free radicals to initiate polymerization.

3. Physical Changes During Setting

When the powder and liquid of an acrylic resin system are mixed, several stages in the setting process occur. These stages can be noticed when a sufficient mass of material is mixed as in the construction of a custom tray. During the initial stages, the changes are physical. The mixed powder and liquid have a "grainy" or "sandy" feel. The powder and liquid are separate phases. As some powder dissolves, the mixed material becomes thicker and less "runny." As more powder is dissolved, the material reaches the "dough" stage. At this point, the material is easy to handle and mold, and up to this point, the changes are mainly physical.

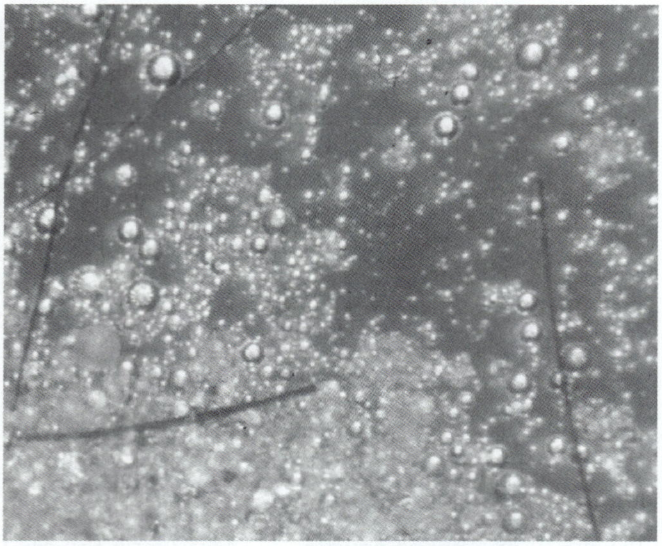

FIGURE 11.2 Low-power magnification photograph of acrylic resin powder. Note the fibers and the various sizes of beads. (Courtesy of E. M. Krouse, Department of Anatomy, West Virginia University, Morgantown, WV.)

4. Polymerization Reaction

A cold-cure or chemically activated system has an activator, typically a tertiary amine, added to the liquid. When the powder and liquid are mixed, the benzoyl peroxide and the tertiary amine react to produce free radicals. The inhibitor in the liquid destroys the free radicals that are initially produced, and working time results. This occurs while the material goes from a grainy to a dough stage.

When the inhibitor is used up, typically during the dough stage, chemical changes occur, and the polymerization reaction proceeds. The doughy material thickens and becomes stiffer. The reaction generates heat as well, and the material becomes warm. Many times when a mass of material is mixed as in the construction of a custom tray, the material becomes hot to the touch. The material becomes rigid and solid as polymerization reaches completion.

5. Residual Monomer

Initially, the set material contains some residual monomer. Any monomer that does not polymerize soon evaporates, leaving little or no monomer or unreacted double bonds in the set material.

6. Cross-Linking

Cross-linking the resin improves mechanical properties. A linear resin without any cross-linking agent is brittle. Addition of a cross-linking agent improves the toughness of the material.

B. Heat-Activated Acrylic Resins

1. Heat-activated acrylic resin systems are very similar to chemically activated systems. The major exception is that no chemical activator is present in the liquid. A minor difference is that less inhibitor is present in the liquid. The inhibitor is not needed to provide working time; it functions as a preservative, reacting with free radicals to prevent polymerization during storage.
2. **Heat-activated** systems are supplied as powder/liquid systems similar to those of cold-cure resins. When the powder and liquid are mixed, they go through the same initial stages of the setting process. Because no chemical activator is present, the mixed material stays in the dough stage for an extended period of time. Therefore, working time is much longer than it is for heat-cure acrylic resins. After the material is formed into the desired shape (to be explained later), the

material is heated in a water bath. The heat breaks down the benzoyl peroxide, forming free radicals. Polymerization proceeds by changing the dough into a rigid material. Products that are properly heat-cured are a bit stronger and tougher than cold-cure acrylic resins.

C. Light-Activated and Dual-Cure Acrylic Resins

Light-activated and dual-cure acrylic resin systems are available, but they are not as popular as light activated and dual-cure composites. Recently, light-activated and dual-cure composite materials for temporary crowns, custom trays, and other uses have been introduced. Because these composite materials are stronger, they are gaining acceptance. As prices decrease, they may completely replace acrylic resins for some uses.

D. Acrylic Resin Systems and Porosity

Regardless of the type of activation of an acrylic resin system, porosity is a major concern. Methyl methacrylate and other monomers evaporate easily at room temperature. If monomer evaporates during handling or processing, the resulting material will be porous, as shown in Figure 11.3. Porosity weakens the material. Also, the denture is likely to collect debris in pores and become foul. A great deal of effort is made to prevent porosity when acrylic resins are processed. Pressure and temperature controls are used to minimize porosity.

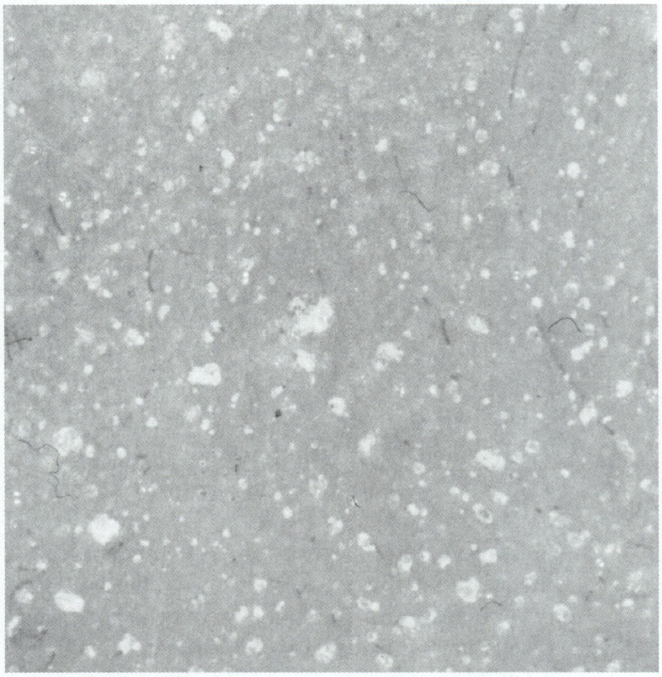

FIGURE 11.3 Close-up photograph showing porosity (*white spots*) in a poorly cured acrylic resin sample.

III. Complete Dentures

A **complete denture** or **full denture** replaces an entire arch of missing teeth, as shown in Figure 1.6. A complete denture also replaces alveolar bone, which is resorbed when teeth are missing. Dentures are made with acrylic materials that are colored to simulate the missing tissues.

Complete dentures are held in place by suction, which is the result of surface tension and atmospheric pressure. Therefore, a complete denture requires precise adaptation to the supporting tissues and a peripheral "seal" for adequate retention (like that of a suction cup). Saliva helps to achieve the seal and improves suction, just as water improves the effectiveness of a suction cup. An impression for a complete denture involves much effort to determine and record the supporting tissues and the proper extension of the denture borders. The borders of the denture that are recorded by the impression are reproduced in the denture. Proper extension of the borders of a denture determines the seal and much of the success of a denture. Most patients function reasonably well with an upper denture. The same cannot be said for lower complete dentures. The peripheral seal of a lower denture is much less effective than that of an upper denture. In addition, an upper denture has a larger surface-bearing area (the palate), and it usually has a better alveolar ridge to support the denture.

A. Components of a Denture

A complete denture has two major components: the white denture teeth and the pink denture base. Denture teeth, as shown in Figure 11.4, are purchased from a manufacturer. The denture base is made in the dental laboratory following the dentist's prescription; it is made on the master cast, which is a positive reproduction of the patient's alveolar ridge.

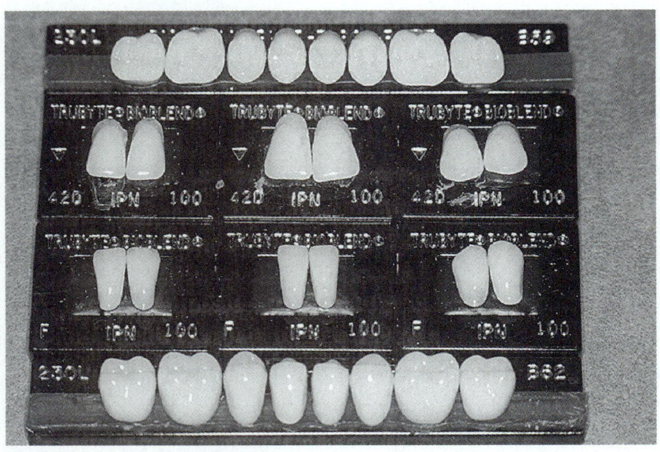

FIGURE 11.4 Photograph of acrylic teeth for maxillary and mandibular dentures (from *top* to *bottom*): maxillary posterior, maxillary anterior, mandibular anterior, and mandibular posterior denture teeth.

B. Denture Teeth

Denture teeth come in a variety of shapes, sizes, and shades. The shape is chosen to match that of the patient's natural teeth, usually as judged from an old photograph. Another technique is to use the shape of the face to select the tooth shape. The size is determined by the size of the patient's arch. The shade of the teeth is chosen to match the patient's natural complexion. Often, the patient desires white teeth and must be counseled as to the true color of natural teeth, because bright white teeth will look artificial.

1. Acrylic Resin Teeth

Today, most denture teeth are made from acrylic resin much like that used to construct the denture base. Denture teeth have more cross-linking agent added. Because the teeth are constructed under tightly controlled conditions at a manufacturing plant, they are stronger than the acrylic material used for the denture base. Acrylic denture teeth are "chemically" bonded to the acrylic denture base during processing of the denture.

2. Porcelain Teeth

Porcelain teeth are made by manufacturers in much the same shapes, sizes, and shades as acrylic teeth. Porcelain teeth are much harder and more stain resistant compared to acrylic teeth. Porcelain teeth are rarely used, however, both because they excessively wear the opposing teeth and because it is generally believed they cause trauma and bone loss in the supporting and opposing alveolar ridges. Porcelain teeth are held in the denture by the mechanical undercuts of pins that are embedded in the back of the denture tooth, as shown in Figure 11.5.

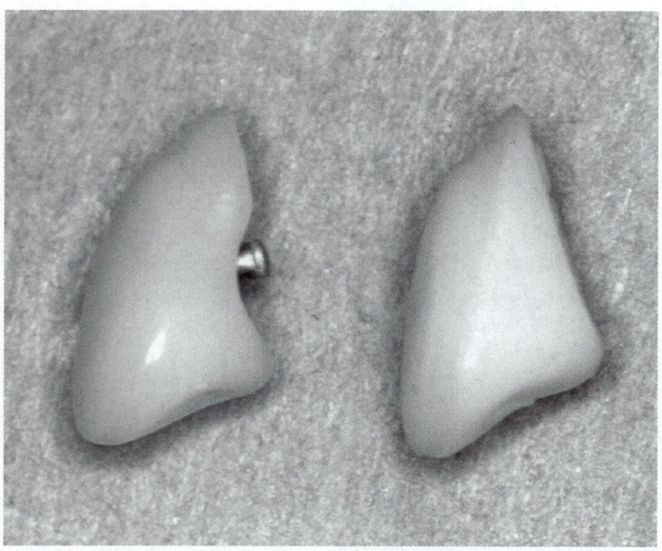

FIGURE 11.5 Photograph of a porcelain (*left*) and an acrylic (*right*) denture tooth. Note the pin protruding from the back of the porcelain tooth. The pin serves to anchor the tooth firmly in the denture base.

C. Denture Base

The **denture base** is constructed on the master cast made from the final impression. The denture base is the pink part of the denture that sits on the alveolar ridge.

IV. Constructing a Complete Denture

A. Impressions and Casts

Typically, denture construction requires a number of dental appointments and laboratory procedures. Many dentists make a preliminary impression, preliminary cast, custom tray, final impression, and master cast (in that order). The denture is directly constructed on the master cast, such as that shown in Figure 11.6*A*.

B. Recording the Maxillary and Mandibular Relationship and Arranging Teeth

The relationship of the maxillary and mandibular ridges, or the "bite of the patient," is very important to the success of the prosthesis. An improper relationship can result in overworked muscles of mastication, poor phonetics, and unsatisfactory esthetics.

1. First, a "baseplate" and "wax rims" are constructed from chemically activated acrylic (or similar material) and baseplate wax, as pictured in Figure 11.6*B*. They are made to precisely rest on the patient's ridge, as shown in Figure 11.6*C*.
2. The wax rims on the baseplates are used to determine the patient's midline, "plane of occlusion," and size of the denture teeth. The plane of occlusion is the plane where the upper and lower teeth meet when a patient bites, as illustrated in Figure 11.6*D*.
3. At the same appointment, the patient's bite is recorded, as shown in Figure 11.6*D*. This bite is used to position the upper and lower casts in the same relationship as the supporting tissues in the mouth (Fig. 11.6*E*).
4. With the aid of baseplates and rims, the casts are mounted on an articulator using dental plaster, as pictured in Figure 11.6*F* and 11.6*G*.
5. The denture teeth are "set" in the wax. Wax is easily softened with a hot instrument to allow the denture teeth to be partially set in wax and then easily moved into the proper position (Fig. 11.6*F*). When all the denture teeth are set in wax, it is called a **denture setup**. A setup simulates the proper bite (relationship of the two arches), the **vertical dimension** (distance between the two arches), and the esthetics of the final denture, as shown in Figure 11.6*G*.
6. Before processing, the setup (the baseplates with the teeth set in wax) is placed in the

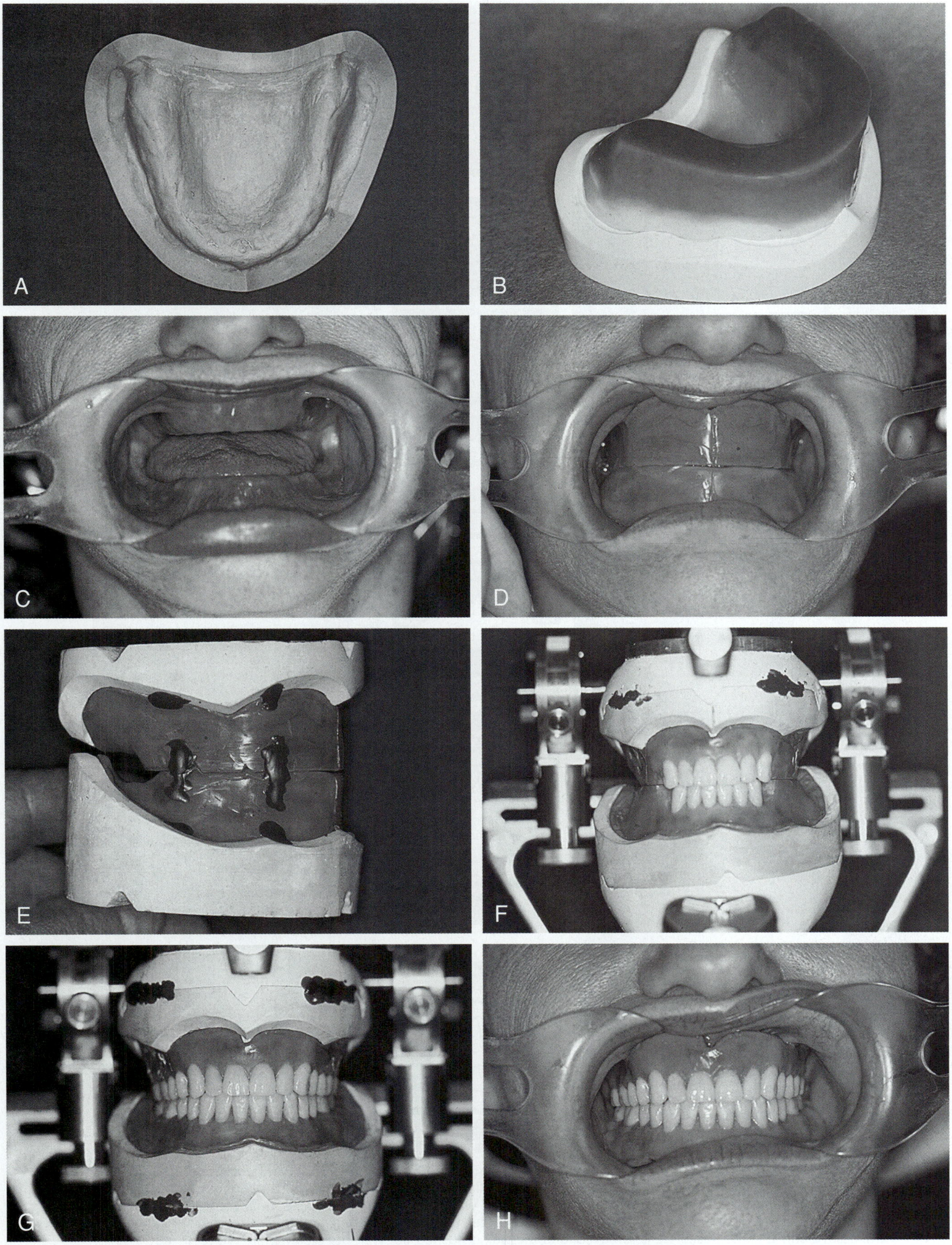

FIGURE 11.6 Steps in the construction of a denture. See text for description. Note that the plastic cheek retractors in **C, D,** and **H** are to aid photography and are not typically used during the dental procedure.

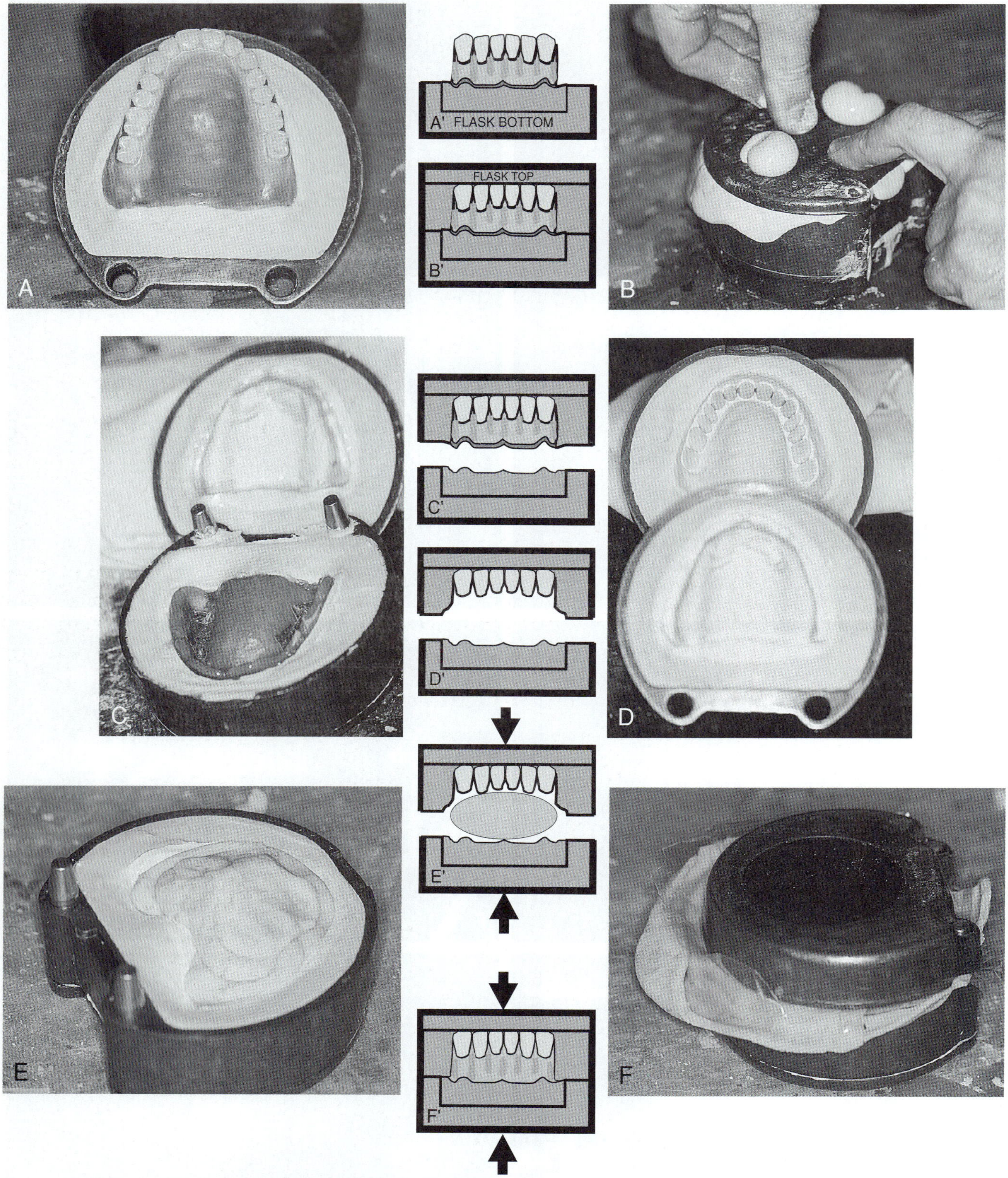

FIGURE 11.7 Processing a denture. First, the master cast and denture setup are embedded in plaster and stone in a denture flask (*dark outside line* in diagram; **A** and **A'**). The first increment fills the lower component of the flask up to the level of the master cast. The rest of the setup is covered with dental stone and plaster until the flask is filled (**B** and **B'**). Second, a mold space is made. After heating in hot water, the flask is opened, and the baseplate is separated from the cast (**C** and **C'**). The baseplate is removed, and the wax is flushed out with hot water while the teeth stay embedded in dental stone (**D** and **D'**). Mixed acrylic resin in the dough stage is then placed in the mold, and the mold is compressed (**E** and **E'**). While under compression, the resin is adapted to the master cast and replaces the baseplate and wax. The teeth stay in proper relationship (**F** and **F'**). Finally, the flask is heated, and the resin polymerizes.

patient's mouth. This procedure is called the "wax try-in" and is pictured in Figure 11.6*H*. The **wax try-in** allows patients to see the arrangement of teeth that their denture will have. It also allows the dentist to check function, occlusion (bite), and phonetics before the actual denture is processed.

C. Processing the Denture

1. Processing a denture involves embedding the master cast and the denture setup in a denture **flask** filled with gypsum materials. It is done in such a way as to create a split mold. The mold is opened, and the wax and the baseplate are removed. Acrylic resin in the dough stage is placed in the mold space. The mold is then closed, and the acrylic resin replaces the wax and base plate, forming the denture base. This process is illustrated in Figure 11.7.
2. The closed mold is heated in a water bath to activate the heat-cure acrylic resin. The heating rate is controlled to reduce porosity. The application of pressure minimizes loss of the volatile monomer. Loss of monomer results in porosity and weak spots.
3. After processing, the denture is removed from the mold by breaking the surrounding gypsum materials. It is then finished, polished, disinfected, and delivered to the patient. Completed dentures are shown in Figure 11.8.

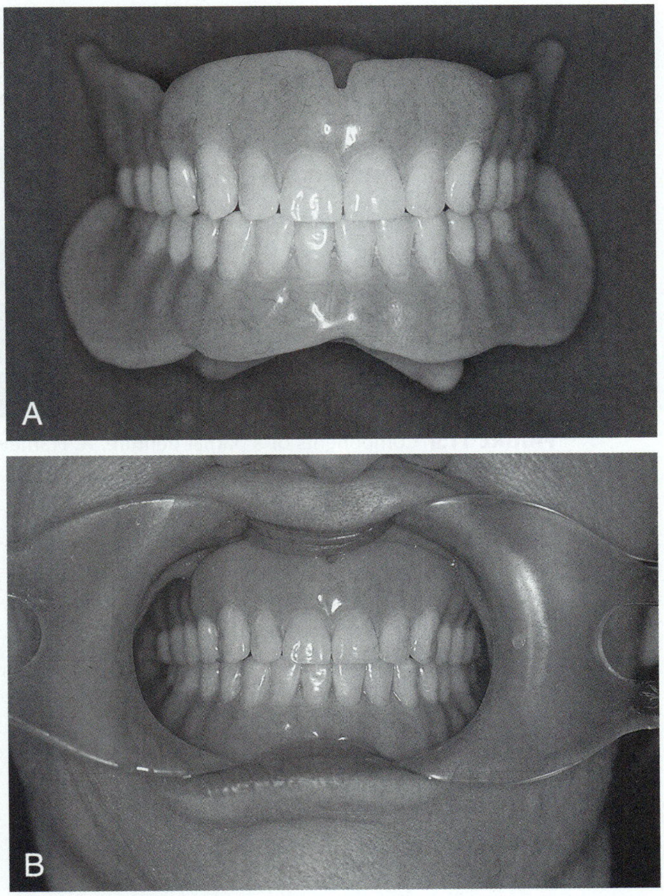

FIGURE 11.8 Photographs of completed dentures as received from the laboratory (**A**) and in place (**B**). (See color images.)

V. Partial Dentures

Many patients are partially edentulous, and the remaining teeth are frequently used to support and retain a prosthesis. If the prosthesis can be removed by the patient, it is called a **removable partial denture** or simply a partial denture. Most partial dentures are supported by both natural teeth and the alveolar ridge, as shown in Figure 1.7. A lower partial denture with a few remaining natural teeth to hold it securely functions far better than a complete lower denture. The dental hygienist should stress to the patient the critical need to maintain the remaining natural teeth so that wearing a mandibular complete denture is avoided.

Patients with a mandibular complete denture often have problems chewing. The mandibular denture will lack suction or retention and will float and move around in the mouth. The lack of stability of a mandibular denture may cause "sore spots" (ulcerations of the oral mucosa) and make speech difficult. Helping the patient to retain several mandibular teeth will allow a patient to wear and use a mandibular partial denture. This is an important preventive responsibility of the dental hygienist.

A. Frameworks

A partial denture uses a cast metal "framework" for retention, as shown in Figure 11.9*A*. The framework is composed of clasps, connectors, and mesh.

1. The framework has clasps that rest on and go around the abutment teeth. A clasp is shown in Figure 11.9*B*. Because the clasps are metal, they can be bent to adjust their fit, as pictured in Figure 11.9*C*.
2. Connectors are the thicker parts of the framework that connect the mesh and clasps together.
3. The framework also has an area of mesh that the acrylic resin flows into and around when the partial denture is processed. This results in the mechanical attachment of the teeth and the denture base to the framework.

B. Denture Base

The denture base is constructed and used in much the same way as a complete denture. However, the mesh areas of the partial denture framework are embedded in acrylic resin.

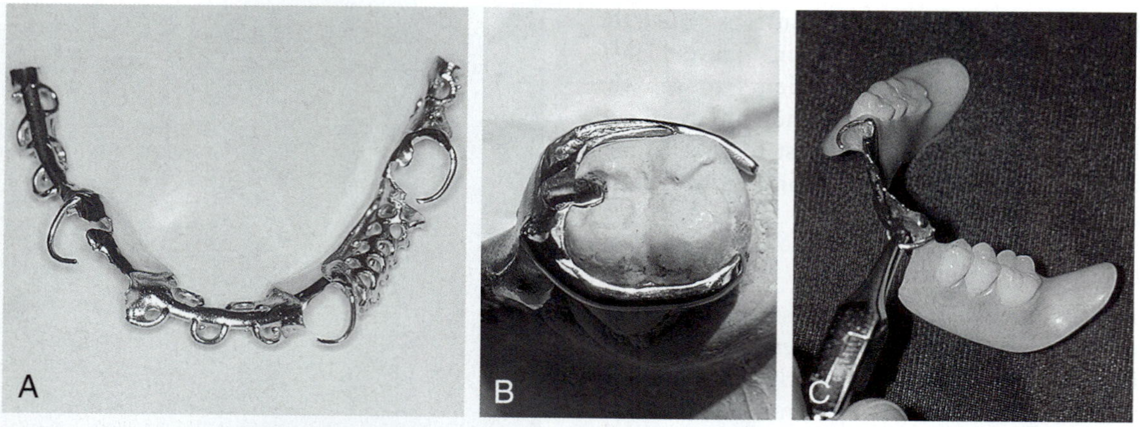

FIGURE 11.9 Components of a partial denture. **A.** Framework. **B.** Clasp. **C.** Denture base. Note the clasp being adjusted or bent.

C. Teeth

The same teeth used to construct complete dentures are used to construct partial dentures. Teeth are chosen with the proper shape, size, and shade to replace the missing natural teeth.

D. Processing a Partial Denture

A partial denture is processed much like a complete denture. However, the acrylic resin must flow through and around the mesh of the framework.

VI. Relining a Denture

Dentures lose their "fit" after a period of time, because the alveolar ridge atrophies and resorbs when teeth are not present. Most resorption occurs when the teeth are first extracted, but resorption continues slowly throughout a patient's life. Therefore, as the alveolar ridge changes, the fit of the denture changes as well.

Indications that a denture is not fitting as well as it should include frequent use of denture adhesives or over-the-counter denture "cushion" materials or liners. Use of these materials makes cleaning the denture difficult and can result in a foul smell. Long-term use of adhesives may cause tissue inflammation. Liners may change the bite or occlusion of a denture, causing trauma to the supporting tissues. The dental hygienist must be aware of these problems and educate patients about the proper use of over-the-counter products and treatment options.

An "old" denture can have its fit improved by a process called relining. **Relining** adds a small amount of new material to the inside tissue area of the denture base to replace the additional ridge that has been lost since the denture was made. Relining a denture can be done either using a dental laboratory or chairside.

A. Laboratory-Processed Reline

A laboratory-processed reline involves making an impression, much like the final impression that is made when a denture is constructed. The existing denture functions as the impression tray. A variety of impression materials are used depending on the clinician's personal preference. The denture containing the impression is sent to a dental laboratory. A cast is poured. The impression and cast are separated, and the impression material is removed from the denture. New acrylic material is added to fill the space between the denture and the cast (the space previously occupied by the impression material). The acrylic material is cured, finished, and polished in the same manner as during the construction of a new denture. The denture is returned to the dentist and given to the patient. A laboratory reline is generally superior to a chairside reline; however, patients must go without their denture for a day or more when the reline is processed at a dental laboratory.

B. Chairside Reline

A chairside reline uses a different material. The same material that functions as the impression material also becomes the added material. The material is mixed, placed in the denture, and then placed in the patient's mouth. The material sets in the mouth and becomes rigid. The excess is trimmed, and the denture is polished and returned to the patient. The advantage is that the patient does not go without his or her denture. The disadvantage is that the new material is more porous and, typically, not as smooth as that of a laboratory reline.

VII. Immediate Dentures

Most dentures are made for patients who have had their teeth previously extracted. An **immediate denture** is a denture that is placed at the same appointment during which the remaining teeth are extracted. Typically, when an immediate denture is constructed, many of the teeth in the arch to receive the denture

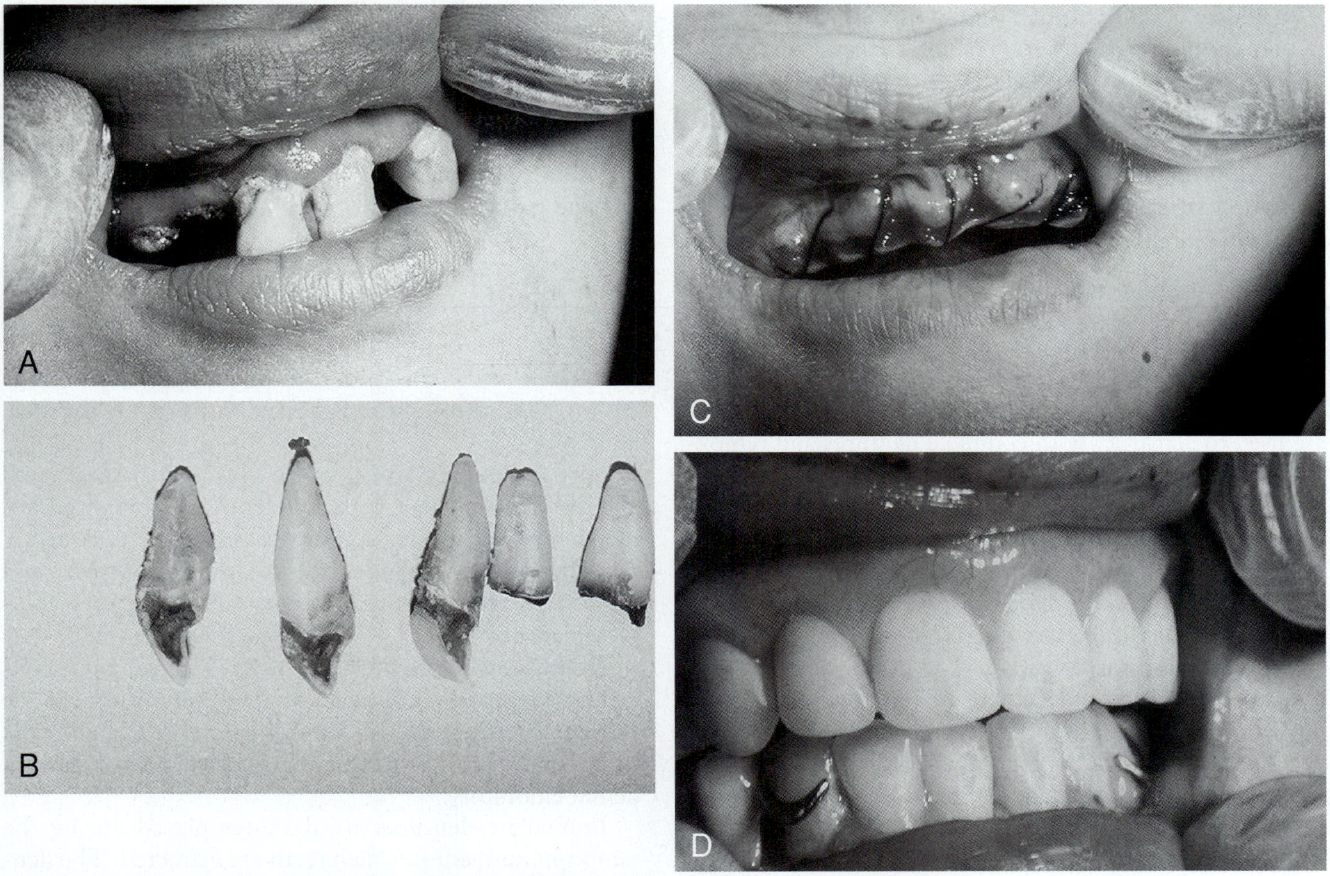

FIGURE 11.10 Photographs of teeth destroyed by caries and periodontal disease (**A**), the extracted teeth (**B**), the alveolar ridge after the extraction (**C**), and the immediate denture in place (**D**).

are already missing and most of the remaining teeth are hopeless. An impression is made by the dentist, and the denture is constructed in the laboratory, similar to a complete denture. At the delivery appointment, the remaining teeth are extracted, the denture is placed, and postoperative instructions are given to the patient (Fig. 11.10). An immediate denture not only restores function and esthetics, it can protect the extraction sites during healing. In most cases, an immediate denture is relined several months after it is placed.

VIII. Repairing Acrylic Prostheses or Appliances

It is not unusual for a denture or other acrylic prosthesis or appliance to fracture. It seems that dogs love to chew on them. Repairs are made by using new, chemically activated acrylic material as a glue to repair the fracture. In many offices, the dental hygienist may be the professional who repairs simple fractures of partial or complete dentures. The process involves several steps.

A. Clean the Surface

First, clean the surfaces being repaired. Often, this involves grinding the surface to remove a thin layer of the surface and any contaminants.

B. Apply Monomer

Next, monomer is applied to the clean surfaces to dissolve some of the set material. One end of some of the polymer chains dissolves in the monomer; the other end remains embedded in the solid acrylic resin.

C. Apply New Material

New material is then mixed, applied to the surface, and allowed to set. The polymer chains of the old material become entangled in the new material. Because no residual double bonds are available for a chemical reaction, the bond is quasi-chemical.

The same process is used to "chemically" bond acrylic denture teeth to the denture base during denture processing.

D. Finish and Polish

Finally, the repaired prosthesis is finished and polished by using acrylic burs, pumice, and other materials as for a complete denture.

IX. Handling Acrylic Devices

It is important that patients regularly clean their dentures. Patients should be instructed to brush their prostheses with a denture cleaner and a denture brush or to use other denture cleaning procedures. Calculus may form on the denture in similar areas as in natural teeth. It is the dental hygienist's responsibility during the recall appointment to remove the calculus in a manner that is not harmful to the acrylic.

Most dentists prefer that their patients do not sleep with dentures in the mouth. Therefore, patients should store their dentures in water at night.

During dental appointments, it is important to store acrylic appliances in water. Do not let them dry out, because they may warp. This applies not only to dentures but also to acrylic orthodontic retainers. The dental hygienist should play an active role during recall visits and educate patients who wear complete and partial dentures.

SUMMARY

This chapter presents the materials and procedures that are used to construct both complete dentures and removable partial dentures. These oral appliances involve the use of acrylic resin. In dentistry, acrylic resins are used for temporary crowns and custom trays in addition to the bases for complete and partial dentures.

Two forms of acrylic resins are used for the fabrication of dentures: chemically activated (cold-cure) and heat activated (heat-cure) resin systems. The chemically activated resin is supplied as a powder and a liquid, the liquid being mostly methyl methacrylate with added cross-linking agent. The powder is polymethyl methacrylate resin with added colorants and benzoyl peroxide. The powder is in the form of very small beads.

Heat-activated resin systems are very similar to chemically activated systems. The major difference is that no chemical activator is present in the liquid. The mixed material also stays in the dough stage for a longer period of time. Heat-activated products are usually stronger than chemically activated resins.

Dentures are composed of two components: the denture base and the denture teeth. Denture teeth may be made of porcelain or acrylic resin. Acrylic teeth are used most often, are bonded to the denture base, and do not excessively wear the opposing natural teeth.

Constructing a denture involves several steps. A resin baseplate is made on a master cast, wax rims are added, and both are mounted on an articulator. Teeth are then embedded in the wax, and the patient approves the wax try-in. Next, the denture is flasked, heat-cured, finished, and polished.

Partial dentures are supported by both natural teeth and the alveolar ridge. A partial denture is composed of a metal framework, the denture base, and denture teeth. The framework includes the clasps, connectors, and mesh. A partial denture is processed much like a complete denture.

Dentures will lose their "fit" as the alveolar ridge continues to resorb; however, an "old" denture can be relined to restore the fit. Resin material is added to the tissue side of the denture either at chairside or using a dental laboratory.

Immediate dentures are dentures placed during the same appointment in which teeth are extracted. The denture serves to restore function as well as to protect the extraction sites during healing. The denture is usually relined several months after it is placed.

Repairing acrylic prostheses or appliances involves grinding a thin layer off the surface, adding monomer, and then applying new mixed material. Once this is set, it is finished and polished.

The role of the dental hygienist in treating patients with complete and partial dentures includes simple repairs and significant patient education on preventing the need for dentures, home care for these oral removable prostheses, and overuse of adhesives.

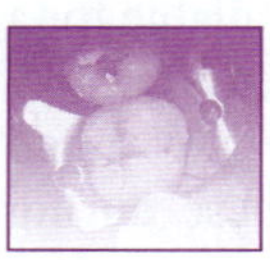

Learning Activities

1. Discuss the periodic dental and dental hygiene care that a patient with complete maxillary and partial mandibular dentures should have.
2. Wet a paper towel, and stick it to a smooth wall or blackboard. What holds it in place?
3. With a dissecting microscope, observe acrylic powders. Note the color of the beads and fibers.
4. Collect several plastic objects of no value. Place a few drops of methyl methacrylate (the liquid from an acrylic system) onto the different plastic materials. What happens to the surface? Can you use the same liquid to remove "permanent marker"?
5. Observe patients in the clinic who have complete and partial dentures. Notice the different shades and shapes of denture teeth. How do these relate to the patient's complexion or the shape of his or her face?

Review Questions

1. The term used when the denture teeth are set in wax is:
a) Denture arrangement
b) Denture setup
c) Articulated setup
d) Articulated arrangement

2. To repair a broken denture, a thin layer is ground off. Next, monomer is applied to the surfaces so that:
a) Some of the set material is dissolved
b) The setting reaction of the repair is accelerated
c) The finishing and polishing of the repair is made easier
d) The color of resin powder does not change

3. Heat-activated acrylic resin systems are very similar to chemically activated systems. The major difference (or exception) is:
a) Heat-activated systems have much less strength than chemically activated systems
b) More inhibitor is present in the liquid of heat-activated systems.
c) Chemical activator is present in the liquid of heat-activated systems.
d) No chemical activator is present in the liquid of heat-activated systems.

4. Most denture teeth used today are acrylic rather than porcelain. Porcelain teeth are softer than acrylic teeth and do not cause excessive wear on natural opposing teeth.
a) The first statement is true; the second statement is false.
b) The first statement is false; the second statement is true.
c) Both statements are true.
d) Both statements are false.

5. Partial denture frameworks usually include:
a) Clasps, denture base, and connectors
b) Teeth, clasps, and connectors
c) Clasps, connectors, and mesh
d) Teeth, denture base, connectors, and clasps

6. Cross-linking of acrylic resins will improve the mechanical properties. The most important or beneficial property it would improve would be:
a) Resilience
b) Toughness
c) Fatigue
d) Creep

7. Mandibular dentures are easier to wear than maxillary. Saliva helps to improve the suction needed to hold a denture in place.
a) The first statement is true; the second statement is false.
b) The first statement is false; the second statement is true.
c) Both statements are true.
d) Both statements are false.

8. The wax rims used for denture construction serve to determine the patient's:
a) Midline
b) Plane of occlusion
c) Size of denture teeth
d) All of the above

9. The acrylic resin of a partial denture is processed the same way as a complete denture EXCEPT:
a) It takes less time because fewer teeth are involved
b) The finishing and polishing technique is much different
c) The acrylic resin must flow through and around the mesh of the framework
d) It takes longer because of the design of the framework

10. Listed below are the steps of constructing a denture. Numbering from 1 to 10, place the steps in sequential order.

_____ Casts and rims are mounted on an articulator.

_____ The master cast and denture setup are embedded in stone within the denture flask.

_____ Acrylic resin is mixed and placed in the mold, and the mold is then compressed.

_____ The patient has the wax try-in.

_____ The mold is created by heating in hot water, the baseplate is removed, the wax is flushed out, and the teeth remain in stone.

_____ The baseplate and wax rims are constructed on the master cast.

_____ The denture is removed from the mold, finished, polished, and disinfected.

_____ The baseplate and rims are fitted on patient; midline, plane of occlusion, and bite determined.

_____ The flask is heated and the resin polymerizes.

_____ Denture teeth are set in wax.

Supplemental Readings

Anusavice KJ. Phillips' Science of Dental Materials. 11th ed. Philadelphia: Saunders, 2003, Chapter 22.

Powers JM, Sakaguchi RL, eds. Craig's Restorative Dental Materials. 12th ed. St. Louis: Mosby, 2006, Chapter 21.

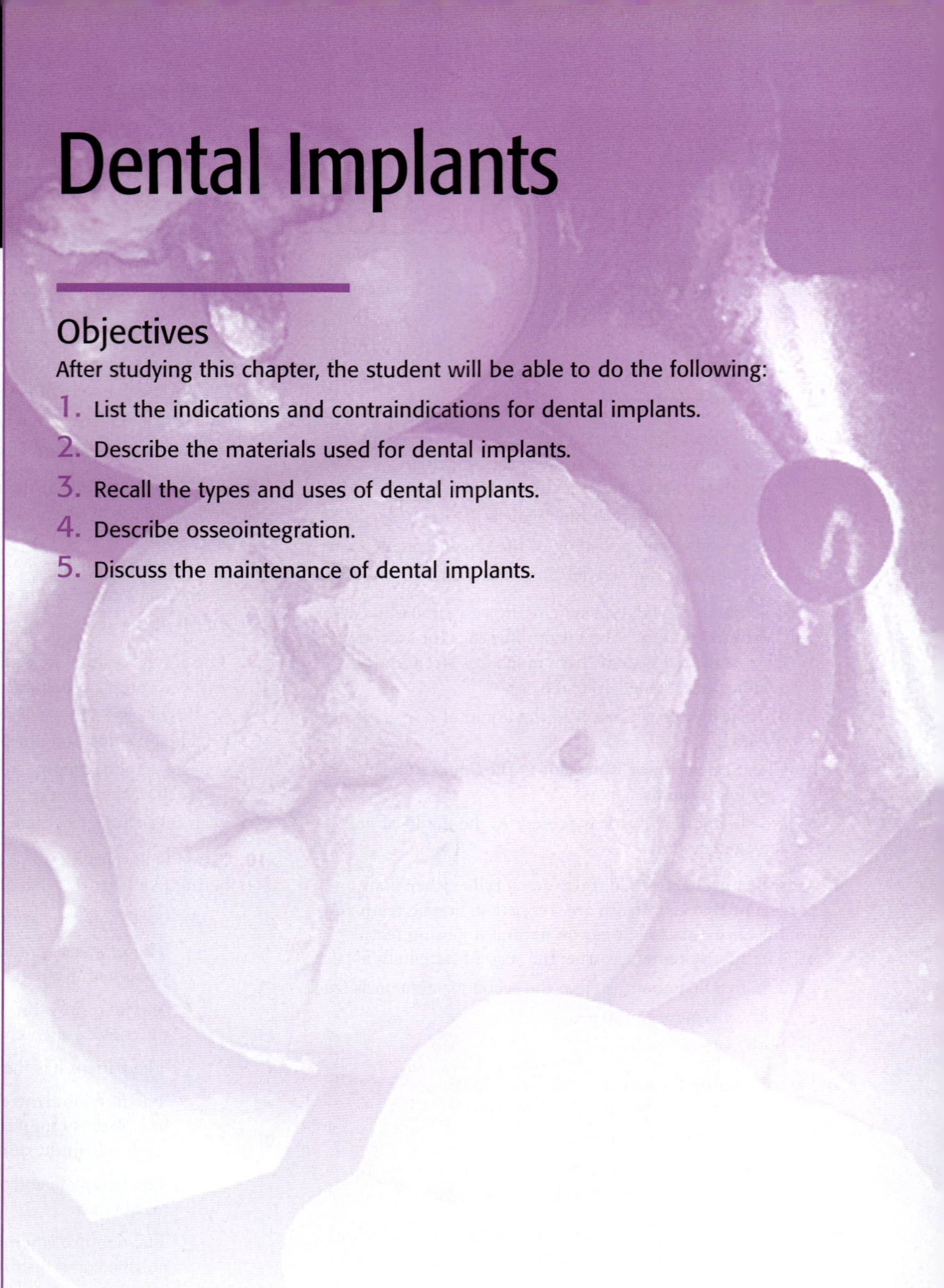

12 Dental Implants

Key Words/Phrases

abutment
atrophic edentulous mandible
dental implant
endosseous implants
hydroxyapatite
osseointegration
subperiosteal implants
titanium
tooth form implants

Objectives

After studying this chapter, the student will be able to do the following:

1. List the indications and contraindications for dental implants.
2. Describe the materials used for dental implants.
3. Recall the types and uses of dental implants.
4. Describe osseointegration.
5. Discuss the maintenance of dental implants.

I. Medical Versus Dental Implants

The typical medical implant is a device that is placed entirely inside the body. The typical **dental implant** exists both inside and outside the body. A dental implant projects through the oral mucosa and, thus, is not completely surrounded by tissues, as with most medical implants (e.g., silicone breast, artificial hip, knee, and lens implants). An implant existing both inside and outside the body is susceptible to infection. The interface of the surface of the implant and the tissues is a potential site for entry into the body of bacteria and other microorganisms.

II. Indications and Contraindications for Dental Implants

A. Indications

1. Restoring an Edentulous Atrophic Mandible

Originally, dental implants were used predominantly for prosthodontic patients in whom no other treatment options were satisfactory. The most common prosthodontic problem has been making dentures for a patient with little or no mandibular ridge. When the teeth are lost, the alveolar bone (bone that supports the teeth) is no longer stimulated. The alveolar bone is resorbed. As the alveolar bone reduces in size or atrophies, the ridge available to support a denture shrinks. This is called an **atrophic edentulous mandible.** Dental implants have greatly improved the treatment of this condition, as shown in Figure 12.1. With the development and success of osseointegrated implants, dental implants are now used as an alternative or adjunct to other conventional prosthodontic treatments.

2. Restoring a Single Missing Tooth

For patients with a single missing tooth, a crown supported by a single endosseous implant is becoming a popular treatment option, as shown in Figure 12.2. The conventional option of a three-unit bridge requires that the two abutment teeth be prepared for crowns, as discussed in Chapter 1 and shown in Figure 1.5. Using an implant and a crown to replace a missing tooth may save previously unrestored (no fillings) abutment teeth from

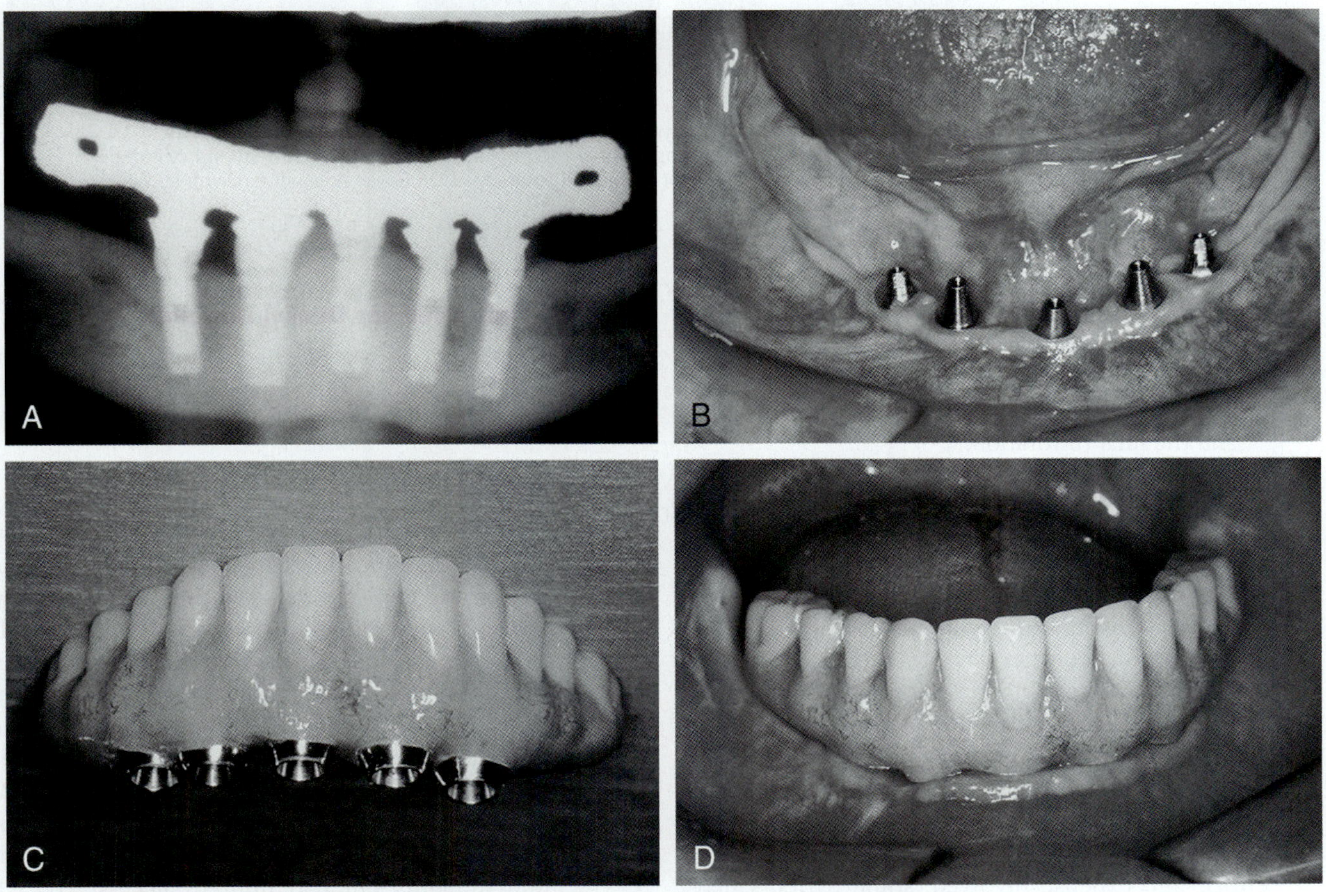

FIGURE 12.1 A mandibular fixed prosthesis supported by implants. Shown are a Panorex of an implant-supported fixed prosthesis (**A**) as well as photographs of the atrophic mandible with five implants (**B**), the prosthesis (**C**), and the implant-supported prosthesis in place (**D**). (See color images.) (Courtesy of Dr. Paul A. Schnitman, Wellesley Hills, MA, and Noble Biocare, Yorba Linda, CA.)

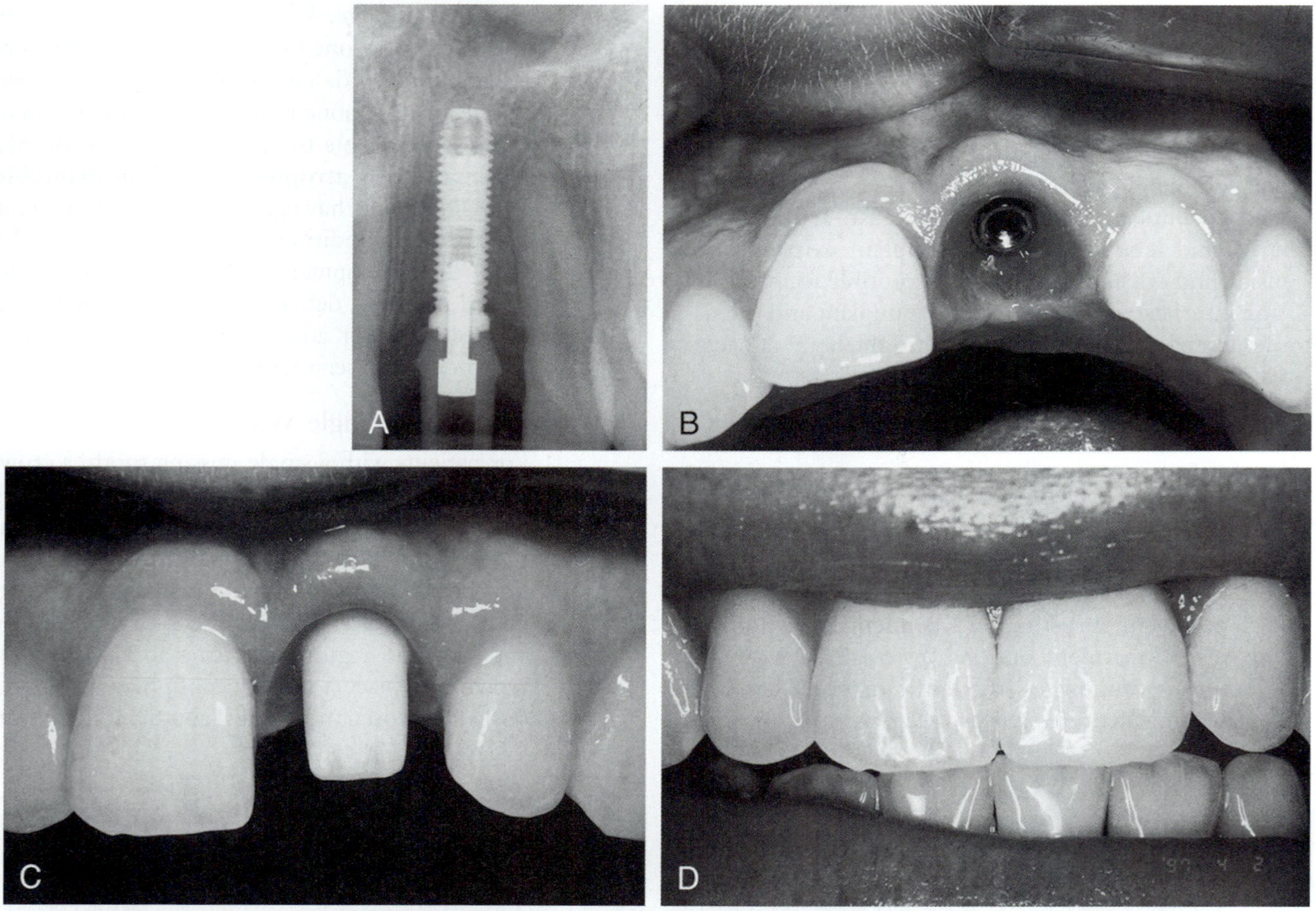

FIGURE 12.2 An endosseous single-tooth implant restored with a crown. Shown are a radiograph of the implant, abutment, and abutment screw (**A**) as well as clinical photographs of the implant (**B**), esthetic abutment and cylinder (**C**), and the crown supported by the implant (**D**). (See color images.) (Courtesy of Dr. Roger A. Lawton, Olympia, WA, and Noble Biocare, Yorba Linda, CA.)

crown preparations. Often, the cost of one implant and a crown is comparable to the cost of a three-unit bridge. The specific cost will depend on the implant chosen, the placement procedures, and the final restoration.

B. Contraindications

Patients with systemic diseases that affect connective tissues are not good candidates for dental implants. The most common of these diseases is diabetes. Smoking is the other major, common contraindication. Another factor to consider is the patient's ability to maintain the implants. Effective plaque control, regular dental prophylaxis, and recall examination are critical to the long-term success of implants. It is also important for the patient to have realistic expectations about the resulting prosthesis. Considering the large amount of time, effort, and expense involved, some patients may expect more than can be delivered. With patients having expectations that cannot be met, it is best to avoid any extensive expensive dental treatment.

III. Materials Used for Dental Implants

It is important to realize that although the implant material is a significant factor, how the material is used is more critical to the success of dental implants.

A. Titanium

Titanium was briefly discussed in Chapter 10. Titanium and titanium alloys are very common implant materials in dentistry and medicine. Unfortunately, titanium is very difficult to cast, and it is commonly manufactured for implants by machining into preformed shapes. The major advantage of titanium is that it will osseointegrate with bone if handled properly. Osseointegration is a kind of biologic bonding of bone to a material. Titanium is used for endosseous and most other types of implants. Numerous early researchers had worked with titanium implants but had limited success. Dr. P.I. Brånemark (an orthopedic surgeon) concurrently developed surgical procedures and implant materials; the results were the first reliable dental implants.

1. "cp Ti," or "commercially pure" titanium, is used for many types of medical and dental implants. As with other pure metals, cp Ti is not very strong, but it is strong enough for many dental implant uses.
2. "Ti-6Al-4V," or titanium with 6% aluminum and 4% vanadium, is a common aerospace alloy that has been used for dental implants. It is stronger and stiffer than cp Ti. Dental and medical versions of this alloy have more restrictive composition requirements compared with other industries.

B. Apatite-Coated Titanium

Another popular implant material is **hydroxyapatite** (HA) bonded to titanium metal. Apatites are a broad class of calcium phosphate materials. The hydroxyapatite of hard tissues, such as teeth and bone, are examples. Hydroxyapatite materials also osseointegrate. Titanium coated with HA is used successfully for many different types of implants. HA-coated implants have had increased clinical success when compared to Ti in certain clinical situations.

C. Other Materials

Dental implants have been made from many other materials. The results were not good; therefore, the search continued until titanium was tried with the proper techniques. These materials included metals, ceramics, and polymers.

1. Metals

Gold, stainless steel, and cobalt-chromium alloys were used with little success.

2. Ceramics

Hydroxyapatite and other calcium phosphate materials are currently used as implant materials. Vitreous (glassy) carbon, pyrolytic carbon, and aluminum oxide (sapphire) have also been tried with little success.

3. Polymers

A variety of polymers, including acrylic resin, have been used. Polymers have had little success as prosthodontic implants, but other uses have been developed. Gortex is a polymer material that is implanted as a "barrier" to tissue growth in periodontics. Gortex is expanded polytetrafluoroethylene, the same polymer as Teflon.

IV. Various Types of Dental Implants

A. Endosseous or Tooth Form Implants

Endosseous implants or **tooth form implants** are screwed or pressed into a hole that is cut into the mandible or maxilla. All the implants shown in the illustrations of this chapter are endosseous implants. They reside inside the bone, thus the name "endosseous."

A variety of shapes are classified as endosseous implants. Some are cylinders, with threads on the surface like a bolt or a screw; others have straight sides. Still others, called blade implants, are shaped somewhat like a blade, with notches cut into it. Current use of implants is dominated by cylindrical endosseous shapes. Endosseous implants are used to support a single crown, multiple crowns, a bridge, or a denture.

B. Transosseous or Staple Implants—Optional

A transosseous implant was used to stabilize a mandibular denture. It consists of a plate and several bolts that transverse the mandible in the anterior region. The plate is placed on the underside of the mandible, and the bolts extend through the bone and gingiva into the oral cavity. The bolts have nuts screwed onto the intraoral side of the mandible to keep the implant in place. An extraoral incision under the chin is required to place a transosseous implant.

C. Subperiosteal Implants—Optionals

Subperiosteal implants were also used to stabilize a mandibular denture. Subperiosteal implants are placed on the mandibular bone below the periosteum and involve two surgical procedures.

1. The first surgical procedure reflects or "flaps" (peels back) the mucosa and periosteum of the mandible, exposing the denture-bearing alveolar bone. An impression is made of this denture-bearing bone. The soft tissue is then sutured back over the bone.
2. Next, a cast is poured, and framework that supports the eventual denture is cast by a dental laboratory. The framework sits directly on the bone and has several posts that extend through the mucosa and support the denture. Chromium-cobalt is the most common alloy used to cast the framework. Chromium-cobalt is not as biocompatible as titanium, therefore, titanium is also used.
3. The second surgical procedure again reflects the soft tissues covering the alveolar bone, and the framework is put into place. The soft tissue is then put back into place and holds the framework in position. At times, surgical bone screws are used to stabilize the implant.
4. Clinical examples of subperiosteal implants can be found with a web search.

V. Osseointegration of Dental Implants

Osseointegration is attachment of molecules, fibers, cells, and tissues to the implant. The outcome is the

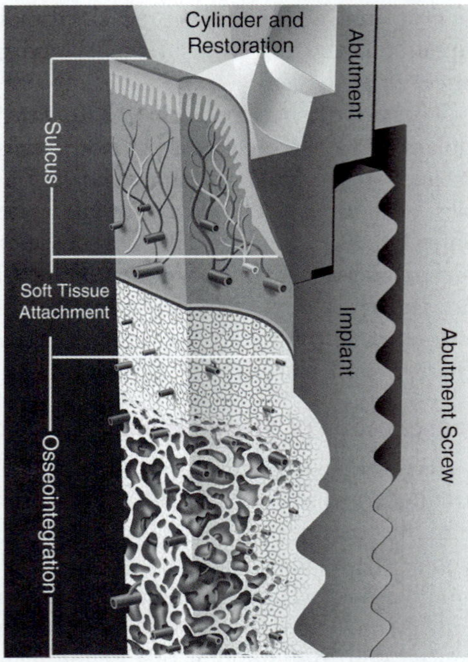

FIGURE 12.3 An artist's rendition of an osseointegrated dental implant. (Courtesy of Nobel Biocare, Yorba Linda, CA. Labels of the implant parts and the tissue/implant interface have been added.)

result of biocompatible materials, kind surgical techniques, and proper healing conditions. Osseointegration is dependent on material biocompatibility, implant surface, status of bone, surgical technique, healing conditions, and biting forces. Successful osseointegration transfers bite forces to bone and stimulates the growth of bone.

A. Tissue Compatibility

The implant must be compatible with bone and must integrate for mechanical stability. The implant must also be compatible with epithelial cells to seal out the oral environment. The implant must be placed so that these two criteria are met.

B. The Interface With Bone

The interface of an implant that is osseointegrated with bone is depicted in Figure 12.3. It includes:

1. Titanium metal
2. Metal surface coated with either:
   - **a)** Titanium oxides, 50 to 100 Å (10^{-10} m) thick (the outer layer is actually TiOH) or
   - **b)** A ceramic coating, usually hydroxyapatite
3. Proteins, 100 Å thick
4. Healthy bone composed of fibers, cells, and hydroxyapatite

VI. Soft-Tissue Attachment to Implants

The attachment of epithelial cells to the implant is called the biological or permucosal seal. This seal forms a barrier, which inhibits microorganisms' entrance into the tissues supporting the implant. Just as teeth may be lost due to periodontal problems, implants may fail if the supporting tissues are not healthy.

VII. Placement of Endosseous Dental Implants

When placing endosseous dental implants, the surgical technique must not injure the bone. Bone-cutting procedures must not heat the bone to greater than 47°C (117°F). Overheating or excessive trauma to the bone prevents osseointegration of the implant; the implant becomes surrounded by poorly organized connective tissue (scar tissue). For a dental implant to succeed, adequate healthy bone is needed to support the implant under an occlusal load. Implants may be placed by using one or two surgical procedures, depending on the location of the implant, the esthetic concerns, and the preference of the surgeon. Either way, the placement technique is nearly identical.

A. Two-Stage Implant Placement Procedures

1. The first surgical procedure cuts the hole into the bone and places the implant. First, a soft-tissue flap is laid, exposing the bone of the implant site. Next, a hole or channel is cut by using a surgical handpiece with special speed and temperature controls. The size and shape of the hole in the bone is matched to that of the implant. The body of the implant is then placed and covered by the soft-tissue flap. The implant is left covered for weeks to several months to allow healing and osseointegration to occur without exposure to oral contamination and mechanical loading, as shown in Figure 12.4*A*.
2. The second stage attaches a healing cap to the body of the implant. The soft tissue covering the implant is removed, and the healing cap held in place with a screw. The healing cap extends out of the mucosa and is exposed to the oral cavity. This allows epithelial tissue to form around a fixed (nonmovable) object. After the soft tissue has healed for several weeks, the prosthodontic phase begins.

B. Single-Stage Implant Placement Procedures

A soft-tissue flap and hole in the bone are created as in the two-stage procedure. The implant is placed with the body extending above the tissue. The soft tissue is repositioned and sutured around the implant. The healing cap is placed. After healing, the prosthodontic phase begins.

C. The Prosthodontic Phase

1. The healing cap is removed, and an **abutment,** as shown in Figure 12.4*B*, is placed on the implant. The abutment functions as an abutment of a bridge; it is attached to and supports the

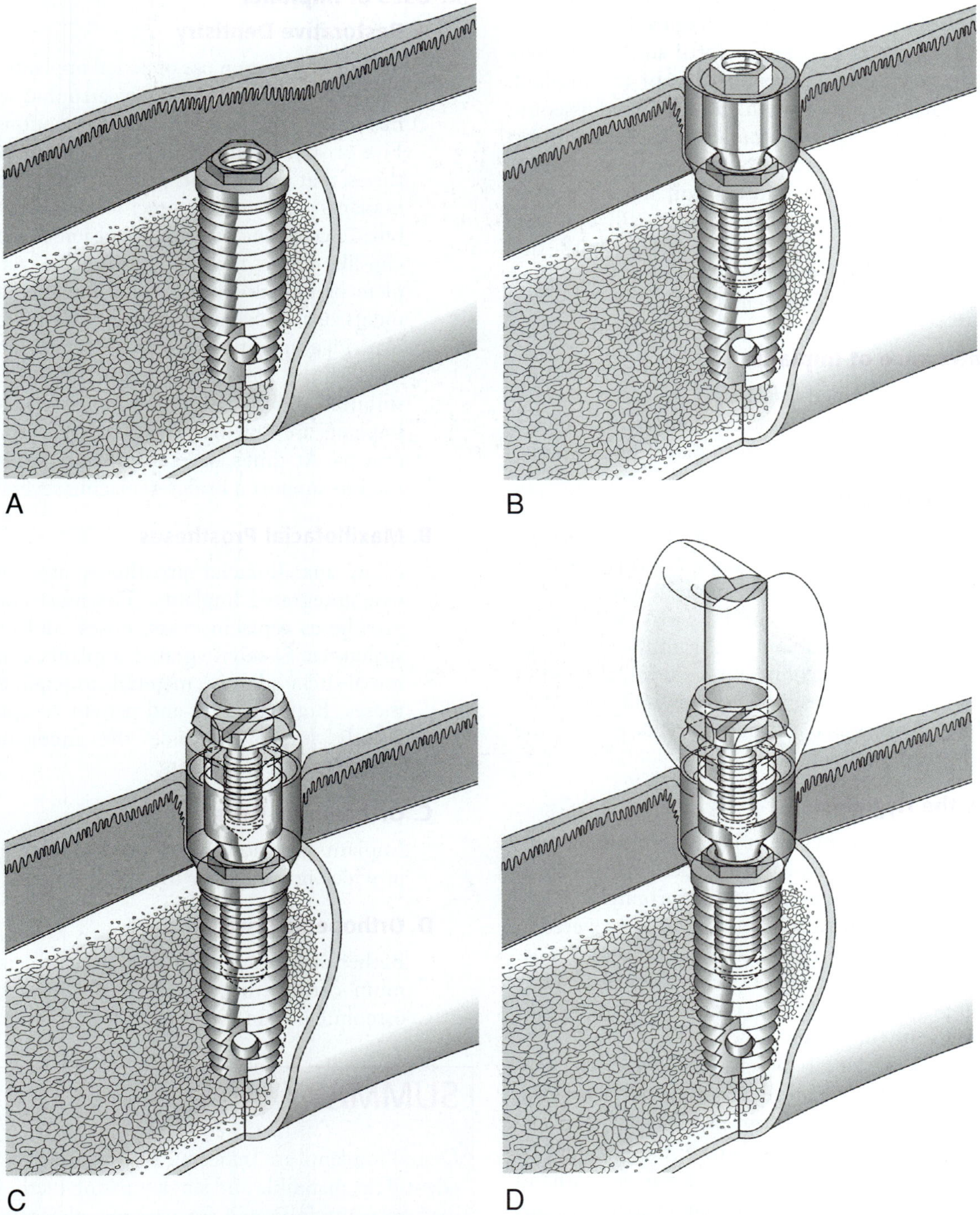

FIGURE 12.4 Placement and restoration of an endosseous implant. See text (*Placement of Endosseous Dental Implants*) for description. (Original artwork, part *D*, is provided courtesy of Noble Biocare, Yorba Linda, CA.)

prosthesis. A precision-fitting cylinder, typically made of gold, is placed on the abutment, as illustrated in Figure 12.4*C*. An impression of the cylinder is used to construct models for crown fabrication.

2. The crown is fabricated on top of the cylinder, as depicted in Figure 12.4*D*. The crown and cylinder become one piece. The fabrication technique for the crown is determined by the restorative material prescribed. The crown may be made of gold, porcelain fused to metal, composite, or ceramic materials.
3. The restoration (crown and cylinder) may be retained on the implant by several means. It may be cemented in the same manner as a tooth-supported crown. Alternatively, it

may be retained with a screw that threads into the abutment, as shown in Figure 12.4*D*.

4. Occlusion is a critical factor if an implant is to be successful. Proper loading of the implant stimulates bone growth and continued osseointegration. Many implants use polymeric restorative materials to cushion biting forces. Overloading the implant will interfere with osseointegration, and mobility will develop. Excessive mobility may interfere with the epithelial attachment. Occlusion and other forces are very important!

VIII. Maintenance of Implants

Maintenance of dental implants is critical so that the epithelial attachment and the biologic seal remain in a state of health and continue to support the prothesis.

A. By the Patient

Effective plaque control must be maintained by the patient along with regular prophylaxis at recall appointments. For single tooth implants, the usual toothbrush and floss may be adequate for plaque removal and health of the surrounding tissue. For a complex prosthesis, the use of interdental brushes, flossing aids, and other auxiliary devices may be necessary as part of the homecare regimen.

B. By the Hygienist

The role of the hygienist in the care and maintenance of dental implants includes patient education, oral hygiene instruction, prophylaxis, and recall appointments. These topics are covered in depth in other texts, such as that of E. M. Wilkins, and in courses on periodontics. Without proper maintenance, the risk of implant failure greatly increases.

From a dental materials perspective, care must be taken not to damage the surface of the implant. Scaling and root planing with conventional instruments will damage the titanium or HA surface. There are now a variety of hand scaling instruments on the market that have tips that are "surface friendly" to the titanium and HA. Power instrumentation, both magnetostrictive and piezoelectric, and reciprocating handpieces, are also indicated providing a low setting is used with the correct tip (or tip covering).

Air-powder polishing with sodium bicarbonate-water slurry does not disrupt the surface characterization or the biologic seal around the implant. The typical rubber cup with a very mild abrasive is commonly used to clean the implant prostheses.

IX. Uses of Implants

A. Restorative Dentistry

The most common use of dental implants was to stabilize a prosthesis for an atrophic edentulous mandible. A variety of restorative options are used. Five or six implants can totally support a fixed prosthesis that restores an entire arch. At times, two implants are used with precision attachments to stabilize a complete denture. Precision attachments are clip-like devices that snap together and retain a complete or partial denture. The implants and attachments keep the denture in place (down), but the alveolar ridge supports the denture against biting forces.

With the long-term success of implants used to stabilize dentures and other prostheses, dental implants are now frequently used to support single crowns. At times, several implants are placed and used to support a bridge replacing several teeth.

B. Maxillofacial Prostheses

Many maxillofacial prostheses are retained by osseointegrated implants. The most common are prostheses replacing ears, noses, and other facial structures. Osseointegrated implants eliminate the use of sticky adhesive materials to retain these prostheses. Both function and patient acceptance have greatly improved since the incorporation of osseointegrated implants.

C. Orthodontic Uses

Implants are now being used in orthodontics to provide anchorage for tooth movement.

D. Orthopedic Devices

Rather than being retained with bone cements, titanium orthopedic devices (e.g., hips, knees) use osseointegration for fixation.

SUMMARY

Dental implants are indicated for restoring an atrophic edentulous mandible and single missing teeth. Implants may be contraindicated for patients who smoke, have diabetes, or exhibit poor oral hygiene.

Titanium is the metal of choice for implants because it will osseointegrate with bone. Osseointegration is a type of biological bonding to a material.

The three types of implants include endosseous, transosseous and subperiosteal. Endosseous implants are quite common and are placed by pressing or screwing them into a hole that is cut into the alveolar bone. Transosseous and subperiosteal implants are used to stabilize dentures.

Endosseous implants may involve a one- or two-stage placement procedure. During the first surgery, a hole is cut into the bone, and the implant is placed. It is then covered by the soft-tissue flap that was cut to expose the bone for implant placement and is left covered for several weeks. The second surgical procedure removes the soft-tissue covering so that a healing cap can be placed. This extends out into the mucosa, and the epithelium tissue heals and forms around it. It is then replaced with an abutment. The one-stage procedure reduces the two-stage procedure into a single surgery. The abutment supports the prosthesis, such as a crown.

Maintenance of implants is critical so that the epithelial attachment and seal are maintained. The dental hygienist will select the necessary auxiliary aides, provide chairside education, establish a home care regimen, and schedule an appropriate recall date.

Learning Activities

1. Review patient charts, and discuss the possible use of dental implants to aid in the restoration of missing teeth.
2. Assume that a student has a congenitally missing maxillary lateral incisor. Discuss the various treatment options.
3. Assume that one of your clinical patients has implants and a prosthesis such as that pictured in Figure 12.1. Discuss your treatment plan for this patient. Include your dental hygiene care, recommended auxiliary aids, home care instructions, and recall schedule.

Review Questions

1. The type of implant that involves cutting a hole into the alveolar bone and then pressing or screwing in the implant is called:
   a) Subperiosteal
   b) Staple
   c) Transosseous
   d) Endosseous
2. Which of the following takes place during the second endosseous implant surgery?
   a) An impression is taken for crown fabrication
   b) An abutment is attached to the body of the implant
   c) A healing cap is attached to the body of the implant
   d) The amount of osseointegration is measured
3. To ensure longevity and function of the implant, the patient is responsible for:
   a) Eventual payment in full of all implant procedures
   b) Plaque control
   c) Application of tray-delivered fluoride
   d) Proper occlusion
4. The surgical procedure for placing implants must not injure the bone. Overheating the bone prevents osseointegration of the implant. Recommended temperatures are not to exceed:
   a) 98.6°F
   b) 47°F
   c) 117°C
   d) 117°F
5. All of the following conditions are contraindications for implant placement except:
   a) Recurrent caries
   b) Poor oral hygiene
   c) Diabetes
   d) Smoking
6. Titanium is very difficult to cast. It is not very strong but is acceptable for implant uses.
   a) The first statement is true; the second statement is false.
   b) The first statement is false; the second statement is true.
   c) Both statements are true.
   d) Both statements are false.

7. A patient who has a very small, or essentially no mandibular ridge, is said to have a (an):
a) Atrophic dentulous mandible
b) Atrophic edentulous mandible
c) Iatrogenic edentulous mandible
d) Dysfunctional edentulous mandible

8. The patient's home care regimen of implant maintenance may consist only of a toothbrush and floss. Without proper maintenance, the possibility of implant failure greatly increases.
a) The first statement is true; the second statement is false.
b) The first statement is false; the second statement is true.
c) Both statements are true.
d) Both statements are false.

9. The prosthodontic phase of implant treatment involves the placement of several "parts" or attachments. A patient who has completed the surgeries and restorative care would receive, in order:
a) cylinder, implant, abutment, crown
b) implant, cylinder, abutment, crown
c) cylinder, implant, crown, abutment
d) implant, abutment, cylinder, crown

10. All of the following should be included in the post-care maintenance of a patient with an implant except one. Which one is the EXCEPTION ?
a) Necessary chairside, home-care instruction
b) Recommended auxiliary aids
c) Selecting the restorative material for an adjacent restoration
d) Specific length of time between recall visits

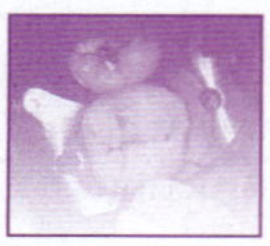

Supplemental Readings

Anusavice KJ. Phillips' Science of Dental Materials. 11th ed. Philadelphia: Saunders, 2003, Chapter 23.

Rapley JW, Swan RH, Hallmon WW, Mills MP. The surface characteristics produced by various oral hygiene instruments and materials on titanium implant abutments. Int J Oral Maxillofac Implants 1990;5:47–52.

Wilkins EM. Clinical Practice of the Dental Hygienist. 10th ed. Baltimore: Williams & Wilkins: 2008, Chapter 30.

Worthington P, Lang BR, Rubenstein JE. Osseointegration in Dentistry—An Overview. 2nd ed. Chicago: Quintessence, 2003, Chapter 9.

13

Specialty Materials

Objectives

After studying this chapter, the student will be able to do the following:

1. Describe the components of a fixed orthodontic appliance.
2. Discuss the caries risk of orthodontic patients and the dental hygienist's role in preventing caries and periodontal disease in these patients.
3. Summarize the procedures involved in root canal therapy.
4. Explain the use of periodontal packs and sutures.

Key Words/Phrases

apicoectomy
appliances
band
bracket
debonding
elastic
elastic ligatures
endodontic files
endodontic sealers
fluoride varnish
gutta percha
irrigants
lateral condensation
lingual arch
obturation
periodontal packs
pulpotomy
retainers
retrofill
root canal therapy
space maintainers
stainless-steel crown
sutures
tube
wires

INTRODUCTION

Dental specialties use many materials in common with the general practice of dentistry. Other materials are unique to one or several specialties. This chapter presents some of the more common materials used by orthodontists, endodontists, periodontists, oral surgeons, and pediatric dentists that the dental hygienist will encounter in a general practice setting.

I. Orthodontic Materials

The specialty of orthodontics seeks to align teeth in their most esthetic and functional position. Orthodontists use a variety of materials and devices. Some are the same materials used in other areas of dentistry; others are unique to orthodontics. Orthodontists use devices called **appliances** to move teeth and to affect growth of the maxilla and mandible. Orthodontists use both fixed and removable appliances. The most common fixed orthodontic appliance consists of brackets, wires, and bands, as shown in Figures 13.1 and 13.2. An orthodontic retainer is a removable appliance and is shown in Figure 13.3.

A. Materials Similar to Those Commonly Used in General Dentistry

1. Impression Materials and Gypsum Products

Impression materials used in orthodontics are the same as those discussed in Chapter 8. Alginate is the most commonly used impression material because orthodontic appliances do not require the precision of a cast restoration. Orthodontists use dental stone to pour casts for the construction of appliances. Orthodontic stone is used for study models. It is not as strong as dental stone because this facilitates model trimming. Whiteners are added to orthodontic stone to improve the appearance of study models.

2. Bonding Materials and Composites

The same bonding materials used in restorative dentistry are used by orthodontists to bond appliances to teeth. Both light-cure and chemical-cure composites are used. Generally, orthodontists use only acid-etched enamel for bonding because no dentin is available. Use of dental bonding primers could improve bonding if contamination of the etched surface is a problem.

Nearly all composite products are strong enough for use in orthodontics when bonding to anterior and premolar teeth. Strength of the bonding material is not a problem, but adhesion is. A macrofilled composite has the advantage in that when fixed appliances are removed at the end of treatment (**debonding**), it is much easier to locate residual composite bonding material. Macrofilled composites are rough and turn gray when abraded with a metal instrument. The filler particles in macrofilled composites are harder than the metal of the instrument; hence, they abrade the instrument and turn gray. General

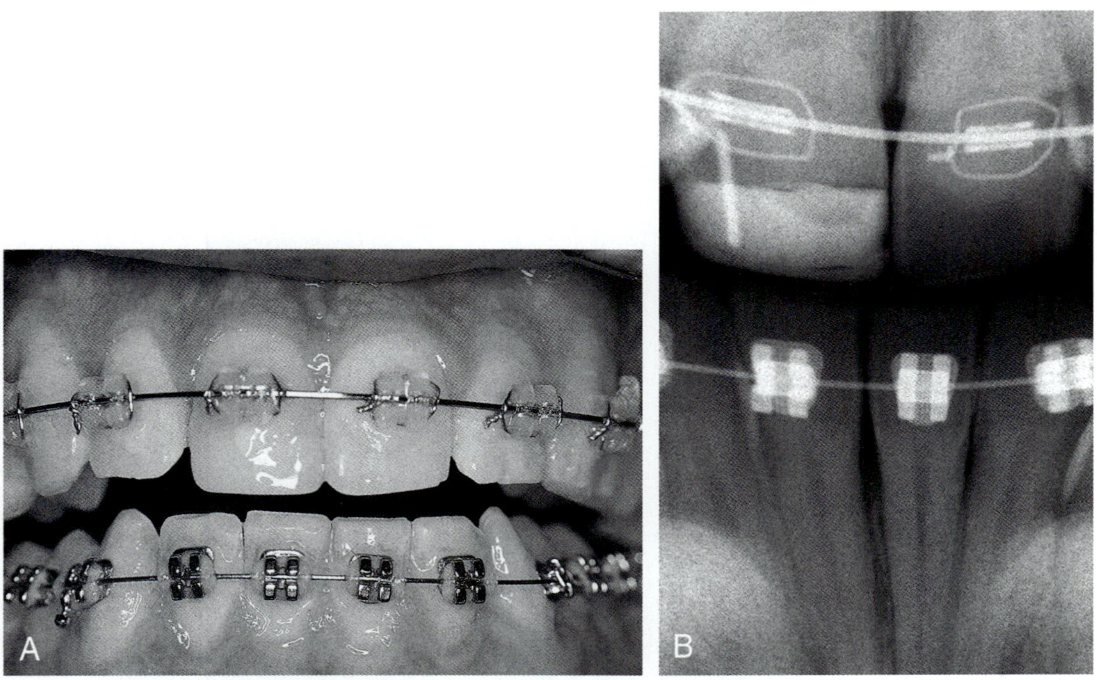

FIGURE 13.1 A. Orthodontic fixed appliance consisting of polycarbonate brackets with metal ligatures and rectangular wire on the upper arch and stainless-steel brackets with elastic ties and a round wire on the lower arch. **B.** Radiograph showing the appliance. Note the composite restoration retained by a pin.

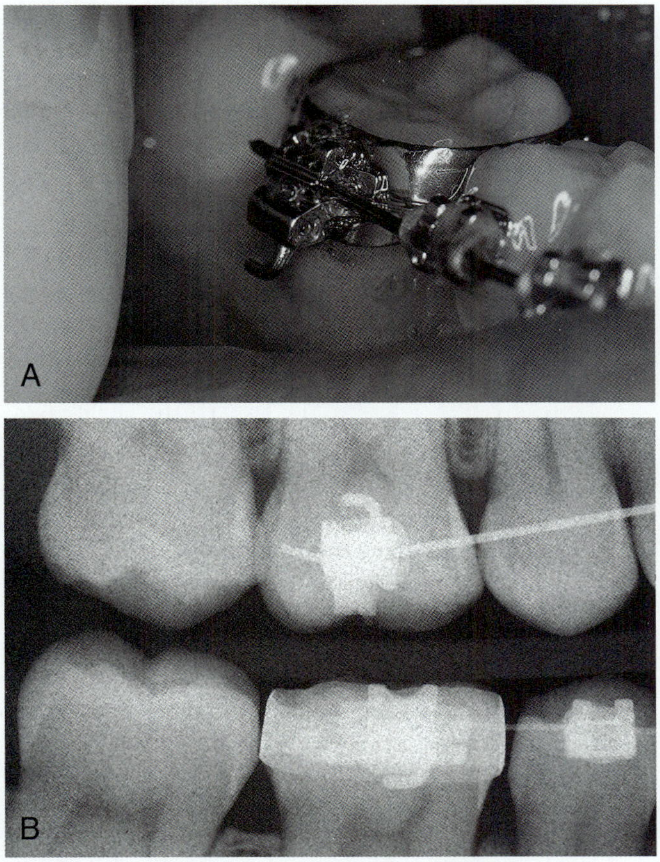

FIGURE 13.2 A. Photograph of a buccal tube that is part of the appliance shown in Figure 13.1. Note the hook for attaching elastics. **B.** A posterior bitewing of the same area. Note that the mandibular tube uses a band, whereas the maxillary tube is directly bonded to the molar.

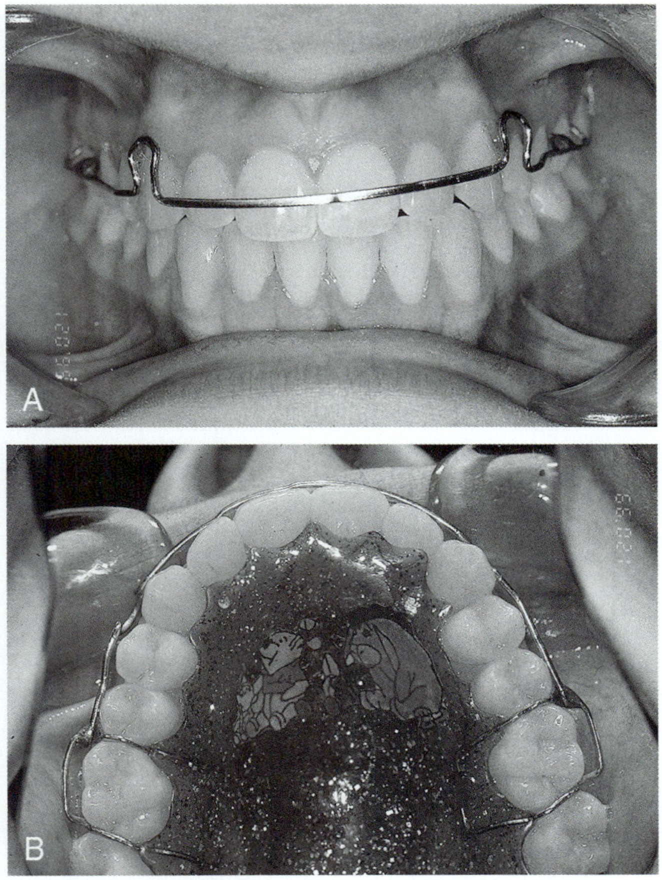

FIGURE 13.3 Photographs of an orthodontic maxillary retainer. **A.** Facial view. **B.** Occlusal view. (Courtesy of Dr. Daniel Foley, Beckley, WV.)

dentists and dental hygienists have spent significant time and effort removing orthodontic bonding material left on teeth after orthodontic treatment. Debonding of orthodontic brackets is presented in Chapter 32.

3. Acrylic Resins

The acrylic resins used to construct orthodontic appliances are the same chemically activated materials as those discussed in Chapter 11. The adolescent patients seen by orthodontists have encouraged the use of colors that stand out rather than match oral tissues. At times, acrylic orthodontic appliances do not blend in with the oral environment but are a fashion statement. Red, green, orange, and even sparkle colors are commonly used.

B. Wires

Wires are used in orthodontics as springs and stabilizers. Many wires are bought preformed to match an ideal archform from the manufacturer. Others are bent by the orthodontist to the desired archform. Wires are attached to the patient's teeth with brackets, ligatures, tubes, and bands. Elastic deformation of the wire (bending) is used to apply force to the teeth, much like with a spring. The force applied by wires pushes, pulls, or rotates teeth into the proper position, as shown in Figure 13.4.

Many metals have been used for orthodontic wires. Stainless steel is the most common. Nickel–titanium wires are also popular because they can store more energy for tooth movement than other wires. Wires are manufactured in a variety of shapes and cross-section sizes. As the size of the wire increases, so does the stiffness of the wire and the force it can apply. Some wires are round; others are rectangular, square, or even several wires braided together.

C. Brackets, Bands, and Tubes

1. Brackets

A **bracket** is a device that is attached to teeth, holds the archwire in place, and is used to transfer the forces of wires, springs, and elastics to the teeth. A variety of materials are used to make orthodontic brackets, as shown in Figures 13.1,

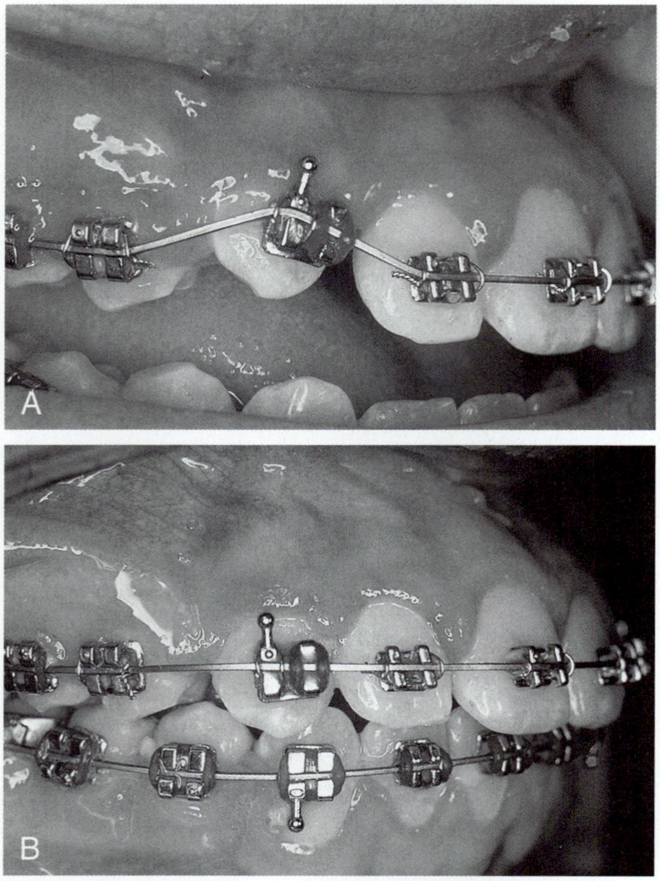

FIGURE 13.4 A. Before a wire is ligated to a maxillary arch with a malposed canine. **B.** After the force of the wire has moved the canine into a more ideal position. (Courtesy of Dr. Daniel Foley, Beckley, WV.)

13.2, and 13.4. Historically, stainless steel has been the most widely used material. A metal mesh is attached to the back of metal brackets. The undercuts of the mesh lock in the bonding material and attach the bracket to acid-etched enamel with composite resin material. Metal brackets have excellent mechanical properties, but they suffer from poor esthetics. They are relatively easy to bond to and remove from teeth.

Other materials used to make brackets are polymers, such as polycarbonate resin, and ceramic materials, such as aluminum oxide. Polymers tend to be too weak for this use, however, and are subject to creep over time. Some manufacturers have added a metal reinforcement to the bracket slot to improve the strength and stiffness of polycarbonate brackets. Ceramic brackets have had mechanical problems as well. Although strong in compression, ceramic brackets are quite brittle. Fracture has also been a problem. On the other hand, the high compressive strength of ceramic brackets has made them difficult to remove from teeth. Many innovations and improvements have been made to both polymeric and ceramic brackets because the esthetic appearance of these brackets is commonly demanded by patients. Bonding polymeric and ceramic brackets to teeth is more technique sensitive than bonding metal brackets, but if directions are followed, success is common.

2. Bands and Tubes

An orthodontic **band** encircles the crown of the tooth. Bands were used to attach brackets to teeth before acid etching became available. Brackets were welded to the bands, and the bands were cemented around each tooth. Current orthodontic practice uses bands only on molar teeth because molars require more force to move compared to other teeth.

Orthodontic bands and tubes are made from stainless steel. An orthodontic **tube** is just that, a tube that allows a wire to slide through it, as shown in Figure 13.2. Most orthodontic tubes are actually a combination of several tubes, both round and square. An orthodontist may use more than one wire at a time. One wire is used to apply force to one or more teeth, and a second wire is used to stabilize the "anchor" teeth. Orthodontic tubes are welded to bands, and the bands are cemented on molars. The cement of choice is glass ionomer cement (because of fluoride release). At times, tubes are bonded to molars by using acid-etched composites.

D. Elastics and Ligatures

The term **elastic** is used in orthodontics for several types of products and thus can be confusing. The "rubber bands" worn by orthodontic patients are used to apply force to teeth. They are called elastics. These rubber bands are changed by the patient several times each day as the force (pull) of the rubber band decays (decreases) over time. They are made from latex rubber and come in a variety of sizes, force levels, and colors.

Other "elastics" are used to secure the archwire into the bracket. These are called **elastic ligatures.** They look like little rubber O-rings and are stretched around the "wings" of the bracket, forcing the wire into the bracket slot. These elastic ligatures are typically made from thermoplastic rubber, such as polyurethane. Other commonly used ligatures are thin, stainless-steel wires that are wrapped around the archwire and bracket wings and twisted to secure the archwire in the bracket. The end of the ligature wire is then cut and tucked in around the bracket, tying the wire into the bracket. Both types of ligatures are shown in Figure 13.1.

E. Retainers

After the teeth are moved into the proper position, the orthodontist removes the bands and brackets. The patient is typically very happy that day. If left alone, however, the teeth would tend to "relapse" or partially return to their original position. To prevent relapse, orthodontists use **retainers** to keep the teeth in the desired position. There are many kinds of retainers, and many are similar to functional removable orthodontic appliances.

The common retainer for the maxillary arch consists of an acrylic palate with several wire clasps (much like a partial denture framework) and a wire that sits on the labial surface of the teeth. A retainer is shown in Figure 13.3. Sandwiched between the acrylic and the wire, the teeth are held in place.

A common mandibular retainer is a **lingual arch.** With this type of retainer, a heavy wire sits on the lingual surface of the lower anterior teeth and is bonded to the canines via a mesh pad with composite. A lingual arch retainer is shown in Figure 13.5.

F. Stainless Steel

Stainless-steel devices are common in orthodontics. Stainless steel typically has a significant nickel content (~8%). Many patients are sensitive to nickel, and orthodontists find themselves in a dilemma with these patients. Until recently, many products were only available as nickel-containing, stainless-steel products. More and more, however, manufacturers are using stainless steel with little or no nickel or other metals. Titanium is a popular alternative to stainless steel.

G. Oral Hygiene and the Orthodontic Patient

All orthodontic patients are considered to be at high risk for caries. Oral hygiene is difficult with orthodontic appliances because food debris is retained after every meal. Many orthodontic patients have "white spots" on their teeth when their brackets are removed. These white spots are the visible sign of initial decalcification (caries). Some orthodontic patients develop cavitated lesions. It is critical that the dental hygienist stress the importance of oral hygiene and proper diet to the orthodontic patient. Poor plaque control frequently results in gingival inflammation. Food debris stuck on the wires and brackets is a continuous source of carbohydrate for acidogenic bacteria. The orthodontic patient's swollen gums quickly heal after the "hardware" is removed, but carious lesions must be restored. It is very frustrating to the general dentist to restore the facial surfaces of anterior teeth in young patients when they know that these carious lesions could have been—and should have been—prevented. Many orthodontists will recommend fluoride rinses and auxiliary oral hygiene aids to their patients in an effort to prevent decay. In addition, orthodontists are using fluoride-releasing bonding materials to reduce the patient's risk of caries.

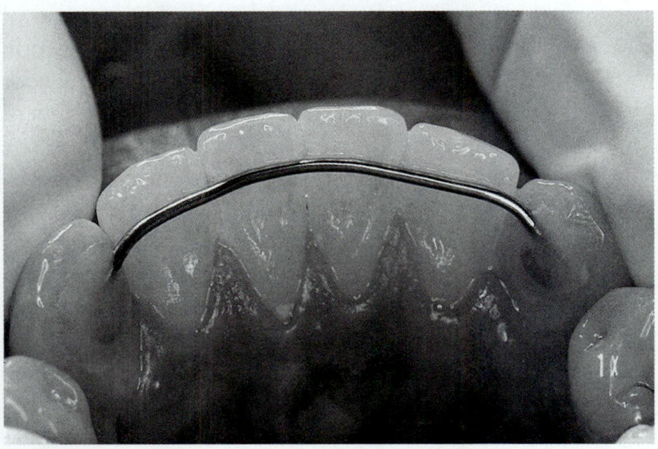

FIGURE 13.5 Photograph of a bonded lingual retainer.

II. Endodontic Materials

A. Endodontics in General

Endodontics is the specialty of dentistry that treats pathology of the pulp and periapical tissues of teeth. Typically, endodontic treatment involves root canal therapy.

1. Diagnosis

Diagnosis involves determining which tooth, if any, requires root canal therapy. The status of the dental pulp and periapical tissues is important to determine the diagnosis. Occasionally, a patient is certain which tooth is causing the pain; other times, the involved tooth is difficult to identify. The clinician must use diagnostic tests to make a definitive diagnosis. Diagnostic tests include percussion tests (tapping the tooth with the handle of a dental mirror), mobility, reaction to hot and cold stimuli, periodontal probing, electric pulp tests, and radiography. A radiograph of tooth #7 with a periapical radiolucency is shown in Figure 13.6*A*. Before root canal therapy is performed, the clinician must determine if the tooth can be restored to adequate form and function. This involves examining the tooth's periodontal health and extent of caries.

2. Root Canal Therapy

Root canal therapy involves removing the contents of the dental pulp space, the pulp chamber, and the canal system. Depending on the status of the pulp, local anesthesia is the first step. The

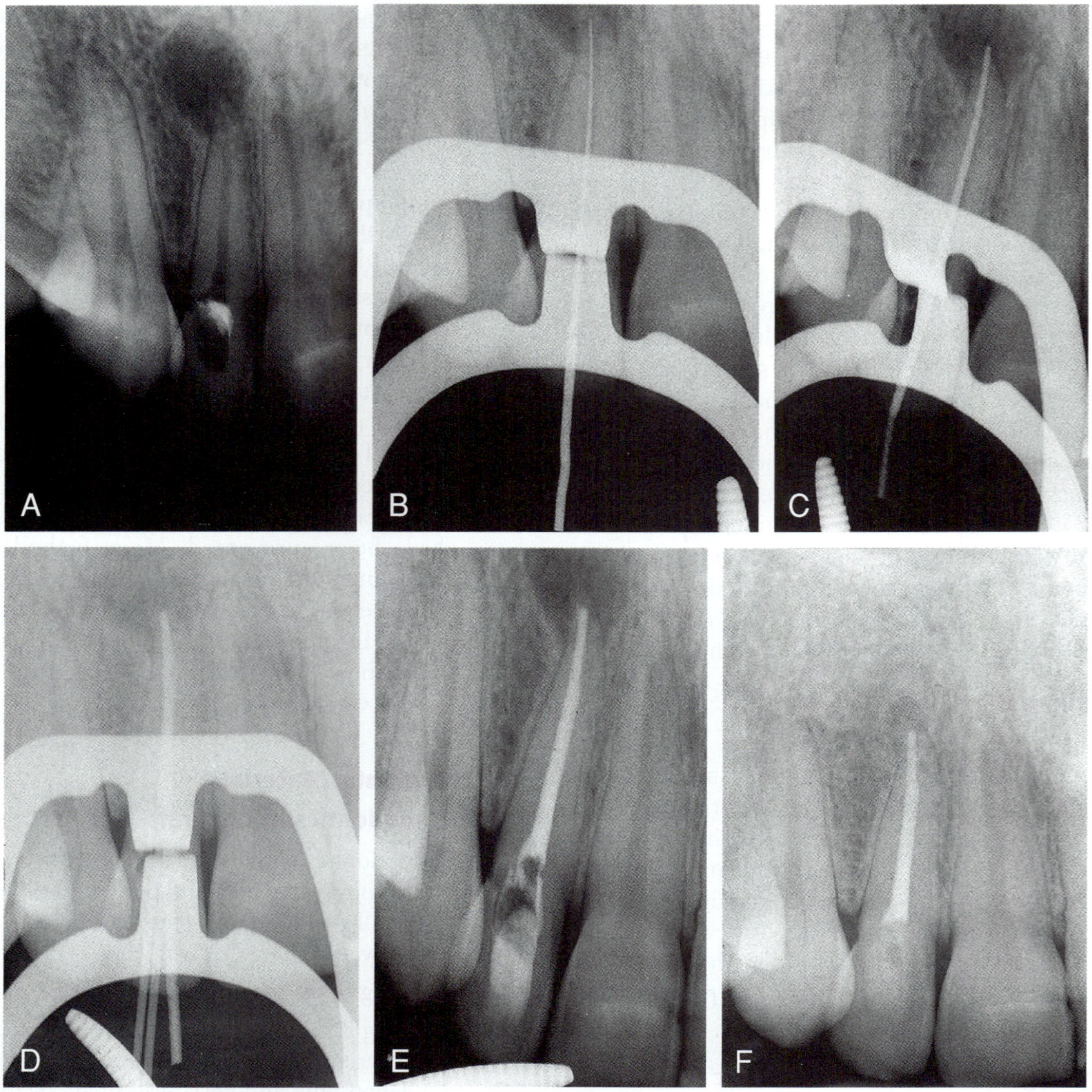

FIGURE 13.6 Radiographs of root canal therapy. **A.** Initial condition with a periapical radiolucency. **B.** Initial working file. **C.** Master apical file. **D.** Master cone and several accessory gutta percha points. **E.** Completed root canal therapy. **F.** One-year recall. Note the decrease in the size of the periapical radiolucency.

pulp may be vital connective tissue, necrotic debris, or a combination of both. Pulp removal is accomplished with files and irrigants, which will be described later in this section. The canal space is prepared to a shape that is designed to receive the filling material. The filling material is gutta percha (a rubber-like material) in combination with an endodontic sealer. The filling material should fill the canal space in three dimensions and prevent leakage of oral fluids and contaminants into the periapical tissues.

3. Restoration

Restoration of an endodontically treated tooth may be as simple as a filling (amalgam or composite) or as complex as a post/core and crown. The complexity of the restoration depends on the location of the tooth and the amount of tooth structure that is missing. The restoration must fill the pulp chamber and protect the root canal–filling material from oral fluids. Current adhesive restorative materials should be employed when restoring endodontically treated teeth to reduce the amount of coronal leakage. Inadequate coronal restoration has caused many well-performed root canal therapies to fail. Many clinicians believe that posterior teeth should receive full coronal coverage to prevent fracture of the tooth. Anterior teeth can be restored with a simple filling if the remaining tooth structure is adequate. Many teeth requiring root canal therapy have lost a large amount of tooth structure. These teeth may require a post, made of stainless steel or dental casting alloy, that is cemented into a canal and supports the core buildup. Core buildups are made of amalgam or composite. They replace the missing tooth structure and retain the crown, as shown in Figure 1.4.

B. Cleaning the Canal Space

1. Preparation of the Access Cavity

After diagnosis, treatment options are discussed with the patient. Local anesthetic is administered, and a rubber dam is placed for isolation. A rubber dam is mandatory when performing root canal therapy to protect the patient from swallowing or aspirating small endodontic instruments or irrigating solutions. Access to the canal space is gained by use of a high-speed handpiece. Each canal is located with an endodontic explorer and endodontic files.

2. Endodontic Files

Endodontic files and other instruments are used to remove the contents of the canal system. Files enlarge and shape the canal to receive the filling material. Files can be divided into two groups: hand files and "handpiece-driven" files. Traditionally, endodontic files were made from stainless steel, but recently, files made of nickel–titanium have become popular. Hand files are moved in a rotational motion or up and down to mechanically clean and shape the canal system. An international standardization for endodontic file sizes has been established (American Dental Organization and International Standards Organization). Corresponding gutta percha and paper points also exist. Files are placed in the canals, and the length of the canal is determined with the use of radiographs, as shown in Figure 13.6*B* and 13.6*C*. As the canal is enlarged, several radiographs are used to determine the exact working length of the canal. The file used to shape the most apical portion of the canal is called the master apical file and is shown in Figure 13.6*C*.

3. Irrigants

Irrigants are aqueous solutions that are used to disinfect the canal system by killing bacteria and dissolving pulpal tissue. Irrigants also flush out debris and lubricate the canal during instrumentation. Common irrigants include sodium hypochlorite (5.25%, or diluted to 2.5%), chlorhexidine gluconate (0.2%), or sterile saline. They are injected into the canal with a syringe and needle. As they flow out of the canal, they are removed with suction.

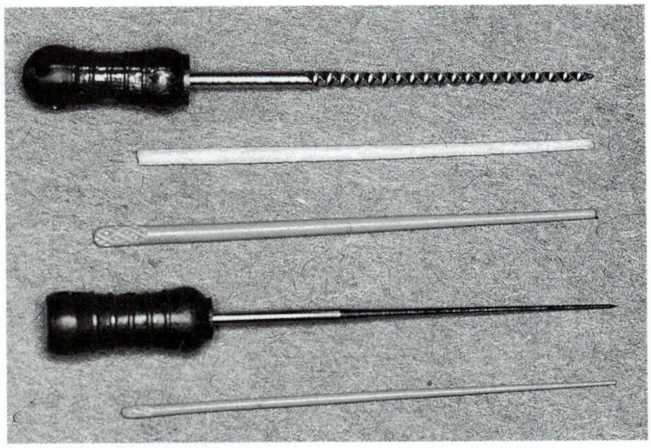

FIGURE 13.7 Photograph of (from *top* to *bottom*) an endodontic file, paper point, gutta percha point, spreader, and accessory gutta percha point. Note that the file, paper point, and gutta percha are all the same shape and diameter.

4. Paper Points

A paper point is shown in Figure 13.7. Paper points are used primarily to dry the canal before it is filled with gutta percha and sealer.

C. Filling the Canal (Obturation)

1. Gutta Percha

Various materials can be used to fill or obturate the root canal. The most common **obturation** material used is gutta percha in combination with an endodontic sealer. **Gutta percha** is a polymeric material that has been used for a variety of purposes for centuries. Dental gutta percha is composed of zinc oxide (~66%); gutta percha (~20%); heavy metal sulfates, such as barium sulfate (~11%); and waxes/resins (~3%). Barium sulfate is added to make it radiopaque, as seen in Figures 13.6, *D–F*. Two gutta percha cones are shown in Figure 13.7. Gutta percha is a flexible material at both room and body temperature; it softens when headed above 65°C (150°F). Gutta percha is used with a variety of filling techniques. It can be softened with heat or a solvent and then placed into the canal space.

2. Lateral Condensation

The most commonly used filling technique is cold **lateral condensation.** In this technique, a master gutta percha cone is selected that matches the size and length of the master apical file. The master cone is coated with an endodontic sealer and placed in the canal so that it reaches the entire length of the prepared canal. An endodontic spreader, as shown in Figure 13.7, is then placed beside the master gutta percha cone and

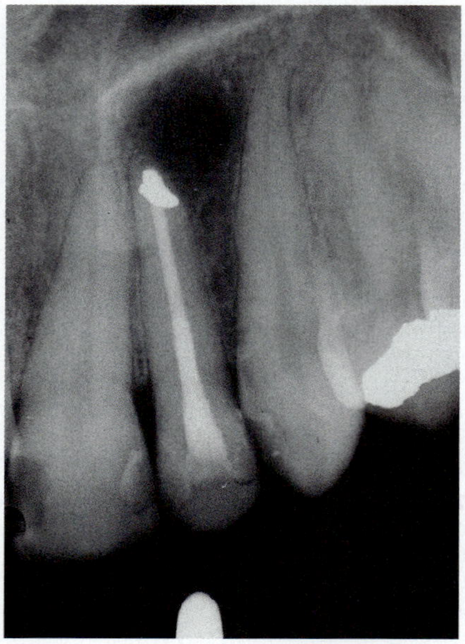

FIGURE 13.8 Radiograph of an apicoectomy and amalgam retrofill. (Courtesy of Dr. C. Russell Jackson, Morgantown, WV.)

pushed into the canal to create a space beside the master cone. The spreader is rotated and removed from the canal, and an accessory gutta percha cone is placed into the space that was created. A radiograph of a master cone with several accessory cones is shown in Figure 13.6*D*. The process of cold lateral condensation is continued until a dense, three-dimensional fill is achieved, as shown in Figure 13.6*E*.

3. Endodontic Sealers

Endodontic sealers are a type of dental cement. Sealers coat the canal space and fill any voids between the canal wall and the gutta percha. Endodontic sealers are predominantly zinc oxide–eugenol (ZOE) products with additives. The most common additives are other essential oils and chemicals, such as barium sulfate or silver, that make the material radiopaque. Calcium hydroxide sealers are also available. Sealers are purchased in either a paste/paste or a powder/liquid system.

D. Restoration and Recall

After root canal therapy is completed, the tooth needs to be restored in a timely manner. Restoration may begin immediately or be delayed until certain symptoms resolve. The patient needs to be informed that placement of a permanent restoration is critical to the success of the root canal therapy. The patient should be informed to return to the office if the temporary filling is lost. Most dentists will take periapical radiographs of teeth with root canals at recall appointments, such as that shown in Figure 13.6*F*, to assess the success of the treatment.

E. Apicoectomy and Retrofills

Root canal therapy is successful in approximately 95% of cases. If failure occurs, treatment options include conservative retreatment, extraction, or an apicoectomy. An **apicoectomy** is a surgical procedure that removes from 1 to 3 mm of the root apex. In addition, the apical portion of the canal is prepared, and a filling is placed to seal the end of the root (**retrofill**). Figure 13.8 shows a radiograph of this treatment. Retrofill materials include amalgam, reinforced ZOE, EBA cement, and mineral trioxide aggregate.

III. Periodontal and Other Surgical Materials

Because periodontics and oral surgery involve the manipulation of soft tissue, it is no surprise that both groups of materials will be discussed in this section. Because dental hygiene programs have significant course work in their curriculums covering periodontics, these materials will not be covered in detail.

A. Periodontal/Surgical Packs

Periodontal packs are used to protect surgical sites and promote healing. Periodontal packs are mixed to a putty-like consistency and then placed over the surgical site. The pack is retained in place by forcing the material into the embrasures of the teeth, as shown in Figure 13.9. The placement and removal of periodontal packs are presented in Chapter 33.

1. Chemistry

Many periodontal packs are based on the typical ZOE formulation described in Chapter 7. When noneugenol temporary cements were developed, noneugenol periodontal packs soon followed. The set material is not as strong as cements and makes them easy to remove when desired.

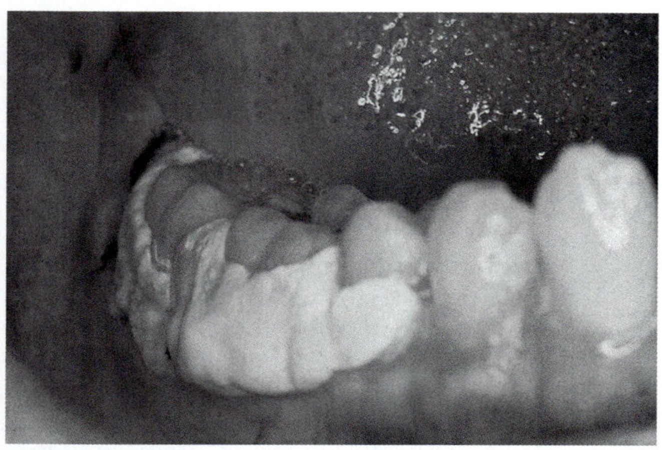

FIGURE 13.9 Photograph of a periodontal pack in place. (Courtesy of Dr. Louise Veselicky, Morgantown, WV.)

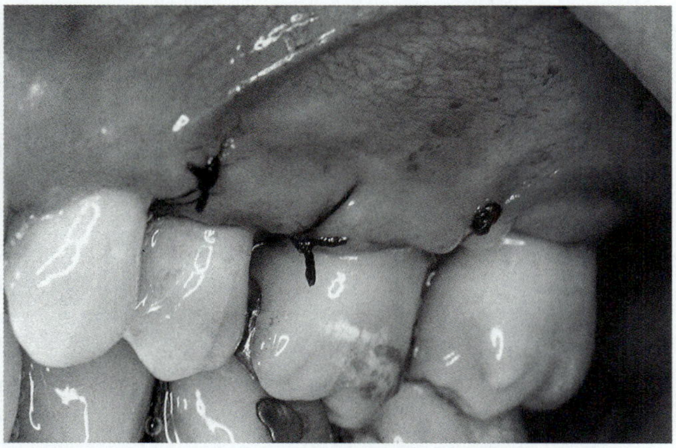

FIGURE 13.10 Photograph of sutures in place. (Courtesy of Dr. Louise Veselicky, Morgantown, WV.)

Light-cure periodontal packs have also been marketed. The setting reaction is the same addition polymerization reaction previously described in Chapter 5. The monomer and resulting polymer are a little different from the usual dental composite. The set material is much weaker than a composite, making it easier to remove.

2. Systems

Most systems are powder/liquid or paste/paste, similar to those of temporary cements. Light-cure materials come as a putty and do not need to be mixed.

B. Sutures

Sutures are threads or filaments that are used to reposition tissues that have been displaced by surgical procedures or trauma. Examples are shown in Figures 11.10*C* and 13.10. A variety of sutures and suture materials are available. They are made from naturally occurring as well as man-made materials. Both absorbable and nonabsorbable sutures are available.

1. Absorbable Sutures

Absorbable sutures are resorbed by the body and, therefore, do not need to be removed at a second appointment. Absorbable sutures include surgical gut, both plain and "chrome," and synthetic polyglycolic acid. Glycolic acid is polymerized via addition polymerization and is formed into fibers. Suture removal is presented in Chapter 34.

2. Nonabsorbable Sutures

Nonabsorbable sutures include surgical silk and other threads, either of natural or synthetic materials. It is important that these sutures be removed at a later appointment. They carry a risk of infection because they exist both inside and outside of the body while they are in place.

3. Physical Characteristics of Sutures

Sutures may be single filaments or twisted or braided, multifilament materials. The size of sutures (diameter) is designated by a number of zeros. The smallest is 0 and is called "ought," 00 is called "double ought," and 3-0 is called "triple ought." The largest size is 8-0, or "eight ought."

4. Needles

Placing sutures requires a needle to pull the filament through the tissue, as when sewing with a needle and thread. Most needles are stainless steel, and they come in a variety of shapes. Most surgeons use swaged needles (needles that do not have an eye). Swaged needles do not use a knot to tie the suture to the needle. Instead, the end opposite the tip is a tube. The suture material is inserted into the tube, and the sides of the tube are crushed or swaged onto the suture, binding it to the needle. Swaged needles pass through the tissues much more easily and cause less tissue damage than needles with an eye and a knot.

C. Bone Replacement Materials

Many materials have been developed to replace bone that has been lost to periodontal disease. Some are natural materials; others are synthetic. Various forms of human and animal bone are available. They are treated with chemicals to prevent transmission of pathogens. Other synthetic materials, typically a calcium phosphate formulation, are used to replace bone. Some of these are resorbable, whereas others are not.

D. Membranes

Polymer membranes are used to prevent the apical downgrowth of epithelial tissue and attachment to cementum at the base of a periodontal pocket after periodontal surgery. Both absorbable and nonabsorbable membranes are available. Placement of a nonabsorbable membrane requires a second surgery to remove it.

E. Antibiotic Devices

Researchers have experimented for more than 20 years with materials that release antibiotics into the gingival crevice and periodontal pockets. New absorbable and nonabsorbable products have received U.S. Food and Drug Administration approval. Examples are Atridox and Arestin. Their use in the treatment of periodontal disease continues to increase.

F. Bone Plates and Screws

Oral surgery is the field of dentistry that treats fractures of the maxilla and mandible as well as other facial structures. At times, a fixation device is used to stabilize sections of bone. Plates and screws or heavy-gauge wires are used. These materials are typically removed after sufficient healing has occurred and are made of stainless steel.

IV. Pediatric Dentistry

Although pediatric dentistry is a recognized specialty, most children are treated in a general dentistry office. A dental hygienist working in such an office will see many young patients. Most of pediatric dentistry can be described as general dentistry for younger patients. A few cases, however, do not quite fit into the typical adult patient restorative procedures. Several are described here.

A. Pulpotomy

A **pulpotomy** is the removal of a portion of the pulp. Usually, this involves removal of only the coronal portion of the pulp of the primary and permanent molars; the pulp tissue in the canals is left in place. After the coronal pulp tissue is removed, various medicaments are placed in the chamber to sterilize or mummify the accessible remaining pulp tissue. The pulp chamber is filled with a dental cement, typically a reinforced ZOE product.

For primary molars, a pulpotomy is a permanent procedure. On the other hand, a pulpotomy is a temporary (frequently emergency) procedure on permanent molars that is followed by root canal therapy (as described earlier). A primary molar with a pulpotomy is typically restored with a stainless-steel crown (Fig. 13.11*A*).

B. Stainless-Steel Crown

In young patients, molars that are badly broken down can be restored with a preformed **stainless-steel crown** (Fig. 13.11, *A* and *B*). The crown is a

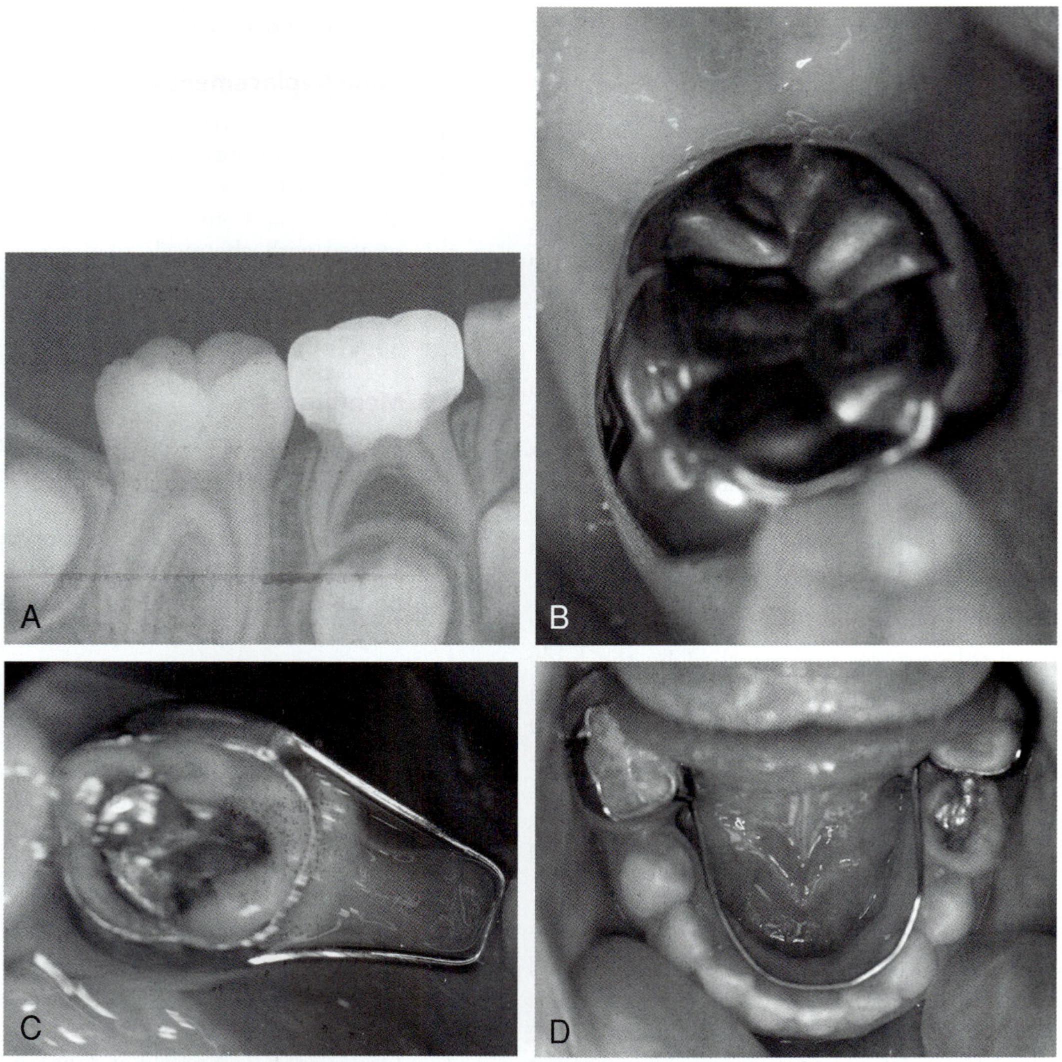

FIGURE 13.11 A. Radiograph of deciduous tooth with a pulpotomy and stainless-steel crown. **B.** Photograph of a stainless-steel crown. **C.** Photograph of a band-loop space maintainer. **D.** Photograph of a lower lingual holding arch. (See color images.) (**A**, Courtesy of Dr. Glenn Boyles, Fairmont, WV.)

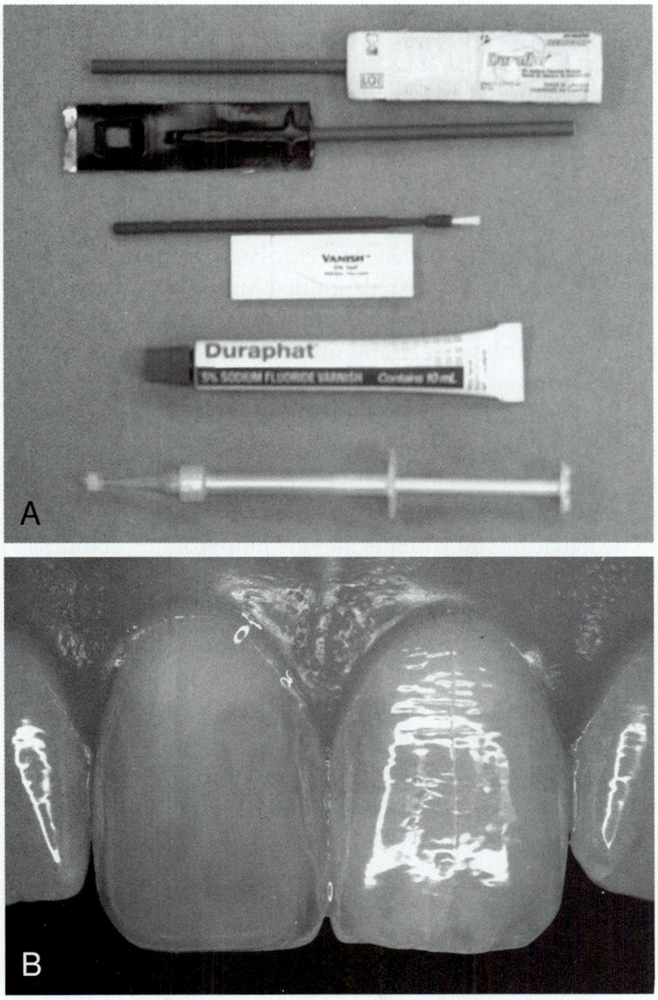

FIGURE 13.12 A. Several fluoride varnish products. **B.** Fluoride polish applied to tooth #8.

metal shell (thin layer) with preformed anatomy. Stainless-steel crowns come in a variety of sizes for each molar. This includes both primary and permanent, maxillary and mandibular, and first and second molars. The tooth is prepared in a manner similar to that for a cast crown. The preformed crown with the proper mesial-distal dimension is chosen. The crown is adapted and then cemented by filling the crown with cement and seating it on the prepared tooth. The excess cement is removed after setting. A stainless-steel crown on a primary tooth is designed to restore the tooth until it is exfoliated. A stainless-steel crown on a permanent tooth is designed to restore the tooth until the patient is older, the tooth is completely erupted, and the risk of caries is more normal.

C. Space Maintainer

Some patients lose primary molars before the permanent tooth is ready to erupt. Teeth adjacent to that space may drift into the space formerly occupied by the lost tooth. Loss of this space for the permanent tooth often results in crowding when the permanent tooth erupts. Orthodontics may be necessary to correct the crowding problem.

Space maintainers are appliances that prevent the drifting of adjacent teeth in such cases. They keep the space open for the permanent tooth to erupt. This reduces the likelihood of orthodontics. When the permanent tooth begins to erupt, the space maintainer is removed. A unilateral band-loop and a bilateral lower lingual holding arch space maintainer are shown in Figure 13.11.

D. Preventive Materials

A variety of preventive materials have been covered in previous chapters. A mouthguard is shown in Figure 1.12. Mouthguards absorb energy and prevent trauma. A sealant is shown in Figure 1.11. Sealants prevent caries by filling caries susceptible pits and fissures with a polymeric material. Pits and fissures are caries susceptible ecological niches of teeth that bacteria colonize and toothbrush bristles cannot clean. The application of dental sealants is presented in Chapter 25. Some may consider glass ionomer materials to prevent recurrent caries. However, definitive supportive research is not available. Several categories of dental products prevent oral diseases. Mouthwashes are available that reduce gingivitis. Fluoridated toothpastes, gels, and rinses have long been known to be effective in preventing caries.

Recently, fluoride varnish has been added to the available products for reducing caries. These products were originally used to reduce root surface sensitivity. They have become a quite popular preventive adjunct for high caries risk patients. They reduce caries by approximately 40% depending on the clinical study. A typical **fluoride varnish** contains 5% (22,600 ppm) NaF, a carrier resin and a volatile solvent. The teeth are dried and painted with the varnish. The patient is instructed to not eat or brush for two hours after placement. Some of the fluoride in varnish is absorbed by the enamel, changing hydroxy-apatite to fluoroapatite, and reducing the solubility of the enamel in an acid environment. Fluoride varnishes are recommended for all ages assuming no medical contraindication is present. A variety of schedules have been used, six months being the most common interval between applications. Several products are shown in Figure 13.12A. Most but not all products result in a temporary yellow tint of the teeth (see Figure 13.12B).

SUMMARY

The dental materials discussed in this chapter include those from the specialties of orthodontics, endodontics, periodontics, oral surgery, and pediatric dentistry. In orthodontics, many of the materials used are the same as those used in general dentistry. These would include impression materials, gypsum products, bonding agents, composites, and acrylic resins. Wires are used in orthodontics to apply force to the teeth. Brackets are bonded to the teeth surfaces and provide a "slot" to hold the archwire. The archwire then extends through many brackets and "connects" all the teeth together. Brackets are made of metal, polymer, or ceramic. Orthodontic bands, which are made of stainless steel, encircle the crown of the tooth. Elastics and ligatures are also orthodontic materials. These materials apply force to the teeth or secure the archwire into the bracket depending on the type of "elastic" used. Retainers are used to prevent relapse of treated teeth.

Root canal therapy uses endodontic files to remove the pulp contents. Some files are used by hand; others are handpiece driven. Gutta percha is a polymeric material that is used to fill the canal space. Barium sulfate is added to gutta percha to make it radiopaque. Endodontic sealers are a type of dental cement that coats the canal space and fills in voids between the canal wall and the gutta percha.

After periodontal surgery, periodontal packs are used to protect surgical sites and promote healing. They are usually supplied in powder/liquid or paste/paste form and are mixed to a putty-like consistency. Sutures are used in many types of surgical procedures to reposition tissues that have been displaced by surgery or trauma. Sutures may be absorbable (do not need to be removed) or nonabsorbable (must be removed). Sutures may be single filaments or twisted/braided multifilament materials. To place a suture, a needle is required. Needles are made of stainless steel and are usually swaged onto the suture material. Other surgical and periodontal materials include membranes, antibiotic devices, bone plates and screws, and those materials used for actual bone replacement.

Dental materials and procedures used in the treatment of pediatric dental patients include pulpotomies, stainless-steel crowns, and space maintainers. Pulpotomies involve removal of a portion of the pulp. It can be a permanent or a temporary procedure depending on the tooth that is involved. Stainless-steel crowns can serve as a functioning restoration until the primary tooth is exfoliated. For permanent teeth, a stainless-steel temporary restoration is replaced when the patient is older. Space maintainers are appliances that prevent the drifting of adjacent teeth until a permanent tooth erupts.

Learning Activities

1. Examine students in the class undergoing orthodontic treatment. Determine what types of materials are being used. Discuss the possible oral hygiene aids these students could use.
2. Examine radiographs of patients who have had endodontic therapy. Discuss the benefits of root canal therapy and the materials used to restore these teeth.
3. Place and remove a periodontal pack on a dentoform.
4. Place and remove sutures in a piece of fabric, an orange, or a piece of chicken.
5. Ask classmates if anyone has ever had a stainless-steel crown or space maintainer. Discuss the treatment that the student experienced.

Review Questions

1. The word "obturation," when used in discussion of root canal therapy, means:
   a) Accessing the canal
   b) Filling and sealing the canal
   c) Placing the final restoration
   d) Removing the contents of the pulp
2. Which type of composite gives the clinician an advantage when removing orthodontic resins?
   a) Microfilled
   b) Macrofilled
   c) Hybrid
   d) None of the above

3. The endodontic surgical procedure that removes 1 to 3 mm of the root apex is called a/an:
a) Endodontic retreatment
b) Retrofill
c) Root resection
d) Apicoectomy

4. What is used to disinfect the canal system by killing bacteria and dissolving pulpal tissue?
a) Endodontic sealers
b) Paper points
c) Irrigants
d) Gutta percha

5. Which orthodontic device prevents "relapse" of the teeth?
a) Archwire
b) Ligature
c) Bracket
d) Retainer

6. The debonding procedure is done after orthodontic treatment is completed. The dental material removed from tooth surfaces is:
a) Composite resin
b) Cold-cure resin
c) Dental cement
d) Ligature material

7. The most commonly used technique to fill a root canal with gutta percha is termed:
a) Direct compression
b) Lateral compression
c) Direct condensation
d) Lateral condensation

8. A pulpotomy usually serves as a ______________ procedure on permanent molars.
a) Temporary
b) Permanent
c) Either temporary or permanent
d) Neither temporary or permanent

9. Which of the following materials used in orthodontic treatment serves to secure the arch wire on the facial surfaces of a tooth?
a) Band
b) Bracket
c) Composite resin
d) Retainer

10. Surgical silk suture is:
a) Another name for surgical gut suture
b) Absorbable and removed at a later appointment
c) Nonabsorbable and removed at a later appointment
d) Absorbable and exist both inside and outside of the body while in place.

Supplemental Readings

Chadwick BL. Products for prevention during orthodontics. Br J Orthodont 1994;21:395–398.

Cohen S, Hargreaves KM, eds. Pathways of the Pulp. 9th ed. St. Louis: Mosby, 2006.

Wilkins EM. Clinical Practice of the Dental Hygienist. 10th ed. Baltimore: Lippincott Williams & Wilkins, 2008, Chapter 40.

14

Clinical Detection and Management of Dental Restorative Materials During Scaling and Polishing

Key Words/Phrases

beveled margin
cavosurface margin
margination
tine

Objectives

After studying this chapter, the student will be able to do the following:

1. Using the criteria listed in Table 14.1, differentiate between porcelain and composite materials.
2. Discuss how the following criteria may help a clinician to distinguish between tooth tissues and restorative materials or between two types of restorative materials:
   - Radiographic characteristics
   - Surface smoothness
   - Tactile and auditory sensations
   - Location
3. Distinguish between other tooth tissues and restorative materials by using the criteria listed in Table 14.1.
4. Describe some common procedures routinely performed by a dental hygienist that could be detrimental to teeth and restorative materials.
5. Verbally compare the expected differences in the surfaces of enamel and a gold crown after polishing with a relatively abrasive agent.
6. Recall the recommended instrumentation technique around the margins of cast restorations.
7. Explain the causes of possible damage to restorations from the use of high-speed instrumentation.
8. Propose a possible scaling-and-polishing protocol for a patient with the following oral findings:
   - 4 mm of recessed gingiva
   - Class V glass ionomer restorations in the maxillary left quadrant
   - Two gold crowns in the mandibular right quadrant
   - Three composite restorations in the maxillary anterior segment

INTRODUCTION

Much has been written about the various techniques, instruments, and materials that are used during scaling and polishing. It is difficult, however, to find adequate references to document potential damage to the surfaces of teeth, restorations, and fixed prosthetic appliances.

In this chapter, the characteristics of restorative materials and tooth structure will be described to aid the dental hygienist in providing the appropriate treatment during scaling and polishing. Criteria will be presented to help identify the various restorative materials that are used most frequently today.

After identifying the patient's restorative materials, the effects of instrumentation and the use of fluorides and polishing agents must be considered. Suggestions will be made as to which cleaning devices, instruments, and agents are acceptable for use on given dental restorative materials.

I. Clinical Detection of Tooth Structure and Dental Restorative Materials

A. Identification of Tooth Structure and Restorative Materials

Many areas of tooth structure and types of restorative materials are easily identified. At times during an examination or scaling, however, it will be difficult to distinguish between exposed dentin and a recent, well-placed composite resin restoration. In such instances, the restorations can be overlooked, and an inappropriate polishing procedure may result.

Table 14.1 was developed as a guide for the hygienist to differentiate between tooth structure and restorative materials and between the different types of restorative materials.

1. An Example

Using Table 14.1 to distinguish between dentin and a glass ionomer restoration, several statements may be made: Both may appear radiopaque. In addition, dentin feels smooth to the explorer, whereas glass ionomer feels rougher.

A detectable margin also differentiates these two materials. If a sharp explorer were to pass over these two surfaces, a variance in sound would be noted, with the dull sound being peculiar to the glass ionomer. The sound referred to as sharp or dull is slight and, in all probability, is a combination of auditory and tactile sensations perceived by the operator. Another way to explain this concept is that most clinicians would agree enamel has a certain hardness and smoothness to it, whereas restorations may have a different texture and feel.

Using only the criteria listed in Table 14.1, rapid identification can be made. If the hygienist is unaware of the presence of the restoration and scales from the dentin surface of the tooth (in an area of gingival recession) onto the composite with heavy pressure, damage could be done to the restoration. A careful analysis of the restorative materials used on the patient must be carried out before initiating any form of treatment.

2. Other Criteria to Aid in Identification

a) Radiographic Characteristics

The shades of gray between the extremes of radiolucency and radiopacity aid the trained clinician in identifying tooth structures and materials. See Chapter 15 for more information.

b) Visual Appearance

Tooth enamel is the only natural material in the oral cavity that is translucent to visible light. Dentin has more color (yellow) and is much more opaque. In recent years, considerable efforts have been made to develop tooth-colored restorative materials that transfer light in a manner similar to that of tooth structure. This was discussed in detail in Chapter 5. These characteristics are evident in both porcelain and resin; the restorations made from these materials are difficult to detect by casual observation.

c) Surface Smoothness

In respect to surface smoothness, it could be stated that all exposed tooth surfaces in the oral cavity should be smooth. When a surface is smooth, it is free of irregularities. An explorer passed over this type of surface will glide freely with the change in contour and will not meet resistance.

One of the goals of the hygienist is to produce smooth surfaces on both natural tooth structure and restorative materials. Less plaque and debris accumulate on smooth surfaces.

d) Sound and Touch

A sharp explorer can be one of the most helpful diagnostic tools available to the astute hygienist. Passage of the tip of the explorer at right angles to the surface with minimal pressure and force will transmit two distinct sensations to the hygienist.

1) The tactile sensation refers to the character of the surface: It will be smooth, as in tooth enamel, or it will be rough, as in a worn composite restoration.
2) Sound also plays a part in the diagnosis. The **tine** (sharp point) of the explorer will be silent on smooth enamel but scratchy or noisy on rough tooth surfaces, worn composite restorations, and residual orthodon-

Table 14.1 Characteristics of Tooth Structure and Restorative Materials

CRITERIA:	*TOOTH*			*POLISHED METAL RESTORATIONS*				*TOOTH-COLORED RESTORATIONS*			*OTHER*	
	Enamel	*Cementum*	*Dentin*	*Amalgam*	*Cast Gold*	*Gold Foil*	*Base Metal Alloys*	*Composite*	*Glass Ionomer*	*Porcelain*	*Pit and Fissure Sealant*	*Cements*
Opaque		X	X	X	X	X	X	1	X	1		X
Translucent	X							X		X	X	
Smooth to Explorer	X		X	X	X	X	X	X		X	X	
Rough to Explorer		X							X			X
Tooth-Colored	X	X	X					X	X	X	2	
Glossy Surface	X		X	X	X	X	X	X		X	X	
Dull Surface		X						X	X			X
*Detectable Margin**					X		X		X	X	X	X
Dull Sound		X						X	X		X	X
Sharp Sound	X		X	X	X	X	X			X		

1. The degree of opacity and translucency for resins and porcelain depends on the thickness of the material and the shade.
2. In many cases, pit and fissure sealants are clear, unfilled resins and difficult to detect. Tints or coloring agents have been added to make them easier to detect; also, it is easier to determine if they need replacement.

*It has been assumed that all restorations are correctly finished and polished.

Modified with permission from Krouse MA, Gladwin SC. Identification and management of restorative dental materials during patient prophylaxis. Dent Hyg 1984;58:456–461. Graphic by C. A. Hoffman.

tic bonding resin. When the tine passes over faulty or worn margins of a restoration, it will produce a "ping" sound.

3) Some restorations will be so well matched to tooth structure that, without the "sound-feel" difference, they may go undetected. The ideal margin of all restorative materials is undetectable by passage of the explorer from tooth to restoration or from restoration to tooth. The tine of the explorer serves as an aid not in identification of the material but in determination of the condition of the restoration at the **cavosurface margin.** The cavosurface margin is the area formed by the cavity wall and the external tooth surface.

e) Location

The location of the restoration can make identifying tooth-colored restorations difficult. Depending on the material used and on the age and marginal integrity of the restoration, the junction of the enamel and the restorative material is often visually indiscernible. For this reason, the clinician should make the most of radiographs and proper transillumination with the mouth mirror to identify the exact location of the restoration before using any instrument.

B. Management of Restorative Dental Materials During Scaling and Polishing

After the dental hygienist has identified the patient's various restorative materials, the selection of cleaning agents, instruments, and specific techniques is made. Polishing agents, instruments, and procedures are designed to aid the clinician in producing highly polished surfaces on the teeth, restorations, and appliances.

Smooth surfaces on tooth structure and restorative materials are less receptive to bacterial colonization and dental plaque formation. Coronal polishing, which may take place after scaling and root-planing, must be accomplished in a way that is not damaging to the tooth and restorative materials. Fairly common examples of detrimental procedures include production of excessive heat during polishing, excessive use of abrasives, damage to the margins of cast restorations, and use of high-speed instrumentation.

1. Production of Excessive Heat During Polishing

Heat is generated when an abrasive, rubber cup and hand piece is used against a natural tooth surface. Rotating a bristle brush, rubber cup, or rubber wheel on a thumbnail readily demonstrates how quickly excessive heat can be generated by speed or pressure. Adding mouthwash, water, or glycerin to make a slurry when abrasives, such as silex or tin oxide, are being used will decrease the amount of heat that is produced.

Prophylaxis pastes supplied in unit doses are moist so that less heat will be produced. It only takes once or twice for a patient to jump during polishing to learn that heat is being generated to make the patient uncomfortable. Either the cup is left on the tooth too long, too much pressure is applied or the clinician is using too much speed.

Temperatures of 140°F or greater will alter the surface characteristics of an amalgam restoration because of a release of mercury. This will result in accelerated corrosion and marginal breakdown.

2. Excessive Use of Abrasives

Excessive use of abrasives can be injurious to patients in several respects. Improper use of an abrasive agent and a rubber cup at the gingival margin can cause trauma to or removal of the surface epithelium in that area.

As will be discussed in Chapter 16, abrasive agents can be harmful because of the following factors:

- Particle size of the polishing agent
- Number of particles applied per unit of time
- Speed of the application
- Amount of pressure applied

It is for these reasons that selective polishing has become an accepted alternative treatment to polishing with abrasives.

A study of the surface roughness of restorative materials after polishing with polishing pastes showed that many restorative materials were rougher after polishing. Gold, amalgam, and microfilled composites were used in this study. It must be remembered that for cast gold restorations, such as inlays, onlays, or crowns, the final polish applied in the dental lab provides the smoothest surface these restorations will have during patient service. Many polishing agents can create fine scratches in several restorative materials because of speed, pressure, and particle size. The hygienist should make a dedicated effort to use a polishing agent containing the smallest abrasive particle that will remove surface stain and attached plaque.

3. Damage to Margins of a Cast Restoration

A third way in which damage could be incurred on a restored surface during scaling is by opening a margin of a cemented casting. This particular type of restoration is likely to have a detectable margin. More so than gold foil or amalgam restorations, cemented castings (inlays, onlays, and crowns) will have a "cement line" margin. A properly mixed cement should have a film thickness of less than 40 microns. The margins of cast restorations are delicate, and they have been adapted to the preparation by the operator. **Margination** is the process of using hand instruments from cast metal to tooth, to adapt the margins of the gold casting to the tooth preparation. Because the longevity of the cast restoration depends, in part, on the condition of the margin, it is critical that the margin be identified. When scaling in the area of a cast restoration, the dental hygienist should alter his or her scaling technique so as not to jeopardize the margin of any cemented casting.

Figure 14.1*A* illustrates the casting in place and a thin, fragile gold edge over the **beveled margin** (the sloping or angled edge of the preparation) of the tooth. A potential position of a curette scaler is shown in Figure 14.1*B*, and Figure 14.1*C* depicts the results of an applied working stroke. Note that destruction of the marginal integrity can lead to recurrent decay, which can be seen in Figure 14.1*D*.

To prevent this damage, use of an explorer and/or a scaling instrument is necessary to first locate the margin of the casting. Once the margin is identified, the working stroke must be kept within an area below the margin. On the facial or

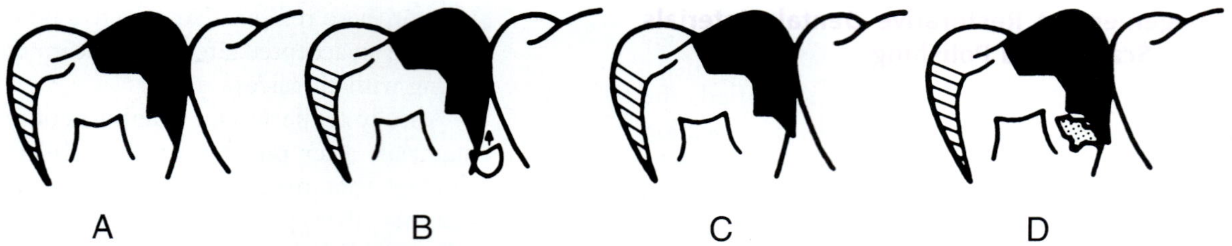

FIGURE 14.1 The cemented casting. **A.** Casting cemented into place. **B.** Curette blade improperly positioned. **C.** Results of an applied working stroke. **D.** Recurrent decay resulting from an opened margin. (Reproduced with permission from Krouse MA, Gladwin SC. Identification and management of restorative dental materials during patient prophylaxis. Dent Hyg 1984;58:456–461.)

lingual surface, a more oblique or horizontal stroke (rather than a vertical stroke) should be used, always keeping in mind the location of the margin of the casting. If a student is in doubt of whether he/she is feeling a cast margin or subgingival deposit when exploring, it is recommended to get the assistance of a clinical instructor to help with this determination.

4. Power Instrumentation

Use of high-speed instrumentation, such as sonic or ultrasonic scalers or air polishers, may cause damage to or removal of several types of restorative materials.

a) Ultrasonic Scalers

The vibrating tips of ultrasonic scalers may harm composite resin restorations, laminate veneers, and titanium implant abutments. Amalgam margins may be altered, and restorations fabricated from porcelain may be fractured.

b) Air Polishers

Dental restorative materials, such as cements, composite resins, and other nonmetallic materials, may be removed or pitted by use of the air abrasive technique. Margins of cast restorations may be significantly damaged with use of this instrument.

5. Application of Fluoride

Some restorative materials may be altered or damaged by the application of topical fluorides.

a) Stannous Fluoride

Tooth-colored restorations and the enamel margins adjacent to the restoration may discolor with the application of stannous fluoride.

b) Acidulated Phosphate Fluoride

The dental hygienist must be aware of the possible deleterious effects of applying acidulated phosphate fluoride to porcelain, composite, and glass ionomer restorations. A 4-minute application may create a loss of reflection or dull the appearance of these restorations. The fluoride will microscopically "etch" the outer surface of these materials.

It is recommended that the hygienist place petroleum jelly over the restoration before application of the acidulated phosphate fluoride. Another option is to apply a 2.0% sodium fluoride (NaF) gel or foam instead of acidulated phosphate fluoride.

II. Suggestions for Polishing Specific Restorative Materials

There are many acceptable methods to finish and polish typical restorative materials. This section will include standard protocols for amalgam, composite, gold, and porcelain.

A. Amalgam

For new or recently placed amalgams, the finishing and polishing consists of using finishing burs with a low-speed handpiece, followed by the use of silex and then whiting mixed in a slurry consistency. Rubber cups or prophy brushes may be used and should be changed when changing to the next abrasive agent.

Another polishing regimen consists of using finishing burs and then brown and green rubber polishing points. These points are impregnated with polishing agents and eliminate the use of liquids and powders. However, it is important to keep the point wet (with saliva). Excessive heat created when these polishing points are being used will cause discomfort for the patient and may injure the pulp. In addition, excessive heat may accelerate marginal breakdown and corrosion of the amalgam restoration. Both methods of finishing and polishing amalgams are described in detail in Chapter 26.

For older amalgams, finishing burs are usually used for a longer period of time to produce a smooth surface. Brown and green polishing points are then used.

B. Composites

As mentioned previously, there are many methods to finish and polish composite restorations.

Interproximal areas may be finished by contouring the surface with a scalpel blade. It can be used to remove overhangs of composite, and shape the line angles. Next, finishing strips may be used from most abrasive to least abrasive grit.

A sequence of aluminum oxide-coated discs may be used for the facial surfaces. For lingual surfaces, an egg-shaped finishing bur is used for finishing. "Enhance" points and cups (by Dentsply/Caulk) are then used to polish. Finally all surfaces may be polished with a composite polishing paste. A technique for finishing and polishing composites is described in detail in Chapter 36.

In recent years, one step diamond micro-polishers have become available in cup and point shapes (Pogo by Dentsply/Caulk), and are recommended for composite, glass ionomer, and compomer restorations.

C. Cast Gold and Gold Foil

To polish gold restorations, either regimen mentioned for amalgam restorations may be used: the brown and green polishing points or a sequence of polishing powders, such as silex, and whiting or tin oxide. Tin oxide produces an excellent result when used as a final polishing agent for gold.

D. Porcelain

For porcelain veneers and crowns, a variety of prophylaxis pastes may be used to clean and polish. Remember that porcelain powders are fired at very high temperatures, which result in a very hard material. For this reason, most prophylaxis pastes may be employed to polish the surfaces of porcelain veneers and crowns.

SUMMARY

It is the professional responsibility of the dental hygienist to determine the composition of the surface being scaled and/or polished. Several criteria aid the in the identification of tooth structure or restorative materials. Once identified, restorations should be managed as follows:

- Temperatures of 140°F or greater are not created when polishing amalgam restorations. Such temperatures accelerate corrosion and marginal breakdown.
- Abrasive agents are not used to excess. Remember that the particle size of the abrasive, the amount of abrasive applied, and the speed and pressure of the rubber cup or brush all play a role in potential trauma to the tissue or creation of a rough surface on tooth structure or restoration.
- Cast margins are not "lifted" from the blades of curettes and scalers. An oblique or horizontal stroke (rather than traditional vertical stroke) should be employed.
- Ultraspeed cleaning devices should be used with caution and only after identifying existing restorative materials.
- Acidulated phosphate fluoride is not used on porcelain, composite, or glass ionomer restorations. This fluoride may etch the outer surface of these materials and create a dull appearance.
- The least abrasive polishing paste is selected to remove stains and plaque.

There are many ways to finish and polish restorations. The last section of this chapter provided suggestions for finishing and polishing specific restorative materials, such as amalgam, composite, cast gold, gold foils, and porcelain.

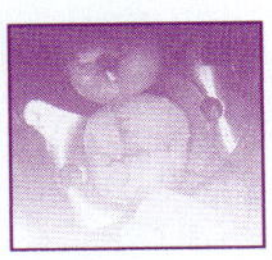

Learning Activities

1. In a clinical setting, attempt to identify restorative materials in the mouths of classmates.
2. List any precautions for managing the materials found in learning activity #1 when scaling or polishing.

Review Questions

1. Which of the following restorative materials may be affected by numerous applications of acidulated phosphate fluoride?
   a) Cast gold
   b) Zinc oxide–eugenol (ZOE) temporary restorations
   c) Glass ionomers
   d) Amalgam

2. Margins of cast restorations can be altered by instrumentation with curettes and explorers. A suggested technique for deposit removal in these areas is to employ:
   a) A vertical stroke, as used on natural tooth structure
   b) A vertical stroke, but with anterior instruments only
   c) An oblique or horizontal stroke, with appropriate instruments
   d) Any stroke, but with ultrasonic scalers

3. A dull sound when an instrument is being used should be evident with which of the following materials?
   a) Gold foil and base metal alloys
   b) Enamel and dentin
   c) Amalgam and cast gold
   d) Composite and glass ionomer

4. Tactile sensitivity and a sharp explorer will aid the clinician in identifying:
   a) Opacities from translucencies
   b) Glossy surfaces from dull surfaces
   c) Dull sounds from sharp sounds
   d) Rough surfaces from smooth surfaces

5. Creating temperatures of 140° F or greater when amalgam restorations are being finished and polished will:
   a) Arrest corrosion and marginal breakdown
   b) Accelerate corrosion and marginal breakdown
   c) Create a roughened surface
   d) Change a sharp sound to a dull sound when using an explorer

6. What are the agents of choice for polishing a gold crown intraorally?
   a) Silex and tin oxide
   b) Brown and green polishing points
   c) A correct sequence of prophylaxis pastes
   d) A sequence of aluminum oxide–coated discs

7. One benefit of a moist polishing agent is:
   a) Heat reduction
   b) Aid in swallowing
   c) Faster stain removal
   d) Ease in rinsing

8. When a cast gold crown has been marginated, it means that the
   a) Casting fits precisely in the preparation
   b) Margins have been closely adapted to the crown preparation
   c) Casting fits within the gingival margin
   d) Casting is in relation to the adjacent marginal ridge

9. When clinically polishing gold and gold foil, the regimen is similar to that of
   a) Composite
   b) Amalgam
   c) Glass ionomer
   d) Porcelain fused to metal crown

10. Acidulated phosphate fluoride is not recommended for the following materials
    a) Composite and porcelain only
    b) Composite and glass ionomer only
    c) Gold, composite and porcelain
    d) Glass ionomer, composites, and porcelain

Supplemental Readings

Darby ML, Walsh MM. Dental Hygiene Theory and Practice, 2nd Ed. St. Louis: Saunders, 2003, Chapter 20.

Krouse M, Gladwin SC. Identification and management of restorative dental materials during patient prophylaxis. Dent Hyg 1984;58:456–461.

Wilkins EM. Clinical Practice of the Dental Hygienist. 10th ed. Baltimore: Lippincott Williams & Wilkins, 2008.

15

Radiographic Appearance of Dental Tissues and Materials

Joan Gibson-Howell, R.D.H., Ed.D.

Key Words/Phrases

attenuation
electromagnetic radiation
radiographic contrast
radiolucent
radiopaque
retrofill

Objectives

After studying this chapter, the student will be able to do the following:

1. Identify various dental tissues and materials on a radiograph.
2. Explain why, radiographically, dental tissues and materials appear radiopaque or radiolucent.
3. Integrate the radiographic appearance of dental tissues and materials with clinical information to assess the patient's status of health or disease.

I. Purposes for Radiographs

Oral radiographs are useful supplements for use in assessing the patient's present oral and dental status. Although many adjunct assessment tools can assist in determining the diagnosis and prognosis of a specific dental disease or condition, the dental radiograph remains an essential component of total patient care. The radiograph provides the diagnostician/practitioner with critical information that cannot be collected by any other method.

II. Essentials for Radiographic Interpretation

It is essential that the dental hygienist be competent in radiographic techniques, patient safety regarding radiation, and proper film handling and processing. It is also imperative that the dental hygienist has a basic knowledge in both general and dental anatomy, periodontics, pathology, and dental materials so that he or she can interpret the processed films.

III. Rationale for Integrating Dental Radiology in a Dental Materials Text

To distinguish dental tissues from dental materials, health from disease, and normal aspects from abnormal aspects, it is essential that dental hygienists competently recognize what is "within normal limits" both clinically and radiographically. When viewing radiographs, the "mind's eye" scans each radiograph looking for normal anatomy, landmarks, and typical restorations. When an unexpected or uncommon area is identified, the dental hygienist's past knowledge and experience assist in the identification and naming of the material, object, or anatomical landmark. The ability to analyze critically what is seen or not seen in regard to oral anatomical structures, dental materials, and objects is essential for an accurate interpretation and/or diagnosis. It is not legally permissible for the dental hygienist to prescribe radiographs or diagnose dental disease. Yet, a critical role of the dental hygienist is to collect the information necessary to assess the need to produce quality radiographs. This information is used not only to educate the patient but also to provide the dentist with accurate data for diagnosis, treatment planning, and treatment.

IV. Producing the Radiographic Image

X-rays are a form of electromagnetic radiation. **Electromagnetic radiation** occurs as waves of photons that vary in wavelength, frequency, and energy. Because electromagnetic radiation may have biologic cellular effects, it is imperative that the dental hygienist be knowledgeable regarding the use and consequences of radiation.

The primary beam of radiation encounters and passes through hard and soft tissue before it reaches the x-ray film. Hard tissues include tooth tissues (enamel, dentin, and cementum) and bone. Soft tissues such as epithelium, muscles, nerves, glands, pulp, and blood vessels also occur in the oral cavity. Tissues and dental materials absorb the x-ray beam according to their thickness and density. As a result, the processed film consists of "darks," "lights," and varying shades of gray (**radiographic contrast**).

This process of reducing the energy of the primary beam as it passes through the differing objects/materials is called **attenuation.** Attenuation results in the respective levels of blacks, whites, and grays on the processed radiograph that assist in distinguishing normal radiographic findings. The thickness and composition (object density) of the tissues and materials contribute to determining the overall radiographic appearance of the processed film. Because of the subtle variations of lights (radiopacities) and darks (radiolucencies), patient information captured on the radiograph can be interpreted and aid in diagnosis.

V. Restorative Materials Categorized by Radiographic Appearance

A. Radiopaque Restorative Materials

Restorative materials that are clearly radiopaque include amalgam, cast gold, cohesive gold, non-precious alloys, and the metal portion of a porcelain-fused-to-metal crown. Two large amalgam restorations including metallic retentive pins are shown in Figure 15.1. Retentive pins are used in several ways and with various materials to increase retention where natural tooth structure is not available. The metal of the ceramometal restorations, as seen in Figure 15.2, is depicted by the white areas. The darker shadows on the incisal surface of these teeth depict the porcelain portion of the crowns. Stainless-steel and aluminum temporary crowns may be radiopaque depending on the thickness of the material.

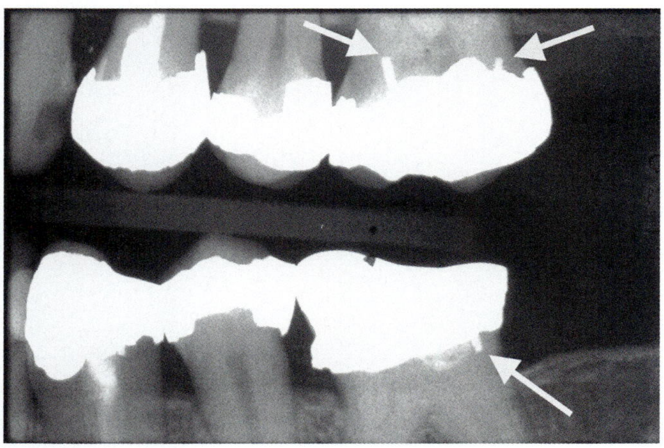

FIGURE 15.1 The amalgam restorations on teeth #14 and #19 include retentive pins (*arrows*) that enhance the resistance and retention of the restorative material.

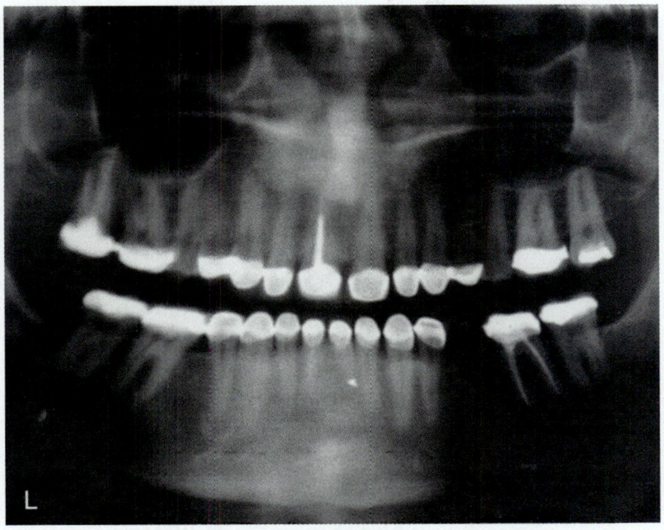

FIGURE 15.2 Numerous porcelain-fused-to-metal crowns are visible on the maxillary and mandibular arches on this panoramic radiograph. The radiolucent shadow at the incisal (#6–11) and occlusal (#2, 3, 14) surfaces is the radiolucent porcelain.

B. Radiolucent/Radiopaque Restorative Materials

Other restorative materials may also appear as varying degrees of gray (darks and lights or radiographic contrast). These materials include composite resins, sealants, cements, bases, and porcelain. Depending on the material, some of these products may appear more radiolucent than opaque, and vice versa. Look at the anterior porcelain and metal restorations shown in Figure 15.2. Depending on the type and amount of the material, varying degrees of radiolucencies and radiopacities are present. Refer to Table 15.1 to recognize the comparative radiographic characteristics of dental materials. Because of varying compositions, cements used for luting and bases may appear darker (radiolucent) or lighter (radiopaque) than the overlying restorations. Radiolucent bases under a metal restoration, particularly amalgam, and excessive adhesive materials under composites may imitate a carious lesion on the radiograph. For example, see Figure 1.9*D*, which shows a base under an existing amalgam restoration (tooth #3).

A dental sealant may be visualized on a radiograph depending on the type and amount of filler in its composition. A posterior composite restoration may also be visualized on a radiograph depending on the type of restorative material and the amount of filler in its composition. In both cases, the radiographic appearance would be radiopaque. Figure 15.3 demonstrates a composite restoration on the occlusal of tooth #28. Although the restoration is opaque, it is less opaque than a metal restoration would appear.

C. Radiolucent Restorative Materials

Some restorative materials may appear more radiolucent because of the lack of fillers or density. These materials include temporary crowns and/or bridges made of acrylic or plastic tooth-colored materials, such as resins and porcelain. Again, refer to Table 15.1 for the radiographic characteristics of the various dental materials. Figure 15.4 demonstrates an older composite resin that is radiolucent. The mesial of tooth #6 shown in Figure 15.4 is not a carious lesion; it is a resin that does not contain radiopaque fillers and therefore appears lucent. The distal of tooth #7 in Figure 15.4 has a radiopaque composite restoration compared to a more radiolucent composite in the mesial of tooth #6.

Table 15.1 Radiographic Appearance of Dental Materials[a]

	Tissues and Materials	Enamel	Dentin	Cementum	Pulp	Amalgam	Cast Gold	Implants	Composite	Glass Ionomer	Cements	Bands	Gutta Percha	Sealants	Porcelain	Other Ceramics
Radiographic Appearance	Radiopaque	X	X			X	X	X	X	X	X	X	X	X		X
	Radiolucent		X		X				X		X			X	X	X

Modified with permission from Krouse M, Gladwin SG. Dent Hyg 1984;58:456.

[a]Certain categories have some products that are radiolucent and other products that are radiopaque.

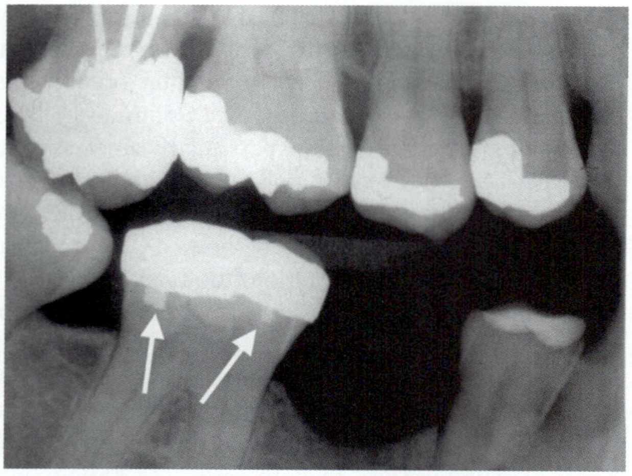

FIGURE 15.3 Note the composite resin restoration on the occlusal surface of tooth #28. Although it is radiopaque, its radiographic appearance is not as opaque as a metal restoration. Also note the retentive pins in tooth #31 (arrows).

VI. Radiographic Descriptions of Dental Tissues, Disease, and Materials

A. Radiographic Description of Tissues and Disease

Radiographically, a variety of dental materials are similar to the natural tooth structure, and others are quite different. Illustrations and a comparative table in this chapter will assist you in distinguishing the radiographic "looks" that are associated with tooth tissue and dental materials.

1. Soft Tissues

Soft tissues are not dense (compact and hard) and do not greatly attenuate the x-ray beam (the beam passes through nearly undiminished). Soft tissues appear black or dark on the processed radiograph and are called **radiolucent.** Therefore, soft tissue is not generally visible on a processed radiograph.

Figure 15.5 illustrates soft-tissue radiolucency. The interdental papilla and pulp canal are both radiolucent. The less dense the tissue or material, the less radiation it absorbs. Therefore, when the primary beam of radiation strikes the x-ray film, it is translated into a dark or radiolucent area on the radiograph.

Some dental materials are radiolucent and so are not visible on the processed radiograph. Such materials transmit the primary beam of radiation so that they are not clearly distinguishable on the processed radiograph. Examples are acrylic resin, porcelain, and most impression materials.

Figure 15.2 illustrates maxillary and mandibular porcelain-fused-to-metal crowns. On this radiograph, the porcelain is a shadow at the incisal and occlusal surfaces of the teeth. Also, note the numerous areas of radiopacities, which denote the metal of the crowns.

2. Hard Tissues

The enamel of the tooth is a very compact tissue. In fact, it is the densest tissue of the body, and it significantly attenuates the x-ray beam. In comparison, bone is slightly less dense than enamel and similarly absorbs the x-ray beam. On the other hand, dentin and cementum are considerably less dense than enamel or bone, and the x-ray beam can penetrate these tissues much more readily. The more dense the tissue or material, the more radiation is absorbed and does not reach the x-ray film to expose the silver halide crystals on the film emulsion. This translates into light or **radiopaque** areas on the film. As a result,

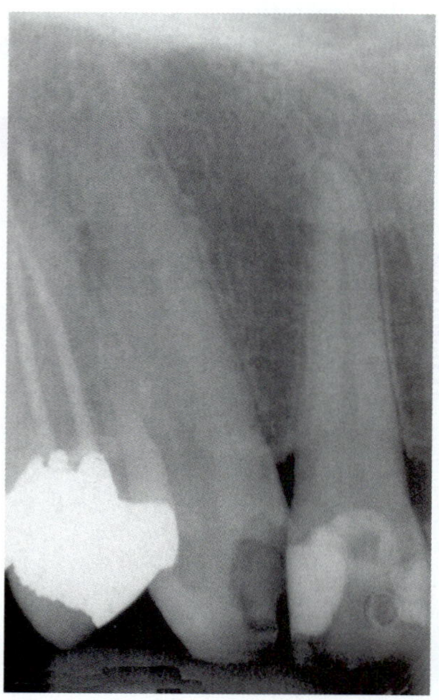

FIGURE 15.4 A radiolucent area is present on the mesial surface of tooth #6. This is not dental decay; it is a composite that appears radiolucent. The distinct outline differentiates it from caries, which would have a more diffuse outline. Root canal therapy is evident in tooth #5. The root canal filling material is gutta percha.

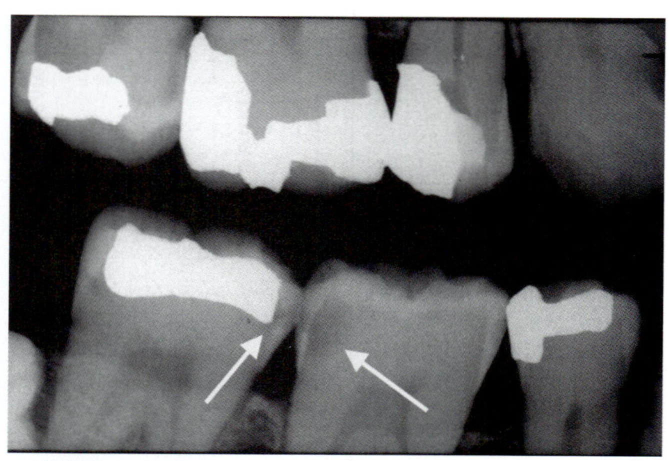

FIGURE 15.5 The radiolucent interdental papillary areas are located between adjacent teeth on this bitewing radiograph. Note the pulp chambers in the crown and root areas. Soft tissue is not visible radiographically and appears radiolucent. Caries are present in the distal of tooth #30 and the mesial of tooth #31 (arrows).

the radiographic appearance of tooth enamel is light. The dentin is less dense and less radiopaque than the enamel. The dental pulp appears dark or radiolucent.

Figure 15.6 illustrates varying hard-tissue radiopacities. Figure 15.2 also depicts numerous areas of radiopacities denoting the metal of porcelain-fused-to-metal crowns.

The alveolar bone is a combination of trabecular bone and compact bone. The trabecular bone consists of shades of gray and a combination of opacities and lucencies. Compact bone is typically more radiopaque than trabecular bone. Some dental materials (metals) are very opaque; others have opacities similar to dentin and enamel. Differentiating a radiopaque dental material from enamel or dentin is accomplished by comparing the shape of the radiopacity with the expected anatomical features of a tooth. Figure 15.7 illustrates the differences between tooth tissues and dental materials. The expected shape of Class II restorations is evident. The same can be said for radiolucencies, but the possibility of caries complicates the identification. Observations from the clinical examination must also be considered when differentiating radiopacities and radiolucencies from normal anatomy. Note the trabecular pattern of alveolar bone of the panoramic radiograph in Figure 15.2. Figure 15.6 depicts the radiopaque crestal bone in proximal areas.

3. Caries

Destruction of the calcified tissues of the tooth (enamel, dentin, cementum) results in dental caries. Radiographically, the carious area is radiolucent when compared to enamel or dentin. It is important that the diagnostician view the radiographs in an appropriate viewing situation and with a critical eye to differentiate between normal tooth anatomy, restorations, and carious lesions. Figure 15.6 illustrates proximal carious lesions (radiolucencies) on the bitewing radiograph. For example, carious lesions can be seen on the mesial of tooth #3, the mesial and distal of tooth #4, and the mesial and distal of tooth #5. In addition, a radiolucency appears on the distal of tooth #28, the mesial and distal of tooth #29, under the MOD amalgam restoration of tooth #30, and on the mesial of tooth #31. Figure 15.7 illustrates a mesial radiolucency on tooth #2.

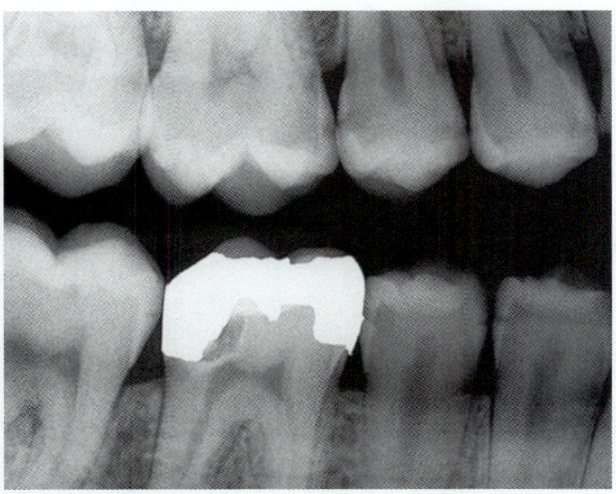

FIGURE 15.6 Radiographically, carious lesions appear radiolucent. The proximal carious lesions on this radiograph are noticeable (mesial of tooth #3, mesial and distal of tooth #4, mesial and distal of tooth #5, distal of tooth #29, and possibly under the large amalgam restoration on tooth #30). The enamel outline is radiopaque because of its density, and the dentin is comparably less opaque than the enamel (more gray). (Courtesy of Dr. Thomas F. Razmus, Department of Diagnostic Sciences, West Virginia University School of Dentistry.)

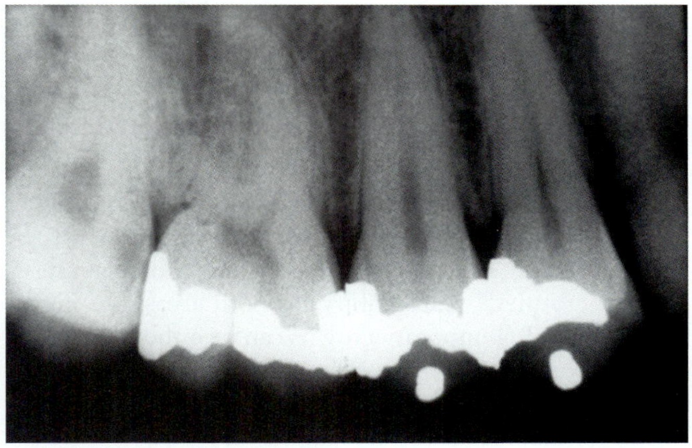

FIGURE 15.7 The carious lesion on the mesial of tooth #2 is radiolucent. The amalgam restorations are radiopaque.

B. Radiographic Description of Dental Materials

1. Dental Amalgam Restorations

As previously described in Chapter 6, dental amalgam is a commonly used direct restorative material. Because of its color, it is used primarily in the posterior teeth and in the pits of lingual surfaces of the anterior teeth. Dental amalgam is an alloy of several dense metals, so it absorbs the primary beam of radiation. The corresponding area of the processed radiograph is radiopaque. Figures 15.1 to 15.3 and 15.5 to 15.8 demonstrate amalgam restorations.

2. Resin Composite Restorations

Resin composite materials are commonly used as direct restorations in anterior teeth. They are also used in posterior teeth. As with other dental materials, both advantages and disadvantages are found when resin composite restorations are used in posterior teeth. For more discussion on this topic, see Chapter 5. Many older resin restorative materials appear radiolucent on radiographs. Figure 15.4 demonstrates a radiolucent resin in anterior teeth. Technology in biomaterials has advanced whereby fillers included in composite resins are now radiopaque to the degree that much less confusion occurs regarding the existence of recurrent caries.

3. Crown and Bridge (Prosthodontic) Materials

Some materials for crown and bridge are radiopaque while others are radiolucent. Metals are radiopaque, Figure 1.5. Porcelain can be either radiolucent or radiopaque. Porcelain fused to metal restorations has both areas, see Figure 15.2. Temporary crowns can be either depending on the material used. Acrylic resins are radiolucent. Bis-arcyl temporary materials can be either radiolucent or radiopaque.

4. Dental Bases

During removal of dental decay and preparation of the tooth for a restoration, the pulp may be traumatized or irritated by the procedure. To reduce pulpal irritation, a dental material called a "base" may be placed in the floor of the cavity preparation to insulate the pulp from thermal stimuli. For the base to be effective as a thermal insulator, it must have sufficient thickness and low thermal conductivity. Thus, the base may be more radiolucent than the overlying amalgam or composite restoration and may imitate a carious lesion. For example, tooth #3 in Figure 1.9, tooth #30 in Figure 15.3, and tooth #19 in Figure 15.8 show a base under an existing amalgam restoration. Refer to Table 15.1 for the radiographic characteristics of the various dental materials.

5. Dental Temporary (Provisional Restorations) Fillings

Some dental procedures cannot be completed in one appointment due to various reasons, i.e., diseased pulp. Between appointments, the tooth preparation must be temporarily sealed to prevent further irritation. Zinc oxide eugenol (ZOE) cement, composite or glass ionomer materials are commonly used. Tooth #19 in Figure 15.9 demonstrated a temporary restoration in the occlusal surface.

6. Endodontic, Orthodontic, Periodontal, and Surgical Materials

Materials used in, on, and around teeth to treat, repair, or restore them are often metallic. Because most metals are dense, they appear on radiographs as radiopaque. Figures 15.10 to 15.14 demonstrate the various metals used in dental specialties.

a) Endodontic Materials

Endodontic therapy is often a portion of the restorative treatment plan. Radiopaque endodontic instruments used during therapy include files, rubber dam clamps, and frame. The radiograph in Figure 15.10 illustrates endodontic files used to clean and shape the pulp canals of the teeth during root canal therapy. Endodontic filling materials include gutta percha, another thermoplastic polymer, or silver points along with an endodontic sealer. Tooth #7 in Figure 15.11 contains a gutta percha root canal filling. Gutta percha is an inert polymer to which barium sulfate is also added for opacity. Tooth #28 in Figure 15.12 shows a silver point. Sealers commonly used are zinc oxide–eugenol materials with barium sulfate added. Other sealers are based on other dental cements or bis-GMA. In certain cases, a retrofill of amalgam or MTA (mineral trioxide aggregate) may also be used. A **retrofill** is a surgically placed

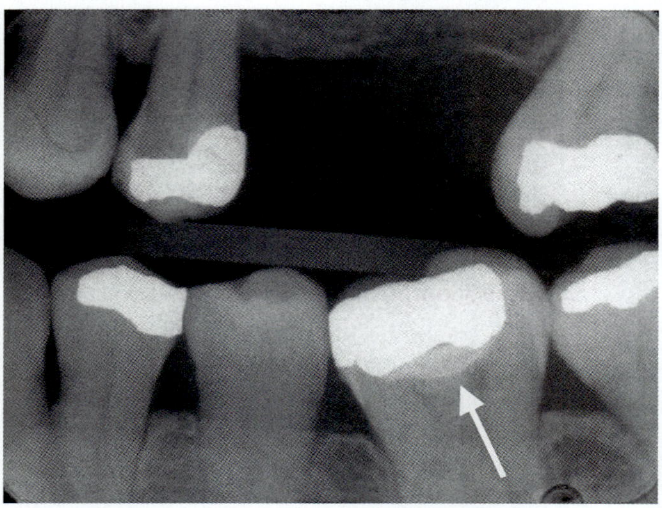

FIGURE 15.8 Amalgam restorations are present on teeth #13, #15, #18, #19, and #21. A base (arrow) is under the amalgam on tooth #19. A mesial radiolucency (carious lesion) is present on tooth #13. The radiopaque crestal bone is clearly depicted on this bitewing radiograph.

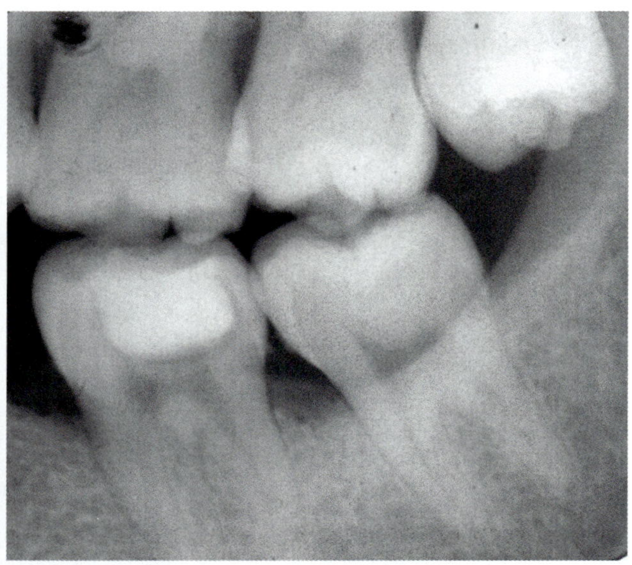

FIGURE 15.9 A temporary restoration exists in the occlusal of tooth #19. It is considered radiopaque, yet more radiolucent than metal. Note the irregular borders. Possible decay (radiolucency) remains between the tooth and restoration.

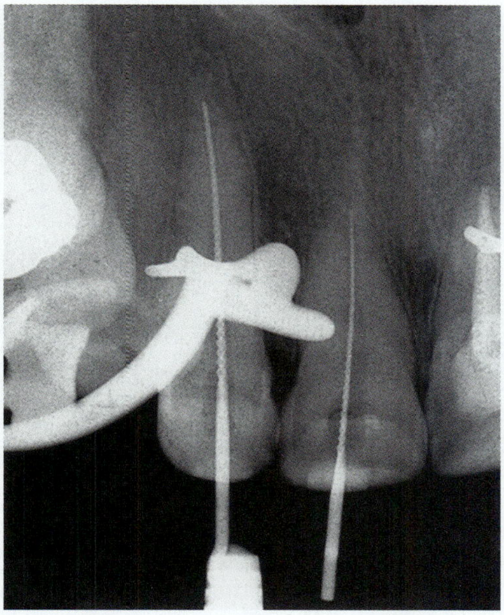

FIGURE 15.10 Teeth #7 and #8. Files are present in the pulp canals to locate the apices during the root canal therapy. (Courtesy of Dr. A.L.C. Kayafas, Akron, OH.)

restoration at the root apex. Figure 15.11 illustrates root canal therapy with an amalgam retrofill. In some instances, a retentive post or dowel pin may be used to strengthen or enhance retention of the tooth's foundation, especially when used for a fixed or removable prosthesis, see tooth #8 in Figure 15.2.

The endodontic files, silver points, retrofill amalgams, rubber dam clamps and frame, metal post materials, and some film-holding devices are metal. These materials appear radiopaque on a radiograph. Although gutta percha is not metal, it contains barium sulfate, which appears radiopaque or as a varying shade of opacity on a radiograph, as illustrated in Figure 15.4 for tooth #5.

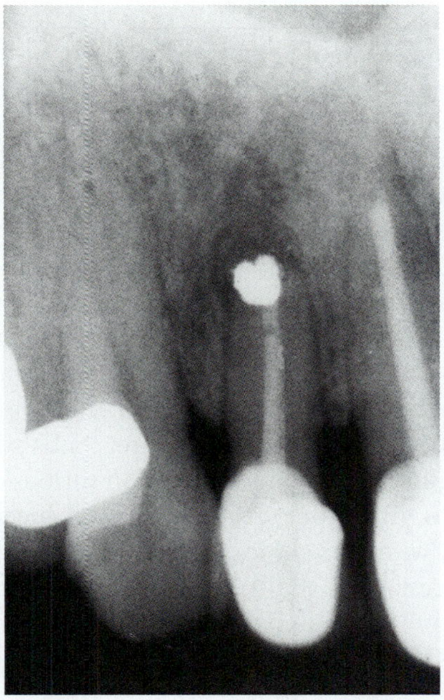

FIGURE 15.11 Tooth #7 exhibits a retrofill amalgam restoration.

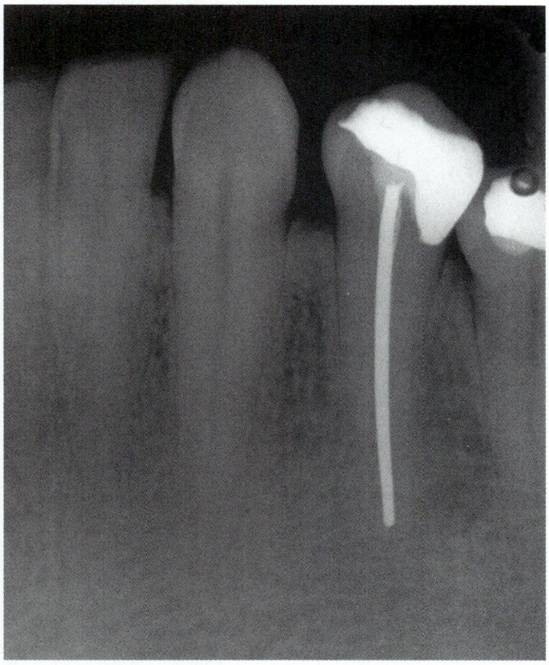

FIGURE 15.12 Tooth #28 has been endodontically treated. A silver point fills the root canal space.

b) **Orthodontic Materials**

Metal orthodontic materials used in dentistry are primarily stainless-steel orthodontic bands, brackets, and wires. Bands interfere with radiographic detection of dental caries. Brackets directly bonded to the tooth are now commonly used, however, and may not interfere. Other frequently used radiopaque orthodontic materials include springs, fixed and removable retainers, space maintainers, appliances that discourage oral habits, and bite planes. Cements and bonding materials may be radiopaque or radiolucent. Refer to Table 15.1 for a comparison of dental materials. Figures 15.13 and 15.14 illustrate a buccal tube, bands, brackets, and stainless-steel ligatures.

c) **Oral and Maxillofacial Surgical Materials/ Objects of Trauma**

The majority of oral and maxillofacial surgical materials are radiopaque. Radiopaque materials can be located on radiographs, whereas radiolucent materials cannot. Surgical items include implants or the implant fixtures, healing caps, and other tissue-replacement materials. Radiographs assist in the continuing assessment of implant healing and stability. Other surgical items that may be used are wires, plates, or screws for stabilization of bone segments during healing.

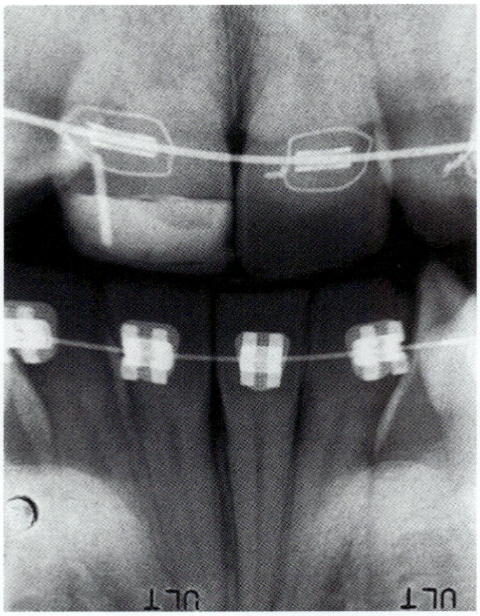

FIGURE 15.13 Anterior vertical bitewing radiograph with brackets, wires, and stainless-steel ligatures. Also note the threaded pin and composite restoring the fractured incisal edge. Bilateral mandibular tori are present and appear radiopaque.

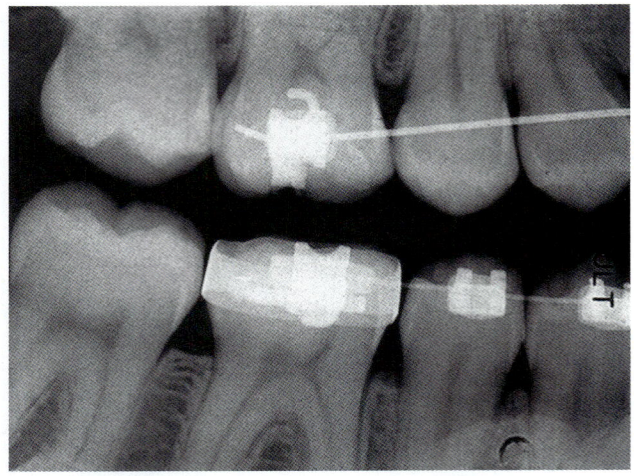

FIGURE 15.14 Posterior bitewing radiograph with orthodontic brackets, bands, wire, and buccal tube.

d) **Periodontics**

The dentist and the dental hygienist view radiographs for changes in the periodontium. Radiographs are an adjunct to the clinical examination. They may illustrate periodontal destruction that has occurred in the past, but they do not demonstrate whether the areas of destruction are currently undergoing periodontal disease activity.

To provide corrective therapy for periodontal disease, periodontists use resorbable and nonresorbable materials to assist in repairing and/or regenerating the periodontium. Periodontists determine which materials to use based on their knowledge, experience, philosophy, location of the therapy, type of defect, and specific therapy to be performed. Nonresorbable materials (e.g., ridge augmentation materials) are visible on a radiograph. Resorbable materials generally are not visible on a radiograph, yet the healing response to these resorbable materials may be visible.

Overhanging restorations, poorly contoured margins, and open contact areas are plaque retentive and contribute to gingivitis and periodontitis. The overhanging restoration in the posterior region of the mouth is most often an amalgam or cast gold restoration. This can be seen as a radiopaque material in tooth #19 in Figure 15.1.

SUMMARY

A patient's dental radiographs are critical components in the decision-making process of a dental hygiene diagnosis or a definitive dental diagnosis. Radiographs are also an important adjunct to the patient's clinical examination. It is essential that the dental hygienist/practitioner be competent in accurately interpreting dental radiographs. The practitioner must be able to distinguish normal radiographic anatomy and landmarks from abnormal and pathological radiographic findings. Radiographic artifacts and errors must be taken into account when interpreting findings as well.

The dental hygienist/practitioner must also be competent in the identification of dental materials used in dental treatment. Products used in dental treatment procedures appear radiolucent to radiopaque on dental radiographs depending on the density or compactness of the materials.

The composition of an object absorbs or attenuates the primary beam of radiation to varying degrees depending on its density. If the object is dense, the beam is absorbed, and the resultant corresponding area on the radiograph is radiopaque. If the object is not dense, the beam passes through the object, and the resultant corresponding area on the radiograph is radiolucent. For example, an amalgam restoration is dense and appears on the radiograph as radiopaque. Resin or porcelain is less dense than amalgam and appears on the radiograph as a gradient of radiolucent.

The dental hygienist must not only be able to consistently produce high-quality radiographs but also to recognize and bring to the dentist's attention various and sometimes subtle gradations of opacities and lucencies that correspond with the clinical examination. With knowledge, a "keen eye," skills, and experience, the dental hygienist serves as an important partner in the oral health team and as the primary patient educator at chairside.

Learning Activities

1. Participate in pairs or groups of three students to explore a full-mouth series of radiographs that include a variety of dental materials. Locate radiolucencies and opacities that correspond with tooth anatomy (i.e., enamel, dentin, pulp) and periodontal structures. Identify and discuss various other types of dental materials in the radiographs. Speculate as to the composition of any restorative material or other dental material that is present.
2. Perform a clinical oral examination on one of your classmates in clinic. Chart the findings: amalgams, composites, gold restorations, prostheses, and so on. After the charting, view the radiographs of your partner to correlate the radiographic appearance of oral findings with the clinical examination findings. Discuss your findings with an instructor.
3. Work in pairs to develop a case-based scenario using various periapical and/or bitewing radiographs with dental materials. Use these cases as discussion in lab sessions or class as a learning activity. Develop an OSCE (objective structured clinical examination) to assess student competency in this area.

Review Questions

1. To integrate dental radiographs into patient treatment, the dental hygienist must be competent to:
   a) Diagnose dental disease from the dental radiographs
   b) Recognize normal anatomy, landmarks, and restorations from abnormalities, pathologies, and artifacts
   c) Prescribe radiographs and determine a dental hygiene diagnosis
   d) Collect data and determine the definitive diagnosis
2. Oral tissues and dental materials in the oral cavity result in radiographic contrast on a processed radiograph. These structures attenuate the primary beam of the x-rays.
   a) The first statement is true; the second statement is false.
   b) The first statement is false; the second statement is true.
   c) Both statements are true.
   d) Both statements are false.
3. The more dense the object/material in the oral cavity, the more radiolucent the area will appear on a dental radiograph. The less dense the object/material in the oral cavity, the more radiopaque the area will appear on a dental radiograph.
   a) The first statement is true; the second statement is false.
   b) The first statement is false; the second statement is true.
   c) Both statements are true.
   d) Both statements are false.
4. An endodontically treated tooth may be sealed with gutta percha. The gutta percha appears radiolucent on the radiograph.
   a) The first statement is true; the second statement is false.
   b) The first statement is false; the second statement is true.
   c) Both statements are true.
   d) Both statements are false.
5. A porcelain-fused-to-metal crown appears both radiolucent and radiopaque on the radiograph. This radiographic appearance is caused by the various types of electromagnetic radiation.
   a) The first statement is true; the second statement is false.
   b) The first statement is false; the second statement is true.
   c) Both statements are true.
   d) Both statements are false.
6. A dentist may decide that it is necessary to place a zinc oxide–eugenol (ZOE) base in a deep cavity preparation before a restoration. Radiographically, how would this base appear compared to an overlying amalgam restoration?
   a) Translucent
   b) Radiopaque
   c) Radiolucent
   d) Similar to a carious lesion
7. The presence of an orthodontic band interferes with the detection of a carious lesion because:
   a) The band encircles the tooth, and its radiolucent appearance prevents the identification of proximal or occlusal decay
   b) The band encircles the tooth, and its radiopaque appearance prevents the identification of proximal or occlusal decay
   c) The band is cemented with zinc phosphate cement and fogs the detection of proximal or occlusal decay
   d) The band is bonded with composite resin and fogs the detection of proximal or occlusal decay

8. Resorbable materials used to repair or regenerate the periodontium are not generally visible on radiographs. The resultant healing of the resorbable material may be identified on the radiograph.
   a) The first statement is true; the second statement is false.
   b) The first statement is false; the second statement is true.
   c) Both statements are true.
   d) Both statements are false.

9. A vertical bitewing radiograph of the maxillary left molar area of a patient demonstrates slight to moderate vertical periodontal bone disease on the mesial of tooth #14. The dental hygienist's clinical examination also detects an overhang on the MODB amalgam restoration which was placed 10 years ago. Which of the following statements best describes the radiographic findings of this area?
   a) The crestal bone on the mesial of tooth #14 no longer exists, the interproximal area is radiolucent, and there is a radiopaque projection of the amalgam restoration in the proximal area
   b) The crestal bone on the mesial of tooth #14 no longer exists, the interproximal area is radiopaque, and there is a radiolucent projection of the amalgam restoration in the proximal area
   c) The crestal bone on the mesial of tooth #14 is intact, and the overhanging amalgam restoration on the mesial of tooth #14 has no bearing on the oral health status of this patient
   d) The radiographic appearance of the crestal bone and the overhanging amalgam restoration are not significant to the oral health status of this patient

10. A base may be placed under a new restoration and act as a thermal insulator to the pulp. Compared to a metal restoration, the radiographically visible base material is:
   a) Opaque
   b) Radiopaque
   c) Radiolucent
   d) Translucent

11. To differentiate a radiopaque dental material from enamel or dentin, one should compare the:
   a) Composition of the material with the anatomical parts of the tooth
   b) Size of the material with the anatomical layers of the tooth
   c) Shape of the radiopacity with the expected anatomical features of the tooth
   d) Amount of the material with the anatomical parts of the tooth

12. In recent years, it has become less confusing to radiographically distinguish composite resin restorations from carious lesions. The reason is that composite restorative material:
   a) Has improved compressive strength
   b) Has coefficients of thermal expansion closer to that of enamel
   c) Contains radiopaque filler particles
   d) Has improved elastic properties

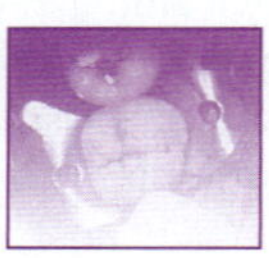

Supplemental Readings

American Dental Association & U.S. Food and Drug Administration. Guidelines for Prescribing Dental Radiographs. http://www.ada.org/prof/resources/topics/topics_radiography_chart.pdf

Ferracane JL. Materials in Dentistry: Principles and Application. 2nd ed. Philadelphia: Lippincott, Williams & Wilkins, 2001.

Haring JI, Lind LJ. Dental Radiography Principles and Techniques. 2nd ed. Philadelphia: Saunders, 2000.

Ingle JI. PDQ Endodontics. London: BC Decker, Inc., 2005.

Langland OE, Langlais RP, Preece JW. Principles of Dental Imaging. 2nd ed. Media, PA: Lippincott Williams & Wilkins, 2002.

Spohn EE, Halowski WA, Berry TG. Operative dentistry procedures for dental auxiliaries. St. Louis: Mosby, 1981.

White SC, Pharoah MJ. Oral Radiology: Principles and Interpretation. 4th ed. St. Louis: Mosby, 2000.

16

Polishing Materials and Abrasion

Objectives

After studying this chapter, the student will be able to do the following:

1. Briefly define the following terms:
   - Cutting
   - Abrasion
   - Finishing
   - Polishing
   - Abrasive
2. Recall six common abrasives that may be used for clinical or laboratory procedures.
3. Summarize factors that may influence the rate of abrasion, and explain why the dental hygienist must have a clear understanding of these factors when providing patient care.
4. Discuss the reasons why tooth structure and restorations are polished.
5. Recall the details of the polishing process. Include the series of steps, scratches produced, and wavelength of visible light.
6. Explain what it means to selectively polish.
7. Describe the characteristics of an acceptable prophylaxis paste.

Key Words/Phrases

abrasion
abrasive
air powder abrasion
aluminum oxide
chalk
cutting
cuttle
emery
finishing
garnet
grit
pumice
sand
selective polishing
Silex
tin oxide
tungsten carbide burs

INTRODUCTION

One of the major responsibilities of the dental hygienist is the cleaning and polishing of teeth and restorations. This responsibility also includes any removable appliances, such as complete and partial dentures.

Before discussing polishing materials and abrasion, it is important to distinguish between the terms "cleaning" and "polishing." Polishing, by definition, involves the abrasion of a surface by an abrasive agent that is harder than the surface to be abraded, or polished. When a dental hygienist is truly polishing, the paste or slurry containing an abrasive agent will microscopically alter the tooth or restorative surface. Section V of this chapter, "The Polishing Process" addresses this topic in greater detail. Cleaning, sometimes referred to as plaque removal, is done with agents that do not contain abrasive particles. The surface being cleaned is not altered or abraded as it would be in polishing.

An abrasive agent chosen to remove an unsightly tobacco stain may not be the best one for polishing a composite resin. The hygienist must carefully select the appropriate abrasive agent for the particular surface to be polished. The agent should clean and polish the surface without causing detrimental effects. For this reason, the hygienist should have a fundamental understanding of the principles of abrasion, finishing, and polishing.

I. Definitions

The topic of polishing materials and abrasion will be easier to discuss if we first define the basic terms that are involved in these procedures.

A. Cutting

Cutting is removing material by a shearing-off process. Examples of cutting would be milling, machining, or drilling. The process results in a somewhat smooth surface. In dentistry, cutting is done with metal burs and hand instruments to create cavity and crown preparations, which receive permanent restorations. An assortment of hand-cutting dental instruments is shown in Figure 16.1. When dental burs are used, the cutting process is affected by:

1. Design of the Bur

Dental burs are available in many shapes that aid the dentist in creating the correct design of the cavity or crown preparation. Examples of typical burs are illustrated in Figure 16.2.

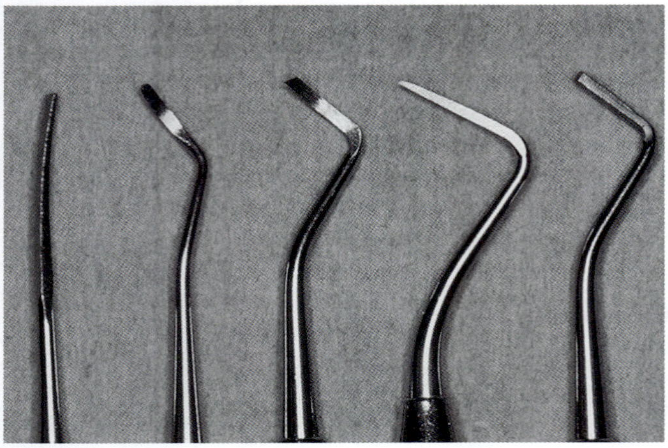

FIGURE 16.1 Examples of hand-cutting dental instruments (from *left* to *right*): Wedelstadt chisel, spoon excavator, gingival margin trimmer, hoe, and hatchet.

2. Sharpness of the Bur

The "lifetime" (or longevity) of a dental bur depends on the material from which it is made. Usually, cutting burs are made of carbon steel or tungsten carbide. **Tungsten carbide burs** are made by packing powdered metal constituents into a mold and then sintering (see Chapter 10) at high temperatures. These burs are harder and maintain a sharper cutting edge than carbon-steel burs. Therefore, they last longer; however, they are more expensive.

B. Abrasion

Abrasion is the wearing away of a surface. It may also be referred to as grinding. Irregular grooves or scratches are produced on a surface as the result of abrasion.

C. Finishing

The process of producing the final shape and contour of a restoration is termed **finishing.** After an amalgam restoration is placed, it may need to be finished and polished at a later appointment. Most

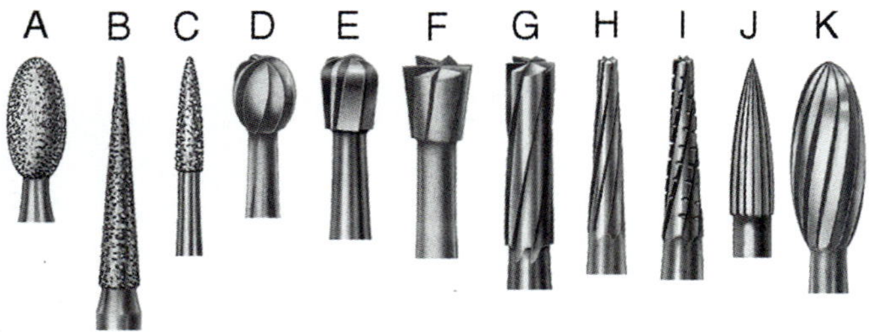

FIGURE 16.2 Names and shapes of dental burs. **A.** Egg or football diamond **B.** Needle diamond. **C.** Flame diamond. **D.** Round. **E.** Pear. **F.** Inverted cone. **G.** Straight-fissure plain. **H.** Tapered-fissure plain. **I.** Tapered-fissure crosscut. **J.** Needle finishing. **K.** Egg or football finishing. (Courtesy of Brasseler USA.)

other restorations are finished and polished when they are first placed. The instruments and armamentarium for finishing differ from those that are used for polishing. Examples used in finishing would be burs and stones.

D. Polishing

Polishing is the process of abrading a surface to eventually reduce the size of the scratches until the surface appears shiny. This concept not only applies to dentistry in regard to tooth structure and restorative materials but also extends into everyday life as well. We know that jewelry is polished, and we "polish" our sinks and bathtubs with certain kinds of cleansers that are recommended for those surfaces. This kind of polishing is different from polishing shoes or furniture. The shoe and furniture polish acts as a surface coat, similar to that of car wax.

E. Abrasive

The material doing the "wearing" (or the abrading) is the **abrasive.** In nature, wind and water carry abrasive particles and can wear away the surface of rocks.

In dentistry, abrasive particles may be bound together onto burs, disks, stones, wheels, or strips, or they may be used with liquids to form a paste or slurry. These are discussed later in this chapter.

II. Types of Abrasives

Many types of abrasives are used in dentistry, and to mention all of them would go beyond the scope of this text. Listed below are some of the more common ones that may be used when performing typical clinical or laboratory procedures:

A. Chalk

A mineral form of calcite is called **chalk.** It is also called whiting or calcium carbonate. Chalk is a mild abrasive and is used to polish teeth, gold and amalgam restorations, and plastic materials.

B. Pumice

Pumice is a silica-like, volcanic glass that is used as a polishing agent on enamel, gold foil, and dental amalgam and for finishing acrylic denture bases in the laboratory. It is the abrasive agent in "Lava Soap" and is used to remove dried or callused skin in the form of a "pumice stone." Both chalk and pumice are illustrated in Figure 16.3.

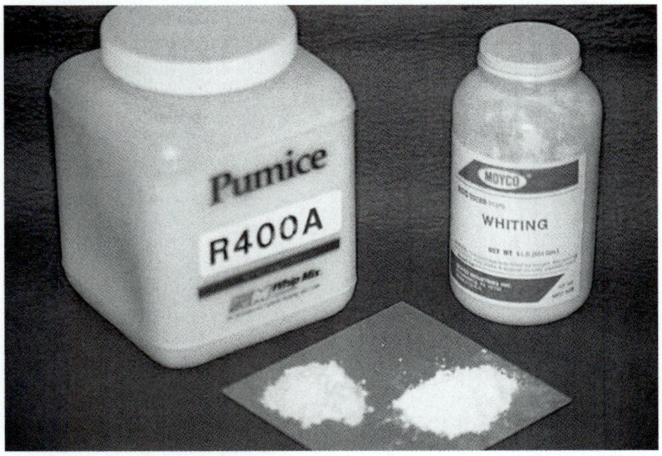

FIGURE 16.3 Chalk (whiting) and pumice in bulk form.

C. Sand

Sand is a form of quartz and may be seen in various colors. Sand particles are rounded or angular in shape. They are typically bonded to paper disks for grinding metals and plastics.

D. Cuttle

As we know it today, **cuttle** is a fine grade of quartz. These particles are also bonded to paper disks and are beige in color. They are available in coarse, medium, and fine grits. In the past, it was manufactured from the inside shell of a Mediterranean marine mollusk. A "cuttle bone" mounted in a parakeet's cage is made of the same material.

E. Garnet

Garnet is usually dark red in color. Because it is very hard, garnet is a highly effective abrasive. It is found on coated disks and is used for grinding plastics and metal alloys. The term **garnet** refers to several different minerals that have similar properties. These minerals are the silicates of manganese, magnesium, iron, cobalt, and aluminum.

F. Emery

Emery is sometimes also called "corundum." We are familiar with this abrasive because of "emery boards," which are used to file our fingernails. **Emery** is a natural form of aluminum oxide, and it looks like grayish-black sand. It is commonly found on arbor bands that attach to a dental lathe for grinding custom trays and acrylic appliances. Sand, cuttle, garnet, and emery disks can be seen in Figure 16.4.

G. Silex

Silex, a commercial product, is a silica-like material such as quartz and is used as an abrasive agent in the mouth. It is supplied as a powder and is mixed with various liquids to form a paste or slurry.

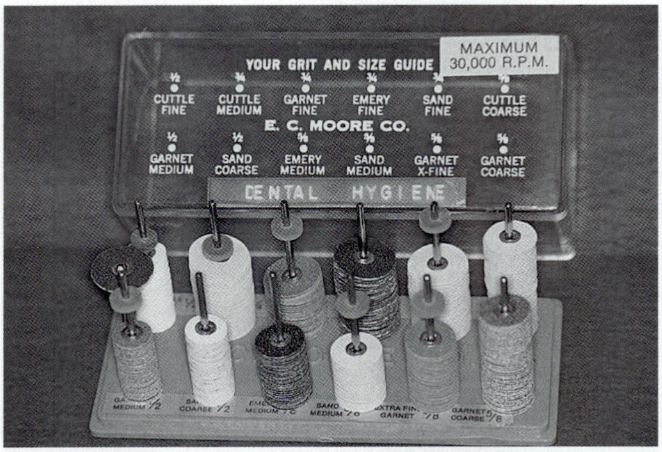

FIGURE 16.4 Kit of assorted disks coated with sand, cuttle, garnet, and emery.

H. Tin Oxide

An extremely fine abrasive, **tin oxide** is supplied as a white powder and is used as a final polishing agent for teeth and metallic restorations. It is used as a paste or slurry in the same manner as Silex. Both Silex and tin oxide are illustrated in Figure 16.5.

I. Aluminum Oxide

Aluminum oxide is a common abrasive used in dentistry, and it has essentially replaced emery for several uses. This abrasive, shown in Figure 16.6, is widely used in the form of disks and strips. It is also impregnated into rubber wheels and points. It is the abrasive used in the popular "white stones" to adjust enamel or to finish metal alloys and ceramic materials.

III. Bonded and Coated Abrasives

To use the abrasives previously discussed, they must be attached to devices that permit an abrasive action. This action is usually rotary-powered, but in the case of finishing strips, it is accomplished by hand. Examples of these items include the following.

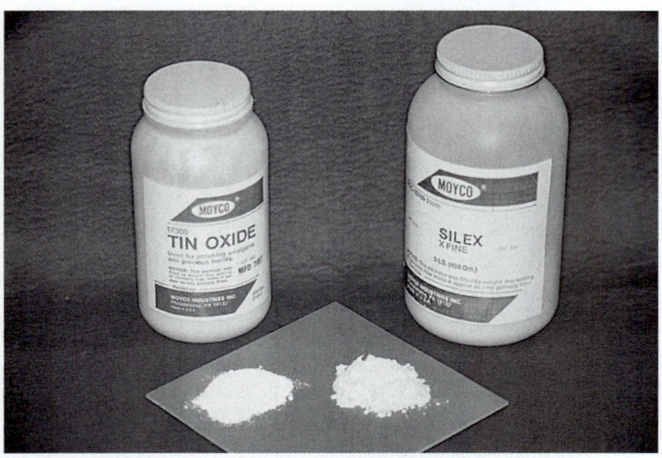

FIGURE 16.5 Silex and tin oxide in bulk form.

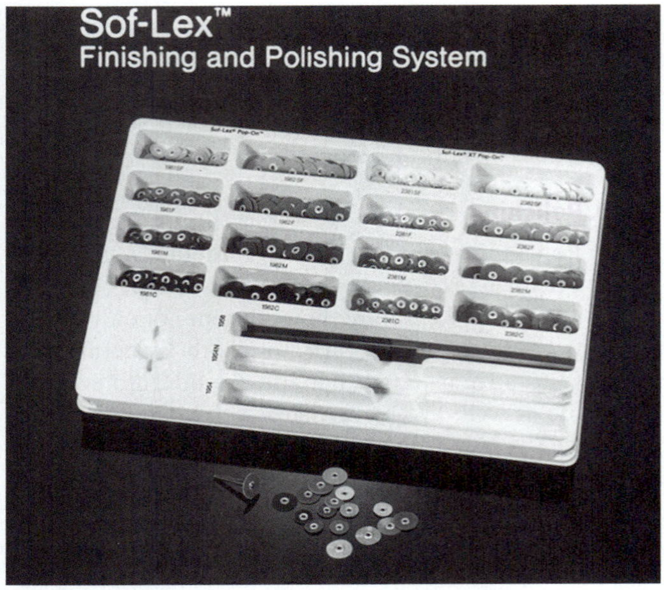

FIGURE 16.6 Aluminum oxide-coated disks and strips. (Courtesy of 3M Dental Products Division.)

A. Diamond Burs

Diamond burs are actually very small diamond chips that are bonded to a shaft. Diamonds are very hard materials and make very good abrasives. Depending on the size of the chips, diamond burs can be used in many dental procedures.

B. Stones

Stones are available in various shapes, sizes, and grits, and they are made from a variety of materials. A "heatless stone" is illustrated on the right in Figure 16.7. Stones are used in clinical and laboratory procedures.

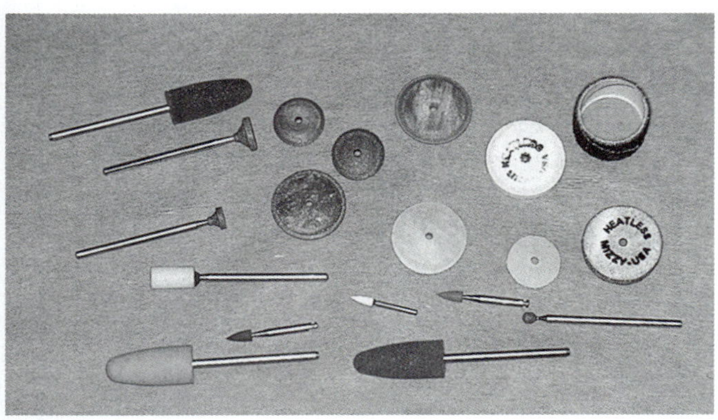

FIGURE 16.7 An assortment of bonded abrasive instruments (stones, rubber wheels, and rubber points) used in dentistry.

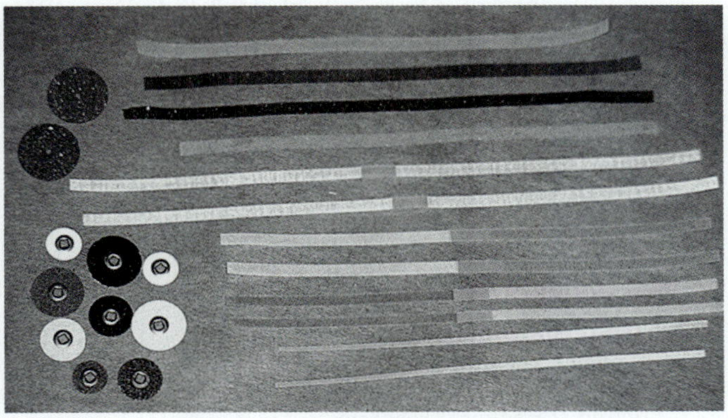

FIGURE 16.8 An assortment of coated disks and strips used in dentistry.

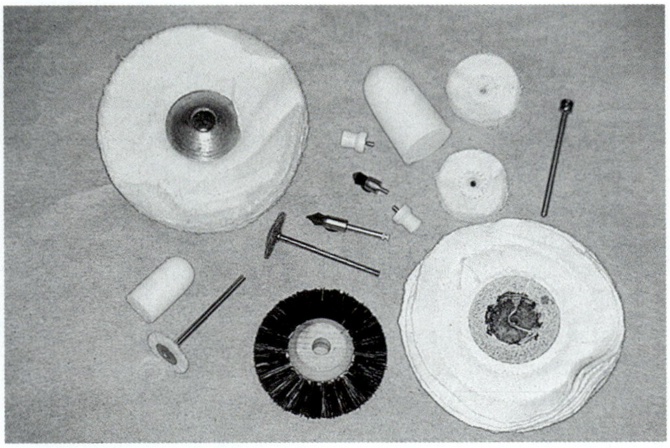

FIGURE 16.9 An assortment of cloth wheels, felt cones and wheels, brushes, and rubber cups used in dentistry.

C. Rubber Wheels or Points

Molded rubber is impregnated with an abrasive into a wheel or point shape. The rubber acts as the matrix (or binder) of the abrasive agent. Examples are shown in Figure 16.7. Rubber wheels and points are designed for both clinical and laboratory procedures.

D. Disks or Strips

Abrasive particles are bonded to a paper, metal, or plastic backing to form disks or strips. Examples of coated disks and strips can be seen in Figure 16.8. They are used for interoral and laboratory procedures.

E. Powders

Powders, such as those illustrated in Figures 16.3 and 16.5, are used in conjunction with other agents and devices. These agents and devices include:

1. "Vehicles," such as water, alcohol, glycerin, or mouthwash, to make pastes or slurries
2. Brushes, rubber cups, felt cones and wheels, and cloth wheels.

Some powders are used for laboratory and clinical procedures, whereas others are used only in the laboratory. Figure 16.9 shows an assortment of cloth wheels, felt cones and wheels, bristle brushes, and rubber cups.

IV. Factors Affecting the Rate of Abrasion

Chances are, even though a class of dental hygiene students is taught to polish the same way, each student probably polishes differently. Depending on how much paste is put into the cup, the amount of pressure used against the tooth, how fast the cup is rotating and what type of abrasive is in the cup, will significantly affect the surface being polished (technically abraded). The following factors affect the rate of abrasion.

A. Hardness

The abrasive particle must be harder than the surface being abraded if an acceptable rate of abrasion is to occur. Otherwise, the abrasive will be worn, and the surface will not be greatly affected. The abrasion rate can be "temperature dependent" (the abrasive heats up during use). The object being abraded could become heated, which may make it softer and affect the rate of abrasion.

Abrasives are usually made of very hard, ceramic materials. Table 16.1 lists Knoop and Moh's

Table 16.1 Moh's and Knoop Hardness Values of Restorative Materials, Abrasives, and Tooth Tissues

Material	Moh's Hardness	Knoop Hardness
Composite (microfill)	2	30
Cementum	2	40
Composite (hybrid)	2–3	55
Dentin	3–4	70
Amalgam	3	90
Gold alloy (inlay)	3	100
Calcite (chalk, whiting)	3	135
Enamel	5	340
Pumice	6–7	560
Porcelain	6–7	590
Sand, quartz, cuttle	7	800
Garnet	8–9	1,400
Tungsten carbide (dental bur)	9	1,900
Aluminum oxide, emery	7–9	2,100
Diamond	10	7,000

Adapted from Handbook of Chemistry and Physics. 64th ed. Boca Raton, FL: CRC Press, 1983; Anusavice KJ. Phillips' Science of Dental Materials. 11th ed. Philadelphia: Saunders, 203:362; Callister WD. Fundamentals of Materials Science and Engineering 2nd ed. Hobokon: Wiley, 2005:217.

hardness of several restorative materials, abrasives, and tooth tissues.

B. Size

Common sense tells us that larger abrasive particles will produce deeper scratches than smaller particles will. Deeper scratches result in a greater amount of surface material removed. **Grit** is a term that is used to describe the size of the abrasive particle. Finer abrasives such as powders or flours are graded F, FF, and FFF as the fineness increases. When the particles are bonded to paper, the grit is designated as O, OO, and OOO in order of increasing fineness. When a prophy paste is labeled "coarse" or "fine," the label is referring to the grit (or particle size) of the abrasive. It is important to note there is no standardization in definition of fine, medium, and coarse grit in prophy pastes among the manufacturers. The "fine" grit paste of one manufacturer may be nearly equal to the "coarse" grit paste of another manufacturer.

C. Shape

Most individuals would agree that a spherically shaped particle would be less abrasive than an irregularly shaped particle. The sharp edges on an irregularly shaped particle tend to dig into the surface rather than roll across it, as a rounded abrasive particle would, thus increasing the rate of abrasion.

D. Pressure

Using excess pressure during finishing and polishing causes a higher abrasion rate because the abrasive particle cuts deeper into the surface. Increased pressure may also result in an increased temperature of the material being polished. An example of this would be using heavy pressure on an amalgam restoration. Raising the temperature of the amalgam could release mercury to the surface, which may increase corrosion and contribute to a marginal breakdown.

E. Speed

The term "speed" refers to the rate at which the polishing device is rotating. Like pressure, the speed at which the abrasive is applied will increase the rate of abrasion. Higher speed also results in an increase in temperature. It is important to control the speed of the polishing cup or brush during polishing so that the abrasion rate and increase in temperature are kept to a minimum.

F. Lubrication

The most frequently used lubricant in dentistry is water. It is used with handpieces and burs to cool the tooth when cavity preparations are being made. During finishing and polishing, lubrication is also recommended to carry the heat that is created by the abrasive action away from the surface being abraded. This is done by mixing lubricating agents, such as water, mouthwash, glycerin, and alcohol, with the abrasive agent, which is usually in powder form. We refer to the resulting mixture as a "paste" or "slurry" depending on the liquid content.

V. The Polishing Process

A. Why We Polish

Tooth structure and restorative materials are polished for several reasons.

1. To Reduce Adhesion

As discussed in Chapter 6, a smooth surface will inhibit adhesion. Plaque, stain, and calculus are less likely to stick to a smooth surface. This is true for both tooth surfaces and restorative materials.

2. To Make the Surface Feel Smooth

Patients will expect a smooth surface on any permanent restoration that is placed in their mouths. In addition, they may comment on the smoothness that is produced after scaling and polishing during a routine dental hygiene recall appointment.

3. To Increase Esthetics

An unpolished amalgam or gold crown is not as attractive as one that appears smooth and shiny. This also holds true for the tooth surfaces of a heavy cigarette smoker before and after polishing. Esthetics play a very important role in dentistry, and polishing helps to create an attractive dentition for the patient.

4. To Reduce Corrosion

When metallic restorations are polished, it reduces the formation of tarnish and corrosion. In turn, this may extend the lifetime of the restoration.

B. What Happens During Polishing

During the polishing procedure, we go through a series of steps. Each step removes a layer of material by abrasion. Because we use a series of finer and finer abrasives, the scratches become smaller and smaller, until they are smaller than the wavelength of visible light (<0.5 μm). With scratches of this size, the surface appears shiny. In short, the smaller the size of the scratches, the shinier the surface.

The same approach should be used when polishing teeth during routine oral prophylaxis. If heavy stains are present, a coarse abrasive, which could be a commercial paste or a powder and liquid mixed at chairside, should always be followed by a different abrasive with a finer grit and a different rubber cup.

Another approach to polishing is to use the same abrasive material in a progression of larger to smaller grits to produce increasingly smaller scratches. This technique is used more commonly in finishing and polishing restorations than it is during prophylaxis.

C. The Polishing Technique

In recent years, it has been determined that it is not necessary to polish all surfaces during every dental hygiene recall appointment. It has been proven that the effects of doing so may be counterproductive. In other words, the clinician may be doing more harm than good to the patients' teeth and restored surfaces. For this reason, the dental hygienist must make sound, professional judgments in deciding when to polish and which teeth to polish. Additional decisions include the appropriate agents and method to use.

When a polishing sequence is employed, it is important to remember that to prevent abrasive contamination, prophy cups and/or brushes must be changed before the next, less abrasive agent is used. The surfaces being polished should be thoroughly rinsed before the next agent is applied. In addition, if the clinician wanted to use a fine abrasive on tooth colored or cast restorations, and one that is coarse on tooth structure, the coarse one should be used first, avoid the restorative materials, have the patient rinse, change the prophy cup, and then polish with the finer agent.

The recommended polishing technique is one of slow speed with light, intermittent pressure. Prophy brushes are suggested for areas such as the occlusal surface because of their abrasive nature and possible trauma to soft tissue.

D. The "Selective Polish Approach"

At this time it would be reasonable to say that most, if not all dental hygiene programs have adopted the selective polishing philosophy. Darby and Walsh have defined **selective polishing** as "the practice of omitting tooth polishing in areas where there is no stain and when polishing could cause damage." It has been documented in the research that polishing may adversely affect the patient's soft tissues, restorations, tooth structure, and the operatory environment.

It is well established that portions of the fluoride-rich layer of enamel (usually 3–4 microns in thickness) can be removed during routine polishing with pumice. The uptake of fluoride that the patient has been accumulating between professional polishings from water, dentifrices, rinses, etc., is removed when tooth structure is polished with excessively abrasive agents. Granted, enamel is in a constant state of "mineralization flux," demineralizing at times and also remineralizing. If a microscopic layer of enamel is removed from polishing with abrasive agents, it will remineralize in time with salivary minerals and exposure to fluorides. But, why subject the patient to that fluoride loss in the first place? Our goal is to create a smooth surface on teeth and restorations with the least abrasive agent to prevent adhesion of deposits.

Demineralized tooth surfaces can be considered as weak tooth structure. Rubber cup polishing may cause a significant amount of surface structure to be removed on demineralized teeth compared to intact enamel.

Polishing restorations may create a roughened surface. Restorative materials such as gold, composite, amalgam and glass ionomer could be affected by the abrasive agents in prophy pastes. The surfaces could be roughened and in some cases the margins of the restoration could be damaged. For implants, there are non-abrasive pastes available for polishing the abutments and pontics.

We must remember that the purpose of polishing is to produce the smoothest possible surface. Whether we are polishing tooth structure or restorative material, we defeat this purpose when we use coarse abrasive agents. Grooves and scratches are created on the surface that may not have previously been there. This uneven surface is now more conducive for the formation and adhesion of plaque, stain, and calculus. These accumulations now occur more rapidly than they did before the surface was improperly polished.

There has been much discussion in the literature regarding patients' acceptance of a selective polishing philosophy. Some accept it after the justification is explained; others do not. If patients insist on rotary polishing, a non-abrasive agent, such as a very mild dentifrice or professional cleaning agent, may be used with a rubber cup. The patient will be pacified, and you will have professionally done "the right thing." A summary of "Dos and Don'ts" when polishing teeth and restorative materials is provided in Table 16.2.

VI. Prophylaxis Pastes

A vast assortment of prophy pastes are available from which the hygienist may choose. In recent years, they have been marketed not only by companies that make toothbrushes but also by those that manufacture disposable and autoclavable prophy angles. There are a few on the market that are supplied in bulk form, such as a jar shown in Figure 16.10. However, most are

Table 16.2 General Summary of "Dos and Don'ts" When Polishing

Do	Don't
Recognize that all materials and devices are potentially harmful to soft tissue.	Don't abuse gingival tissue.
Avoid pulpal trauma and amalgam deterioration by using slow speed, moderate to light pressure, and adequate coolant when necessary.	Don't generate excessive heat.
Remember that cementum and dentin abrade much easier than enamel.	Don't overlook potential damage to root surfaces, especially on tooth-colored restorations.
Use high-polish, low-abrasion prophylaxis pastes.	Don't use excessively abrasive prophylaxis pastes.
Employ selective polishing procedures where indicated.	Don't polish every patient's teeth with the same polishing agents.

supplied in unit-dose cups as shown in Figure 16.11. Prophy paste is manufactured in a variety of colors, textures, flavors, grits, and formulations. Prices also vary depending on the brand and the quantity purchased.

In 1982, a journal article published by research associates Putt, Kleber, and Muhler from Indiana University addressed enamel polish and abrasion by prophylaxis pastes. This article became a "keystone" publication for this topic because it provided the hygienist with important information about polishing. It also rated 10 commercial prophy pastes for their enamel polish and abrasion properties. Unfortunately, this was more than 25 years ago. Most of the pastes rated in this article are no longer on the market. A few of the major points follow.

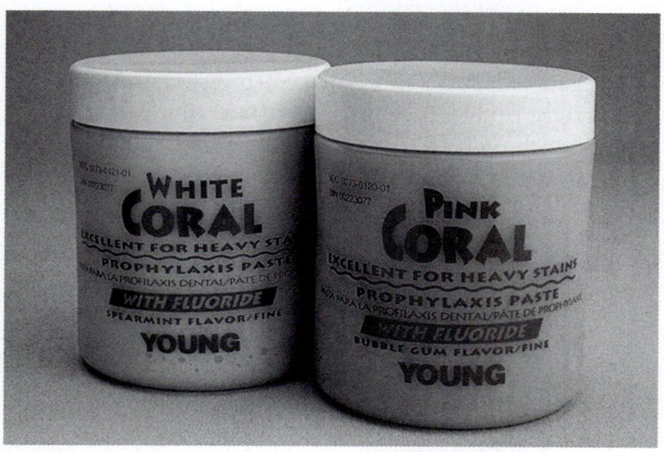

FIGURE 16.10 Prophylaxis pastes supplied in bulk form. (Courtesy of Young Dental Mfg.)

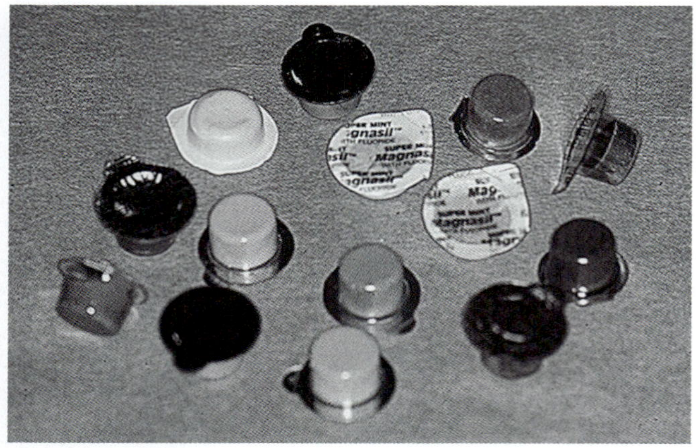

FIGURE 16.11 Assorted unit-dose cups of prophylaxis paste.

A. Polishing Ability

A polishing agent should not create deep scratches and grooves, as discussed earlier. Instead, it should produce very fine, shallow scratches and grooves so that light may be reflected, and therefore, "shine." In recent years, a prophylaxis paste has been developed that has both cleaning (abrasive) and polishing abilities in one paste. This product is illustrated in Figure 16.12. Sheet-shaped particles, known as "Perlite," convert from coarse to fine with 15 seconds of use. Figure 16.13 presents the particle shape and conversion after 15 seconds of polishing.

B. Abrasive Properties

The abrasive particle used in the paste should not produce a detrimental effect on the surface. It must, however, remove the stain.

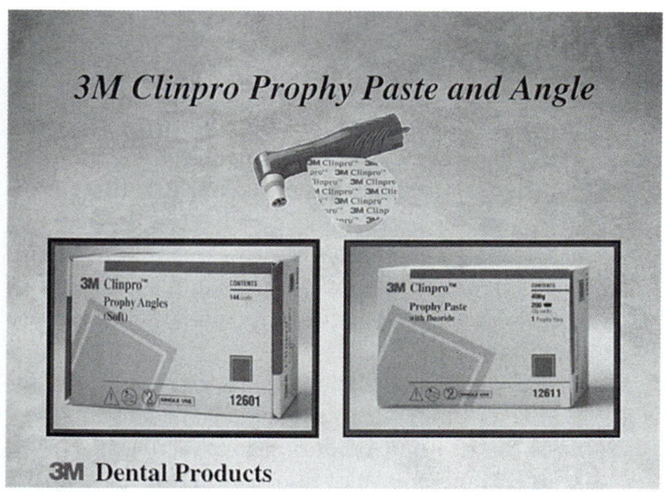

FIGURE 16.12 "Clinpro" prophylaxis paste. (Courtesy of 3M/ESPE Dental Products.)

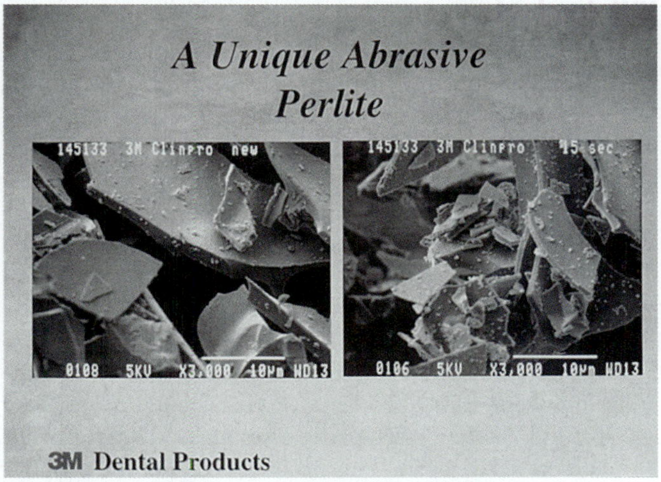

FIGURE 16.13 "Perlite" abrasive particle (in Clinpro): coarse (*left*) and resulting fine (*right*). (Courtesy of 3M/ESPE Dental Products.)

An acceptable prophy paste will possess properties of both a high-polish rate and a low-abrasion rate. The Putt, Kleber, and Muhler publication identified a few pastes that exhibit these qualities, as well as some that produced a low-polish and a high-abrasion rate.

The Putt, Kleber, and Muhler researchers also commented on the use of polishing agents in areas of gingival recession. It must be remembered that dentin will abrade 25 times faster than enamel. Cementum, which is only temporarily present in areas of gingival recession, will abrade 35 times faster than enamel because of its thin layer and "softness." Common practice would dictate that abrasive polishing agents be contraindicated in gingivally recessed areas.

C. "Specialty" Prophylaxis Pastes

Manufacturers have developed prophy pastes that do more than clean and polish. The dental hygienist may typically have an assortment of products on hand that contains a prophy paste as well as a therapeutic agent. Some pastes, such as Clinpro (3M/ESPE) will transition from coarse to fine. This product was discussed in Section VI. A. and is shown in Figure 16.12 and 16.13. Others may contain various amounts and types of fluoride such as "D-Lish" (Young Dental), "Topex" (Sultan Healthcare, Inc.), and "Enamel Pro" (Premier), to name a few. Yet others, such as "NuCare" (Sunstar Americas, Inc.) and "Proclude" (Ortek Therapeutics), have been reported to reduce sensitivity. Clinpro, NuCare, and Enamel Pro are pictured in Figure 16.14.

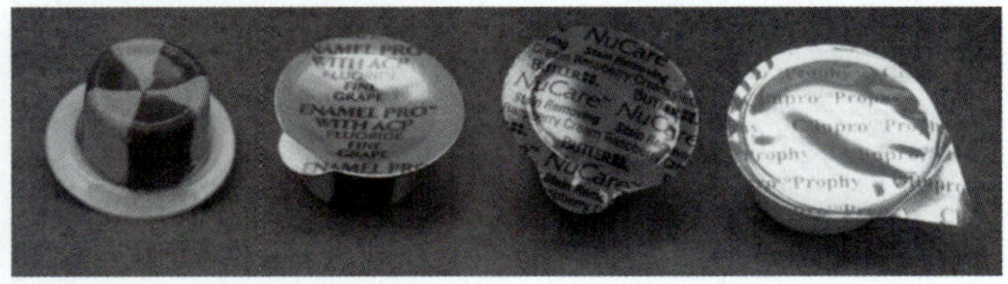

FIGURE 16.14 Assorted "specialty" prophylaxis pastes in unit dose packaging.

D. Prophy Pastes for Esthetic Restorations

In recent years there has been a great demand by patients for esthetic restorations. The typical ones include microfills, hybrids, and compomers. Due to their "softer composition" many traditional prophy pastes should not be used on these restorations since they may create a very rough surface. Instead, prophylaxis pastes formulated for esthetic restorations are recommended. These contain abrasives such as Perlite, aluminum oxide, or diamond powder, just to name a few.

If the hygienist knows the brand name of the restorative material, it is important to follow the manufacturer's recommendations for polishing. In many cases, one of their own products will be recommended for polishing. These polishing agents contain very fine abrasives and are available in the form of pastes in unit doses and dispensing syringes, cups, points, and disks. Examples of these products are shown in Figures 16.15, 16.16, and 16.17.

Identifying the types of materials used for these restorations (Chapter 14, Table 14.1) and using the correct agents to polish them will indeed require some planning and time. But it is our responsibility as a professional to use the appropriate agents on teeth and restorations. The end result is a smoother, longer lasting restoration, and your extra

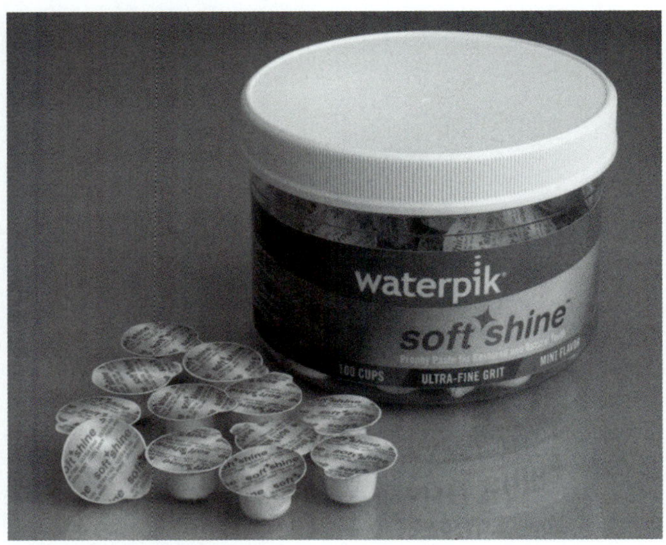

FIGURE 16.15 "Soft Shine" cosmetic restorative paste for restored and natural teeth. (Courtesy of Water Pik, Inc.)

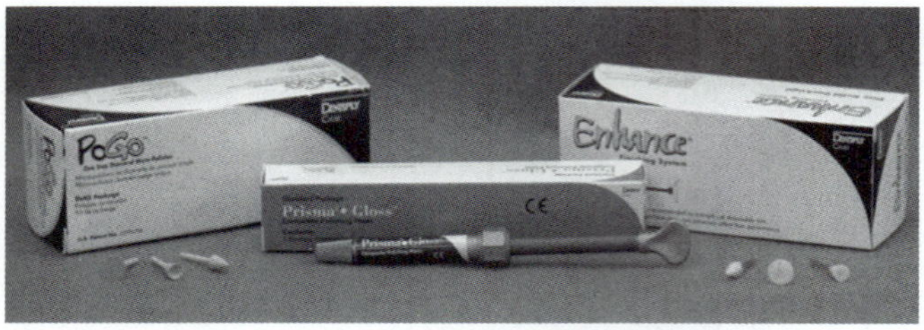

FIGURE 16.16 An assortment of pastes, cups, points and disks for polishing esthetic restorations.

care and effort will be greatly appreciated by your patient.

VII. Air Powder Polishing

Air powder polishing combines air, water, and sodium bicarbonate (or aluminum trihydroxide) into a spray that propels the polishing particles to the tooth surface. It is indicated for removal of tobacco and chlorhexidine-induced stains on teeth as well as stain and biofilm on orthodontically banded and bracketed teeth, and dental implants. At this writing, it is not yet determined if aluminum trihydroxide is compatible with dental implants. Also at this time another air polishing powder is being developed that is designated as a low abrasive material. It has yet to be released on the market. The technique and contraindications for the air powder cleaning method are described in detail in dental hygiene clinical practice textbooks.

Air powder polishing should not be confused with air abrasion systems. Air abrasion involves "sandblasting" the tooth surface with a high velocity stream of air that carries a very hard abrasive particle (aluminum oxide) as part of a restorative procedure. Air abrasion systems were discussed in more detail in Chapter 5.

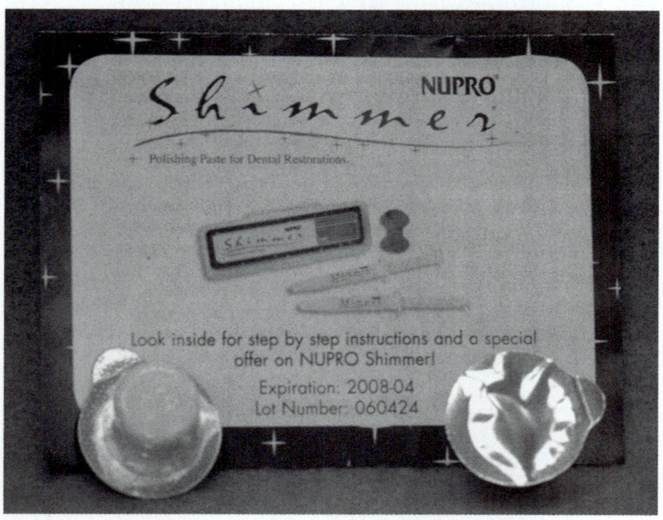

FIGURE 16.17 A cleaning and polishing agent for dental restorations.

VIII. Implants

As mentioned previously, dental implants may be cleaned with the "Prophy Jet" or air powder polishing, but plaque and biofilm may be removed with a rubber cup and an appropriate cleaning agent. When polishing, the incompatibility of titanium with other metals and some chemicals must be taken into consideration during the prophylaxis appointment. True polishing agents are contraindicated for dental implants because the goal is not to alter (abrade) the surface integrity of the titanium.

An ideal agent for removing soft debris is a cleaning agent called Pro Care (Young Dental Mfg.). The round, "softer," flat particles in this powder are not described as a grit. This product is one of the prophylaxis pastes that researchers Putt, Kleber, and Muhler (described previously in this chapter) found to possess low abrasion and high polishing properties. The powder and liquid that are combined for this prophylaxis paste are pictured in Figure 16.18. Needless to say, to remove hard deposits from implants, special plastic hand instruments have been developed as well as plastic sheaths for ultrasonic scaling instruments.

IX. Denture Cleansers

Full and partial dentures will accumulate plaque, stain, and calculus in the same manner as natural teeth. It is the dental hygienist's responsibility not only to examine the condition of removable appliances but also to return them to the patient in a deposit-free condition at the end of the appointment.

Denture base materials and denture teeth are, indeed, dental materials for which the hygienist provides professional services. Dentures may be cleaned and polished in several ways, and textbooks devoted to the clinical practice of dental hygiene discuss these in detail.

The goal in cleaning and polishing dentures, as when cleaning and polishing natural teeth and other restorative surfaces, is to remove deposits in a manner that is not detrimental to the surface. Care must be taken so that abrasives, rotary devices, or caustic ultrasonic solutions do not damage the surface of the removable denture appliance.

X. Dentifrices

As with denture cleansers, dentifrices are discussed in detail in clinical practice textbooks. From a dental materials standpoint, the most important constituent in a dentifrice is the abrasive agent.

A. Abrasive Content and American Dental Association Acceptance

One of several types of abrasives may be added to the dentifrice formulation. Several years ago, dentifrices

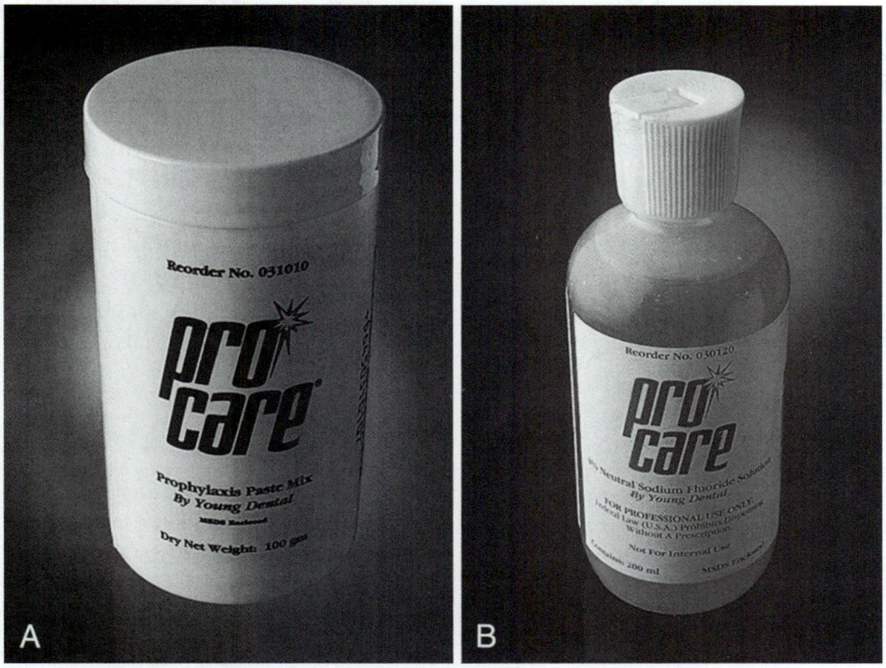

FIGURE 16.18 For this bulk form of prophy paste, powder (**A**) must be mized with liquid (**B**) before use. This is considered a cleaning agent, and is recommended for implants and esthetic restorations.

were on the market that were considered to be very abrasive, such as those recommended for smokers. To reassure the consumer today, the American Dental Association (ADA) evaluates dentifrices in their Acceptance Program. This was discussed in more detail in Chapter 1. A dentifrice is "ADA Accepted" if it meets the specific requirements set forth by the ADA. In summary, these requirements are:

1. Safety and Efficacy

The dentifrice must be safe and effective. In past ADA guidelines, abrasivity could not exceed a value of 250. This number is obtained from standardized testing that involves irradiating dentin specimens, brushing them with test and reference dentifrices, and then calculating a ratio by comparing the amounts of radioactive phosphorus released by each dentifrice. This number is then multiplied by 1,000 to yield an abrasivity score. Currently, the U.S. Food and Drug Administration (FDA) regulates dentifrices and their abrasivity.

2. Scientific Data

The manufacturer of the dentifrice must provide scientific data to the ADA to support any claims made in advertisements and on the packaging of the product. These data are usually the result of extensive clinical trials.

B. Abrasives Used in Dentifrices

There are three major categories of dentifrice abrasives:

1. Phosphates

These contribute to a whiter look and cleaner "feel" to the teeth. Two phosphates used in dentifrices are dicalcium phosphate dihydrate and calcium pyrophosphate.

2. Carbonates

Carbonates have been used for almost 100 years to make products and environments smell better in addition to their abrasive properties.

a) Sodium bicarbonate

This is also known as baking soda. In the 1920s it was used to clean silver; in the 1940s it was the deodorizer for refrigerators. The 1970s saw baking soda used as a laundry detergent and carpet deodorizer. In the past 20 years it has been used as a dentifrice abrasive. In addition, research studies have shown that "sodium bicarbonate is compatible with fluoride, bactericidal against most periodontal pathogens, safe, as well as low in abrasivity and cost. It may be said that sodium bicarbonate is the consummate dentifrice ingredient."

b) Calcium carbonate

As discussed previously, this abrasive is also known as chalk. It is one of the most economical mechanical abrasives available. Sodium monofluorophosphate is used with calcium carbonate.

3. Silicas

These are available in many particle sizes and characteristics. They are largely nonreactive with other toothpaste ingredients, and have become the most frequently used abrasive in recent years. Silicas are compatible with soluble fluorides.

Information for Section IX. B. came from: "Dentifrice Abrasives: Heroes or Villains?", Hefferren, JJ, Li, N, Academy of Dental Therapeutics and Stomatology, Chesterland, Ohio, 4 CEUs, 2005.

C. Factors Affecting Abrasion Rate by Dentifrices

Intraoral and extraoral factors will influence the rate of abrasion from a dentifrice. Extraoral factors include the type, size, and amount of abrasive in the dentifrice as well as the quantity of dentifrice used. The type of toothbrush, method of use, amount of force delivered, and frequency of brushing are other extraoral factors.

Intraoral factors include xerostomia, saliva consistency and quantity, exposed root surfaces, quality and quantity of deposits, and presence of certain restorative materials.

SUMMARY

The dental hygienist should have a fundamental understanding of the terms associated with the cleaning and polishing of teeth and restorations. Cutting is removing material by a shearing-off process. Abrasion is the wearing away of a surface. Finishing is the process of producing the final shape and contour of a restoration, whereas polishing is the abrasion of a surface to eventually reduce the size of the scratches until the surface appears shiny. The material doing the wearing or abrading is the abrasive.

The chapter includes descriptions of several abrasives commonly used in the practice of dental hygiene. To use these abrasives, they must be attached to devices that permit abrasive action. These devices include diamond burs, stones, rubber wheels or points, disks, strips, and powders.

The factors of hardness, size and shape, pressure, speed, and lubrication may affect the rate of abrasion. Polishing with a very dry abrasive and a hard-bristle prophy brush with significant pressure and speed is likely to produce an excessively abraded surface on tooth structure and restorative materials. In contrast, when the hygienist uses a wet, fine-grit paste or powder and a rubber prophy cup with gentle pressure and slow speed, a surface of high polish and low abrasion is more likely to be produced.

Reasons for polishing include reducing adhesion to discourage deposits, creating a smooth surface, increasing esthetics, and reducing corrosion of metallic restorations. During the polishing procedure, progressively finer scratches are produced as abrasives are used in a sequence from coarse to fine. However, a decision must be made regarding whether to polish at all. Many dental hygiene programs have instituted "selective polishing" as a recommended protocol.

Prophylaxis pastes are supplied in a variety of colors, textures, flavors, grits, and formulations. Recommended pastes are those with high polish and low abrasion levels. There are prophy pastes that now contain fluoride and desensitizing agents as well as one that transitions from a coarse to a fine abrasive agent. Yet others are formulated to contain a very mild abrasive or no abrasives to essentially be cleaning agents.

Denture base materials and denture teeth are dental materials that deserve attention during the dental hygiene recall/maintenance appointment. Plaque and calculus must be removed in a manner that is not detrimental to the prosthesis.

An important constituent in dentifrices, from a dental materials standpoint, is the abrasive agent. A U.S. FDA approved and "ADA accepted" dentifrice must meet requirements concerning level of abrasion and have scientific data to support any claims regarding effectiveness.

Air powder polishing uses air, water, and an abrasive to remove stain and biofilms on teeth, orthodontic bands and brackets, and implants. Because the surface of titanium implants must not be altered, only cleaning agents, not abrasive agents, should be used for polishing.

There are three major categories of dentifrice abrasives: phosphates, carbonates, and silicas. The carbonates include sodium bicarbonate, which is compatible with fluoride, bactericidal, safe, and low in abrasivity and cost. Silicas have become the most frequently used abrasive in dentifrices in recent years.

Learning Activities

1. Take a small piece of brass or Plexiglas, a slow-speed handpiece, and a few prophy cups or brushes. Use three different grits of abrasive agents to polish as follows:

a) Using the abrasive with the largest grit, finish the entire surface of the brass plate with scratches going in one direction only (see **A** at right).

b) Change the cup or brush, use the second most abrasive agent, and rotate the surface 90° so that the new scratches are perpendicular to the previous scratches. Polish approximately two-thirds of the surface (see **B** at right).

c) Change the cup or brush again, use the finest-grit agent, rotate surface 90° back to the original position, and polish one-third of the surface (see **C** at right).

d) With the same cup and agent, polish the entire bottom half of the surface going across all the previously polished areas (see **D** at right).

Evaluate your specimen, and describe the results. Note the appearance of scratches in the various areas. What does this tell you about polishing in proper sequence? Now compare the bottom and top halves. What is the result of polishing with the finest abrasive directly over the rougher sections?

2. Squeeze a long sample of composite restorative material onto a resin strip. Fold the strip over, and flatten the sample. Light cure until set. Divide the strip into three sections, and polish in the same manner as described in learning activity #1, using Sof-Lex aluminum oxide discs in sequence from coarse to fine. Evaluate your sample in the same manner as the brass plate or Plexiglas.

3. Polish a classmate's teeth, using different polishing materials, such as:

a) Toothpaste

b) Silex

c) Tin oxide

d) Whiting

e) Pumice

f) Various brands of commercial prophy pastes

Notice the consistency, tendency to splatter, and grit. Have the "patient" report to you on the differences in grit, taste, and texture.

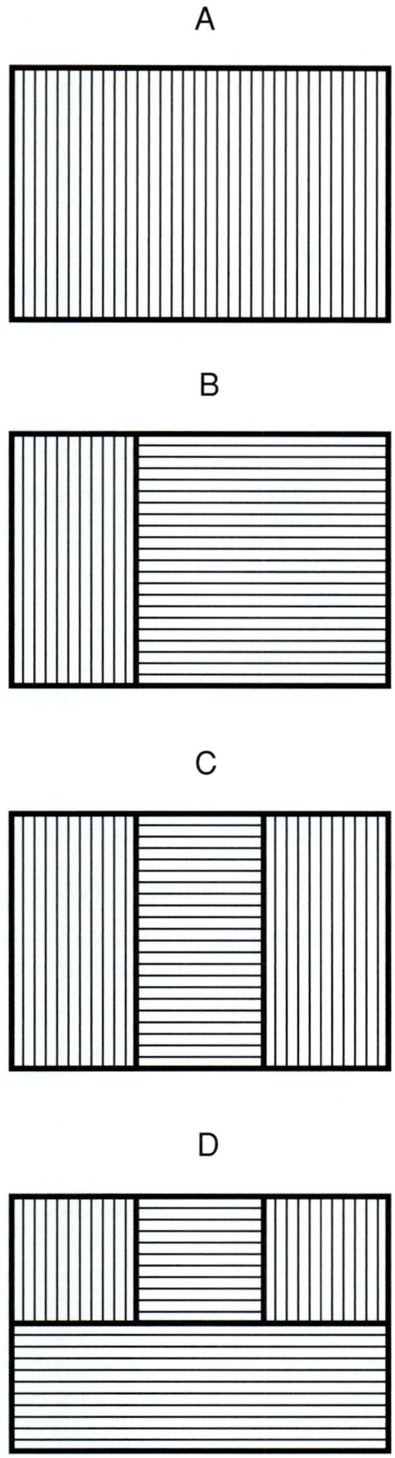

Review Questions

1. Which type of abrasive looks like a grayish-black sand and is sometimes called "corundum"?
a) Tin oxide
b) Garnet
c) Pumice
d) Emery
e) Tripoli

2. Which type of abrasive is produced from volcanoes and is used in the laboratory and on restorative materials, such as gold, amalgam, and gold foil?
a) Aluminum oxide
b) Pumice
c) Zirconium silicate
d) Sand

3. Which abrasive is used as a slurry to polish amalgam restorations and is also called calcium carbonate?
a) Silex
b) Whiting
c) Pumice
d) Aluminum oxide

4. When an abrasive on a dental restorative material is used, the abrasive action must be ____________ the surface you are abrading.
a) Harder than
b) Softer than
c) Equal to
d) Any abrasive material will be effective

5. All of the following factors affect the rate of abrasion except one. Which one is the EXCEPTION?
a) Pressure
b) Speed
c) Size of particle
d) Bonded and coated abrasives

6. The process of producing the final shape and contour of a restoration is termed:
a) Cutting
b) Abrasion
c) Polishing
d) Finishing

7. An example of a "vehicle" to be used with powders would be:
a) Rubber cups
b) Felt cones
c) Glycerin
d) Prophy brushes

8. Polishing involves using a series of finer and finer abrasives. It can also be accomplished by using the same abrasive material in a progression of larger to smaller grit.
a) The first statement is true; the second statement is false.
b) The first statement is false; the second statement is true.
c) Both statements are true.
d) Both statements are false.

9. During routine polishing with pumice, ________ μm of the fluoride-rich layer can be removed.
a) 1–2
b) 3–4
c) 5–6
d) 7–8

10. The recommended prophylaxis pastes possess the properties of:
a) High polish and high abrasion
b) Low polish and high abrasion
c) Low polish and low abrasion
d) High polish and low abrasion

11. Which of the following is harder than enamel?
a) Pumice
b) Amalgam
c) Composite
d) Gold alloy

12. Air powder polishing is designed to remove:
a) Biofilm
b) Biofilm and stain
c) Calculus and stain
d) Plaque and calculus

13. The most frequently used abrasive in dentifrices is:
a) Carbonates
b) Pumice
c) Silica
d) Phosphates

14. Which of the following abrasives would most likely be found in a polishing agent for esthetic restorations?
a) Pumice
b) Calcium carbonate
c) Diamond powder
d) Emery

15. Mrs. Smith presents for her prophylaxis appointment after a year, rather than the 6 month prescribed time. She has: tobacco stain on the linguals of her natural teeth, two gold alloy crowns and several esthetic restorations. Which combination of cleaning/polishing agents should be chosen?
a) Traditional prophy paste, tin oxide, and a polishing agent for esthetic restorations
b) Pumice, traditional prophy paste, and a polishing agent for esthetic restorations
c) Traditional prophy paste, pumice, and tin oxide
d) Silex, tin oxide and a traditional prophy paste

Supplemental Readings

ADHA Board of Trustees. ADHA position on polishing procedures. Educ Update 1996;16 (Fall/Winter):2.

Anusavice KJ. Phillips' Science of Dental Materials. 11th ed. Philadelphia: Saunders, 2003:351–377.

Barnes CM, Covey DA, Walker MP, Johnson WW. Essential selective polishing: the maintenance of aesthetic restorations. J Pract Hyg 2003;12:18–24.

Barnes CM, Toothaker RW, Ross JA. Polishing dental implants and implant restorations. J Pract Hyg 2006;15:28–29.

Ferracane JL. Materials in Dentistry—Principles and Applications. 2nd ed. Baltimore: Lippincott Williams & Wilkins, 2001:293–308.

Hefferren JJ, Li N. Dentifrice Abrasives: Heroes or Villains? CE Course Booklet: Academy of Dental Therapeutics and Stomatology, Chesterland, Ohio, 4 CEUs, 2005.

O'Hehir TE. The definition of polishing: science, myth & new technology. Hygienetown 2007;3:10–13.

Putt MS, Kleber CJ, Muhler JC. Enamel polish and abrasion by prophylaxis pastes. Dent Hyg 1982;56:38–43.

Wilkins E. Clinical Practice of the Dental Hygienist. 10th ed. Baltimore: Lippincott Williams & Wilkins, 2008: Chapter 43.

17

Tooth Whitening

Michelle R. Sweeney, R.D.H., M.S.D.H.*

Key Words/Phrases

amelogenesis imperfecta
calcium peroxide
carbamide peroxide
dentinogenesis imperfecta
dicalcium phosphate dihydrate
extrinsic stain
fluorosis
gutta percha
hydrated silica
hydrogen peroxide
intrinsic stain
laser whitening
neutral sodium fluoride
nightguard vital whitening
nonvital tooth
potassium nitrate
power whitening
precipitated calcium carbonate
reversible pulpitis
root canal
sodium perborate
sodium percarbonate
tetracycline staining
tooth whitening/tooth bleaching
vital tooth
vital tooth whitening
walking bleach

Objectives

After studying this chapter, the student will be able to do the following:

1. Define tooth whitening, and explain the difference between vital and nonvital tooth whitening.
2. Explain the difference between intrinsic and extrinsic stains, and list examples of each.
3. Identify two chemical agents used for vital tooth whitening, and explain the process by which whitening agents whiten teeth.
4. Identify two chemical agents used for nonvital tooth whitening.
5. List the factors that affect the success of tooth whitening.
6. Compare and contrast patient-applied and professionally applied vital whitening.
7. List contraindications for both patient-applied and professionally applied tooth whitening procedures.
8. Discuss measures to prevent or alleviate tooth whitening side effects.

*The original chapter contributor for the 1st and 2nd editions was William R. Howard, D.D.S., M.P.H., Western Kentucky University, Bowling Green, Kentucky.

INTRODUCTION

Teeth that are naturally discolored or have become stained can be treated with a whitening agent. Depending on the cause of the discoloration or the type of stain, one of several whitening techniques may be used. The procedure is often referred to as **tooth whitening** or **tooth bleaching.**

A nonvital tooth is treated differently than a vital tooth. A **nonvital tooth** gives no response to temperature change or electrical stimulus. The pulp in this tooth is no longer living, hence the term "nonvital." The pulp cavity within a nonvital tooth may contain necrotic pulp, no pulp, or an inert material placed when an endodontic procedure known as a **root canal** was completed.

The terminology used when vital teeth are treated is **vital tooth whitening.** A **vital tooth** (a tooth with living pulp tissue) can be whitened in the dental office by the dental team or at home by the patient. When the whitening treatment is done at home by the patient, it is frequently called **nightguard vital whitening** because the whitening agent is applied to the teeth inside a custom tray resembling a nightguard appliance. Recently, a trayless tooth whitening system has been introduced. This trayless system uses flexible, adhesive, polyethylene strips that are coated with a whitening agent.

Tooth whitening is a cosmetic procedure—and the most frequently performed of all cosmetic dental procedures. A patient's perception regarding his or her appearance is critical in determining whether tooth whitening is sought and/or accepted. The dentist and dental hygienist may be satisfied with the results of a prescribed whitening treatment, but the patient may or may not be satisfied, again depending on his or her perception.

I. Treatment Options: Restoration or Whitening

A. Restoration

Occasionally, tooth whitening fails to achieve the desired cosmetic result. When the discoloration or stain is severe, restoration of the tooth may be the treatment of choice. Full crowns, either all porcelain or porcelain bonded to metal, require a significant amount of tooth removal from all surfaces. Facial veneers, either porcelain or composite, are a more conservative restorative option because less tooth removal is required. In some clinical situations, restoration of teeth may not be the preferred treatment because of the need to conserve tooth structure. A treatment plan may include whitening of some teeth and restoration of others. When restoration of teeth is planned in conjunction with whitening, whitening is usually accomplished first so that the esthetic restorations can then be matched to the resulting shade of the whitened natural teeth. An immediate relapse in the whitening effect occurs immediately after the treatment is completed. For this reason, esthetic restoration of teeth should be delayed for 2 weeks after the completion of tooth whitening.

Restorative treatment that involves bonding to enamel, such as facial veneers, must be delayed for a minimum of 2 weeks after whitening is completed, because recently whitened tooth enamel produces a weaker bond to restorative materials.

B. Whitening

Whitening is the most conservative treatment option for the esthetic improvement of discolored or stained teeth. No tooth structure is sacrificed in the preparation of vital teeth for whitening. In the treatment of nonvital teeth, an opening into the pulp chamber, either from the lingual surface of anterior teeth or from the occlusal surface of posterior teeth, is necessary. Many factors potentially affect the outcome of the whitening procedure. The success of the procedure depends on the following factors:

- Cause or type of discoloration or stain
- Degree or intensity of discoloration or stain
- Whitening agent selected
- Strength of the whitening agent
- Length of exposure of the tooth to the whitening agent
- Whitening technique
- Vitality of the tooth
- Presence of a restoration in the tooth

II. Causes of Tooth Discoloration

A. Nonvital Teeth

A tooth with a necrotic pulp or one that has been endodontically treated has a tendency to darken with the passage of time. Significantly darkened teeth should be noted during clinical examination, and the cause of the darkening should be investigated.

An injury to a tooth may cause the pulp tissue to become necrotic, with no sign or symptom of necrosis other than a noticeable darkening of the tooth. The decomposition of pulp tissues, especially the hemoglobin of the red blood cells, produces a dark stain that penetrates the dentinal tubules.

After a tooth has been diagnosed as nonvital, appropriate endodontic treatment must be performed. The most common endodontic procedure is root canal therapy. When a root canal procedure is performed, the contents of the pulp cavity, including both the root canal(s) and the coronal pulp chamber, are removed. The pulp chamber and root canal(s) are then filled with an inert material, such as **gutta percha** (a natural resin). The entire procedure is performed under aseptic conditions and usually requires multiple appointments. After a nonvital tooth has been successfully treated, a full crown is usually recommended to strengthen the tooth. If an endodontically treated tooth is not restored with a crown, a nonvital whitening treatment may be performed to lighten the color (shade) of the darkened tooth.

B. Vital Teeth

Teeth are naturally white and bright, with a translucence that contributes to their brightness. Teeth vary in color or shade from person to person, and as teeth age, they also darken. Some patients may ask if the natural shade or color of their teeth can be changed to improve their appearance. Whitening may be an effective treatment option for the esthetic improvement of healthy natural teeth.

C. Stain

Both vital and nonvital teeth are subject to staining. There are two types or classifications of stain: extrinsic stain and intrinsic stain.

1. Extrinsic Stain

An **extrinsic stain** occurs on the surface of the tooth. Causes of extrinsic staining include foods and drinks, such as coffee and tea, and tobacco, both smoked and smokeless. Some extrinsic staining can be removed, at least partially, by the patient using a toothbrush and dentifrice. Some dentifrices are formulated and marketed to aid in extrinsic stain removal, but they have limited effectiveness in removing severe staining. Extrinsic staining that is resistant to removal by the patient may be removed with scaling and polishing by the dentist or dental hygienist. Extrinsic stains that are resistant to complete removal can be effectively removed by whitening treatments. Whitening treatments are more effective against extrinsic than against intrinsic stains.

2. Intrinsic Stain

An **intrinsic stain** occurs within tooth structures (enamel or dentin).

a) Post-eruptive Stain

Some intrinsic stain occurs after the tooth erupts. Causes for this type of stain include:

1) Amalgam Restorations
   Stains caused by silver amalgam cannot be successfully removed by the whitening process.
2) Caries
   Caries should be removed and the tooth restored before whitening is attempted.
3) Endodontic Treatment (Root Canal Therapy)
   Stains resulting from endodontic treatment can be successfully whitened.

b) Pre-eruptive Stain

Other intrinsic stains occur before tooth eruption, when the teeth are in the formative or calcification stage. These stains include:

1) Tetracycline Stain
   Tetracycline antibiotics that are ingested during tooth calcification may cause an intrinsic **tetracycline staining** of both dentin and enamel. Tetracycline binds chemically with the hydroxyapatite crystals of dentin and enamel. When tetracycline-stained dentin or enamel is exposed to a black light, the tetracycline crystals produce a fluorescent glow. Under natural and artificial light, tetracycline stains appear as gray or brown stains of varying intensity, usually occurring in horizontal bands within the tooth. Tetracycline-stained teeth are difficult to whiten. The milder the staining, the more successful the result.
2) Fluorosis
   High levels of fluoride (>1 ppm) consumed in the drinking water during tooth formation and calcification may cause staining known as **fluorosis.** Fluoride-containing dentifrices and mouthwashes are potential sources of excessive systemic fluoride. Parents should be cautioned to supervise children who use a fluoride dentifrice or mouthwash to prevent accidental or intentional swallowing. In its milder form, fluorosis appears as white spots in the enamel, with no pitting. In more severe cases, fluorosis causes brown spotting and pitting of the enamel. Teeth with fluorosis are difficult to whiten. The milder the fluorosis, the more successful the result.
3) Dentinogenesis Imperfecta and Amelogenesis Imperfecta
   Dentinogenesis imperfecta and **amelogenesis imperfecta** are inherited conditions that result in defective dentin and enamel formation, respectively. Whitening

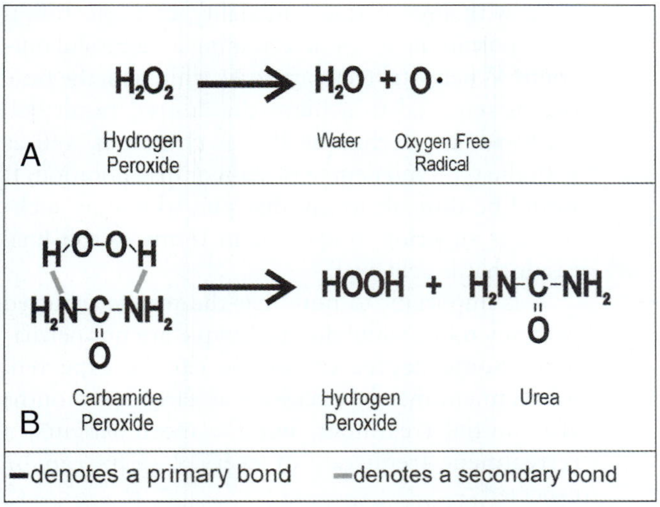

FIGURE 17.1 Decomposition of hydrogen peroxide. **A.** Hydrogen peroxide, a strong oxidizing agent, breaks down into water and free radicals of oxygen. Free radicals of oxygen oxidize the pigments in both extrinsic and intrinsic stains, producing the bleaching effect. **B.** Carbamide peroxide, a weaker oxidizing agent, breaks down into hydrogen peroxide and urea.

will not significantly improve the appearance of teeth that are affected by dentinogenesis or amelogenesis imperfecta.

III. Whitening Agents

A. Hydrogen Peroxide

Hydrogen peroxide (H_2O_2) is a strong oxidizing agent that readily decomposes into water and oxygen. The decomposition of hydrogen peroxide releases free radicals of oxygen that react with pigments in both extrinsic and intrinsic stains, producing the whitening effect. Free radicals of oxygen contain an unpaired electron and, therefore, are highly reactive. Figure 17.1*A* illustrates the decomposition of hydrogen peroxide into water and free radicals of oxygen.

Hydrogen peroxide can penetrate enamel and dentin and may produce a **reversible pulpitis,** which is a temporary inflammation of the pulp tissue. Tooth sensitivity resulting from pulpitis is the most frequently reported side effect of the whitening process. Precautions must be taken to protect the patient's eyes, face, and intraoral soft tissues (lips, cheeks, and tongue), as well as the patient's clothes from hydrogen peroxide solutions.

Hydrogen peroxide is applied to the teeth in either a liquid or a gel form and in strengths varying from 5% to 35%. Figure 17.2 shows an example of a hydrogen peroxide tooth whitening agent (Zoom, Discus Dental).

B. Carbamide Peroxide

Carbamide peroxide ($CH_6N_2O_3$) is a weaker oxidizing agent and is more stable than hydrogen peroxide. It is applied to the teeth in either a liquid or a gel form and in strengths varying from 10% to 20%. Figure 17.3 shows examples of a carbamide peroxide gel (Rembrandt; Dent Mat, Santa Monica, CA) and paste (Colgate Platinum; Colgate Palmolive, New York, NY).

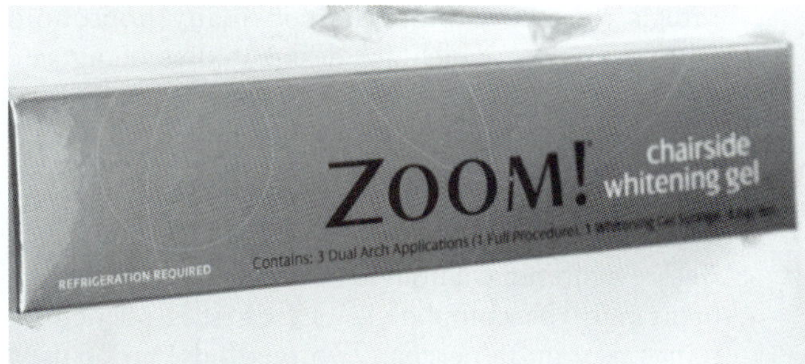

FIGURE 17.2 A Hydrogen Peroxide whitening agent. Zoom™ chairside whitening (Discus Dental).

Carbamide peroxide is a complex (secondary bonds) of urea and hydrogen peroxide. It decomposes into hydrogen peroxide, which then breaks down into water and oxygen (Fig. 17.1*B*). A 10% carbamide peroxide solution is equivalent to 3% hydrogen peroxide, whereas a 15% solution is equivalent to 5% hydrogen peroxide. Most carbamide peroxide whitening gels contain Carbopol (BF Goodrich, Richfield, OH), which is a thickening agent that increases adhesion of the gel to the tooth, thereby prolonging exposure to the whitening agent.

C. Sodium Perborate

Sodium perborate is another weak oxidizing agent. It is sometimes used together with hydrogen peroxide to whiten nonvital teeth. Sodium perbo-

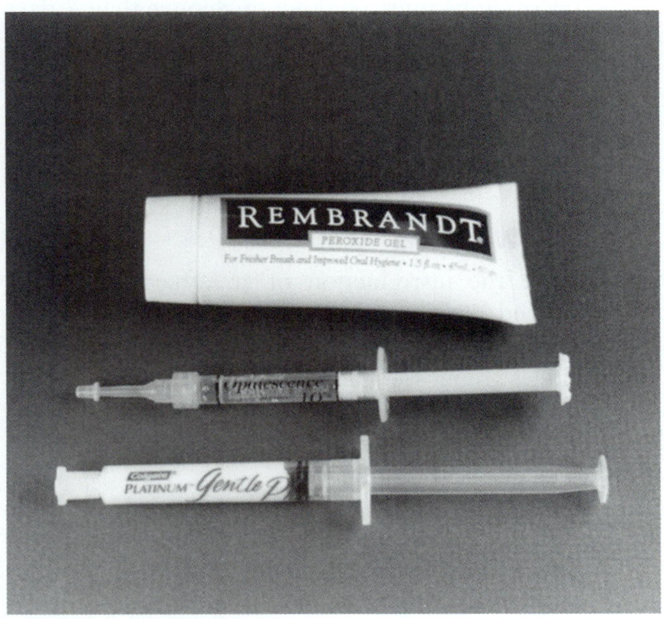

FIGURE 17.3 Carbamide peroxide whitening gels.

rate is the active ingredient in many household fabric bleaches, which are designated as being safe for colors.

IV. Whitening Techniques

A. Nonvital Whitening

Before whitening, a nonvital tooth endodontic treatment must be completed. The canal is opened by removal of gutta percha. Two methods can be used to attain bleaching: a power (heat and light activated) whitening or a walking bleach method.

The power whitening would be done similarly to the vital tooth bleaching. Once the pulp chamber is cleared of debris, a bur may be used to clear the canal. The canal is sealed and the tooth is isolated with a resin dam. An in-office heat-, light-, or laser-activated bleaching material may be applied to the coronal surface of the tooth. Once activated and whitening is attained, the canal may be filled with an esthetic restorative material. Research has shown that bond strength of materials is weakest immediately after bleaching. With the weak bond post-bleaching, esthetic restorations must be placed at least 7 days after the whitening procedure.

Nonvital walking bleach is a second method of lightening endodontically treated teeth. Sodium perborate mixed with 35% hydrogen peroxide or one of the commercial in-office bleaches is placed in the cleared canal. The canal is packed with a cotton pellet and sealed with zinc phosphate or IRM®. The endodontic patient will retain the bleach within the canal for 3 to 7 days; at that time the patient will be reevaluated for results. The method can weaken the bond between tooth surface and esthetic restorations. Therefore restorations must be done no sooner than 7 days after bleaching. Walking bleach can also lead to increased hydroxyl free radical formation at the apex of the nonvital tooth. Because of these side effects, the walking bleach method is not done as frequently.

B. Vital Whitening

Since the introduction of an effective patient-applied technique in 1989, tooth whitening has grown rapidly in popularity. Two whitening techniques are most popular:

1. A professionally applied, in-office technique.
2. A patient-applied (at-home), professionally supervised technique.

Over-the-counter whitening products are also available to the public. Most of these are not recommended, however, because they are used without professional supervision. These will be discussed later in this section.

As with any treatment modality, case selection is an important factor in determining a successful outcome. When vital teeth are to be whitened, the time that is required to achieve the desired result will vary with the technique that is chosen as well as with the type and degree of stain or discoloration. It would be difficult to say that one whitening technique is superior to another in terms of the final result that is achieved.

It is important to note that the results achieved with any tooth whitening technique are not permanent. Some degree of relapse can be expected. Retreatment may be necessary as early as 6 months after initial treatment, but for most patients, a retreatment frequency of every 2 years can be expected.

1. Professionally Applied, In-Office Whitening

The professionally applied, in-office whitening technique is often referred to as **power whitening**. As power whitening uses higher concentrations of hydrogen peroxide (15%–35%), all soft tissues and eyes must be protected. Teeth to be whitened are isolated with a rubber dam or a paint-on liquid resin dam. Often a light- or heat-activated method of accelerating the bleaching process is utilized, but their effectiveness has been questioned.

The paint-on resin dam (e.g. Liquid Dam™ or Pulpdent Kool Dam™) has become popular and is replacing the use of the conventional rubber dam. The paint-on resin dam may be autocure or light-cure. When using a paint-on resin dam, the gingiva, tongue and facial mucosa are protected with a coat of a petroleum-based lubricant. Figure 17.4 illustrates proper isolation for the power whitening procedure. In addition, the

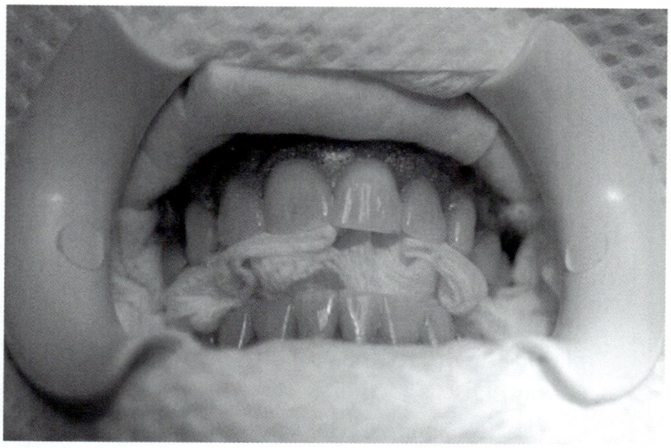

FIGURE 17.4 Patient isolated with retractors, cotton rolls, gauze, and paint-on resin dental dam awaiting power (light/heat activated) whitening procedure.

patient's eyes are protected with appropriate safety glasses.

Hydrogen peroxide is usually supplied in a gel form and delivered to the teeth from a syringe. The hydrogen peroxide is then activated with heat using a variety of lights, some being resin-curing lights. Many in-office bleaching products have a chemical added to absorb light and warm the bleaching material. To avoid damage to the vital pulp, care must be taken not to apply too much heat to the teeth. In addition, the teeth must not be anesthetized with local anesthesia because this would prevent the patient from responding to painful stimulation produced by excessive heat.

The latest innovation in professionally applied techniques is **laser whitening.** In this technique, a laser beam, either argon or carbon dioxide, is applied to the teeth to activate the whitening agent. In addition to activating the whitening agent, the argon laser interacts directly with dark stains to neutralize them, but it becomes less effective in directly neutralizing stains as the tooth whitens.

Laser whitening is the most rapid whitening technique that is currently available; however, extra caution must be exercised. Both the patient and the dental team must wear special safety glasses to protect the eyes from the energy of the laser beam. Laser whitening is usually completed in one appointment. Laser whitening must be used with caution. Compared to other lights used to activate bleach, the laser is the only one that can increase intrapulpal temperature and cause dental pulp necrosis. Lasers should never be used at full power for vital bleaching.

Aqueous Cleaning Technology, a product of GRINrx Corporation, has been introduced as a pre-bleaching procedure used to clean and remove stains before the power bleaching procedure. The system combines the elements of time and action with solvents, surfactants, chelators, and saponifiers. The material elements are available in a convenient swab. The tooth is swabbed to remove debris and stain, enhancing the overall whitening procedure. Some evidence suggests the procedure hydrates the tooth before the bleaching procedure that subsequently dehydrates tooth structure.

2. Patient-Applied, Professionally Supervised Whitening

Either hydrogen peroxide or carbamide peroxide may be used in the patient-applied, professionally supervised technique. Results of patient-applied whitening depend primarily on the strength of the whitening agent and the length of the treatment.

a) Hydrogen Peroxide

Hydrogen peroxide gels in strengths varying from 2% to 10% are dispensed by the patient into custom-made resin trays. The trays are worn over the teeth for multiple treatment sessions of 30 minutes each. The resin trays are commonly made by the dental hygienist. This procedure includes making alginate impressions, fabricating gypsum casts, and trimming the tray. Chapter 31 provides a step-by-step procedure to fabricate resin trays for the patient-applied, professionally supervised technique.

Another whitening technique in this category was introduced by Procter and Gamble (Cincinnati, OH) in 2000. Crest "Whitestrips" are available to the patient both over-the-counter and professionally; the difference between the two products is the strength of the hydrogen peroxide contained in the strip. The strips adhere to the facial surfaces of the anterior teeth. No tray is needed. The professional Whitestrips contain 6.5% hydrogen peroxide and are worn twice a day for 30 minutes each. Figure 17.5 shows the "Professional Whitestrips" for both upper and lower arches.

In 2004, Proctor and Gamble introduced an even higher concentration of whitestrip, Whitestrips Supreme. The hydrogen peroxide concentration is 14%. Whitestrips

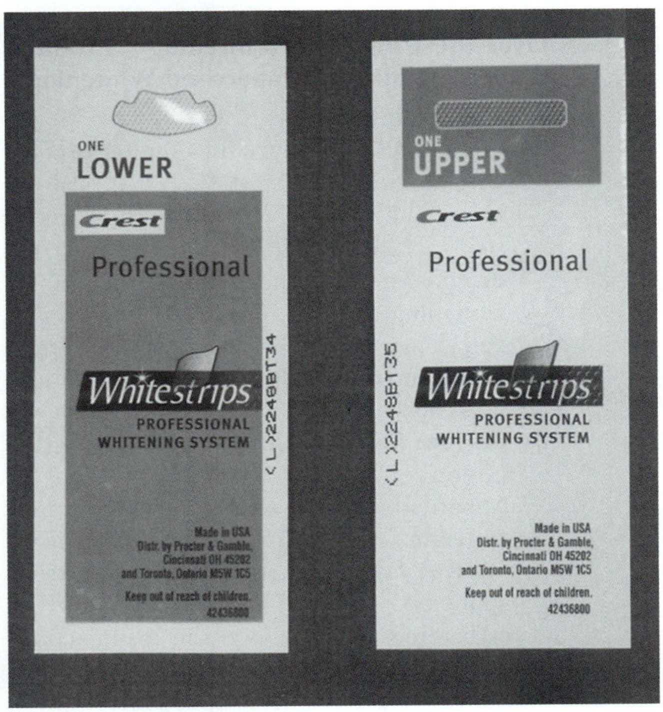

FIGURE 17.5 Crest Professional Whitestrips.

Supreme is only available via a dental professional. The 14% strips are applied in the same manner as the lower concentrations. Strips are applied over the facial smile line of the dentition's upper and lower arches and worn for 30 minutes twice per day. The concentration allows these strips to work faster. The patient should be monitored by their dentist throughout the procedure.

b) Carbamide Peroxide

Carbamide peroxide gel in strengths from 10% to 22% is dispensed by the patient into custom-made resin trays. The trays are worn during the day for multiple treatment sessions of 2 hours each. Alternatively, the patient may choose to wear the trays for 8 hours while sleeping.

The American Dental Association (ADA) discourages the use of any whitening that is not approved by the ADA Council of Scientific Affairs. The Seal of Acceptance on the product packaging indicates ADA approval, as shown in Figure 1.1.

c) Professional Whitening and Stain Removing Swabs

Aqueous Cleaning Technology manufactured by GRINrx, introduced as a prebleaching procedure, may be used to clean and remove stains at home. The product can also be used for touchup bleaching. In the future, the convenient swab may find its way into hospitals, restaurants, and cafes as an alternative to tooth brushing.

3. Over-the-Counter Whitening Products (Patient-Applied, Unsupervised Whitening)

a) Crest Whitestrips

To date, the only over-the-counter product with demonstrated safety and efficacy is Crest Whitestrips. The over-the-counter strips are identical to the professional strips, except that they contain a less concentrated whitening agent (5.3% hydrogen peroxide gel). They are applied to the facial surface of the anterior teeth twice daily for 30 minutes each.

b) Colgate Simply White and Simply White Night

A patient-applied whitening gel is now available. The gel is painted on the facial surface of the teeth, much like nail polish is applied to fingers. The gel contains 18% carbamide peroxide, and the manufacturer claims it delivers 6% hydrogen peroxide. Simply White Night is applied once daily at night.

c) Whitening Dentifrices

The effect of whitening dentifrices is achieved primarily through the mechanical removal of extrinsic stain by an abrasive. Common abrasives include **hydrated silica, precipitated calcium carbonate,** and **dicalcium phosphate dihydrate.** Some whitening dentifrices contain a peroxide that also contributes to the whitening effect. Among the peroxides are hydrogen peroxide, **calcium peroxide,** and **sodium percarbonate.**

Whitening dentifrices, although somewhat effective in maintaining whitened teeth, are not as effective as whitening agents applied in the office or by the patient in a tray or on a strip. Examples of whitening dentifrices are shown in Figure 17.6.

d) Additional Products

With consumer demand at an increasingly high level, many additional whitening products are available. Chewing gum, floss, mouth rinses, pens, flexible waxlike strips, and even bleaching trays with light systems claim to whiten or brighten the dentition, Figure 17.6. Many of the products do not have any solid scientific studies to substantiate their whitening capabilities or their safety to the dentition. Dental patients must be

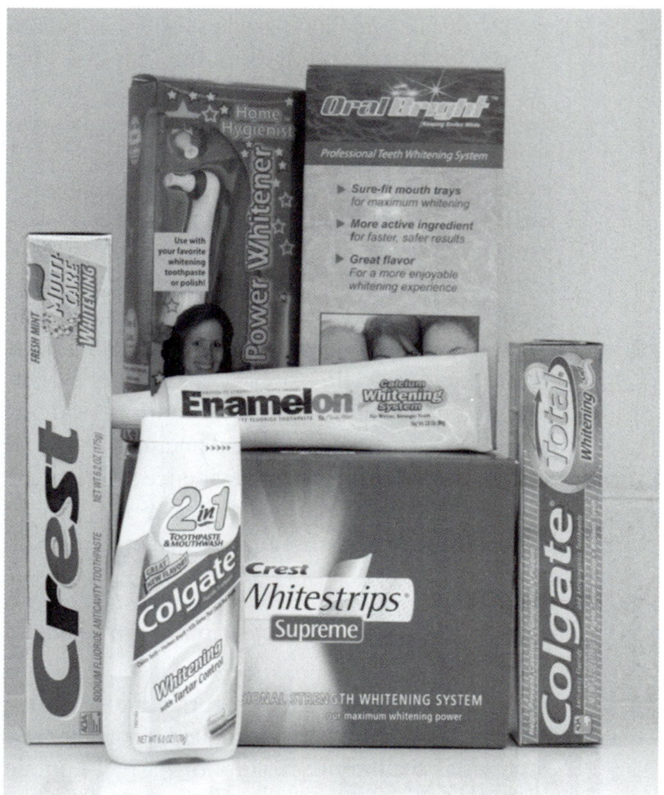

FIGURE 17.6 A variety of over-the-counter tooth whitening products.

aware that many of these products do not have ADA approval.

V. Side Effects of Whitening

Tooth sensitivity and gingival irritation are the most frequently reported side effects of whitening. Both side effects are transient, usually lasting no more than a few days after treatment is discontinued. Gingival irritation may occur when a whitening agent exudes out of the tray or when accidentally leached onto the tissue during a power whitening procedure. Care must be taken to protect the gingival tissues completely with a conventional rubber or paint-on resin dam during in-office procedures. With patient-applied trays, the tray should be trimmed to produce a scalloped border that ends on the teeth rather than on the gingiva. Tooth sensitivity occurs either from pressure by a tray that is too rigid or from the whitening agent itself. If the whitening agent alone is suspected, tooth sensitivity is effectively treated by discontinuing treatment and, if necessary, topical application of either **neutral sodium fluoride** or **potassium nitrate.** The desensitizing agent can be applied in the whitening tray for 30 minutes twice daily until sensitivity is controlled.

Use of a potassium nitrate toothpaste two weeks prior to and during bleaching has been documented as an effective method of preventing sensitivity during the whitening process. An increase in intrapulpal temperature during heat, light, or laser-activated bleaching may result in reversible pulpitis. Lasers should be used at the lowest setting for bleaching to avoid pulpal necrosis.

Any bleaching procedure using peroxides will produce free radicals. Free radicals have been linked with cancers. With time, more severe consequences may be discovered with long-term overuse and abusive bleaching procedures. Patients with other risk factors for oral cancer, tobacco and excessive alcohol use, should be cautioned to follow instructions.

VI. Concerns for the Dental Hygienist

Patients tend to rely on recommendations and advice from their dental hygienist. With the increasing demand for tooth whitening from the dental professional, the hygienist must educate their patient about the procedure. Patients must be informed of both contraindications and side effects of whitening.

A. Contraindications for Whitening

1. Patients with aesthetic anterior restorations must be informed that whitening is ineffective on those restorations. Unless the patient is willing to replace those restorations 2 weeks after the bleaching they should not bleach.
2. Patients with cracked or hypoplastic enamel should not bleach.
3. Patients with carious lesions should not bleach.
4. Patients with cervical abrasion or tooth sensitivity should not bleach.
5. Patients undergoing radiation or chemotherapy must not use light-activated systems.
6. Patients with melanoma must not use light-activated systems.
7. Patients using photosensitive drugs or photosensitive herbal remedies must not use light-activated systems.
8. Patients considering nonvital bleaching must not bleach if tooth was extensively restored. Nonvital teeth are inherently weaker and the bleach creates an even weaker tooth structure so only nonvital teeth with minor restorations should be considered.
9. Patients with amalgam stains in dentinal tubules must not undergo nonvital bleaching since the product will not whiten those areas.

B. Factors to Consider When Tray Whitening

1. Gingival sensitivity may be prevented with the use of a dentifrice containing potassium nitrate two weeks prior to, during, and after the whitening procedure.
2. Gingival sensitivity may be prevented by using scalloped trays. Patients must not dab more than one dot of bleaching material to the facial surfaces of the tray. More material does not result in faster bleaching. Apply and wipe any bleach from gingival surfaces.
3. Gingival sensitivity may warrant discontinuing the procedure for 1 to 2 days. If upon resuming sensitivity remains see your dental professional.
4. Reversible pulpitis may occur. Patients may need to discontinue whitening for 1 to 2 days or see their dentist if sensitivity continues.
5. Sensitivity can be reduced by use of neutral sodium fluoride or potassium nitrate twice daily for 30 minutes in night guard tray.
6. Remind patients using over-the-counter systems to search for products with the ADA seal of approval.

C. Factors to Consider When Power Whitening

1. Gingival sensitivity or irritation may occur. Use of a Vitamin E oil may soothe the tissues.
2. Prophylactic use of nonsteroidal anti-inflammatory drugs may prevent effects of reversible pulpitis before and after procedure.
3. Patient should avoid foods that stain (tea, coffee, mustard, red sauces) for 24–48 hours.

4. Use of neutral sodium fluoride or potassium nitrate twice daily for 30 minutes can help reduce sensitivity.
5. Additional nightguard bleaching can enhance power bleaching procedure; do not use if gingival irritation or tooth sensitivity occur.
6. Mouth rinses, dentifrices, and night guard bleaching can be used to maintain whitening or for touch up of whitening.
7. Dentist must be notified if sensitivity lasts more than 2 days after the whitening procedure.

D. Overbleaching

Overbleaching one's dentition could be a sign of body dysmorphic disorder (BDD). BDD is a disorder where one is never satisfied with their looks. Just as this disorder applies to shapes and body sizes, the disorder now includes tooth whiteness. Patients who whiten become obsessed with the color and too light or too white does not seem to be in their vocabulary. Although dental hygiene professionals are not psychiatrists or psychologists, they must try to identify such patients. Recognizing a patient's obsessive need to overbleach and prevent further abuse may save the dental health of that patient. Be aware of those patients already using an at-home whitening procedure and seeking higher strength peroxides. Evaluate the dentition for an overly white and chalky look. Advise these patients of dental health consequences such as sensitivity, pain, and pulpal necrosis.

SUMMARY

Tooth whitening has become the most popular esthetic procedure and the most requested dental procedure. Teeth can be whitened in the office by the dentist or staff (dental hygienist) or at home by the patient. To enhance safety of whitening, professional supervision is recommended. Side effects of whitening include tooth sensitivity and gingival irritation, which are usually mild and abate within a day or two after treatment is discontinued. Patients must be made aware that in rare cases pulpal necrosis could occur. Any bleaching procedure using peroxides could produce hydroxyl free radicals. Hydroxyl free radicals have been linked to cancers. With time more severe consequences may be discovered with long-term use, overuse, and abusive bleaching procedures. The dental hygienist plays an important role in identifying who may benefit from whitening and those who may be harmed by whitening.

Learning Activities

1. Find a coffee or tea cup that is stained inside from use. Fill the cup one-quarter full with 3% hydrogen peroxide, which can be found on the shelf of your local pharmacy. Let the cup stand uncovered for 24 hours. Empty the cup, and rinse with cool water. Note the difference in the appearance of the bleached and unbleached inner surfaces of the cup.
2. Hard-boil two white eggs, and brew a cup of strong tea. Completely immerse both eggs in the tea, and let them stand for 24 hours. Remove both eggs from the tea, and note the dark stain. Place one egg in a cup half-filled with 3% hydrogen peroxide, and let it stand for 24 hours. Remove and dry the egg, and compare the whitened egg to the tea-stained egg.
3. Visit the household cleaning products section of a grocery store. Select several fabric bleaching products, including laundry detergents with bleach. Read the ingredients list on the labels. Which ingredients are responsible for the bleaching effect that is claimed for the product? Is there one common ingredient in most of the "color safe" products?

Review Questions

1. The term "nonvital" may be used to describe a tooth that has:
  a) Been treated with a root canal procedure
  b) A necrotic pulp
  c) No pulp tissue in the pulp cavity
  d) All of the above

2. Which of the following esthetic tooth treatments requires no removal of tooth structure?
  a) Nonvital tooth whitening
  b) Vital tooth whitening
  c) Facial veneer
  d) Porcelain-bonded-to-metal crown

3. Which of the following statements is the most accurate?
  a) Hydrogen peroxide is more stable than carbamide peroxide
  b) Carbamide peroxide is used in the nonvital tooth whitening technique known as a walking bleach
  c) Hydrogen peroxide decomposes into water and free radicals of oxygen
  d) Carbamide peroxide is most often applied to teeth as a gel at a 35% concentration

4. Which of the following variables is not a factor in the success of a vital tooth whitening treatment?
  a) Number of teeth to be treated
  b) Strength of the whitening agent
  c) Type and intensity of discoloration or stain
  d) Length of exposure of the tooth to the whitening agent

5. Teeth with a moderate degree of ______________ are the most difficult to successfully whiten.
  a) Extrinsic food and beverage stain
  b) Yellow intrinsic discoloration
  c) Extrinsic tobacco stain
  d) Tetracycline stain

6. Which of the following statements is NOT true regarding tooth sensitivity from vital tooth whitening?
  a) It is a common side effect
  b) It is not reversible
  c) It can be treated by topical application of potassium nitrate
  d) It may be caused by a tray that is too rigid

7. Which of the following is the most common esthetic procedure in dentistry?
  a) Facial veneer
  b) All-porcelain crown
  c) Porcelain-bonded-to-metal crown
  d) Tooth whitening

8. Brushing with a potassium nitrate containing dentifrice before and after bleaching is advised. During power bleaching a patient must be anesthetized.
  a) The first statement is true; the second statement is false.
  b) The first statement is false; the second statement is true.
  c) Both statements are true.
  d) Both statements are false.

9. When should a bleached tooth be restored with a composite restoration?
  a) Immediately
  b) 1–2 days
  c) 3–4 days
  d) 1–2 weeks

10. All of the following are contraindications to light-activated bleaching procedures except:
  a) Use of photosensitive drugs
  b) History of melanoma
  c) Undergoing radiation therapy or chemotherapy
  d) Previous use of night guard bleaching system

Supplemental Readings

American Dental Association, Council on Dental Therapeutics. Guidelines for acceptance of peroxide-containing oral hygiene products. J Am Dent Assoc 1994;125: 1140–1142.

Aqueous Cleaning Technology™ A disruptive new technology promoting oral health and smile aesthetics. GRINrx Corporation NY, NY; 2006.

Buchalla W, Attin T. External bleaching therapy with activation by heat, light or laser—A systematic review. DentMat 2006;23(5):586–596.

Christensen GJ. The tooth-whitening revolution. J Am Dent Assoc 2002;133:1277–1279.

Dam that's Kool Tech Specifications from the Manufacturer Contemporary Esthetics and Restorative Practice. January 2004. retrieved March 14, 2007 from http://www.pulpdent.com/studies/Kool_Dam_Glazer.pdf

Farmer D, Burcham P, Marin P. The ability of thiourea to scavenge hydrogen peroxide and hydroxyl radicals during the intra-coronal bleaching of bloodstained root-filled teeth. Aust Dent J 2006;51(2):146–152.

Goldstein RE, Garber DA. Complete Dental Bleaching. Chicago: Quintessence, 1995.

Haywood VB. Night guard vital bleaching: current concepts and research. J Am Dent Assoc 1997;128(suppl):19S–25S.

Haywood V, Cordero R, Wright K, et al. Brushing with a potassium nitrate dentifrice to reduce bleaching sensitivity. J Clin Dent 2005;16(1):17–22.

Marcato et al. University of Nice. Laser Assisted Non Vital Tooth Whitening in One Step: Comparison of Two Wavelengths. Retrieved March 14, 2007 from http://fotoan.sitedesign.net/files/clinicalpapers/pdf/poster_la_non_vital_whitening_Marcato_ISLD_o6.pdf

Sagel P, Landrigan W. A new approach to strip based tooth whitening: 14% hydrogen peroxide delivered via controlled low dose. Compen Contin Educ Dent 2004;8:9–13.

Shinohara M, Peris A, Rodrigues J, Pimenta L, Ambrosano G. Effect of non vital bleaching on shear bond strength of composite resins. J Adhes Dent 2004;6(3):205–209.

Sulieman M, Addy M, Rees J. Surface and intra-pulpal temperature rises during tooth bleaching: a study in vitro. Br Dent J 2005;199:37–40.

Sulieman M, Addy M, Rees J. Surface and pulp temperature rises during tooth bleaching using a diode laser: a study in vitro. Br Dent J 2006;200:631–634.

Turkin M, Turkin L. Effect of nonvital bleaching with 10% carbamide peroxide on sealing ability of resin composite restorations. Int Endo J 2004;37(1):52–60.

Ziempa S, Felix H, Ginger M, Ward M. Randomized Prospective Effectiveness of Zoom^{2TM} Dental Whitening Lamp and Light-catalyzed peroxide gel. Clinical White Paper. Discus Dental Inc. Feb 2005.

18

Oral Appliances

Christine Nathe, R.D.H., M.S.

Objectives

After studying this chapter, the student will be able to do the following:

1. List the different oral appliances used in dentistry.
2. Describe the reasons for the use of oral appliances.
3. Name the different thermoplastic materials used in the fabrication of oral appliances, and discuss the properties of these materials.
4. Explain the steps involved in fabricating an oral appliance.
5. Describe the proper maintenance of oral appliances.
6. Prepare a script or dialogue that may be used for patient education regarding oral appliances.

Key Words/Phrases

athletic mouthguard
bleaching tray
custom-made mouthguard
fluoride custom trays
mouth-formed mouthguard
obstructive sleep apnea
oral appliances
stock mouthguard
thermoplastic
thermoset
vacuum former

INTRODUCTION

Oral appliances are made from a variety of materials: thermoplastic polymers, thermoset polymers, wires, bands, and other prefabricated parts. Thermoplastic materials have an advantage over other types of materials in that they are easily used to construct an oral appliance. They simply are heated and molded into the desired shape. Thermoplastic materials are increasingly used in the dental office to serve a variety of needs.

As dental hygienists, it is our responsibility to inform the patient of the need for an oral appliance, the care that is required to maintain it, and any possible side effects. **Oral appliances** currently available to patients include athletic mouthguards, bleaching trays, fluoride custom trays, orthodontic appliances, nightguards, periodontal stints, space maintainers, and appliances for the treatment of obstructive sleep apnea (OSA) and snoring as well as nonnutritive (thumb) sucking. These appliances, along with their purposes, are listed in Table 18.1. Two different oral appliances are illustrated in Figures 18.1 and 18.2.

Some oral appliances, such as athletic mouthguards and custom fluoride trays, are relatively easy to make in the laboratory area of a typical dental practice. This chapter will discuss several types of oral appliances and provide a summary of the fabrication procedure for fluoride trays and mouthguards.

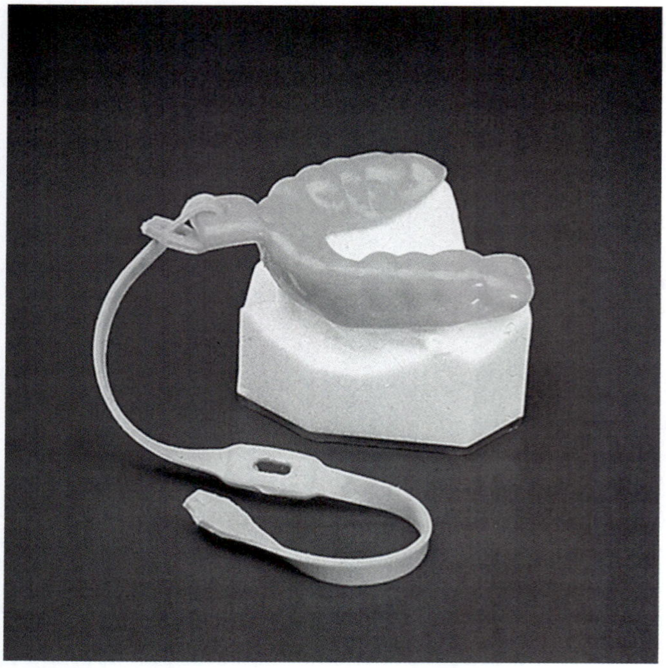

FIGURE 18.1 Athletic mouthguard. (Courtesy of Great Lakes Orthodontics, Ltd.)

I. Types of Oral Appliances

A. Athletic Mouthguards

An **athletic mouthguard** is a removable oral appliance that protects the teeth and surrounding tissues during contact sports (see Figs. 18.1 and 18.3). The athletic mouthguard, which is sometimes referred to as a mouth protector, provides protection against injuries to the teeth and supporting structures by absorbing energy. The force of the blow is spread over many teeth, and contact between maxillary and mandibular teeth is prevented. The mouthguard is dually capable of realigning and repositioning the jaws so that the condyles of the mandible do not contact the soft tissues of the joints, thus avoiding injury to these areas. Mouthguards are used to prevent orofacial trauma during contact sports and other recreational activities.

Table 18.1 The Purpose of Oral Appliances

Appliance	Purpose
Appliances for nonnutritive sucking habits	To help stop the habit of sucking thumb/fingers
Athletic mouthguards	To prevent orofacial injury
Bleaching trays	To hold bleaching solution in close proximity to dentition to "whiten teeth"
Fluoride custom tray	To hold prescription fluoride gel trays in close proximity to dentition; to decrease the occurrence of demineralization and increase remineralization
Orthodontic retainers	To stabilize teeth after movement
Nightguards	To alleviate tooth surface wear
Periodontal stints	To hold anesthetic and antiseptic materials after periodontal surgery and/or to hold gingival flaps during surgery
Snoring/sleep apnea appliances	To advance the mandible, which will decrease airway obstruction during sleep, thus alleviating snoring and mild to moderate cases of sleep apnea
Space maintainer	To temporarily hold teeth in position
Tooth positioners	To provide minor tooth movement

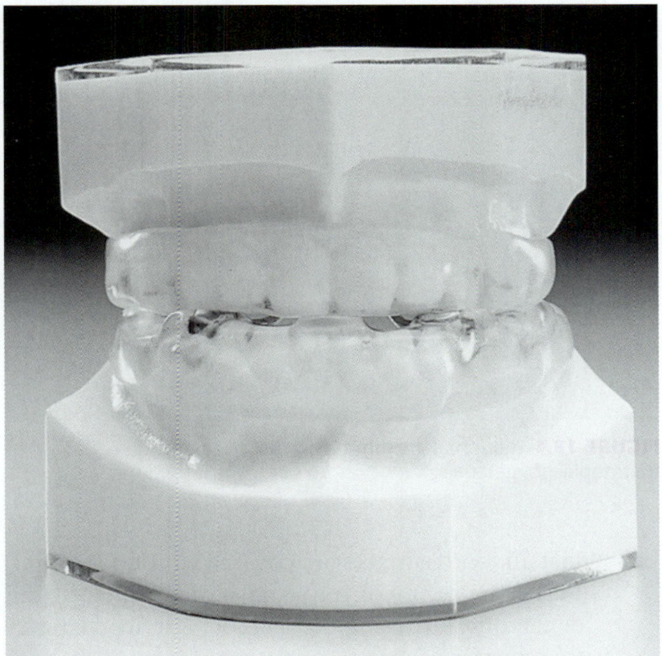

FIGURE 18.2 Klearway appliance for the treatment of snoring and obstructive sleep apnea. (Courtesy of Great Lakes Orthodontics, Ltd.)

1. Advantages

Research has shown a significant decrease in injuries when a mouthguard is used. Injuries that can be decreased by wearing an athletic mouthguard include tooth avulsion, fractured teeth, gingival and/or mucosal injuries, jaw fractures, neck injuries, and even concussions.

2. Popularity

Mouthguards have been used since the 1950s. Many athletic associations, including the National Collegiate Athletic Association (NCAA), mandate their use. Interestingly, most professional sports do not require the use of mouthguards, but most professional athletes wear them voluntarily.

3. Wide Application

Mouthguards are recommended for a variety of contact sports and recreational activities. These are listed in Table 18.2.

4. Encouraging the Use of Mouthguards

Many patients are unaware of the necessity for wearing an athletic mouthguard when playing contact sports or enjoying recreational activities. Dental hygienists are responsible for educating patients on the importance of the athletic mouthguard and the need to use it in all situations. Research suggests that the earlier a child starts wearing a mouthguard during amateur

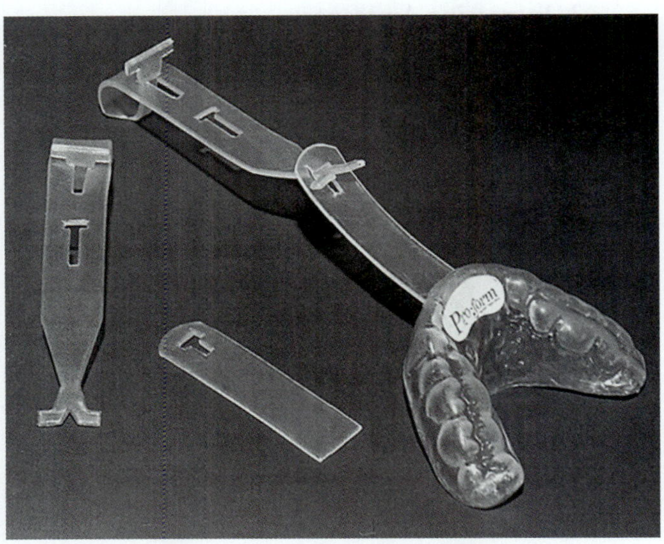

FIGURE 18.3 Athletic mouthguard. (Courtesy of DR Dental Resources, Inc.)

Table 18.2 American Dental Association Recommended Activities for Use of Athletic Mouthguards

Acrobatics
Baseball
Basketball
Bicycling
Boxing
Equestrian events
Field events
Field hockey
Football
Gymnastics
Handball
Ice hockey
In-line skating
Lacrosse
Martial arts
Racquetball
Rugby
Shotputting
Skateboarding
Skiing
Skydiving
Soccer
Softball
Squash
Surfing
Volleyball
Water polo
Weightlifting
Wrestling

sports, the higher the compliance rate will be when he or she is playing in more organized, competitive sports. In fact, younger, inexperienced children are more likely than older athletes to sustain orofacial injuries. Therefore, the importance of wearing a mouthguard is greater for these young participants.

5. Types

Three types of athletic mouthguards exist.

a) The **stock mouthguard** is available in different sizes. It is not custom-made, nor is it preferred (because of poor fit and excess bulk).

b) A **mouth-formed guard,** which is generally referred to as a "boil-and-bite" style, can be heated in water and then placed in the mouth. The athlete bites into the guard, and an inexact fit is produced. This type of mouthguard can become distorted and does not accommodate an individual athlete's unique oral features.

c) The most effective mouthguard is the **custom-made mouthguard.** This type of mouthguard is custom fabricated and fits precisely over the individual athlete's dentition. Because it is more comfortable and better fitting, compliance is increased; therefore, the custom-made mouthguard is better at reducing injuries. This type of mouthguard does need to be replaced, however, when changes occur to the athlete's dentition. See Table 18.3 for information on ideal mouthguard properties.

B. Fluoride Custom Trays

Fluoride custom trays are ideal for patients who have a high prevalence of dental caries or high caries risk (see Fig. 18.4). These trays are custom-made to fit the particular individual's dentition so that all tooth surfaces are covered with fluoride gel. Furthermore, these trays can be fabricated in the dental office by using the method described later in this chapter.

Table 18.3 Ideal Mouthguard Properties

To provide adequate protection a mouthguard should:

- be properly fitted to the wearer's mouth and accurately adapted to his or her oral structures;
- be made of resilient material approved by the U.S. FDA and cover all remaining teeth on one arch, customarily the maxillary;
- stay in place comfortably and securely;
- be physiologically compatible with the wearer;
- be relatively easy to clean;
- have high-impact energy absorption and reduce transmitted forces upon impact.

Adapted from American Dental Association. Using mouthguards to reduce the incidence and severity of sports-related oral injuries. J Am Dent Assoc 2006;137(12):17712–17720.

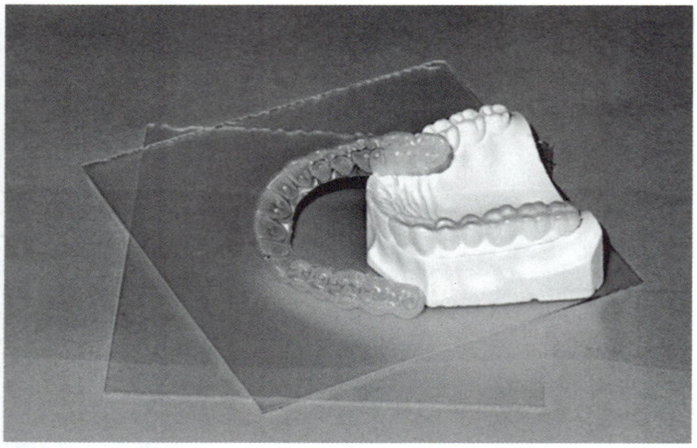

FIGURE 18.4 A fluoride custom tray, gypsum cast, and thermoplastic materials.

1. Qualifying Conditions

Use of fluoride custom trays is indicated for the following oral conditions:

- A high incidence or risk of dental caries, including rampant enamel or root caries
- Xerostomia
- Overdentures
- Hypersensitivity
- Radiation therapy

2. Compatible Gels

Types of fluoride gels that may be placed in the custom-made tray include:

- Acidulated phosphate fluoride (0.5%)
- Sodium fluoride (1.1%)
- Stannous fluoride (0.4%)

3. Increasing Awareness

It is advantageous to educate patients about the causes of dental caries and the role that fluoride plays in the remineralization of teeth.

4. Latest Developments

Latest developments include the use of desensitizing agents in the fluoride custom tray for the treatment of dentin hypersensitivity. Remineralization is the process of restoring mineral ions to the tooth structure. There are new calcium phosphate products available that claim to aid in the remineralization process when placed in a custom tray. These are used for caries prevention and dentinal hypersensitivity.

C. Orthodontic Appliances (Tooth Positioners)

Orthodontic appliances may be used to correct overbites, overjets, spacing problems, and slight

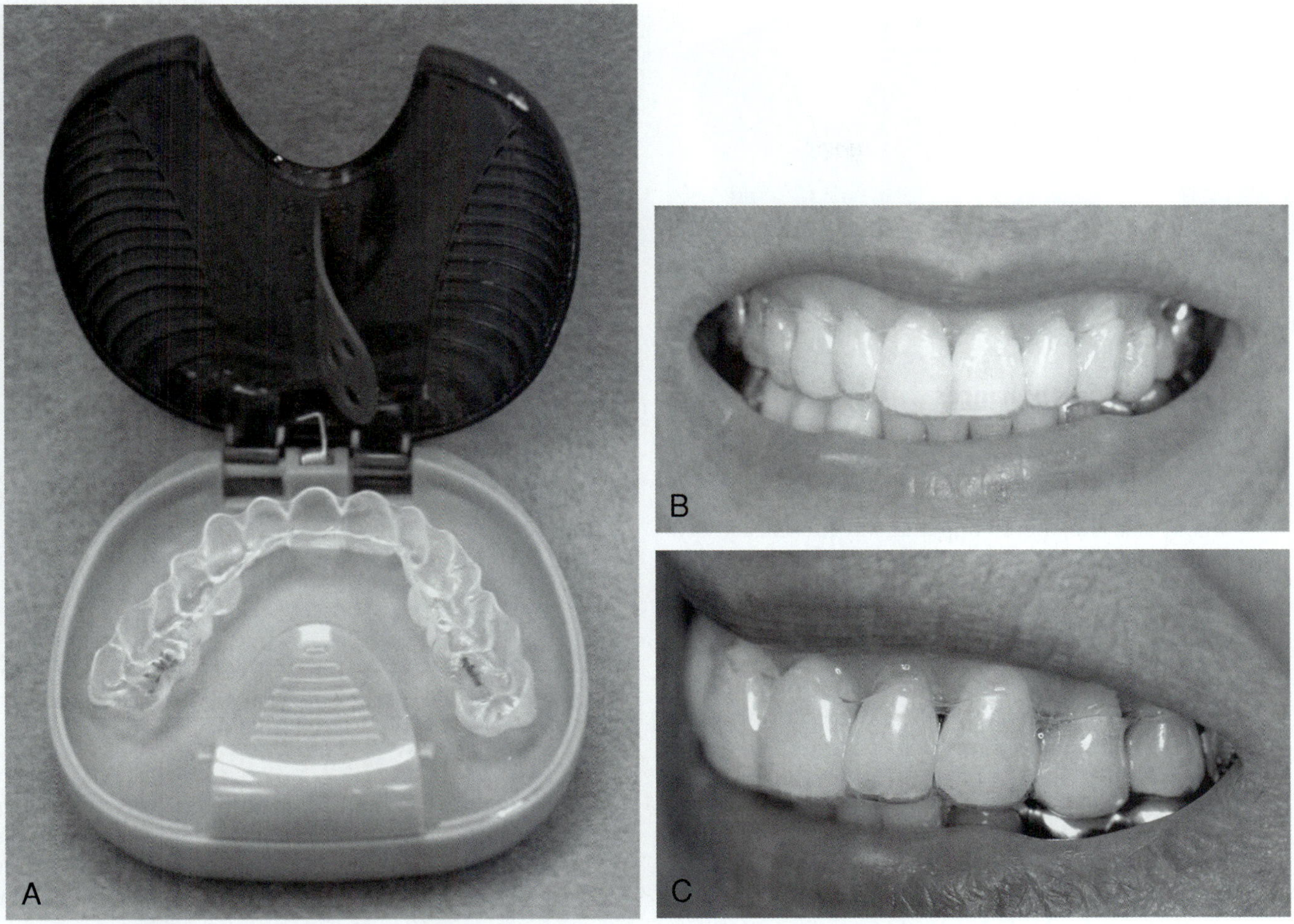

FIGURE 18.5 Invisalign appliance. **A.** Appliance in storage case, **B.** Appliance in place, **C.** Lateral view.

malocclusions. Several types of thermoplastic orthodontic appliances are used. During the final stages of orthodontic treatment, tooth positioners are used to attain the final, precise position of the teeth. In cases involving only minor movements of the dentition, an oral appliance such as the Invisalign system (Align Technologies, Inc., Santa Clara, CA) can be used (Figure 18.5).

During fabrication of both types of appliances, the teeth on the study model are removed. They are repositioned into their proper alignment with a hard baseplate wax used to hold the teeth in place. An impression of the corrected study model is then taken, and both a cast and an oral appliance are fabricated from this second impression. The patient may need to wear the appliance at night and possibly during the day as well.

Other orthodontic appliances include retainers and active appliances. They are fabricated from wires, bands, and thermoset resins. Several were discussed in Chapter 13, Specialty Materials.

D. Nightguards

Nightguards are prescribed for patients with bruxism. The function of the nightguard is simply to absorb the forces of clenching, thereby alleviating wear on the dentition. It is more cost-effective to periodically replace the appliance than to repair the damage to the dentition. Most patients will need to wear a nightguard only during sleep, but in extreme cases, it may also be worn during the day (Figure 18.6).

E. Space Maintainers

A space maintainer is a temporary appliance that is used when primary teeth have been lost prematurely (Figure 13.11). The purpose of this appliance is to prevent the adjacent teeth from drifting and closing the space before the eruption of the succeeding, permanent teeth. Thus, crowding and the need for orthodontics are reduced. Both removable and fixed space maintainers are available.

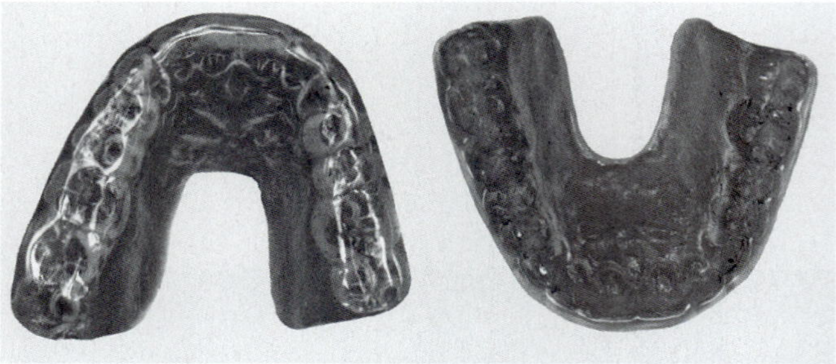

FIGURE 18.6 Nightguard. (Courtesy of Dr. James Foor, Morgantown, WV)

F. OSA/Snoring Appliances

Oral appliances are also currently being used to treat obstructive sleep apnea (OSA) and snoring. OSA is thought to be caused by a reduced upper airway size and altered upper airway muscle activity. The rationale for the use of oral appliances is that they advance the mandible, thus reversing some of these conditions.

Many different types of oral appliances have been developed to treat this condition. Patients with mild to moderate OSA and/or snoring wear this oral appliance during sleep hours. Research suggests that these appliances have no significant effect on either the periodontium or the occlusion.

G. Bleaching Trays

Recently, great emphasis has been placed on cosmetic dentistry. Included in this emphasis is tooth whitening or "bleaching," which was discussed in detail in the previous chapter. Figure 18.7 shows a **bleaching tray** designed for patient application at home. Bleaching trays appear very similar to fluoride trays.

H. Acrylic and Bis-Acryl (TRIAD) Appliances

Acrylic and bis-acryl materials are used for custom trays, provisional bridges, and denture relines and repairs. Bis-acryl appliances closely resemble traditional acrylic appliances. Both materials are considered to be thermoset polymers. The TRIAD System from Dentsply International uses light-activated polymerization and results in a faster curing time. Also, no methyl methacrylate monomer odor or hazard is involved. The TRIAD system, as shown in Figure 18.8, can also be used to fabricate orthodontic retainers and nightguards. Fabrication of a custom impression tray using the TRIAD system is explained in Chapter 29.

II. Material Used in Fabrication

A. Definition

A variety of thermoplastic materials are used for the production of oral appliances. These are illustrated

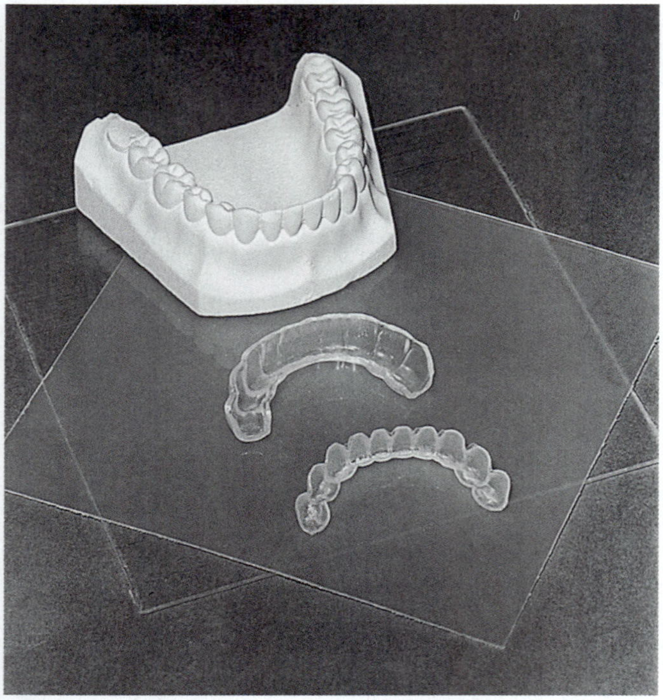

FIGURE 18.7 Bleaching trays, a gypsum cast, and thermoplastic materials. (Courtesy of DR Dental Resources, Inc.)

in Figure 18.9 and listed in Table 18.4. The term **thermoplastic** implies that a polymer softens on heating and then hardens into the final shape upon cooling. This is a desirable property for an oral

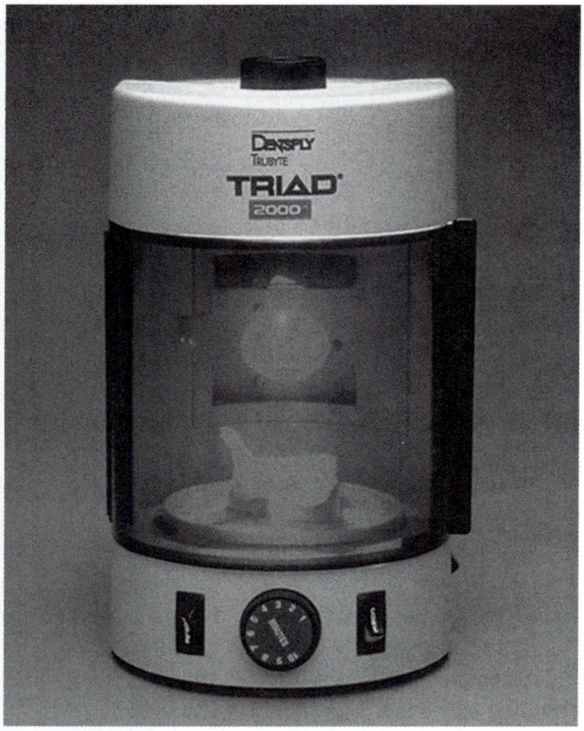

FIGURE 18.8 TRIAD 2000 visible light curing unit. (Courtesy of Dentsply.)

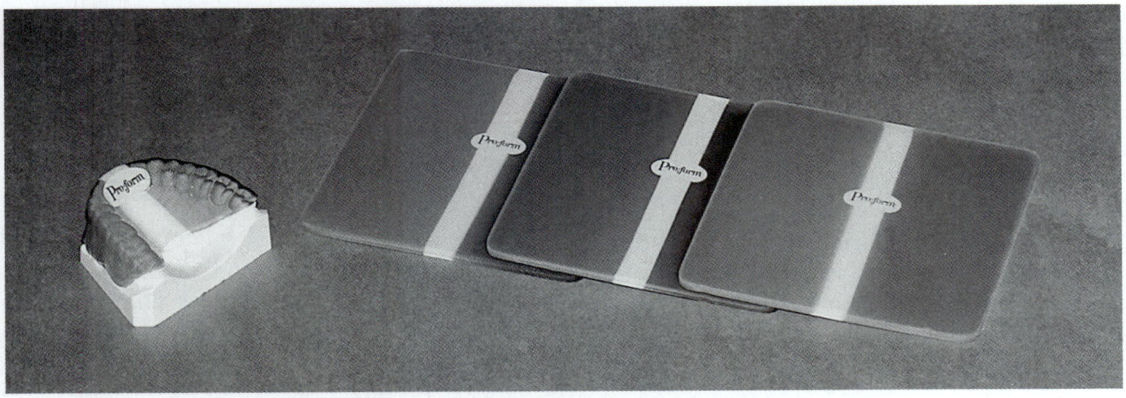

FIGURE 18.9 Thermoplastic materials. (Courtesy of DR Dental Resources, Inc.)

appliance because the final shape can be individualized for each case by using a study model. Occasionally, thermoset materials are used instead of thermoplastic materials for oral appliances. **Thermoset** materials are molded and then polymerized in the final shape. They are resistant to change when heated. Thermoplastic and thermoset polymers were discussed in Chapter 5.

B. Types

Most of the plastics that are used in the fabrication of simple oral appliances are thermoplastics. Polyethylene, polyvinyl chloride, polypropylene, polystyrenes, and polycarbonates comprise the majority of the thermoplastic materials that are used in the fabrication of oral appliances. In particular, polyethylene is used for the majority of oral appliances that may be made by the dental hygienist.

Table 18.4 Use of Thermoplastics

Material	Application
Polycarbonates	Temporary crowns and bridges Orthodontic retainers
Polyethylene	Mouthguards Tooth positioners Nightguards Space maintainers Fluoride custom trays Stints
Polypropylene	Temporary crown and bridge molds
Polystyrenes	Custom impression trays Denture bases
Polyvinyl chloride	Splints Dual laminates Temporary removable partial denture (Flipper) Ortho retainers

C. Properties

Each thermoplastic material has a specific polymer component. Individualizing the addition of polymers can affect the processing characteristics, the end performance, or the coloring. These are desirable properties because an oral appliance can thus be made for a variety of uses.

III. Fabrication of an Oral Appliance

This summary of the basic fabrication technique applies to most of the oral appliances that dental hygienists may fabricate "in-house." For a more complicated oral appliance, the hygienist may need to contact a laboratory. Figure 18.10 shows the necessary equipment.

The cast must show characteristics specific to the individual dentition, such as gingival margins and

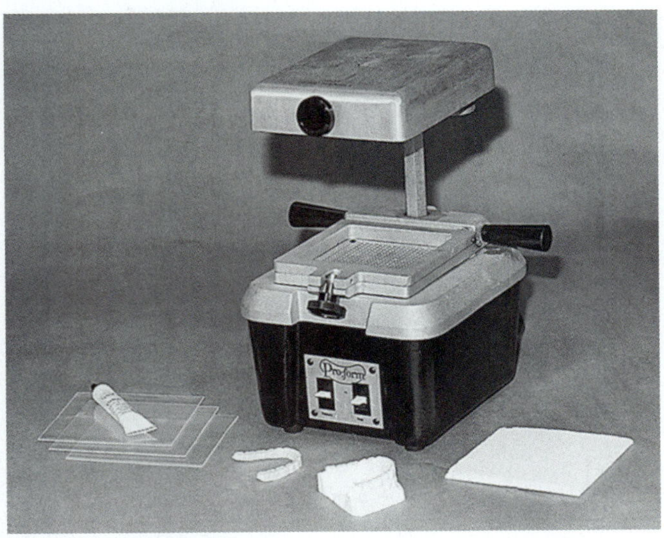

FIGURE 18.10 Vacuum former machine. (Courtesy of DR Dental Resources, Inc.)

tooth anatomy. The model height must be vertical to maintain occlusal characteristics. Because it is porous, plaster is recommended for the model. Therefore, it is easier to create suction directly through the model. When using a suction type of vacuum former, drill a hole in the palatal or lingual area of the model to allow suction into these vacuum pockets.

After a model has been poured and trimmed, turn on the heating element of the **vacuum former** and preheat the machine for 2 to 3 minutes. The fabrication then proceeds as follows:

1. Select the appropriate thermoplastic material indicated for the particular appliance.
2. Spray the model and frame with a silicone spray to reduce sticking. Place the selected thermoplastic material into the frame, and latch it shut. Raise the frame to the heater, and allow the material to heat.
3. Each material has different thermal properties, so heating times will vary between plastics.
4. Let the material heat and sag. Thin materials will sag only a small amount (0.25–0.5 inch), and thicker materials, such as mouthguard material, will sag a greater distance (0.5–1.0 inch) before they are ready. Thus, the further the material slumps, the thinner the material becomes.
5. After the material has heated and slumped, lower the frame onto the model, and switch on the vacuum former. For the best adaptation, allow the suction to run for 20 to 30 seconds. For further adaptation, use a wet paper towel, and press the material around the model while the vacuum motor is still on (Fig. 18.11).
6. Allow the material to cool on the model. Cooling times will vary between materials. To speed the cooling process, place both the molded plastic and the model in cold water.

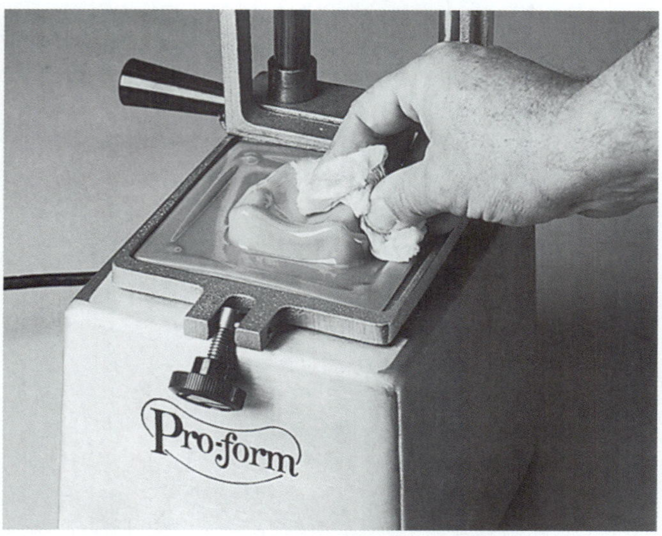

FIGURE 18.11 Oral appliance during fabrication procedures. (Courtesy of DR Dental Resources, Inc.)

Table 18.5 Appropriate Technique for Finishing Appliance

Oral Appliance	Technique
Athletic mouthguard	Remove palatal area from model. Trim around the central frenum and lateral frena.
Bleaching trays	Trim material along gingival margin.
Fluoride custom trays	Trim material along gingival margin.

7. Remove the appliance from the model.
8. Trim the appliance by using crown and bridge scissors for thinner materials and an acrylic bur for thicker and harder materials.
9. Finish the appliance by using the appropriate technique described in Table 18.5. When trimming the appliance, the gingival margin should be replicated so that it fits properly and retention is ensured.

A criteria sheet for a bleaching tray is included in Appendix 2. Construction of a bleaching tray is presented in Chapter 31.

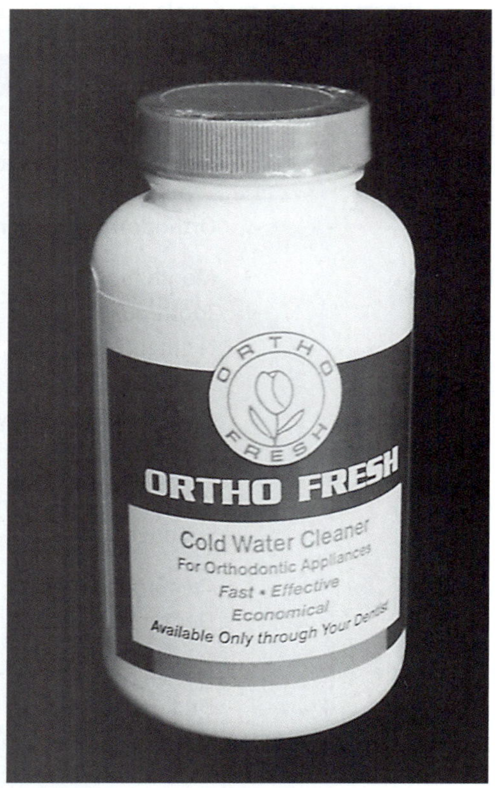

FIGURE 18.12 Ortho Fresh oral appliance cleaner. (Courtesy of Distar, Inc.)

IV. Maintenance of an Oral Appliance

The dental literature suggests daily rinsing and brushing of appliances with a soft-bristled, wet toothbrush. Some oral appliances are supplied with brushes that can be used.

Professional cleaners are also available for soaking appliances. Cleaners generally are available for specific appliance materials. A sample of a commercial cleaner is shown in Figure 18.12.

Some oral appliances, particularly the "boil-and-bite" and stock appliances, should not be cleaned in hot water. This could lead to distortion.

With proper construction and maintenance, the custom-made oral appliance should last its recommended useful life, which is usually a minimum of 2 years.

SUMMARY

Oral appliances are frequently used for a variety of reasons, ranging from treating OSA to whitening the teeth. Dental hygienists should be able to discuss with patients the reasons for using oral appliances and the proper procedures for maintaining oral appliances. Thermoplastic materials are used in the fabrication of most oral appliances and usually require a cast of the patient's dentition. Dental hygienists should be familiar with the maintenance of each appliance and specific oral hygiene care for each patient.

Learning Activities

1. Before fabricating an oral appliance for a student partner, practice on a study model. This provides time to learn the proper technique without encountering problems with model inconsistencies.
2. Fabricate an oral appliance on a student partner with close faculty supervision to clinical competency before completing appliances on patients.
3. Participate in role-playing activities regarding patient education for an athletic mouthguard, bleaching tray, and fluoride custom tray.
4. Divide the class into several groups of approximately three to five students each, and assign each group an area high school in which to research the following. Have the groups present their findings to the class.
   - The sports that require mouthguards
   - The kind of mouthguards used
   - If any injuries have occurred with their use
   - Any other comments coaches or players provide regarding mouthguards

Review Questions

1. The purpose of wearing an oral appliance for OSA is to modify the position of upper airway structures so that:
   a) The airway is enlarged
   b) The airway is reduced
   c) Collapsibility is reduced
   d) Both a and c
   e) Both b and c
2. Patients wearing an oral appliance during sleep have demonstrated a/an:
   a) Increase in periodontal diseases
   b) Decrease in periodontal diseases
   c) Frequent periodontal abscesses
   d) No changes in periodontal health
3. Athletic mouthguards may prevent a concussion. However, they must be worn correctly and consistently.
   a) The first statement is true; the second statement is false.
   b) The first statement is false; the second statement is true.
   c) Both statements are true.
   d) Both statements are false.
4. Nightguards are worn to:
   a) Prevent dental caries
   b) Alleviate tooth surface wear
   c) Provide minor tooth movement or stabilization
   d) Temporarily hold teeth in position

5. Dental professionals fabricate stock mouthguards. Custom-made mouthguards can be purchased at most athletic and drug stores.
   a) The first statement is true, the second statement is false.
   b) The first statement is false, the second statement is true.
   c) Both statements are true.
   d) Both statements are false.
6. Thermoplastic materials will _____ on heating and _____ on cooling.
   a) Soften, reharden
   b) Harden, soften
   c) Harden, stay hard
   d) Soften, melt
7. Patients may clean oral appliances with a soft-bristled, wet toothbrush. No commercial products are available in which to soak oral appliances.
   a) The first statement is true, the second statement is false.
   b) The first statement is false, the second statement is true.
   c) Both statements are true.
   d) Both statements are false.
8. Mouth protectors can be:
   a) Custom-made
   b) Stock
   c) "Boil-n-bite"
   d) All of the above
9. Space maintainers are used to:
   a) Alleviate bruxism
   b) Hold the tongue in proper position
   c) Temporarily hold teeth in position
   d) Alleviate OSA
10. Athletic mouth guards should be properly fitted, stay in place comfortably, be made of resilient material approved by the United States Food and Drug Administration and:
    a) Be physiologically compatible with the wearer
    b) Have a fresh scent
    c) Increase the amount of force placed on the occlusion
    d) Be worn on the mandibular arch
11. When fabricating an oral appliance, it is necessary to replicate which of the following oral anatomical structures?
    a) Sulcus
    b) Periodontal ligament
    c) Gingival contours of the teeth
    d) Soft palate
12. Fluoride custom trays are recommended for which of the following patients?
    a) Elderly patient with severe periodontal disease
    b) Three-year-old patient with early childhood caries
    c) Adult patient undergoing head or neck radiation therapy
    d) Adolescent patient with severe halitosis

Supplemental Readings

American Dental Association Report. Using mouthguards to reduce the incidence and severity of sports-related oral injuries. J Am Dent Assoc 2006;137(12):1710–1720.

Chalmers J. The evolving technology of amorphous calcium phosphate. 2006. Dimensions of Dental Hygiene Web site. Available at: www.dimensionsofdentalhygiene.com/dimensionsCE.asp, Accessed Jan 15, 2007.

Kielbassa AM. Dentine hypersensitivity: Simple steps for every day diagnosis and management. Int Dent J 2002;52:394–396.

Kleyman M, Vigil A. Use of mouthguards: review of the literature. JNMDHA 1996;3:4–19.

Nathe C. Athletic Mouthguards. ACCESS 2005, 19:22–24.

Nathe C, Logothetis D, Schmidt-Nowara W. Oral Appliances for the treatment of obstructive sleep apnea. J Pract Hyg 2001;10:28–32.

Nupro White Gold Doctor's Instructions Directions for Use. Pamphlet. York, PA: Dentsply, 2006.

Roe S. Treatment recommendations for nonnutritive sucking habits. J Pract Hyg 1998;9:11–15.

Schmidt-Nowara W, et al. Oral appliances for the treatment of snoring and obstructive sleep apnea: a review. Sleep 1995;18:501–510.

The Klearway Appliance. Pamphlet. Toward, NY: Great Lakes Orthodontic, 1996.

The Vacuum Forming Booklet. Pamphlet. 4th ed. Delano, MN: DR Dental Resources, 1992.

TRIAD 2000. Brochure. York, PA: Trubyte/Dentsply, Inc., 2002.

19

Instruments as Dental Materials—Care and Maintenance*

Objectives

After studying this chapter, the student will be able to do the following:

1. Explain the basic differences between carbon-steel and stainless-steel instruments.
2. Discuss the processes of passivation and electropolishing.
3. Summarize the problems or conditions that can affect instruments, including corrosion, rust, pitting, spotting, and stains.
4. Explain why it is important to inspect instruments.
5. Explain the reasons for sharpening instruments, and determine the appropriate time and frequency of sharpening.
6. Discuss the cleaning of instruments, both immediately after use and when timely cleaning is not possible.
7. Recall the advantages and disadvantages of the four methods of sterilizing instruments.
8. Design an instrument maintenance schedule or cycle that could be used routinely in a private-practice office setting.

Key Words/Phrases

carbon-steel instruments
corrosion
electropolishing
passivation
pitting
rust
spotting
stainless-steel alloy
tarnish

*Note: The information in this chapter is provided courtesy of Hu-Friedy Manufacturing Co., Inc.

INTRODUCTION

The previous chapters have discussed dental materials such as gypsum, cements, and impression and restorative materials, all of which are typically used in a dental practice. Other dental materials that are important to the dental hygienist but often overlooked are those that comprise dental instruments. It is a rare workday for a dental hygienist when a dental instrument goes unused. A hygienist's instruments are some of the most important items necessary to fulfill his or her professional responsibility.

Dental instruments represent a significant financial investment. For this reason alone, it would benefit the student to have a clear understanding of the materials from which they are made and what is necessary to keep them in good working condition. The amount of care that is given to dental instruments directly affects the lifetime of those instruments. The longer an instrument lasts, the greater return it yields on the financial investment.

This chapter will address the composition, undesirable conditions, inspection, and care of instruments.

I. Composition of Instruments

Dental instruments are usually made of either carbon-steel or stainless-steel alloys. Some instruments have resin handles.

A. Carbon-Steel Alloy

Carbon-steel instruments are known for their hardness and ability to hold sharp, cutting edges. They are more sensitive than stainless-steel instruments to chemicals and susceptible to corrosion, and they require special handling.

B. Stainless-Steel Alloy

The major components of **stainless-steel alloy** are iron, chromium, and nickel. The amount of carbon in a stainless-steel alloy is directly related to the alloy's hardness and ability to hold a sharp, cutting edge. The addition of chromium enhances corrosion resistance, and nickel improves the mechanical properties of the metal. The problems with stainless-steel instruments are discoloration, constant necessity of sharpening, and corrosion when exposed to certain chemicals. Some instruments are made with two kinds of stainless steel. One is hard and maintains a sharp edge; this is used to make the cutting edge or tip. The second is more resistant to corrosion and is welded or soldered to the first to form the handle.

The carbon in the alloy, which is necessary for hardness and a sharp edge, is the culprit that causes corrosion or rusting. Instrument manufacturers reduce surface corrosion by using two processes:

1. **Passivation**

   Passivation is a chemical process that creates a thin layer of chromium oxide on the surface of the instrument. This layer is transparent but tough, and it protects the underlying metal. After passivation, the instrument is much less likely to corrode.

2. **Electropolishing**

   Electropolishing produces a smooth, highly polished finish. A highly polished surface is less likely to corrode. Electropolishing is an efficient method for polishing complex shapes.

C. EverEdge™ Technology

A new stainless steel alloy for instruments has been developed by Hu-Friedy Mfg. Co. Inc. This new technology in metallurgy, heat treatment, and cryogenics is used in the manufacture of instruments. Blades stay sharper 50% longer compared to other instruments. These instruments are not coated, but the long-lasting wear is present throughout the entire instrument tip. If the instrument stays sharper longer, there is less sharpening, and less hand fatigue. An EverEdge instrument is illustrated in Figure 19.1.

D. Resin Handles

Some instruments may have resin handles. Inside the resin is a full-length, steel inner core for added strength and tactile sensitivity. The handles may have grooves and knurling to increase rotational control and to provide a light (but secure) grasp. Resin instruments and items require specific care.

E. Separation of Stainless-Steel and Carbon-Steel Instruments

Stainless-steel and carbon-steel instruments should be kept separate throughout the cleaning and sterilization process. If processed together, the carbon-steel instruments may create cross-corrosion on the stainless-steel instruments.

Carbon-steel instruments should be thoroughly dried before sterilization to prevent rusting or corrosion. Use of a protective rust-inhibitor solution is recommended before sterilization.

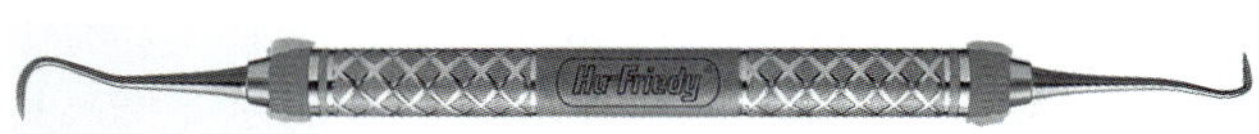

FIGURE 19.1 A EverEdge™ scaling instrument. (Courtesy of Hu-Friedy Mfg. Co., Inc.)

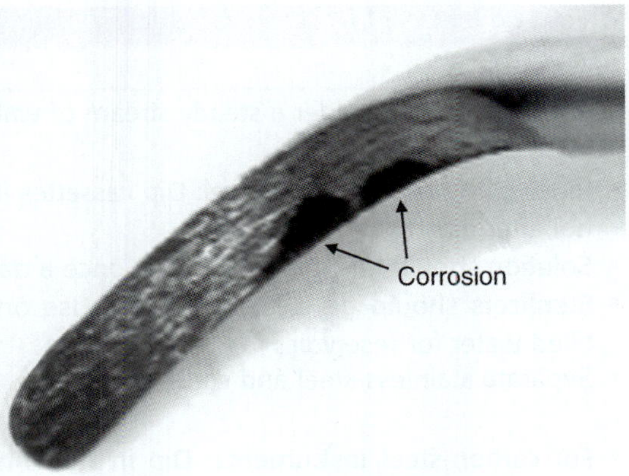

FIGURE 19.2 Photograph of a corroded curette tip. (Courtesy of Hu-Friedy Mfg. Co., Inc.)

II. Problems of Instruments

A. Forms of Corrosion

1. Corrosion

Corrosion is a process in which a metal is changed to a metal oxide. A common example is when iron is changed to iron oxide, or rust. Corrosion occurs because the metal oxide is the lower-energy form of the metal. Corrosion is increased in a warm, wet environment, such as in the mouth or an autoclave. An example of a corroded curette tip is shown in Figure 19.2.

2. Tarnish

Tarnish is a chemical or electrochemical attack on a metal surface. Many times, corrosion starts as a surface discoloration called tarnish. If tarnish is a continuous film, it will protect the metal from the environment (like paint on metal) and prevent corrosion. Many films on metals are transparent and unseen, but they may still protect the surface from corrosion. If the film is not continuous and the surface not protected, corrosion may proceed, and loss of material will occur.

3. Galvanic Corrosion

Corrosion in a wet environment, such as saliva, is an electrochemical process called galvanic corrosion. Galvanic corrosion is the same process that produces electricity in a battery. In a battery, two dissimilar metals cause a current to flow. Corrosion may be caused by two dissimilar metals contacting, such as carbon steel and stainless steel, or by the same metal existing in two different environments. The two environments could differ in humidity, pH, oxygen concentration, or other chemical concentrations. As corrosion proceeds, material is lost, and the instrument becomes discolored and weakened.

Corrosion does not always occur uniformly over a metal surface. Many times, corrosion aggressively attacks small areas; and surface staining and pitting result. The base of a pit of a metal restoration or an instrument may have a different pH and oxygen concentration compared to the rest of the surface. The different environments of the base of the pit and the surface will encourage corrosion. Corrosion will continue in the pit, and the pit can become deeper and deeper. Therefore, removing pits and other surface defects by polishing reduces corrosion.

4. Galvanism

When two dissimilar metals are present in the mouth, galvanic corrosion may occur. Sometimes, this is called oral galvanism. The closer the two metals are physically, the greater the likelihood of galvanism. Several authors have stated that one should not place an amalgam restoration in contact with a gold crown, and vice versa. Galvanism is the alleged reason. However, such adjacent restorations frequently occur in patients with little or no ill effect on either restoration. Galvanism has been blamed for numerous health problems, but without a scientific basis.

5. Preventing Corrosion

In dentistry, we protect metallic restorations and instruments from corrosion by using two techniques.

a) The first technique is to make restorations with noble metals. Noble metals do not corrode; but they are expensive—too expensive to use for instruments.

b) The second technique is to use metals that form a tough, adherent oxide layer on the surface. This is called passivation, and it protects the metal surface from the environment. Stainless steel works this way. Unfortunately, the chromium oxide layer that protects stainless steel can break down in the presence of chloride ions. It is important to rinse off chloride-containing cleaning agents before sterilizing instruments. Residual cleaning chemicals can attack the protective film, and instruments may then corrode, rust, stain, and pit.

6. Pitting

Pitting is caused by a chemical and electronic attack on surfaces. **Pitting** is localized corrosion, and it is prevented by:

- Rinsing instruments thoroughly after use
- Avoiding long exposure to chlorides and acids
- Avoiding detergents with high pH
- Not mixing metals in ultrasonic cleaners

Table 19.1 Hu-Friedy Troubleshooting Guide for Instruments

Problem	Cause	Prevention
Spotting	• Insufficient rinsing after ultrasonic cleansing	• Rinse thoroughly under a steady stream of water for 30 seconds.
	• Insufficient drying after ultrasonic cleaning	• Rinse with hot water. Optional: Dip cassettes in alcohol after rinsing.
	• Not changing ultrasonic solution	• Solution should be changed at least once a day.
	• Sterilizer has not been cleaned	• Sterilizers should be cleaned weekly. Use only distilled water for reservoir.
Rust	• Corrosion from carbon-steel instruments spreads to stainless-steel instruments.	• Separate stainless-steel and carbon-steel.
		• For carbon-steel instruments: Dip in rust-inhibiting solution as suggested by sterilizer manufacturer.
Pitting	• Chemical attack on instruments	• Rinse and dry instruments thoroughly.
		• Use approved cleaning and sterilization solutions only.

Courtesy of Hu-Friedy Mfg. Co., Inc.

7. **Spotting**

Slow or improper drying leaves mineral deposits that cause **spotting.** To prevent this, check the operation of the autoclave, and use chloride-free solutions for sterilizing, disinfecting, rinsing, and cleaning.

8. **Summary**

Table 19.1 summarizes several of the instrument problems discussed above.

B. Stains

Stains can either be deposited onto the instrument, as in the case of spotting caused by contaminated water in the autoclave, or develop from within the alloy, as in the case of rust. Identifying the source of the stain is important in solving instrument staining problems. Most stains occur during the sterilization cycle. Possible causes of stains include:

- An inadequately maintained sterilizer
- Instrument contact with harsh detergents and chemicals
- Processing dissimilar metals together during cleaning and sterilization cycles

C. Rust

Rust is iron oxide that forms when iron or steel alloys corrode. Rust can be black, brown, or reddish in color. Severe rust appears as pits in the surface or as blisters, which eventually flake off the surface.

1. Without proper care, dental instruments may corrode. Rust, in the form of stains and pits, may appear on instruments as a result.
2. Rust can also be deposited on instruments when water containing dissolved rust evaporates, leaving behind a rust stain. This process is similar to what happens when drinking glasses are left to air-dry after washing, resulting in water spots.
3. If solid rust is suspended in the water of an autoclave, it can be deposited on instruments during sterilization. A properly maintained autoclave with clean water will minimize this problem.

III. Instrument Inspection

In every dental hygiene practice setting, a regular routine should be established for inspecting instruments between uses. The purpose of instrument inspection is to determine aging of the instruments or other compromising conditions. Several instruments in optimum condition are shown in Figure 19.3. Instruments should be inspected for the following conditions:

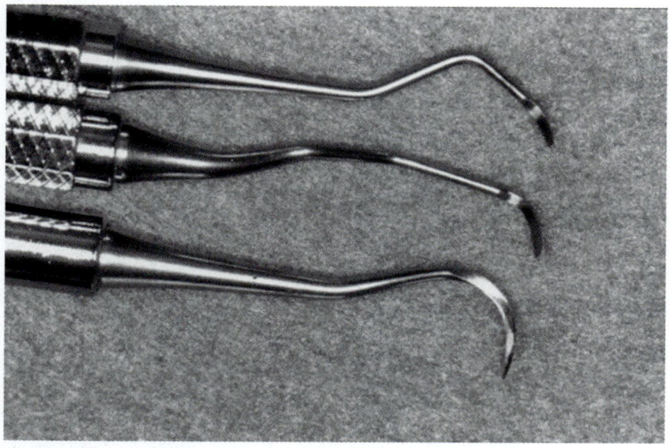

FIGURE 19.3 Photograph of two curettes and a scaler in optimum condition.

- Corrosion
- Pitting
- Discoloration
- Broken, loose, or bent tips or components
- Cracked handles
- Dull or oversharpened edges
- Damaged blades

IV. Retipping

Instrument retipping services are available from many sources. However, having new tips inserted into an older instrument handle involves risks.

A. Detachment

The handle may develop small cracks when the tip is removed, creating a weakened point of attachment. Repeated retipping increases the chance for cracked handles to develop and the possibility of the tip to fall out during treatment.

B. Contamination

Small cracks in the handle may collect debris and interfere with proper sterilization.

C. Imbalance

Retipping often results in an unbalanced instrument.

D. Wear Rates

Stainless-steel blades may vary from lot to lot. Therefore, the cutting edge may wear at a faster rate and dull more easily.

V. Sharpening Instruments

A. Why Sharpen Instruments?

Instruments should be kept sharp and true to their original design so that quality care may be provided to the patient. Properly sharpened and maintained instruments make dental procedures easier for both patient and clinician. The additional benefits of sharp instruments include:

1. Reduced Clinician Fatigue

Fewer strokes and less pressure per stroke are needed when the blade is sharp. This is less demanding on the clinician's hand, muscles, and tendons.

2. Improved Removal of Calculus

As you may have experienced by now, a dulled, or blunt cutting edge is difficult to control because it will slip and slide off of the tooth surface. It is incapable of cleaving under a deposit to remove it. Instead, it slides over the outer surface, which results in burnished calculus. A sharp instrument will remove the entire deposit, as shown in Figure 19.4.

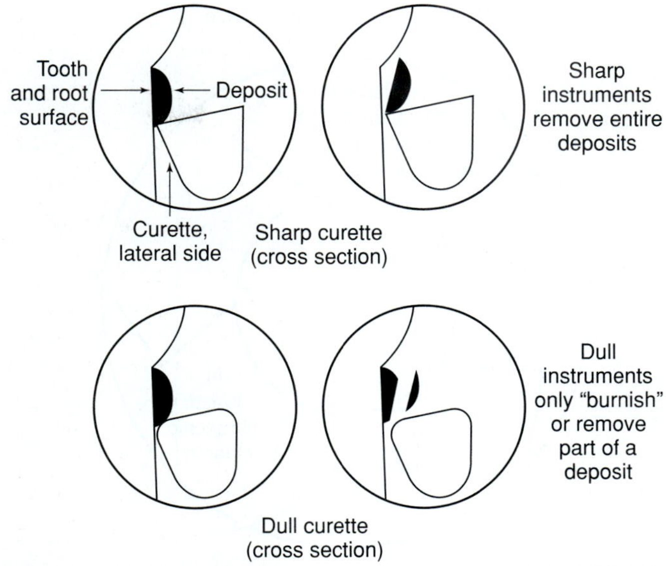

FIGURE 19.4 Dull versus sharp instruments for removal of calculus. (Courtesy of Hu-Friedy Mfg. Co., Inc.)

3. Less Chair Time

Sharp instruments decrease chair time for patient and clinician.

4. Improved Tactile Sensitivity

A sharp edge allows the clinician to feel the deposit more easily.

5. Less Patient Discomfort

Fewer strokes and less pressure will be needed in the same area, thus increasing overall patient comfort.

B. When Should Instruments Be Sharpened?

The safest time to sharpen instruments is after sterilization, immediately before use. This requires the availability of a sterile stone that can be used for additional chairside sharpening and then processed with the instruments. Do not wait until an instrument is seriously dull and ineffective before sharpening it. Maintain instruments daily on a regular schedule to protect your financial investment.

The maintenance cycle, as shown in Figure 19.5, represents a maintenance routine that can be easily adapted to your own practice setting. Sterilization should be done again after sharpening if electric honing equipment is used. The honing stone and its plastic mounting cannot be sterilized because the plastic portion would melt in the autoclave. Therefore, sterilized instruments would no longer be sterile with use of a honing machine.

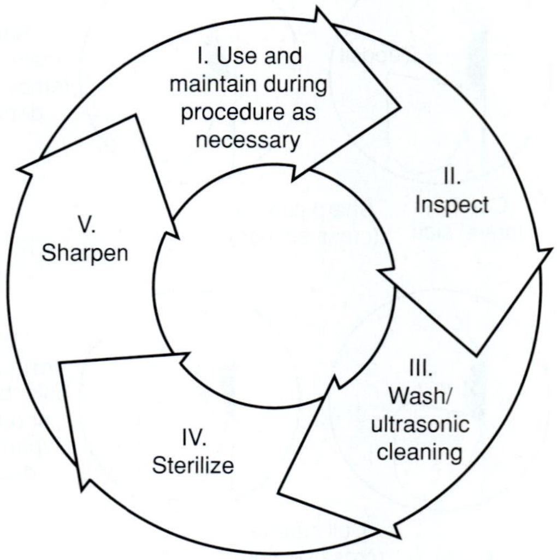

FIGURE 19.5 Instrument maintenance cycle. (Courtesy of Hu-Friedy Mfg. Co., Inc.)

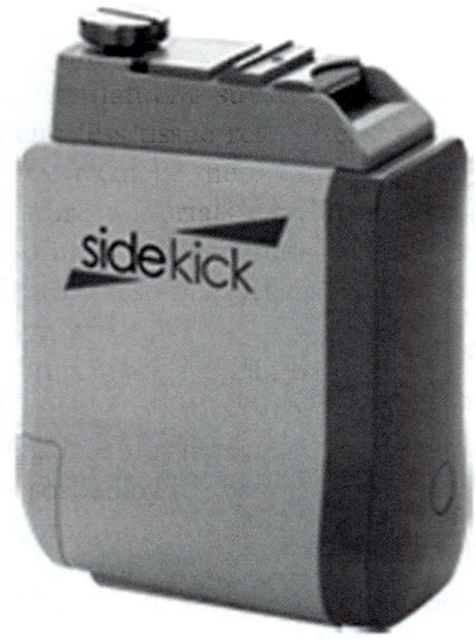

FIGURE 19.6 Hu-Friedy's "Sidekick" sharpening device. (Courtesy of Hu-Friedy Mfg. Co., Inc.)

C. How Often Should Instruments Be Sharpened?

You can answer this question by looking at your appointment book and asking three simple questions:

1. How many times a day did I, or will I, use a specific instrument?
2. What degree of difficulty did I, or can I expect to, encounter while using this instrument?
3. For what procedures did I, or will I, use the instrument?

Using the answers to these three questions, you will be able to design the most effective sharpening schedule for your own day-to-day requirements.

D. Sharpening Devices

Several manufacturers have developed sharpening devices that eliminate the margin of error that may occur in the traditional freehand method of sharpening. Each device operates differently and it would be important to follow the written instructions carefully so that instruments are not damaged. They range in expense from one to several hundred dollars. One such device is pictured in Figure 19.6.

VI. Cleaning of Instruments

When cleaning instruments, special gloves that protect the skin from possible puncture wounds are recommended.

A. After Patient Care

Before they are sterilized, all instruments should be cleaned (ultrasonic cleaning is recommended) with a noncorrosive, low-sudsing detergent. Enzymatic cleaners maximize cleaning for surgical and periodontal instruments by digesting blood proteins, tissues, and other debris faster than ordinary cleaners. These specific cleaners also eliminate the need for hand scrubbing, which decreases the risk of hand injuries and spread of contamination because of splatter. Phenols, glutaraldehyde, and iodophors are contraindicated for resin instruments.

B. When Timely Cleaning Is Not Possible

If the instruments cannot be cleaned immediately, place them in a presoak solution. Dried debris can result in instrument staining and inadequate sterilization. The presoaking liquid should completely cover the instruments.

VII. Sterilization of Instruments

Proper sterilization can extend the life of instruments and keep the need for costly replacements to a minimum. Sterilization of instruments may be accomplished by using the following methods.

A. Steam Autoclave

Steam autoclaving is regarded as most effective for destroying pathogenic organisms or vegetative forms. It is achieved at 270°F and 27 pounds per square inch (psi) for at least 6 minutes; this is for a Station-type autoclave (rapid steam heat) only. Check with autoclave manufacturers for correct cycle times. Cycle time should be closer to 15 minutes depending on whether the unit is hot or cold at the start of the cycle. Also, times for both ultrasonic cleaning and sterilizing differ if instruments are bagged or are in cassettes. Use of a steam autoclave is recommended for resin instruments.

B. Unsaturated Chemical Vapor

Unsaturated chemical vapor is effective for all metal instruments. It is best suited for carbon-steel instruments, however, because chemical vapors contain less water, which causes rust and corrosion in certain instruments, compared to other sterilization methods. It is achieved at 270°F and 20 to 40 psi for at least 20 minutes. Disadvantages include odor and the need for ventilation.

C. Dry Heat

Dry heat sterilization is achieved when the internal temperature of the unit is maintained at 320°F for approximately 2 hours (temperatures >350°F may cause premature instrument failure). This method is used for items that will not withstand compressed steam conditions. Less corrosion occurs with this method, and tips and cutting instruments stay sharper.

D. Chemical Solutions

Several chemical solutions are available for sterilization. However, the American Dental Association and the Centers for Disease Control and Prevention recommend their use only for materials that cannot withstand a heat sterilization process. These solutions are not recommended for sterilization of metal dental instruments. To be effective, the solution must come in direct contact with an organism for the appropriate length of time for that organism to be destroyed. This length of time may extend to several hours.

SUMMARY

Dental instruments are also considered to be a dental material. Because a dental hygiene student invests a significant amount of money for his or her instruments, it is beneficial to have a good understanding of instrument care and maintenance.

Dental instruments are made of carbon-steel alloy or stainless-steel alloy. Some instruments may have resin handles. Surface corrosion of stainless-steel instruments may be reduced during manufacturing by passivation and electropolishing. Stainless-steel instruments should be kept separate from carbon-steel instruments during cleaning and sterilization so that cross-corrosion does not occur. Within this chapter, problems of instruments such as corrosion, tarnish, galvanic corrosion, pitting, spotting, stains, and rust are discussed.

Instruments should be inspected for a variety of conditions. The purpose of inspection is to determine aging or other compromising conditions. Retipping of instruments is not recommended because of the risk of detachment, contamination, imbalance, and wear.

Instruments should be sharpened to reduce clinician fatigue, improve calculus removal, save time, improve tactile sensitivity, and increase patient comfort. The safest time to sharpen instruments is after sterilization and before use. An instrument maintenance cycle is recommended.

All instruments should be cleaned before sterilization; ultrasonic cleaning is recommended. If timely cleaning is not possible, a presoak solution should be used. Methods to sterilize instruments include steam autoclave, unsaturated chemical vapor, dry heat, and chemical solutions. Not all methods are appropriate for all instruments. The recommended method for each instrument composition (resin, carbon steel, and stainless steel) is discussed.

Proper care and maintenance of instruments will enhance their function. This, in combination with clinical expertise, will result in quality care for patients.

Learning Activities

1. Divide into small groups, and examine used instruments. Look for the conditions discussed in the chapter. Review the causes and prevention of these conditions.
2. With gloves, select some extracted teeth with calculus (or paint on artificial calculus), and scale it with both sharp and dull instruments. Discuss any differences between the two.

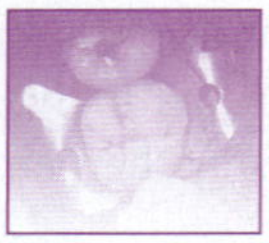

Review Questions

1. A uniform corrosive attack that produces a film or surface layer on the metal is termed:
a) Corrosion
b) Tarnish
c) Electrochemical corrosion
d) Concentration cell corrosion

2. A beneficial chemical process in manufacturing that creates a thin layer of chromium oxide on the surface of the instrument to protect it from corrosion is called:
a) Manufacture of alloy
b) Tarnish
c) Passivation
d) Electropolishing

3. The standard protocol for chemical vapor sterilization is:
a) 270°F at 27 psi for at least 6 minutes
b) 320°F for approximately 2 hours
c) 270°F at 20 to 40 psi for at least 10 minutes
d) 270°F at 20 to 40 psi for at least 20 minutes

4. Risks are involved when retipping instruments. One of these risks is frequent breakage between the shank and tip.
a) The first statement is true; the second statement is false.
b) The first statement is false; the second statement is true.
c) Both statements are true.
d) Both statements are false.

5. To determine when instruments should be sharpened, this chapter provides __________ questions to ask when looking over the appointment book so that you may develop an effective sharpening schedule.
a) 2
b) 3
c) 4
d) 5

6. The major components of stainless-steel alloy are:
a) Tin, chromium, and nickel
b) Iron, silver, and nickel
c) Iron, aluminum, and nickel
d) Iron, chromium, and nickel

7. The major disadvantage of using noble metals for the fabrication of instruments is:
a) Cost
b) Corrosion
c) Wear rate
d) Pitting

8. The dry heat method of sterilization is used when:
a) Ventilation is not adequate
b) Items cannot withstand temperatures greater than 270° F
c) Items cannot withstand compressed steam conditions
d) Items are needed for the next patient

9. Which of the following sequence of steps is correct for the instrument maintenance cycle?
a) Use and maintain, sharpen, sterilize, inspect, wash/ultrasonic clean
b) Sharpen, inspect, use and maintain, sterilize, wash/ultrasonic clean
c) Use and maintain, inspect, wash/ultrasonic clean, sterilize, sharpen
d) Use and maintain, inspect, wash/ultrasonic clean, sharpen, sterilize

10. The name of the procedure that produces a smooth, highly polished finish on an instrument is:
a) Passivation
b) Electropolishing
c) Heat treatment polishing
d) Cryogenic polishing

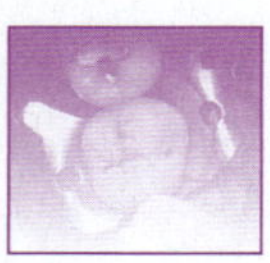

Supplemental Readings

Burns S, Bendit JZ. The sharper edge of instrument technology. J Pract Hyg 2006;15:31–32.

Gilmore HW, Lund MR, Bales DJ, Vernetti J. Operative Dentistry. 3rd ed. St. Louis: Mosby, 1977, Chapter 4.

Hu-Friedy Mfg. Co. Inc. EverEdge Technology Pamphlet. Chicago: Hu-Friedy, 2006.

Hu-Friedy Mfg. Co., Inc. Longer Life for Dental Instruments. Booklet. Chicago: Hu-Friedy, 1990.

Hu-Friedy Mfg. Co., Inc. Resin Eight. Pamphlet. Chicago: Hu-Friedy, 2001.

Parker P, Groya L. Dental surgical instruments: care and maintenance. Dent Surg Products 1997;April:12–16.

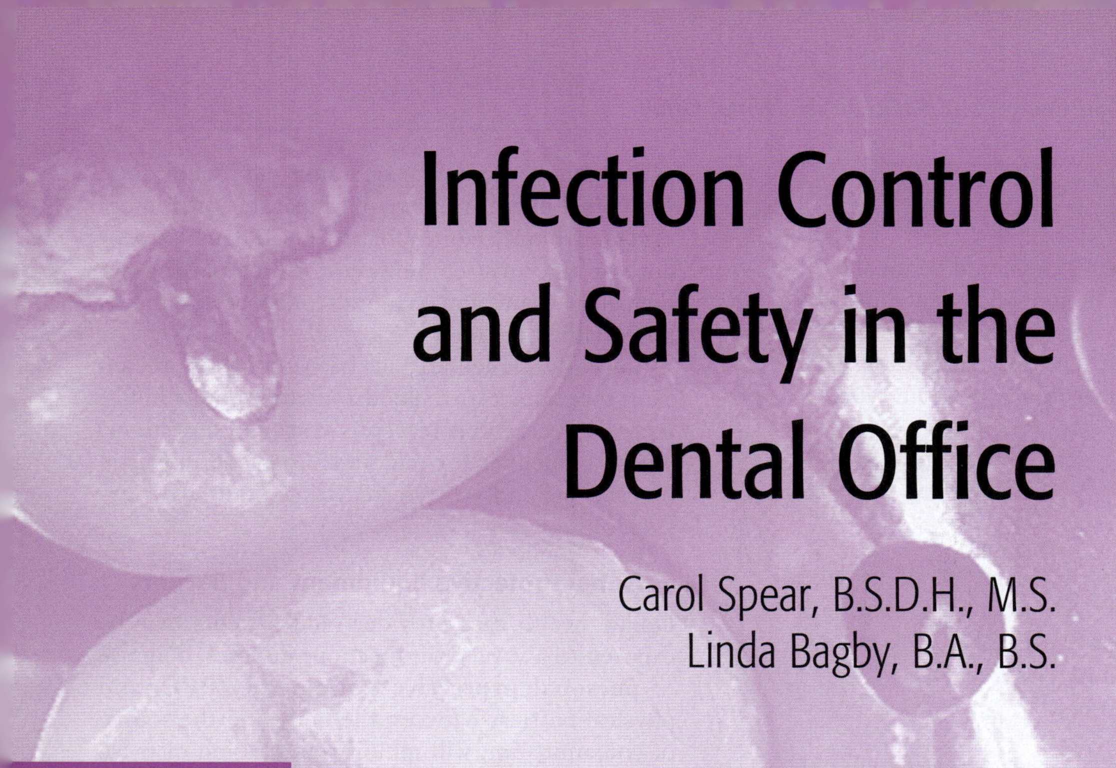

20

Infection Control and Safety in the Dental Office

Carol Spear, B.S.D.H., M.S.
Linda Bagby, B.A., B.S.

Objectives

After studying this chapter, the student will be able to do the following:

1. Describe safety and risk in terms of common hazards in everyday life and work in a dental office.
2. Define and appreciate the practice of universal precautions in dentistry.
3. Identify the types of personal protective equipment (PPE) that must be used for the practice of dentistry in the operatory and laboratory.
4. Explain the criteria for selection of PPE during dental procedures.
5. Determine the methods of sterilization or disinfection that can be used to decontaminate each type of instrument or item in the dental operatory or laboratory.
6. Evaluate surface disinfectants that may be used in the dental office.
7. Recall the methods that may be used to prevent cross-contamination during distribution of dental supplies.
8. Describe effective ways to manage contamination caused by aerosols and splatter.
9. Discuss safe handling and disposal of sharp items contaminated with blood or saliva.
10. Appreciate the significance of an office exposure control plan and protocol for managing exposure to bloodborne pathogens.
11. Describe the infectious, physical, and chemical hazards in a dental office.
12. Recognize office and laboratory housekeeping practices that contribute to infection control and safety.

Key Words/Phrases

critical objects
ergonomics
erythema
exam gloves
exposure control plan
ground fault circuit interrupter (GFI)
high-efficiency particulate air (HEPA) masks
high-level disinfectants
hydrophilic
intermediate-level disinfectants
lipophilic
low-level disinfectant
nitrous oxide
Material Safety Data Sheet (MSDS)
noncritical objects
Occupational Safety and Health Administration (OSHA)
overgloves
personal protective equipment (PPE)
risk
safety
semicritical objects
Spalding classification of inanimate objects
spray, wipe, spray
standard precautions
surgeon's gloves
time-weighted average (TWA)
universal precautions
utility gloves
unit dose
urticaria

INTRODUCTION

What kind of health and safety issues could be involved in working at a dental office? In general, a dental office is a very safe place to make your livelihood. However, some hazards do require that you take precautions to minimize the risk of accident or injury, either to yourself or to those around you.

A. Risk

Risk is the probability of harm. All of us take chances in everyday life. Do you wear your seat belt? Some people enjoy the thrill of risk taking. Others do not and avoid it.

B. Safety

Safety is the opposite of risk; it is the probability of no harm. In reality, nothing is completely safe. People are injured in car accidents every day. Lightning strikes. Bees sting. Some days, it even seems that trouble comes looking for us. In fact, there is a real chance (albeit very, very small) that an airplane will fall from the sky and kill us when we are "safe" in our bed at night. (And you thought passing the next dental materials exam was your biggest worry!) We can reduce the hazards of work and play by using common sense, avoiding excessive risk, and using safety equipment. This chapter will discuss many of the risks that are present in the dental office and the ways to reduce the likelihood of harm.

I. Ionizing Radiation

Ionizing radiation, such as that produced by x-ray machines, could potentially involve some risk if it is not handled properly. Precautions for the safe use of ionizing radiation are normally addressed in radiology classes and are not covered in this text.

II. Infectious Diseases

Some of the potential risks in a dental office involve exposure to infectious agents borne in bodily fluids, such as blood or saliva. Taking precautions to protect yourself from these fluids and from those objects contaminated by these fluids will minimize risk.

A. Infection Control

Since the inception of the Standard for Occupational Exposure to Bloodborne Pathogens by the **Occupational Safety and Health Administration (OSHA),** the practice of "universal precautions" has been mandated for dentistry. Universal precautions must be followed by the dental profession when a potential exists for exposure to bloodborne pathogens in the dental operatory and laboratory. **Universal precautions** require that the same infection control procedures for any given dental procedure or task must be followed for each patient and that all patients and materials must be treated as potentially infectious.

Recently, guidelines have been issued for precautions for contact with blood and other bodily fluids, including secretions (except sweat) and excretions. These guidelines include and supersede universal precautions and are referred to as **standard precautions.**

B. Personal Protective Equipment and Barriers

Dental health care providers and patients may be exposed to a variety of infectious diseases. The use of **personal protective equipment (PPE)** and physical barriers between the body and the source of contamination will inhibit transmission of these infections. Under its Bloodborne Pathogen Standard, OSHA requires that the dental care provider wear appropriate PPE (gloves, masks, eye protection, and clothing) during all patient care activities involving contact with saliva and blood. The PPE should not be worn out of the clinical treatment area or room. An example of a dental care provider wearing PPE is shown in Figure 20.1.

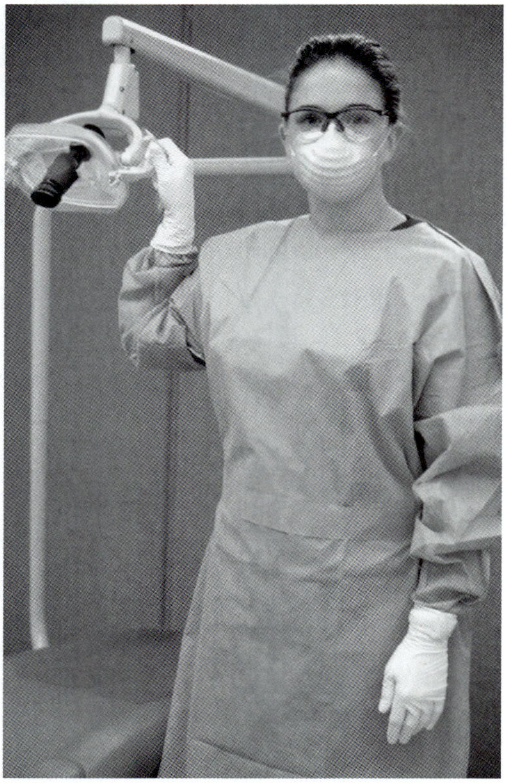

FIGURE 20.1 Dental care provider wearing required eye protection, gloves, mask, and cover gown.

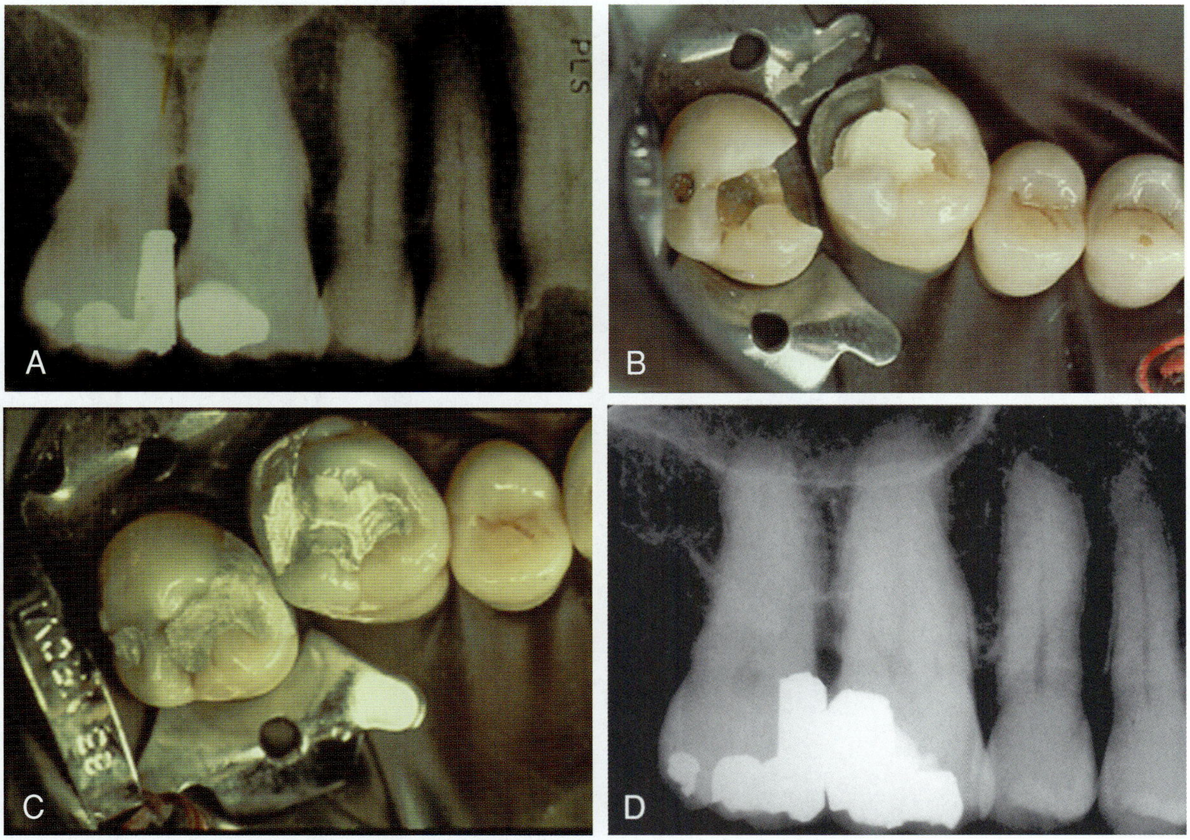

FIGURE 1.9 (A-D) (page 12) & FIGURE CS2.1 (A-D) (page 394)

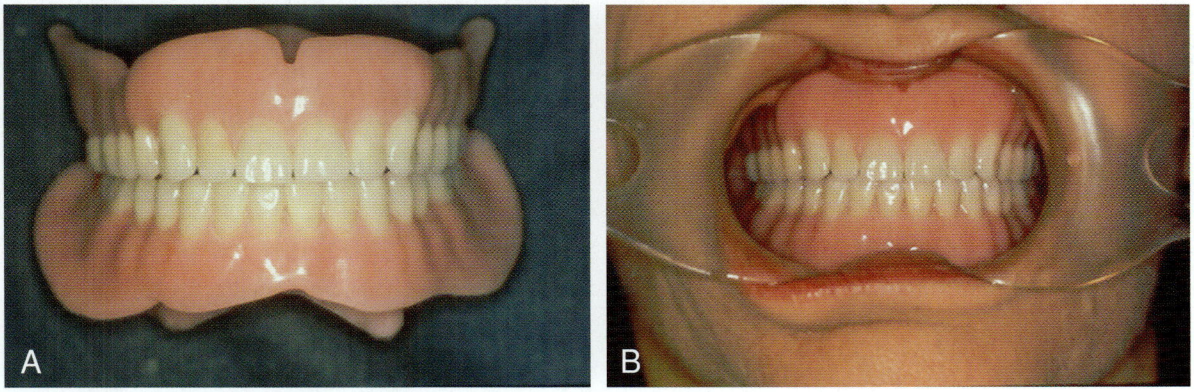

FIGURE 11.8 (A, B) (page 153)

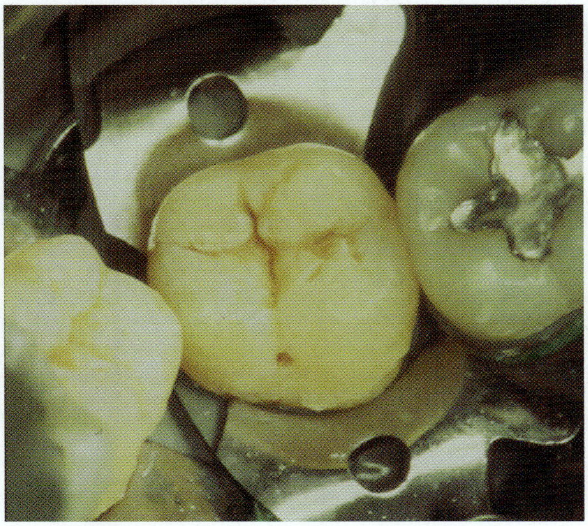

FIGURE 4.4 (page 47)

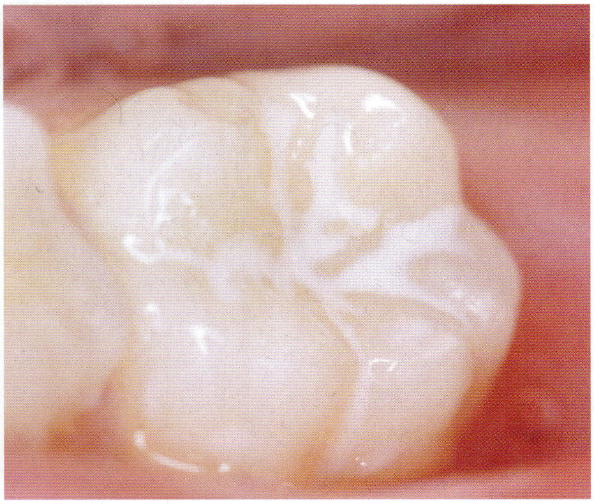

FIGURE 1.11 (page 14)

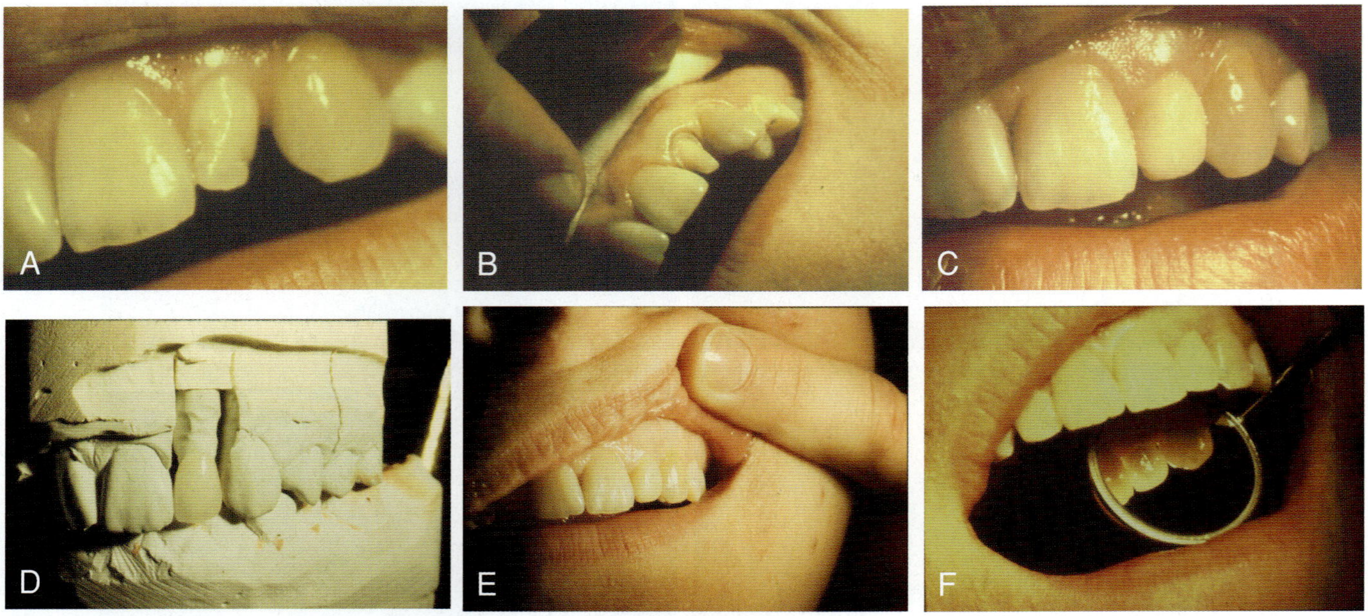

FIGURE 1.10 (A-F) (page 13) & FIGURE CS3.1 (A-F) (page 396)

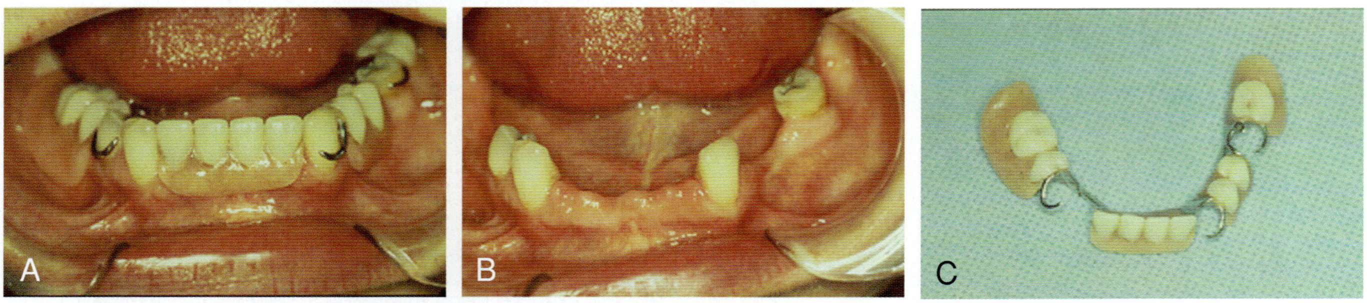

FIGURE 1.7 (A-C) (page 10) & FIGURE CS1.1 (A-C) (page 393)

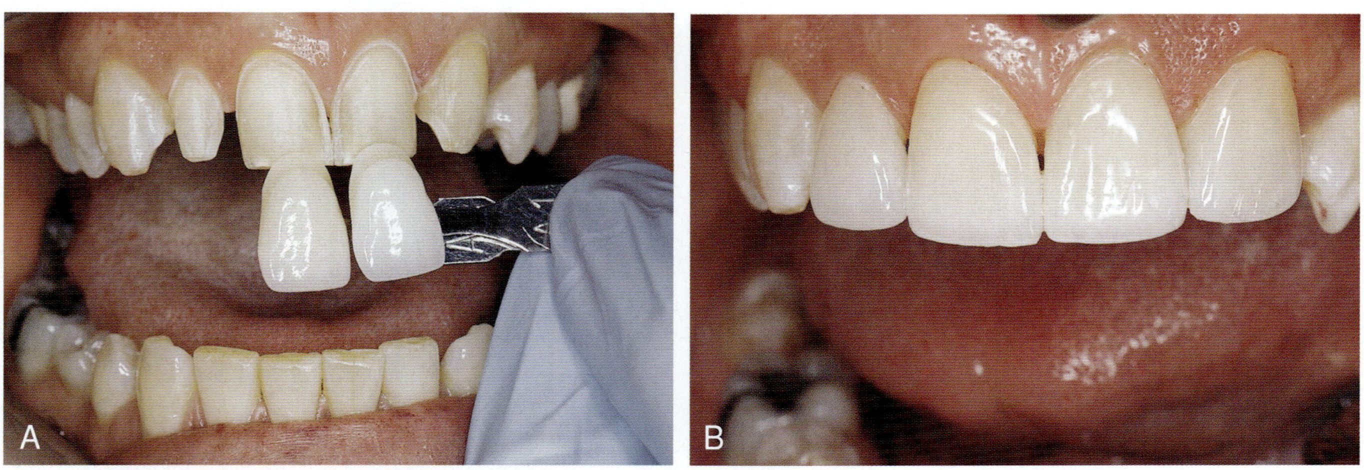

FIGURE 10.2 (A, B) (page 132)

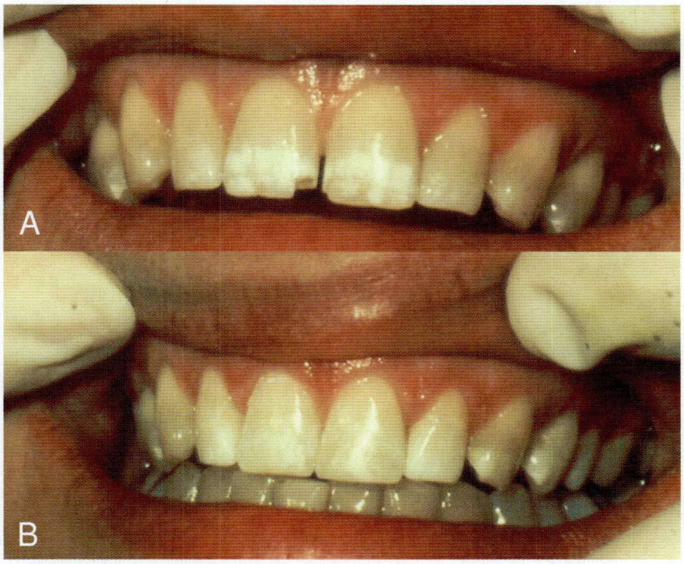

FIGURE 5.9 (A, B) (page 65)

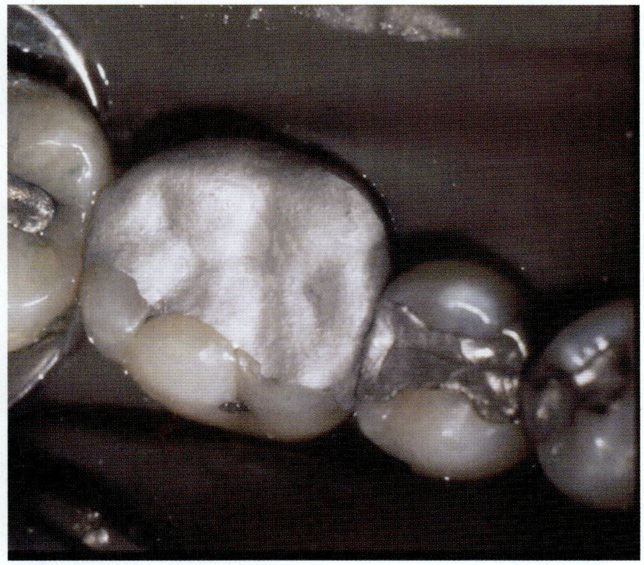

FIGURE 6.11 (page 83)

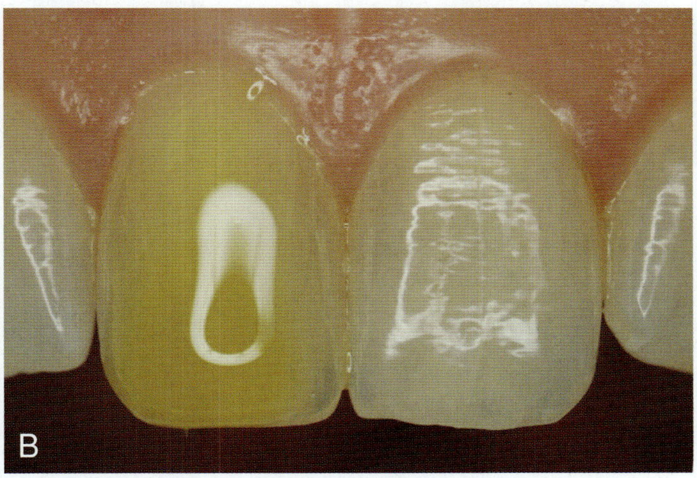

FIGURE 13.12B (page 177)

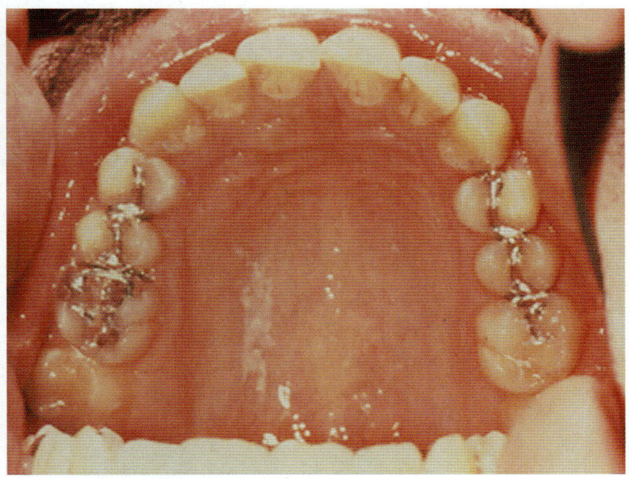

FIGURE 6.10 (page 82)

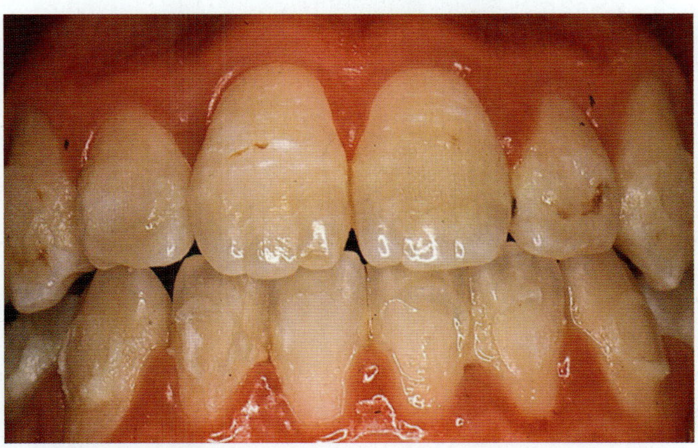

FIGURE 32.1 (page 357)

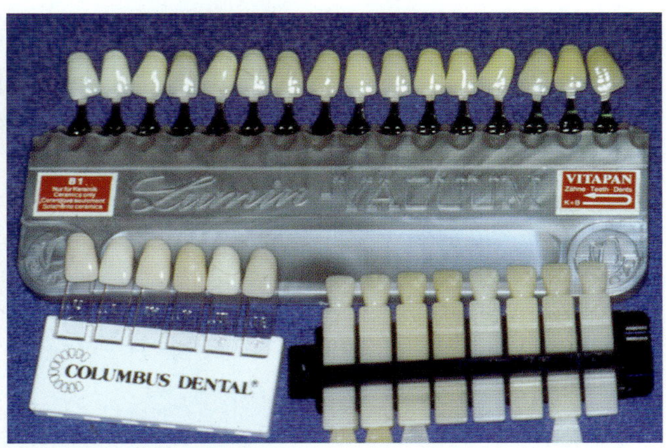

FIGURE 3.4 (page 35)

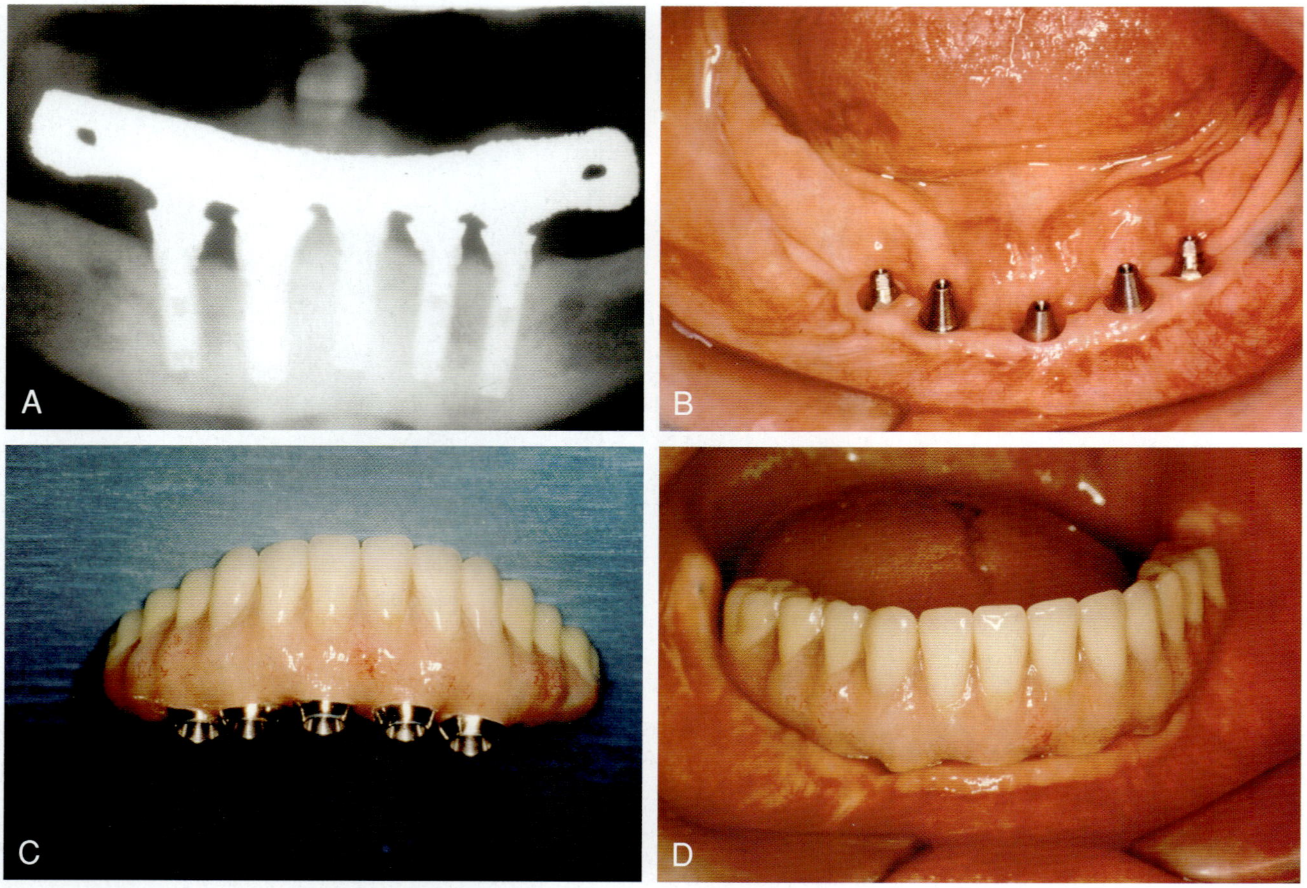

FIGURE 12.1 (A-D) (page 159)

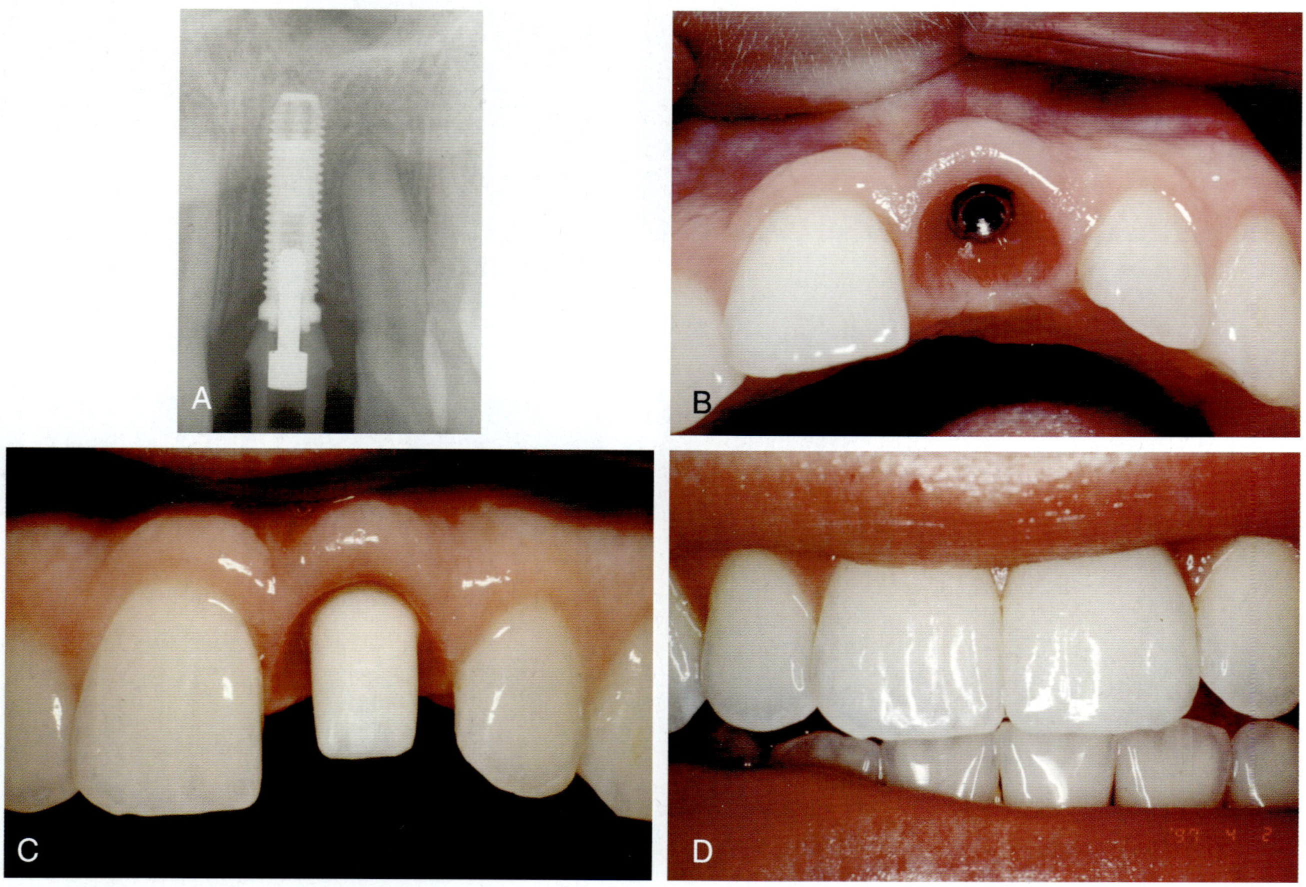

FIGURE 12.2 (A-D) (page 160)

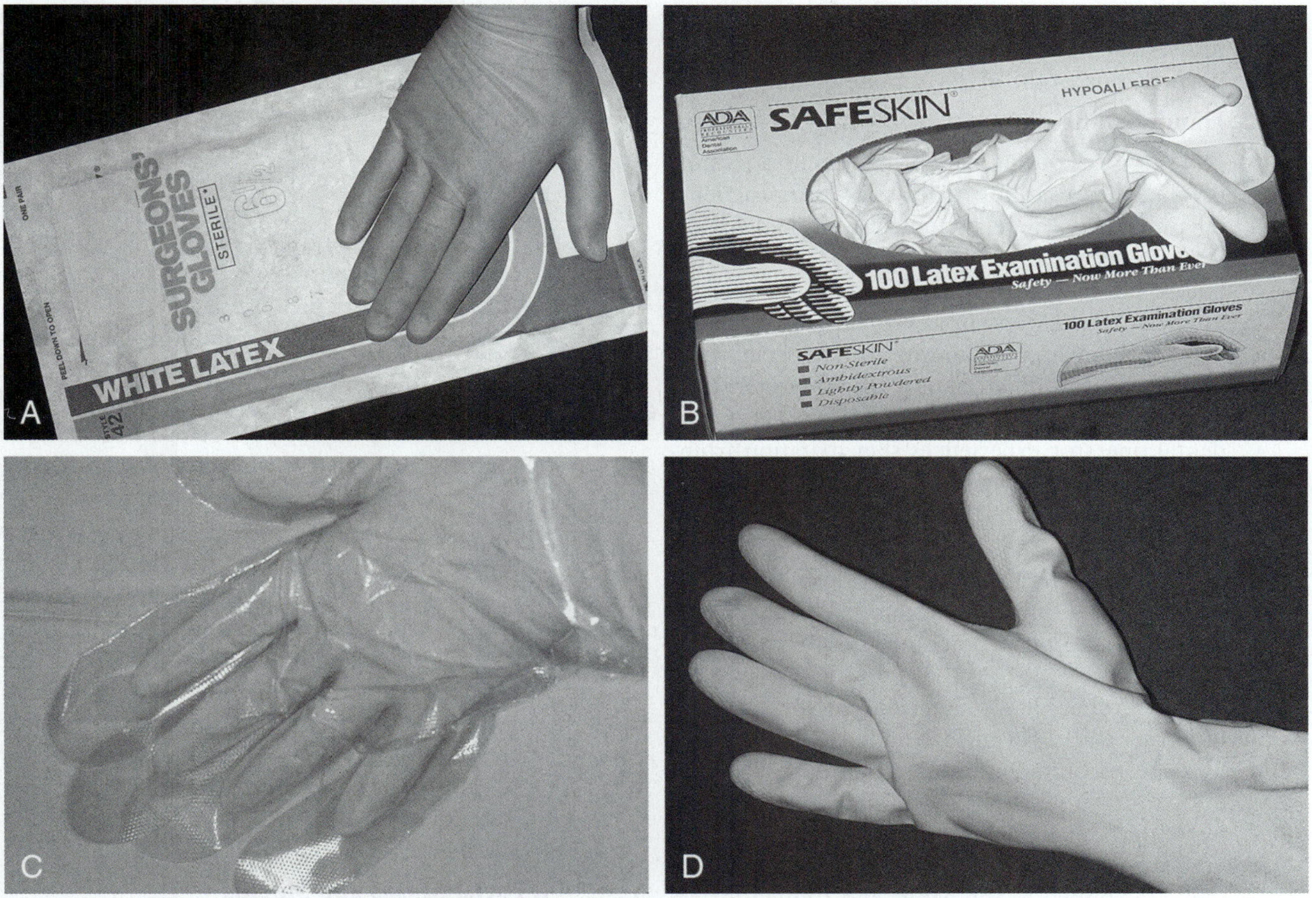

FIGURE 20.2 Types of gloves. **A.** Sterile surgeon's glove. **B.** Nonsterile exam glove. **C.** Overglove. **D.** Utility glove.

1. Gloves

Appropriate gloves must be worn for each specific dental task that involves direct contact with blood or saliva and when handling items that may be contaminated with these bodily fluids. Types of gloves include sterile surgeon's gloves, nonsterile exam gloves, overgloves, and utility gloves, as shown in Figure 20.2.

Sterile **surgeon's gloves** are recommended for use during invasive procedures, which include surgery and involved periodontal scaling. They are the most expensive type of glove because of their sterility and the high degree of quality control used during their manufacture.

Nonsterile **exam gloves** may be worn for examination and nonsurgical procedures that are not invasive and when handling most contaminated objects (instruments, impressions, and dental appliances). They are not subject to the same quality-control standards as sterile surgeon's gloves. Exam gloves are not available in specific sizes, such as size 7. Instead, they come in small, medium, large, and so on. They are the suggested gloves for use by dental personnel during most procedures.

Overgloves are thin copolymer or plastic "food handler" gloves that may be worn over nonsterile exam gloves when it is necessary to touch objects not in the oral cavity, such as patient charts, during patient treatment. However, it is difficult to don overgloves without contaminating the exam gloves. In most instances, therefore, a better alternative is to remove exam gloves and then replace them with new gloves when resuming patient treatment. Overgloves are discarded after use on each patient.

Utility gloves are heavy, nonsterile, puncture-resistant gloves that should be worn during cleaning and processing of contaminated instruments, cleaning and disinfecting of contaminated surfaces, and handling of chemicals. They must be cleaned and disinfected after each use.

Gloves used for treatment (exam and surgeon's gloves) are available in both natural latex and synthetic materials, such as vinyl, nitrile, and neoprene. In addition, they may be powdered or powder-free. Both exam and surgeon's gloves must be changed for each patient—or more often if the texture of the glove is modified during use.

2. Handwashing

Use of gloves during patient treatment does not preclude handwashing. Prior to nonsurgical dental procedures, hands should be washed for at least 15 seconds, rinsed, and dried thoroughly before donning and after removing gloves. Do not wash the gloves, however, because wicking and breakdown of composition may occur. Use of an antimicrobial handwash is preferable, although a milder cleanser may be used if the dental operator experiences skin irritation from the hand-cleansing agent. Avoid long fingernails or wearing rings under treatment gloves, which may contribute to holes or tears in gloves. They can harbor bacteria and prevent thorough cleaning of hands during handwashing. This may contribute to the occurrence of allergic reactions under rings.

In October 2002, the Centers for Disease Control and Prevention added to its hand hygiene recommendations an endorsement of 60% to 95% alcohol-based (ethyl alcohol preferred) products for hand cleaning. These products are available as foams, gels, or rinses, and they are applied to the hands and rubbed for at least 15 seconds until the agent is dry. These products are not appropriate, however, when hands are visibly contaminated or soiled. They also must be used and stored away from high temperatures because they are highly flammable.

3. Preventing or Managing Latex Irritation

An awareness of hypersensitivity to latex or other irritants by either the patient or the operator is extremely important so that allergic reactions can be avoided.

a) Latex Allergy in Dental Staff

Gloves worn to protect the hands may cause skin problems. In one study, 15% of dental students developed nonallergic irritation or contact dermatitis from the disposable latex gloves that are commonly worn. Sometimes, this results from the talc or cornstarch with which many gloves are dusted, and in some cases, prolonged exposure may result in either immediate or delayed hypersensitivity immunologic reactions. Immediate hypersensitivity is indicated by **urticaria** (hives) and **erythema** (redness) at the points of contact with the skin minutes after the exposure. The severity of this immediate hypersensitivity may range from a rash to systemic reactions, even including life-threatening bronchospasm, hypotension, anaphylaxis, and death. Contact dermatitis, which occurs from 6 to 72 hours after exposure, is the manifestation of delayed hypersensitivity. If hypersensitivity develops, a nonlatex glove made of synthetic material should be worn. However, it is important to determine if a true latex allergy exists; therefore, one should see an allergist and get an accurate diagnosis.

b) Latex Allergy in Patients

An awareness of latex allergy in patients is extremely important. This knowledge can be gained by questioning the patient during the medical history review before beginning any dental treatment. Risk factors for latex allergy include a history of allergies, multiple surgeries, and frequent contact with latex. For treatment of a patient with known latex allergy, schedule the patient early in the day to minimize exposure to airborne latex powder and residue. In addition, those involved in direct patient care must wear nonlatex gloves, and other dental personnel should wear powder-free gloves. During the dental procedure, avoid the use of any latex-containing items. Common dental products that may contain latex are listed in Table 20.1.

4. Facial Masks and Shields

A mask must be worn by the dental operator during any treatment in which splatter or aerosol is created. The mask should be changed for each patient because its outer surface becomes contaminated either with splatter and aerosol or from the operator touching the mask during dental procedures. Likewise, the mask should be changed during treatment of one patient if it becomes wet from exhaled air and, thus, ceases to act as a filter.

Face masks are available in various styles, as shown in Figure 20.3. Acceptable face masks are composed of synthetic material that filters out at least 95% of small particles that contact the

Table 20.1 Latex Dental Products
Ambubags
Elastic waistbands and wristbands
Gloves
Mask neck/ear loops
N_2O/O_2 analgesia masks
Orthodontic elastics
Rubber dams
Prophy cups
Syringe tips

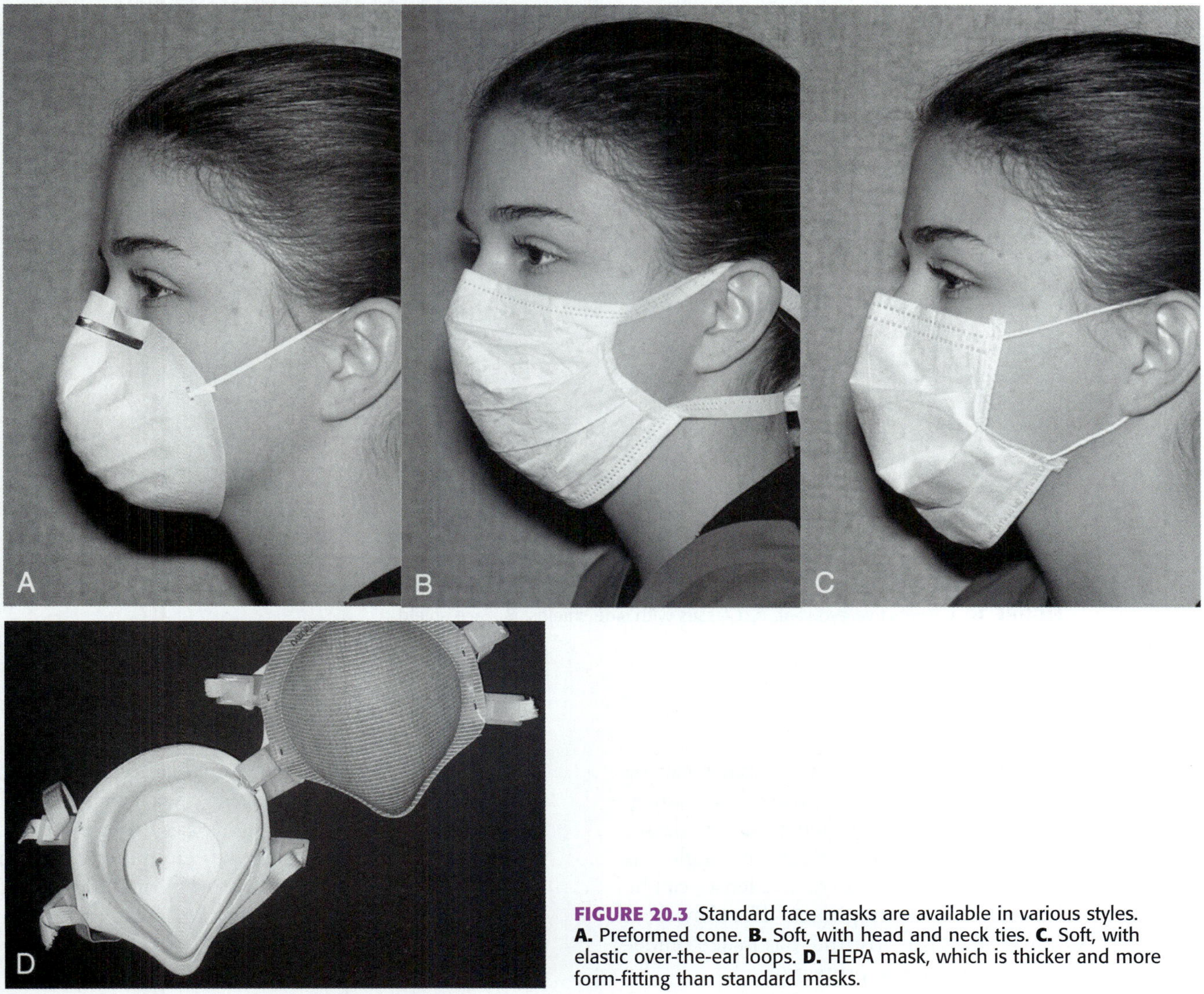

FIGURE 20.3 Standard face masks are available in various styles. **A.** Preformed cone. **B.** Soft, with head and neck ties. **C.** Soft, with elastic over-the-ear loops. **D.** HEPA mask, which is thicker and more form-fitting than standard masks.

mask. Standard masks are not intended to protect health care providers against inhalation of highly infectious aerosols, such as those containing *Mycobacterium tuberculosis*. In such instances, **high-efficiency particulate air (HEPA) masks** must be worn. These masks are designed to filter out small particles and are more form-fitting to the face.

A complete face shield, as shown in Figure 20.4*B*, protects the face from splatter, but not from aerosol, because of the potential for suction of aerosol up under the shield. Therefore, a mask must be worn under a face shield. If worn, a shield must be cleaned and disinfected between use with each patient.

5. Eye Protection

Protective eyewear with side shields must be worn by the dental care provider during any patient treatment or procedure in which aerosol, splatter, or projectiles may be generated. This is not only for protection against infectious disease agents but also for protection against objects and chemicals that could damage the eyes.

a) Hazards

Hazardous chemicals, such as acids, stannous fluoride, disinfectants, and silver nitrate, can be splashed into the eyes. Ultrasonic and high-speed equipment create a spray of aerosols during use; particulates from broken teeth, amalgam, calculus, pumice, gold, or pieces of burs can be thrown out of the mouth at speeds of nearly 60 mph. In the laboratory, personnel are exposed to hazards from rotary equipment, such as grinders; hazardous chemicals, such as disinfectants and developers; and high temperatures. To minimize the consequences of a chemical splash, eye wash equipment should be available, especially in the laboratory.

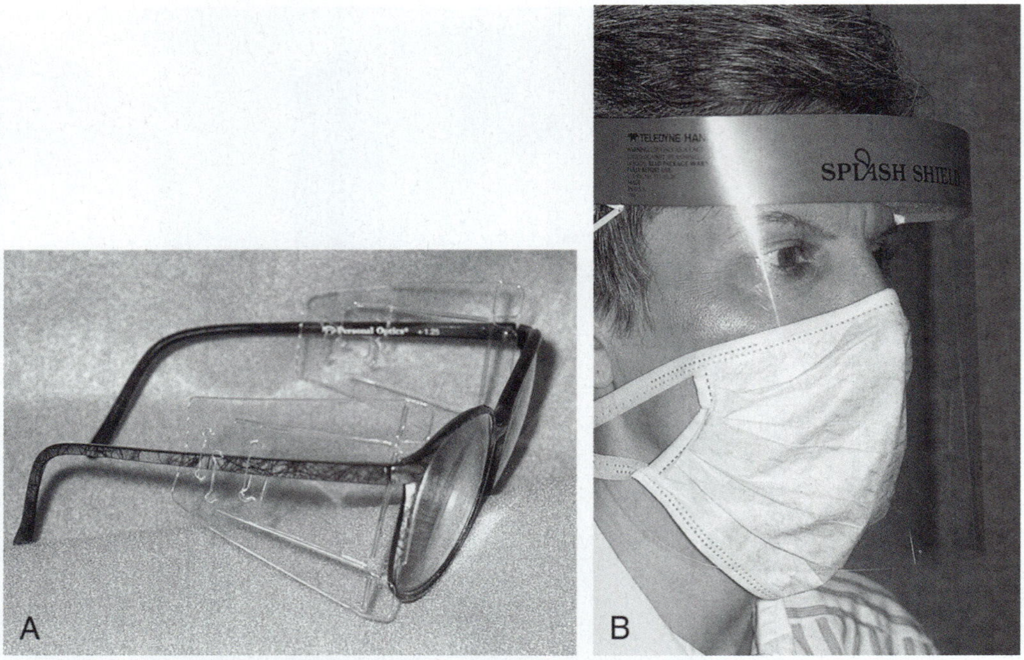

FIGURE 20.4 Protective eyewear. **A.** Glasses with side shields. **B.** Face shield.

b) Equipment
Most potential injuries of these types can be avoided if appropriate eye protection is worn. Acceptable eyewear can include safety glasses with side shields, a face shield, or goggles, as shown in Figure 20.4. Corrective lenses can be incorporated in safety glasses. The American National Standards Institute has issued guidelines for selecting eye protection.

c) Patient Protection
This type of potential hazard not only places the dental personnel but also the patient at risk. When being treated in a reclining position, the patient is exposed not only to the same hazards as the dental personnel but is also at risk from instruments, syringes, or materials that drop from the practitioner's hand or off the delivery tray. Although not mandated, protective eyewear should be worn by the patient as well. Unless disposable glasses are provided to the patient, eyewear should be cleaned and disinfected between each use.

d) Curing Light Hazards
Today, dental personnel also face eye hazards from several types of light: ultraviolet (UV) light, visible blue light, and lasers. Especially in wavelengths between 320 and 400 nm, UV light can cause cataracts and retinal damage. At one time, UV light was used to activate addition polymerization, but visible blue light (400–500 nm) has now replaced UV light in most polymerization applications. Although blue light is not inherently hazardous, the high intensity of curing lights can cause injuries to the retina. Protective equipment recommended by manufacturers includes safety shields or specially tinted glasses.

e) Lasers
When lasers are used, it is important not to direct the laser at any nontarget tissue, especially the eyes, or toward any reflective surface. Special eye protection is required for both the operator and the patient. This eye protection must be matched to absorb the specific wavelength of the laser that is used. Nonreflective instruments and personnel shields are available for use with lasers. Signs are also required in any area where a laser is being used.

6. Protective Attire

Protective attire is the outer layer of clothing worn over underlying clothes. The type and characteristic of protective clothing depend on the exposure that is anticipated. A convenient approach is to use disposable gowns with long sleeves, a high neck, and sufficient length to cover street clothes. This outerwear may be disposable or reusable, and it includes uniforms, clinic jackets, lab coats, and gowns. By OSHA mandate, contaminated reusable attire cannot be laundered at home; it must be laundered in the office or by a commercial laundry service. Protective clothing should be changed daily (or sooner, if it becomes visibly soiled) and should be worn only in the clinical area.

C. Instrument Sterilization and Surface and Equipment Disinfection

1. Degree of Decontamination

The degree of decontamination of dental instruments or equipment depends on its risk of transmitting infection or disease. To determine which method of decontamination to use, categorize the object as either critical, semicritical, or noncritical according to the **Spalding Classification of Inanimate Objects.**

2. Critical Objects

Critical objects must be heat sterilized in either steam, dry heat, or saturated chemical vapor. This category includes items that may penetrate or touch broken mucous membranes or skin. Examples include all instruments, handpieces, and burs. Before wrapping for sterilization, all instruments must be cleaned either ultrasonically or by scrubbing. Follow the manufacturer's guidelines for cleaning and preparing handpieces for sterilization. Store sterile instruments in their sterile wraps, and unwrap them just before use.

3. Semicritical Objects

Semicritical objects include items such as radiographic film holders, shade guides, and mouth props that contact, but do not penetrate, mucous membranes. Heat or chemical liquid sterilization **(high-level disinfectants)** is required for these objects. Heat sterilization is preferred, although chemical liquid sterilization may be necessary for items that may be damaged by heat. Liquid chemicals for sterilization include glutaraldehyde, hydrogen peroxide, and peracetic acid. The long sterilization time (6–10 hours), potential for corrosion, and maintenance of sterility during storage are disadvantages of liquid chemical sterilization.

4. Noncritical Objects

Noncritical objects are those items that do not come in contact with mucous membranes but that are touched or contaminated during dental treatment. These items include the dental unit, switches, handles, radiographic tube heads, the dental chair, and plaster bowls and spatulas.

Intermediate-level disinfectants should be used for the disinfection of noncritical objects. Acceptable disinfectants are those that are registered with the U.S. Environmental Protection Agency (EPA), tuberculocidal, and virucidal. These disinfectants must be virucidal against both lipophilic and hydrophilic viruses. **Lipophilic** viruses, which are enveloped by lipids, are much easier to kill than are **hydrophilic** viruses, which are coated with protein. Properties of acceptable surface disinfectants are summarized in Table 20.2.

Table 20.2 Properties of Acceptable Surface Disinfectants

Property	Type of Microorganism Destroyed
Tuberculocidal	Mycobacterium tuberculosis
Lipophilic	Hepatitis B virus
	Human immunodeficiency virus
	Herpes simplex virus
	Herpes zoster virus
	Influenza virus
Hydrophilic	Adenovirus
	Rotavirus
	Coxsackievirus
	Poliovirus

Acceptable surface disinfectants include hydrogen peroxide, citric acid, iodophors, phenols, quaternaries, sodium hypochlorite and sodium bromide and chlorine. Products for surface disinfection are summarized in Table 20.3. Because of their instability, some of these disinfectants must be mixed fresh daily; however, some are premixed and have a 2-year shelf-life. You should inquire about all the aforementioned features before selecting the product that is most appropriate for use in your office.

Low-level disinfectants are actually detergents or cleaning agents. Some disinfectants contain detergents, but many do not. This information must be obtained from the manufacturer of the disinfectant. The cleaning agent, whether it is a component of the disinfectant or a separate product, must be used during the initial step in the process of disinfecting surfaces.

Surface disinfectants may be applied by sprays or wipes (see examples in Figure 20.5). Application from bottled surface disinfectants involves a **spray, wipe, spray** procedure. The initial spray may be completed with a cleaning agent or a disinfectant that contains a detergent. The surface is then wiped (cleaned), usually with a disposable paper towel. This is followed by a final, light spray with the surface disinfectant, after which the surface is allowed to air dry for a minimum of 10 minutes. The spray, wipe, spray procedure is shown in Figure 20.6. If

Table 20.3 OSAP Surface Disinfectant Reference Chart–2006

PRODUCT CLASSIFICATION	PRODUCT BRAND INFORMATION				
Category	**Brand (packaged as)**	**EPA #**	**Dilution**	**TB Claim**	**Manufacturer or Distributor**
Accelerated Hydrogen Peroxide	**Optim 33 TB**	74559-1-83259	RTU	5 min	SciCan
Citric Acid Citric acid, hydroxyacetic acid, dipropylene glycol n-butyl ether	**Lysol IC Ready to Use Disinfectant Cleaner**	675-55	RTU	10 min	Sultan Healthcare
Iodophors Alpha- (p-nonylphenyl)-omega-hydroxypoly (oxethylene) iodine	**IodoFive Surface Disinfectant/Cleaner**	4959-16-50611	1:213	10 min	Certol International
Phenolics (Dual) Water-Based Phenylphenol and benzylchlorophenol or tertiary amylphenol	**Birex SE Concentrate**	1043-92-51003	1:256	10 min	Biotrol International
	DisCide Germicidal Foaming Cleaner	33176-6	RTU	10 min	Palmero Health Care
	ProSpray C-60 Conc. Surface Disinfectant	46851-1-50611	1:32	10 min	Certol International
	ProSpray Surface Disinfectant Spray	46851-5-50611	RTU	10 min	Certol International
	ProSpray Wipes	46851-10	RTU	10 min	Certol International
Phenolics (Dual) Alcohol-Based Tertiary amylphenol and/or phenylphenol + ethyl alcohol or isopropyl alcohol	**Coe Spray II (Pump)**	11694-98-10214	RTU	6 min	GC America
	DisCide Disinfectant Spray	706-69-10492	RTU	10 min	Palmero Health Care
Quaternaries Dual or Synergized Plus Alcohol Diisobutylphe-noxyethoxyethyl dimethylbenzyl ammonium chloride; isopropanol or ethanol; alkyldimethyl benzyl ammonium chloride	**CaviCide Spray**	46781-6	RTU	5 min	TotalCare/ Pinnacle/Metrex
	CaviWipes	46781-8	RTU	5 min	TotalCare/ Pinnacle/Metrex
	Cetylcide II Broad Spectrum Disinfectant	61178-1-3150	2 oz/gal	NOL	Cetylite Industries
	Clorox Disinfecting Spray	67619-3	RTU	10 min	Harry J. Bosworth Company
	DisCide ULTRA Spray	10492-5	RTU	1 min	Palmero Health Care
	DisCide ULTRA Wipes	10492-4	RTU	1 min	Palmero Health Care
	DisCide V Detergent Disinfectant	1839-83-10492	RTU	5 min	Palmero Health Care
	GC Spray-Cide	1130-15-10214	RTU	6 min	GC America
	Lysol IC Disinfectant Spray	777-72-675	RTU	10 min	Sultan Healthcare
	Maxispray Plus	46781-6-10597	RTU	5 min	Sullivan-Schein Dental
	Maxiwipe Germicidal Cloth	9480-4-10597	RTU	5 min	Sullivan-Schein Dental
	Opti-Cide-3 Spray	70144-1	RTU	3 min	Micro Scientific Industries
	PDCare Surface Disinfectant Spray	46781-6-43100	RTU	5 min	Patterson Dental

Table 20.3 OSAP Surface Disinfectant Reference Chart–2006 (continued)

PRODUCT CLASSIFICATION	PRODUCT BRAND INFORMATION				
Category	**Brand (packaged as)**	**EPA #**	**Dilution**	**TB Claim**	**Manufacturer or Distributor**
Quaternaries Dual or Synergized Plus Alcohol (continued)	**PDCare Wipes**	46781-8-43100	RTU	5 min	Patterson Dental
	Sanitex Plus Spray	1130-150-64285	RTU	6 min	Crosstex International
	Sanitex Plus Wipes	9480-4-64285	RTU	5 min	Crosstex International
	Sani-Cloth HB Wipes	61178-4-9480	RTU	NOL	PDI International
	Sani-Cloth Plus Wipes	9480-6	RTU	5 min	PDI International
	Super Sani-Cloth Wipes	9480-4	RTU	2 min	PDI International
	Clorox Germicidal Spray	67619-13	RTU	30 sec	Harry J. Bosworth Company
Sodium Hypochlorite	**Clorox Germicidal Wipes**	67619-12	RTU	2 min	Harry J. Bosworth Company
Sodium Bromide & Chlorine	**Microstat 2 Tablets**	70369-1	2 tabs/qt water	5 min	Septodont

IMPORTANT INFORMATION: Listing does not imply endorsement, recommendation or warranty. Other products are available. Only OSAP member *Hospital Disinfectants* are represented in this chart. Purchasers are legally required to consult label and package insert for changes in formulation and recommended use. Check compatibility of material before use on dental/medical equipment.

KEY: RTU = Ready to Use; NOL = Not on label, e.g., one or both of the HIV/HBV claims is not provided on the label. OSAP is using the CDC guidelines. Be sure to use a disinfectant with a TB claim if there is any blood or OPIM present.

The interactive chart may be found at www.OSAP.org, then Infection Control Issues, then OSAP Surface Disinfectant Reference Chart.

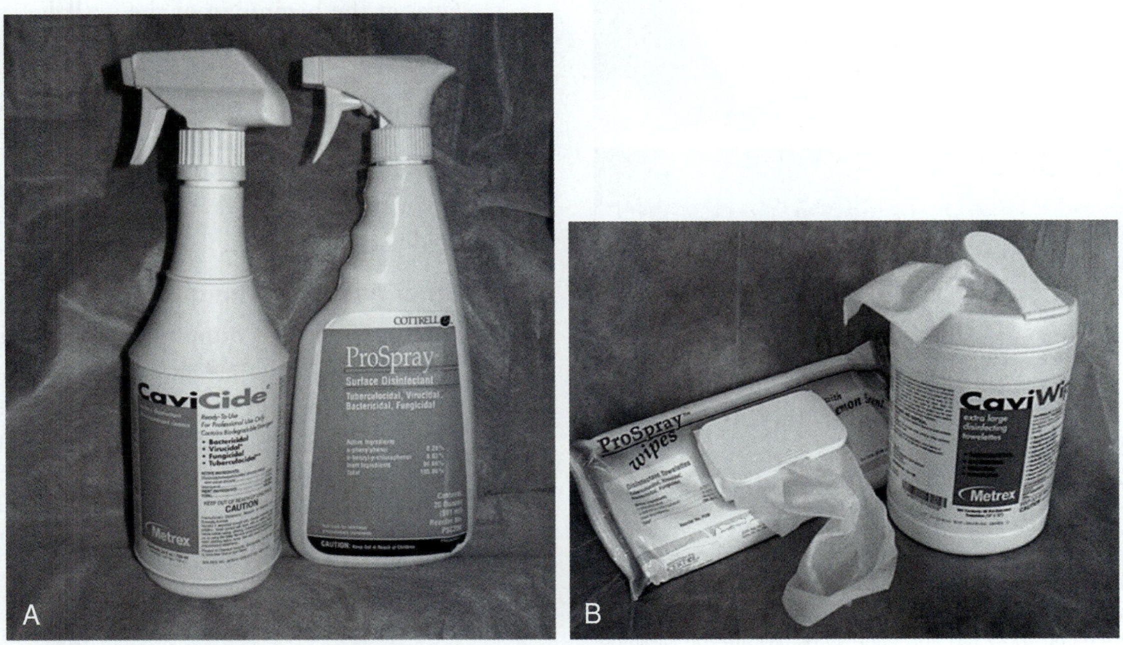

FIGURE 20.5 Examples of surface disinfectant. **A.** Sprays. **B.** Wipes.

disinfectant wipes are used, use one soaked wipe to first clean the surface. Then, with a new wipe, wipe again to disinfect the surface and let air dry for 5–10 minutes, depending on the disinfectant (check the label).

D. Protective Barriers

An effective way to maintain surface disinfection is to cover cleaned and disinfected surfaces with disposable protective barriers. This involves proper placement of a surface cover before there is an opportunity for contamination of the surface after disinfection, as shown in Figure 20.7. Surface covers should be impervious to fluids, and they include clear plastic wrap, bags, or tubes. These plastic covers are available in preformed shapes that fit over specific items or as plain sheets that must be wrapped around items. Choose the type of barrier that is most economical and appropriate for your office.

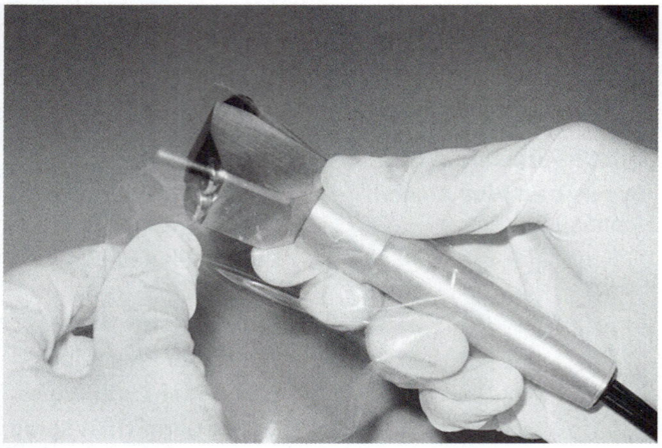

FIGURE 20.7 Protective barriers or covers may be placed over surfaces after they are disinfected and before there is an opportunity for contamination.

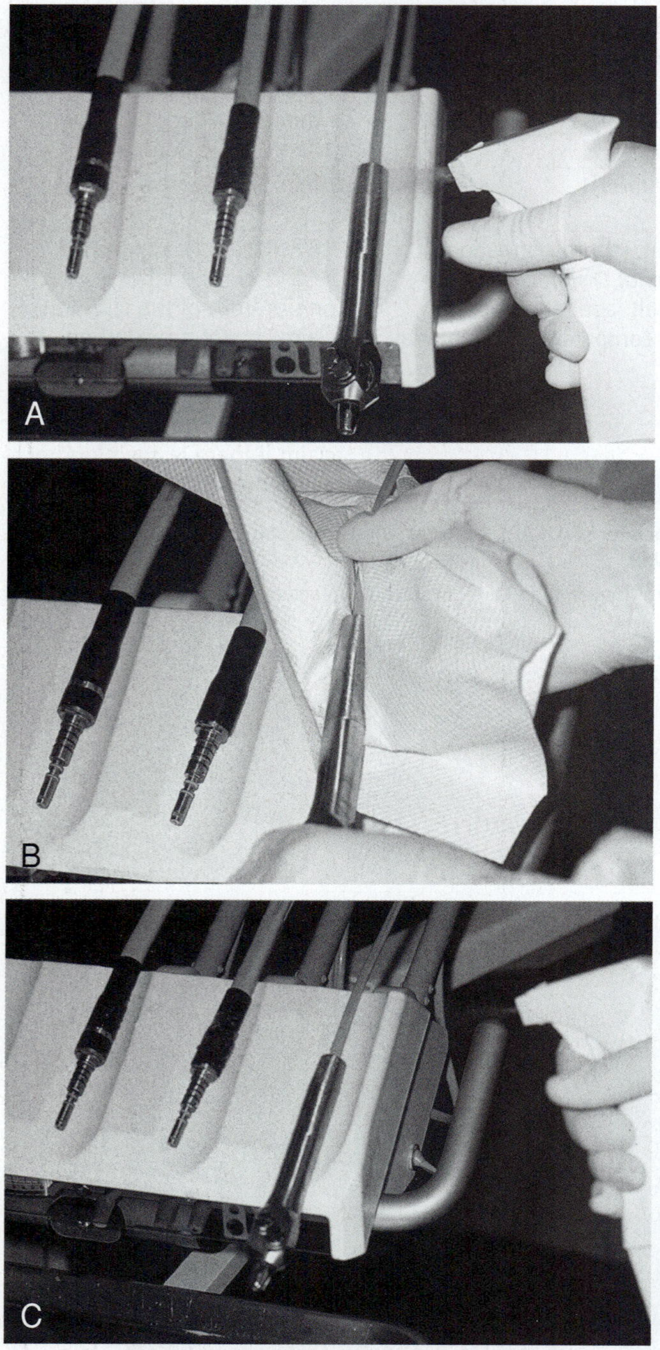

FIGURE 20.6 Surface disinfection includes a "spray, wipe, spray" procedure. The initial spray (**A**) and wipe steps (**B**) are the cleaning phase and are followed by the final spray with a disinfectant (**C**).

Use of protective barriers on surfaces does not preclude surface disinfection; rather, these barriers are used in combination with it. If you choose to use protective barriers, clean and disinfect surfaces at the beginning of the workday, then cover these surfaces with clean barriers between patient treatments. Remove contaminated barriers with gloved hands, and replace clean barriers carefully so that the disinfected surfaces are not contaminated. Use of protective barriers is especially advocated for surfaces that contain buttons, knobs, and crevices.

E. Other Aseptic Techniques

1. Distribution of Supplies and Materials

Numerous supplies and materials are used for patient care, and their proper storage and distribution must be of primary concern so that cross-contamination is avoided. Examples include gauze, cotton rolls, articulating paper, prophy paste, impression materials, and other restorative materials.

a) Bulk Supplies

To avoid contamination of supplies stored in bulk, sterile retrievers (forceps) must be provided for aseptic removal of items. Extreme care must be taken by all office personnel when obtaining these items.

b) Kits

Kits of restorative materials, such as dentinal bonding systems that are used at chairside on more than one patient, must be cleaned and disinfected between each patient. The box may be covered with a clean barrier for each patient; however, any bottles or tubes that are contaminated must be disinfected before being returned to the box or cabinet for storage.

c) Unit Dose

Many types of supplies or materials can be supplied as a **unit dose,** as shown in Figure 20.8, so that cross-contamination can be avoided. This is accomplished by packaging small amounts of materials or supplies in individual packets for use on individual patients. Unit dosing can be more expensive, but it is very effective in the prevention of cross-contamination and also reduces labor costs.

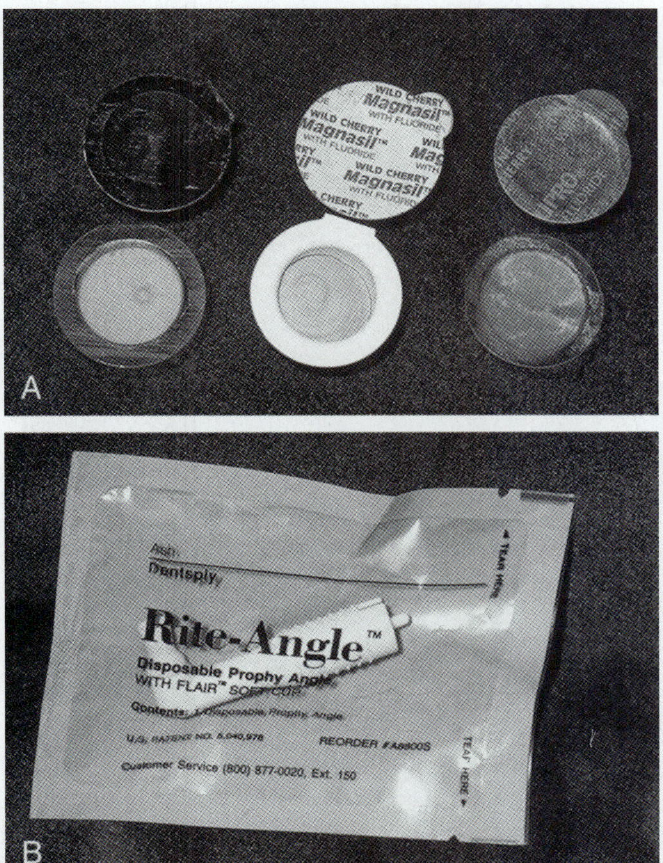

FIGURE 20.8 **A.** Unit-dosed prophy paste. **B.** Disposable prophy angle.

2. Use of Disposable Items

Disposable items are usually manufactured from inexpensive materials, such as plastics, and are designed to be disposed of after use. Examples include the saliva ejector, evacuation tip, air/water syringe tip, impression trays, and prophy angles. Other items include treatment gloves, cover gowns, surface covers, facial masks, and anesthetic syringe needles. Use of disposable items also reduces labor costs.

It is important to properly dispose of these items after use. Avoid any attempt to clean, sterilize, or disinfect them for reuse.

F. Managing Aerosol and Splatter

Aerosol and splatter that are generated and propelled from the patient's oral cavity during dental treatment create the potential for microbial contamination of the dental operator and the adjacent environmental surfaces. The amount of aerosol and splatter can be controlled, however, by using the following practices.

1. Rubber Dam

Whenever possible, use a rubber dam to reduce the amount of saliva at the operative site. Simultaneous use of high-speed evacuation along with a rubber dam provides optimum reduction of dental aerosol and splatter.

2. Pretreatment Mouthrinse

Provide the patient with a pretreatment mouthrinse, such as an American Dental Association (ADA)–approved mouthrinse containing chlorhexidine gluconate or essential oils. These significantly reduce the number of microorganisms that may escape in splatter or aerosol.

3. Pretreatment Toothbrushing

A simple but effective way to reduce the potential for microbial contamination from aerosol and splatter is to have the patient brush his or her teeth with an ADA-approved dentifrice before any treatment begins.

G. Safe Handling and Disposal of Sharp Items Contaminated with Blood or Saliva

1. Sharps Containers

Extreme safety precautions should be followed when handling any sharp instrument, orthodontic wire, anesthetic needle, irrigating syringe, or other item that may be contaminated with bloodborne pathogens. These precautions include avoiding punctures or cuts during the use of these sharp items and proper disposal of these items into hard "sharps" containers. An example of a "sharps" container is shown in Figure 20.9.

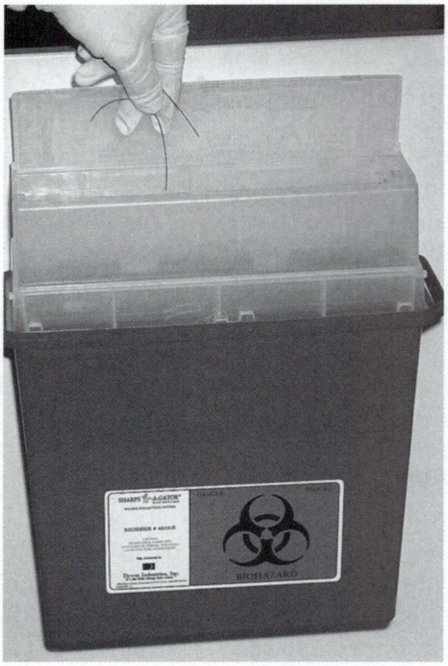

FIGURE 20.9 Dispose of all sharp items into a hard "sharps" container.

2. Recapping Needles

Recapping of anesthetic needles should never be performed as a two-handed technique. The two-handed technique greatly contributes to needlestick accidents. One of the following practices can greatly reduce the potential for accidental needlesticks: the one-handed scoop technique, use of a barrier cap-holding device, or use of a disposable self-capping "safe" syringe (Fig. 20.10).

H. Office and Laboratory Housekeeping Practices

To minimize the potential for infection of the dental care provider by cross-contamination, the following housekeeping practices should be observed.

1. Eating and Cosmetics

Do not eat, drink, apply cosmetics or lip balm, or place (or remove) contact lenses in the treatment area, dental laboratory, or sterilization and radiograph processing area. Use disposable tissues rather than handkerchiefs.

2. Food Storage

Do not store food or drink in refrigerators or freezers that are also used to keep dental products or other potentially infectious or hazardous materials.

3. Separate Contaminated Items

Keep two separately designated areas in the laboratory for receiving contaminated items and for storing or handling clean or sterile items.

4. Infectious Wastes

All infectious wastes must be disposed of according to local, state, and federal regulations. As a

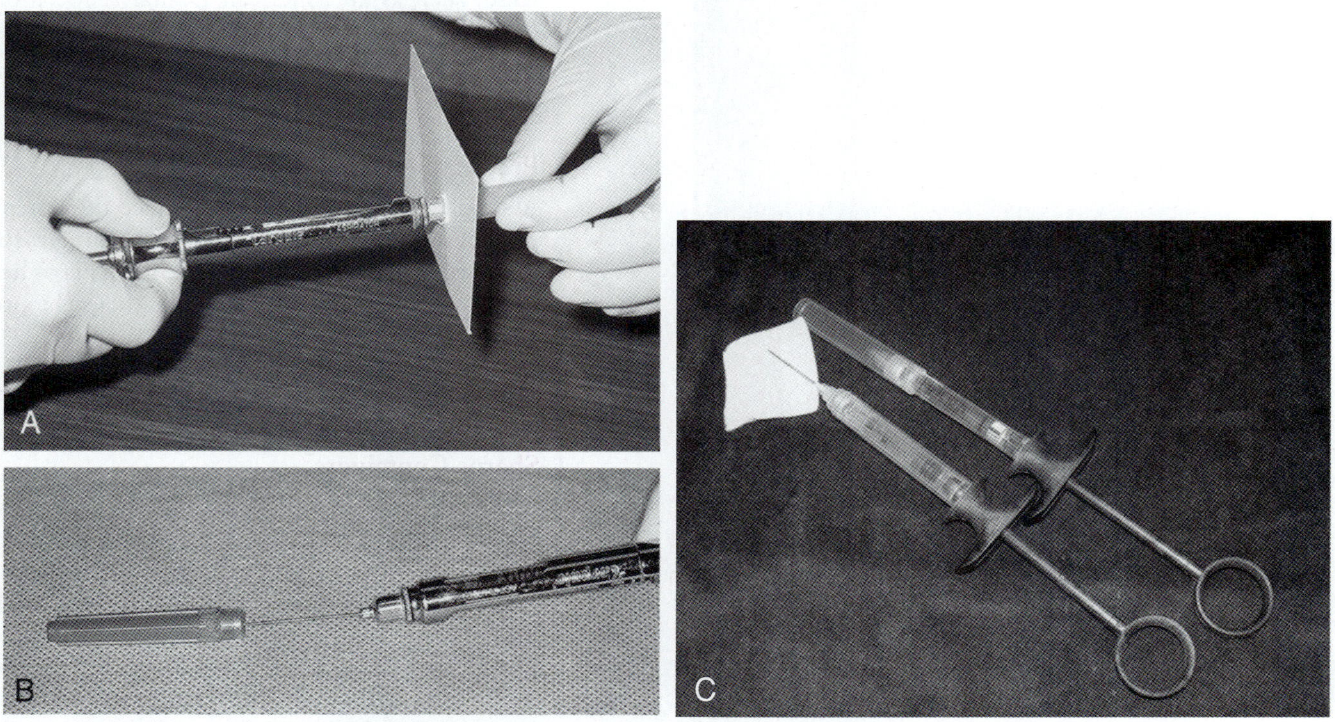

FIGURE 20.10 Two acceptable methods for recapping needles. **A.** Use of a barrier cap-holding device. **B.** A one-handed scoop technique. **C.** Self capping "Safe Syringe."

general rule, blood-soaked items as well as hard and soft tissue are considered to be infectious waste and must be placed in appropriately marked biohazard infectious waste containers (boxes, plastic bags) and disposed of by specified agencies.

I. Exposure Control Plan

The dental office or laboratory must have a written **exposure control plan** that includes all steps necessary to prevent exposure to bloodborne pathogens for each dental procedure that is performed. The plan must also include the protocol to follow if an exposure to a bloodborne pathogen occurs. You must familiarize yourself with the exposure plan, and you should review it at least annually. Someone in the office should be designated to update this plan each year.

III. Physical Hazards

Many common sense things can be done to minimize possible accidents. Arrange the work area to allow enough room for people to pass and safely get around each other and any equipment.

A. Trips, Slips, Hits, and Spills

1. Floors

Use no-skid absorbent rugs at doorways and in areas likely to get wet, such as near the sink. Use only low matte rugs because wrinkled throw rugs can be the cause of trips, especially for the elderly. Mobile equipment often has cords and tubes that can also be a trip hazard; keep these out of traffic areas. Spills on smooth floors are an important concern as well and should be cleaned up as soon as possible. Some powders used in dentistry, such as plaster and acrylic powders, can make a smooth floor very slippery.

Open cabinet drawers and doors can cause injuries. A lower drawer, left open, can be a trip hazard. One can walk into an open upper cabinet door when looking down or hit one's head when rising after bending over. Cabinet drawers and doors should not be left open, especially in a high-traffic area.

2. Patients

When patients have been reclined for an appointment, it is a good idea to sit them up when giving them postoperative instructions. If they stand up immediately after they are moved to an upright position, fainting or light-headedness may occur. Raising patients to an upright position for a few minutes will reduce such problems. For some patients, it is advisable to have them turn in the dental chair and sit with their feet on the floor for a few additional minutes. One may want to stand near certain patients in a supportive position should they feel light-headed when they stand up. In addition, one must move the operatory light and other equipment out of the patient's way to avoid head injuries. Patients with impaired vision are a special concern; if necessary, they should be escorted into and out of the dental operatory.

B. Lifting Injuries

Back injuries are a major problem in many types of work. Although this may not be a frequent problem in the dental office, boxes of files, disinfectant, or developing solution may be heavy. The general rule is to bend the legs instead of the back when lifting heavy items. This may include patients who need help to get in or out of the chair.

C. Lathes

It is very easy to get loose items stuck in the rapidly spinning parts of a lathe and other equipment. Be sure to contain long hair securely, and do not use the lathe while wearing loose jewelry, ties, scarves, or loose-fitting gloves. These loose items can get caught and drag the hand—or, worse, the head—into the rapidly spinning shaft or cutting device. Eye protection is a must when a lathe is being used, and a mask is also recommended.

D. Model Trimmers

When a model trimmer is used, it is important to make sure that a slip will not result in a finger or a hand being thrust into the cutting disk. Use a "palm rest," where the palm of the hand rests on the front of the table of the model trimmer (see Chapter 28). The fingers should hold the cast in the area most distant from the cutting disk. Use flexure of the fingers to push the cast toward the cutting disk rather than pushing the cast with an unstable hand or fingers. If the flexure method is used and the part of the hand that is pushing slips off the cast, the fingers will only straighten and extend over the cast, not into the cutting disk.

E. Burns, Scalds, and Fires

1. Sterilization Equipment

Removing items from a hot autoclave has been the cause of numerous burns and scalds. Be sure that items have adequately cooled before taking them out of an autoclave, or use heat-resistant gloves. Follow the manufacturer's directions for opening an autoclave or other heat sterilization equipment. Remember, hot items do not look different from cold items.

2. Personal Protection Equipment

Loose-fitting gloves are a hazard when a lighter is used to heat an instrument or light a Bunsen burner. If the tip of the glove extends into the flame, it will melt onto the finger. Lighters with extended tips are available for lighting grills and candles. These are much safer to use than the typical disposable lighter. Also, use only flame-resistant or flame-retardant disposable cover gowns.

3. Flammables

Many of the chemicals used in dentinal bonding systems are flammable. Luckily, they are packaged in small containers and are used in very small quantities. They do not present a great hazard.

Acrylic monomers are also flammable but are packaged and used in much greater quantities. Do not use them around open flames, and clean up any spills immediately. Acrylic monomers and any alcohol that is used as a fuel should be properly stored. Do not leave an open flame unattended. It is important to know where the fire extinguishers are located, and all employees should know how to use them. Smoke detectors should also be present. Remember, if a fire should occur, the first priority is to get people to safety, not to fight the fire.

4. Oxygen

Oxygen is used in every dental office that uses nitrous oxide. Oxygen should be present in the emergency kits in a dental office. If one remembers that fire requires oxygen, the danger of pure oxygen is obvious. If an oxygen leak occurs in any equipment, a spark could mean disaster. Also, the metal tanks that are used to supply oxygen and nitrous oxide are heavy and need to be securely fastened in place. If they were to fall over, serious injury could occur.

F. Electrical Hazards

1. Outlets Near Sinks

To minimize the chance of electrocution, current standards for electrical safety require that outlets near a sink incorporate a **ground fault circuit interrupter** (**GFI,** or GFCI), either in the outlet itself or in the electrical box. Should equipment plugged into a GFI outlet become immersed in water, the resulting short circuit would trigger the GFI. Electricity is then rapidly cut off to the circuit so that anyone touching the item would avoid serious injury. Keep portable electrical equipment away from sinks to minimize the hazard of the equipment falling into water.

2. Maintaining Equipment

When performing maintenance on equipment, such as replacing a bulb in a curing unit, it is important to unplug the unit. Repairing or maintaining equipment that is plugged into an electrical outlet presents a significant risk and should be avoided. Depending on the nature of the task, it may be wise to unplug some equipment during cleaning.

3. Pacemakers

Pacemakers may be affected by an electromagnetic field that is given off by some dental equipment. Electrosurgery and ultrasonic units should not be used on patients with an older, "unshielded" pacemaker. If the patient or the patient's doctor cannot ensure that use of such equipment is safe for the patient with a pacemaker, do not use this equipment.

G. Hearing Protection

1. Harmful Noise Levels

For many years, noise from dental equipment has been suspected of contributing to hearing loss. Dental professionals as a group experience hearing losses. Many studies of the dental environment have been done, but the results have been contradictory. In the dental office, exposure to noise should be controlled in accordance with OSHA standards. The occupational exposure limit is given in terms of an 8-hour, time-weighted average of 85 decibels (dBA). Harmful noise levels can be encountered from a variety of sources, many of them not work-related. Examples of noise sources that have been measured to generate sound levels above 85 dBA include a vacuum cleaner, lawn mower, car radio, hair dryer, and TV commercials. To protect hearing from all sources, the U.S. EPA specifies that exposures should not average more than 70 dBA during a 24-hour period.

2. Protection

The susceptibility to hearing loss varies from person to person. Noise-induced hearing loss is subtle and, eventually, irreversible. Usually, it first affects a higher frequency range than is normally used in conversation, so it may go unnoticed for some time. To determine if a person has a hearing loss, he or she can be tested by an audiologist. Measurements of noise levels in the dental office can be made by hearing conservation companies. Hearing protection, in the form of ear plugs or ear covers, can be effective in reducing exposure, but it may also affect a dental practitioner's ability to converse with a patient. Some practitioners have earplugs connected by a cord that they can hang around their neck when talking but have easily available for use when needed. With all the noise present both in and out of work, it may be prudent to take preventive measures to reduce exposure to excessive noise from any source.

H. Respiratory Hazards

1. Aerosols, Dusts, Allergies, and Asthma

In the dental office, there is the potential for injury to the respiratory system from a number of different sources, including infectious agents. Occupational asthma, pneumoconiosis (an example is silicosis), and chronic bronchitis may occur from the inhalation of fine particles into the respiratory tract. Some of the dusts generated in a dental office can include amalgam, asbestos, beryllium-containing alloys, cobalt, dentin, gold, gypsum, pumice, and silica. Various size particles and aerosols are produced from grinding and polishing techniques, and some of the fine particles may be suspended in the air for hours or even days.

Spray disinfectants are another source of aerosol. They may irritate the respiratory system or aggravate asthma. A mask and eye protection should be worn when spray disinfectants are used. Lasers produce aerosols of tissue debris that are not always sterile.

2. Allergic Sensitization

Exposure to acrylic dusts has been related to allergic sensitization of the respiratory tract. Occupational asthma has occurred from exposures to persulfates (found in many plastics), stainless steel, nickel, cobalt, chromium, tungsten carbide, formaldehyde, solvents such as toluene, oil of orange, xylene, and various epoxy compounds. The respiratory hazards of mercury are considered in a later section.

3. Protection

To minimize the distribution of these particulates and aerosols, a high-velocity vacuum system with filters should be used. The practitioner should also wear a mask that is capable of filtering out these particles. The types of masks currently worn to protect from infectious material (for particles 1–2 μm in diameter) will not filter out many of the dusts and aerosols that have been noted. Masks designed to filter out respirable dusts are available, however, and are recommended, especially for use when grinding composite materials and porcelain.

In general, the use of volatile materials and the performance of activities that produce dusts and aerosols should be carried out in an area that is equipped with proper dust collection equipment. In the operatory, good general ventilation is also essential. Although standards may not be specified for operatories, those for laboratories would probably be appropriate. A rate of six air exchanges per hour is recommended. To minimize energy costs, replacement air could be heated with an air-to-air heat exchanger, which can usually be incorporated into the existing furnace/air conditioning system.

I. Dermal Hazards

The skin on the hands of a dental care provider can be subject to many different types of abuse. Irritants can include soaps and detergents, germicides, adhesives, essential oils, filling materials, metals, organic solvents, and radiograph processing chemicals.

1. Allergic Contact Dermatitis

Allergic contact dermatitis can be caused by a number of dental materials. Examples include acrylic monomers (among them, methyl methacrylate), ethylene glycol dimethacrylate, eugenol, bisphenol A (an epoxy resin compound), and disinfectants. Acrylic monomers and glutaraldehyde can penetrate latex and polyvinyl chloride gloves. See the Material Safety Data Sheet, as shown in Figure 20.10, or contact the manufacturer for information on appropriate alternatives to latex gloves.

2. Latex Gloves

As previously discussed, gloves that are worn to protect the hands may be the cause of problems. Latex sensitivity should be considered when any dermal irritation occurs on the hands. Powderless latex gloves cause fewer problems than powdered gloves.

J. Musculoskeletal Problems

Although it does not directly relate to dental materials safety, another health concern for dental care providers is that of musculoskeletal disorders. Recent studies have shown a large increase in the number of occupationally related disorders involving the musculoskeletal system, particularly among dental hygienists. These disorders are also known as cumulative motion trauma, repetitive motion disorders, and/or cumulative trauma disorders. They result from repetitive insults to the muscles, bones, and related structures. Musculoskeletal disorders can occur in any part of the body, but the areas most often noted as being problems for dental care providers were the lower back, neck, shoulders, arms, wrists, and hands. Carpal tunnel syndrome is a disturbingly common problem and is discussed in most dental hygiene texts.

1. Ergonomics

Dental professionals can be at risk for injuries because of the nature of their work. Experts in **ergonomics** (also known as biomechanics or human factor engineering) seek to assess the best way for a person to perform a task. Ergonomics takes into consideration the physical dimensions and capabilities of the human body as well as the optimal design of equipment and the work area to promote the comfort and efficiency of the worker.

Following are recommendations for improved musculoskeletal health.

2. General Recommendations

- **a)** Good lighting is important to avoid eyestrain. Good light and the use of magnification will reduce slouching over the patient and associated problems.
- **b)** Use good posture. Keep the back and neck in line without tipping forward or twisting.
- **c)** Use a chair that provides good lumbar support and has a seat width that allows for shifting and movement. The height of the seat should be adjusted so that the feet can be flat and the thighs parallel to the floor. Casters on the chair should make it easy to move without twisting.
- **d)** Get up and move around between patients. This gives a break to the muscles used during sitting and takes the pressure off some of the discs between the vertebrae.
- **e)** Ask patients to change their head position instead of leaning or twisting for a better view or work angle.
- **f)** Use indirect vision with a dental mirror to view hard-to-see areas of the mouth. Avoid leaning and twisting to use direct vision.
- **g)** Do exercises that promote flexibility and strengthen the hand, back, abdominal, hip, and leg muscles.
- **h)** Consider limiting off-the-job activities that contribute to musculoskeletal problems. These include certain sports, excessive computer use, and repetitive finger activities, such as knitting or crocheting.

3. Hand and Wrist Recommendations

- **a)** Use gloves that fit well.
- **b)** Use a neutral hand position and finger rests. Less pressure will be exerted on the median nerve in the wrist if flexion and extension can be minimized.
- **c)** Lower the vibration components when using vibratory instruments. Vibration can contribute to carpal tunnel syndrome.
- **d)** Rest and exercise hands. Stretch the hands when changing instruments and between patients.

4. Instrument Recommendations

- **a)** Use the proper instrument for the task.
- **b)** Use lightweight and evenly balanced instruments. Consider using hollow instruments.
- **c)** Choose instruments with a textured grip. They are easier to hold and require less "pinching" when in use.
- **d)** Larger-diameter instruments, when being used, also minimize the need to pinch.
- **e)** Keep the cutting edges of instruments sharp to make them effective with a minimum amount of force and fewer deliberate strokes. This recommendation is discussed in more detail in Chapter 19.

5. Preventing Injuries

Having a coworker watch or videotape you while you work can be helpful. Another person can often spot potential ergonomic problems that are overlooked when the dental care worker is concentrating on patient care. At present, OSHA is working with organized dentistry to address ergonomic issues in the workplace. Even without such a standard, dental professionals should take steps to prevent musculoskeletal disorders and the discomforts they cause.

IV. Chemicals

The term "chemical" may sound scary to many people. We do not want chemicals in our water or our food. On the other hand, water is a chemical, and most foods are a complex mixture of many chemicals. (Try reading the label on a cereal box.) Here, we are interested in the hazardous chemicals and materials in the dental office. We need to know what chemicals we are using and how to avoid injury from them.

A. Material Safety Data Sheets

Manufacturers usually send a **Material Safety Data Sheet (MSDS)** with products that meet the OSHA definition of a hazardous material. A MSDS is shown in Figure 20.11. The MSDS will list the hazards of the material, precautions that should be employed when the material is used, and procedures to take in emergencies. If you do not have a MSDS for a particular product, call the manufacturer. Most will be happy to send one. All dental personnel should know where the MSDSs are stored. They should be available to be read by anyone who might come in contact with the material in question.

The information in a MSDS is for worker safety as directed by OSHA. Only hazardous chemicals are included. Chemicals added to a product that are "generally recognized as safe" are not detailed in the MSDS, nor are they listed as ingredients in a product unless directed by the FDA. Many additives that flavor or sweeten are not listed on professional dental products' labels or package inserts. This lack of information can be a problem for patients or personnel with unusual allergies or metabolic problems. Obtaining complete information from a manufacturer about all ingredients in a professional product such as a fluoride gel or prophy paste can be difficult. Manufacturers regard such information as proprietary. What is the dental

MATERIAL SAFTEY DATA SHEET	PARKELL, INC. 155 SCHMITT BLVD. FARMINGDALE, NY 11735 631-249-1134	24-HOUR EMERGENCY TELEPHONE 1-800-535-5053

SECTION I - PRODUCT IDENTIFICATION

PRODUCT NAME: SNAP MONOMER — STOCK NO: S441
DOT HAZARD LABEL: Flammable Liquid — UN NUMBER: UN2283
PROPER SHIPPING NAME: Isobutyl Methacrylate, Inhibited — DATE PREPARED: 09/01/99
NFPA CODES: HEALTH - 2 FLAMMABILITY - 2 REACTIVITY - 2

SECTION II - HAZARDOUS INGREDIENTS/IDENTITY INFORMATION

HAZARDOUS COMPONENTS	CAS NUMBER	PEL	TLV	%
Isobutyl Methacrylate	97-86-9	100 ppm	100 ppm	
4-Methoxyphenol	150-76-5	5 mg/m^3	5 mg/m^3	.01%

SECTION III - PHYSICAL & CHEMICAL CHARACTERISTICS

BOILING POINT: 311° F — SPECIFIC GRAVITY (H_2O = 1): .889
VAPOR PRESSURE: 3 mm HG — PERCENT VOLATILES: 90%
VAPOR DENSITY (Air = 1): 4.9 — EVAPORATION RATE (Butyl Acetate = 1): 0.5
APPEARANCE AND ODOR: Pale yellow liquid; acrid fruity odor

SECTION IV - FIRE AND EXPLOSION HAZARD DATA

FLASH POINT (TCC): 111°F (44°C) FLAMMABLE LIMIT (air, % by vol) UPPER: NE LOWER: NE
EXTINGUISHER MEDIA: Chemical foam, carbon dioxide, dry chemicals.
SPECIAL FIRE FIGHTING PROCEDURES: Wear self contained breathing apparatus, and full protective gear. Use water spray to cool containers. EXPLOSION HAZARD - Fight fire from protected location.
UNUSUAL FIRE & EXPLOSION HAZARDS: Vapors may travel to source of ignition and flash back. Heat can cause polymerization with rapid release of energy which may rupture container explosively. (Spontaneous polymerization may occur on prolonged storage). EXPLOSION HAZARD - Fight fire from protected location.

SECTION V - REACTIVITY DATA (PHYSICAL HAZARDS)

STABILITY: [X] STABLE [ ] UNSTABLE
CONDITIONS TO AVOID: Heat and ignition sources, aging and contamination.
INCOMPATIBILITY (Materials to avoid): Reducing and oxidizing agents and UV light.
HAZARDOUS DECOMPOSITION PRODUCTS: None under normal conditions; oxides of carbon when burned.
HAZARDOUS POLYMERIZATION: [X] MAY OCCUR [ ] WILL NOT OCCUR
CONDITIONS TO AVOID: Temperatures above 40° C, oxidizing/reducing agents, peroxides, amines.

MATERIAL SAFETY DATA SHEET (continued)

PRODUCT NAME: SNAP MONOMER — STOCK NO: S441

SECTION VI - HEALTH HAZARD DATA

PRIMARY ROUTE(S) OF ENTRY: [X] EYES [X] SKIN [X] INHALATION [ ] INGESTION
HEALTH HAZARDS (Acute & Chronic): Over exposure from liquid or high vapor concentration can irritate eyes, respiratory system and cause skin rashes. Prolonged exposure can lead to headaches, nausea, drowsiness and unconsciousness.
SIGNS & SYMPTOMS OF EXPOSURE: Irritation of eyes and respiratory system; skin rash; headaches; nausea; drowsiness and unconsciousness.
CARCINOGENICITY: [No] NTP? [No] IARC MONOGRAPHS? [No] OSHA?
EMERGENCY AND FIRST AID PROCEDURES:
INHALATION: Remove to fresh air. Get medical help if discomfort persists.
EYES: Flush with water for 15 minutes, including under eyelids.
SKIN: Wash with soap and water.
INGESTION: Induce vomiting, obtain prompt medical attention.

SECTION VII - SPECIAL PRECAUTIONS AND SPILL OR LEAK PROCEDURES

PRECAUTIONS TO BE TAKEN IN HANDLING & STORAGE: Store in cool dry place. Ground all metal containers when transferring. Use explosion-proof equipment. Check inhibitor levels every three months.
OTHER PRECAUTIONS: NA
STEPS TO BE TAKEN IN CASE MATERIAL IS RELEASED OR SPILLED: Evacuate area. Eliminate sources of ignition. Use self-contained breathing apparatus and protective clothing. Dike and absorb with inert material. Transfer to proper containers for disposal, use non-sparking tools. Keep spills out of sewers and open bodies of water.
WASTE DISPOSAL METHODS (Consult federal, state, and local regulations): Incinerate liquid and diking material after addition of excess inhibitor, in accordance with Federal, State, and Local regulations.

SECTION VII - SPECIAL PROTECTION INFORMATION/CONTROL MEASURES

RESPIRATORY PROTECTION: Use self-contained breathing apparatus when needed.
VENTILATION: Use local ventilation with a minimum capture velocity of 100 ft/min. (30 m/min.) at point of monomer release.
PROTECTIVE GLOVES: Impervious, neoprene
EYE PROTECTION: Safety glasses or goggles.
OTHER PROTECTIVE CLOTHING OR EQUIPMENT: Provide eyewash station.
WORK/HYGIENIC PRACTICES: Wash hands and face before eating, drinking and/or smoking.

The information accumulated herein is believed to be accurate but is not warranted to be whether originating with the company or not. Recipients are advised to confirm in advance of need that the information is current, applicable, and suitable to their circumstances.

FIGURE 20.11 An MSDS for an acrylic monomer.

professional to do? We must assess patient risk on an individual basis and provide the best treatment possible.

B. Labels

It is very important that chemicals be properly labeled. The name of the chemical and other important information should be on each and every chemical container. Chemicals must not be stored in the same refrigerator as food.

C. Disinfectants

Disinfectants can be very irritating to the skin. Many disinfectants are corrosive; that is, they can cause a chemical burn if they come in contact with bare skin. Some disinfectants may penetrate some types of glove material; it is important to pay attention to the manufacturer's instructions for handling a material. Some disinfectants may react with other chemicals used in the office. Avoid such mixing, unless it is known to be safe.

D. Mercury

Mercury is used in the making of dental amalgams, as was discussed in Chapter 6. For many years, concern has been raised about the hazards to patients and dental professionals from exposure to mercury. Mercury was observed to be related to neurological problems even before *Alice in Wonderland* was published in the 1860s. The "Mad Hatter" character was based on hatmakers of the time who became "mad" from their use of inorganic mercury salts to soften fur to make felt hats.

1. Mercury Toxicity

Most forms of mercury can be toxic. The degree of toxicity is related to the chemical form of mercury. Organic forms, such as methyl mercury, are particularly hazardous. These forms are not used in dentistry. Inorganic mercury salts are toxic and are also not used in dentistry. The mercury in dental amalgam is an intermetallic compound and has very low or no toxicity. The most hazardous form of mercury in the dental office is metallic or elemental mercury. In this "quicksilver" form, it becomes volatile, especially if heated. When mercury vapor is inhaled, most is absorbed through the lungs. If liquid mercury or freshly mixed amalgam is handled without gloves, it can be absorbed through the skin. Chronic mercury toxicity affects the central nervous system. In addition, muscle tremors, mouth inflammation, irritability, and decreased kidney function can result from chronic exposure to unsafe levels of mercury. Acute mercury poisoning affects the kidneys.

2. Dental Personnel

Studies have found some dentists to have elevated mercury levels in their blood and urine compared to nondentists. Some dentists have demonstrated early signs of neurological damage. Their offices were found to have poor mercury hygiene habits.

A dental office contains many potential sources for exposure to mercury. Spilled mercury will roll off countertops, hide within cracks in tile floors, or be absorbed by carpets. It is very important that mercury spills be cleaned immediately. Spill kits are available specifically for mercury. Amalgam alloy (the powder) will absorb and react with mercury. Precapsulated amalgam has reduced the need to handle mercury and greatly simplified mercury hygiene. The ADA has published guidelines for mercury hygiene. If good mercury hygiene is practiced in a dental office, then exposure and risk of toxicity are greatly reduced. In fact, this risk is small when compared to the risk posed by infectious agents.

E. Nitrous Oxide

Nitrous oxide (also known as laughing gas) is used as an analgesic in some dental offices. Exposure of dental personnel to nitrous oxide most often occurs during its administration to the patient (if protective measures are not used). Some effects that have been associated with exposure to high levels of nitrous oxide include spontaneous abortion and reduced fertility. Other effects include neurologic, hematologic, immunologic, liver, and kidney problems as well as certain kinds of malignancy. Most data supporting the relationship between nitrous oxide exposure and the occurrence of these problems were obtained before the use of protective measures had been widely implemented.

1. Reproductive Problems

The use of scavenging equipment seems to lessen the risk of spontaneous abortion. In a study published in 1995, women who worked in offices where they were exposed to unscavenged nitrous oxide for 3 hours or more per week had a substantially higher rate of spontaneous abortion than an unexposed group. Those women who worked in offices using scavenging equipment showed no significantly different rate of spontaneous abortion compared to unexposed women. Another study showed that men as well as women were affected by exposure to the gas. Male dentists exposed to high levels of nitrous oxide were also subject to reduced fertility. The mechanism(s) by which nitrous oxide produces these effects is still being investigated.

2. Exposure

Debate exists regarding how much exposure is too much. As of the writing of this chapter, OSHA has not issued regulations about exposure to nitrous oxide. The National Institute of Occupational Safety and Health (NIOSH), the group that researches the hazards of materials and makes recommendations to OSHA, has recommended limiting exposures to a **time-weighted average (TWA)** level of 25 ppm for dental personnel. A TWA measures the average exposure to a chemical over a period of time, and NIOSH has publications giving advice on practical ways to reduce exposures for dental personnel.

3. Measures to Reduce Exposure to Nitrous Oxide

a) Check and maintain the delivery system to prevent leaks. Any leaks must be repaired before the equipment is used again.

b) Employ a scavenging system to reduce the amount of waste gas that is released in the room. Vent the system to the outdoors.

c) Make sure the scavenging system's mask fits the patient.

d) Monitor periodically to determine exposure levels. Commercially available monitoring devices can be used to estimate personnel exposure.

e) Use local exhaust near the patient's mouth to capture excess nitrous oxide.

f) Ensure good room ventilation. The supply and exhaust vents should be well separated to prevent intake of contaminated air.

F. Disposal of Chemicals

Some chemicals can be poured down the drain. For many chemicals, however, it is illegal to do so because they may harm the environment. Proper disposal is required. Unused materials and chemicals may need to be disposed of as hazardous waste. Some, such as amalgam scrap, can be recycled. Radiology wastes, such as developer, film (Ag), and lead foil, can also be recycled. Unfortunately, it is beyond the scope of this text to cover this subject in detail.

V. Emergencies

Emergencies can happen even in the safest and most conscientious dental office. It is important to know what to do in the event of a medical emergency, fire, or other accident. Some state boards require first aid and cardiopulmonary resuscitation training for dentists and dental hygienists. Such training should be considered for all dental personnel. Phone numbers for emergency services, such as "911," local hospitals, poison centers, and so on, should be posted by a phone. Emergency exits and escape routes should be posted as well. Emergency lighting and fire extinguishers should be properly maintained. There is no substitute for training in the event of an emergency. Remember, the most likely person to have a heart attack in the dental office is the dentist. First aid kits, emergency drug kits and emergency equipment, including a defibrillator, should be properly maintained or restocked.

Children in the dental office could be described as trouble waiting to happen. They should not be allowed in office and laboratory areas. They should not be left unsupervised in the clinic and waiting rooms while a patient receives treatment. The waiting room should be childproofed in the same manner as a home. Unused electrical outlets should be covered. Toys should not have small parts that may cause choking. Children should not be allowed to climb on the furniture and disrupt the waiting room. An area with entertainment such as books and puzzles should be provided for young children. Many "kids' movies" are enjoyed by both children and adults.

VI. Putting Risk in Perspective

By now, you might be thinking, "Wow! There are a lot more hazards in this job than I realized. It might be safer to be a stunt double or a rodeo clown!" It is true that many safety issues need to be considered in the dental profession. However, it is also important to remember that the existence of a risk does not automatically result in an injury or an illness.

We face many potential hazards all the time in our daily lives. We routinely cook our food, drive our cars, cut our lawns, and so on without giving too much thought about the risks we take in doing these activities. Most of the time, our daily activities do not result in accidents because we take the necessary precautions to avoid problems as a natural part of performing the task. In general, what precautions should you take to reduce your risk of injury or illness in the dental office?

- Keep yourself informed. Learn about hazards and how to protect yourself. Some information has been provided under specific topics in this chapter, but research continues. Professional groups often are aware of the latest studies and may be a good source of information.
- Use proper procedures and equipment to minimize the chance of injury.
- Be prepared to deal with accidents or emergencies.
- At least annually, or more frequently if problems arise, do a self-audit. Take the time to examine what you are doing, and consider if it could be done better or more safely, not only regarding your own safety but also that of your patients and coworkers.

VII. Acknowledgement

The authors thank Dr. Daniel Della-Giustina, Professor of Industrial and Management Systems Engineering at West Virginia University, for his review of this chapter.

SUMMARY

Universal precautions must be followed for each patient. By OSHA mandate, dental care providers must wear appropriate gloves, mask, eye protection, and clothing during patient care activities involving saliva and blood. Patient treatment gloves are available in a variety of materials. Use of gloves does not preclude hand washing.

Facial masks are available in various styles and should be changed for each patient. For protection against inhalation of highly infectious aerosols, HEPA masks must be worn. Protective eyewear with side shields must be worn during procedures that may generate aerosol, splatter, or projectiles.

Dental instruments and equipment are categorized as critical, semicritical, or noncritical to determine the required method for decontamination. Intermediate-level disinfectants should be used for disinfecting noncritical items. Acceptable surface disinfectants are registered with the U.S. EPA. They are tuberculocidal and kill both lipophilic and hydrophilic viruses. An effective way to maintain surface disinfection is to cover the cleaned and disinfected surface with protective barriers.

Precautions must be taken to avoid punctures when handling sharp objects. Housekeeping practices must also be followed to protect the patient and dental care providers from cross-contamination. Each dental office and laboratory must have a written exposure control plan that includes the necessary steps to prevent exposure to bloodborne pathogens. This plan must be updated annually and be reviewed by all dental care workers in the facility.

Physical hazards in a dental office include the typical trips and falls that are risked in everyday life. Injuries from chemicals and equipment are also a concern. Flammable materials and oxygen increase the risk of fire, and autoclaves can be another cause of burns. Latex gloves, disinfectants, and other chemicals can cause skin problems. Ergonomics, for obvious reasons, are a particular concern for dental hygienists. Proper posture, lighting, and instrumentation reduce the likelihood of musculoskeletal problems. Chemicals should be properly stored and labeled. Mercury and nitrous oxide are known hazards in the dental office, but following proper procedures will reduce their risk. Preparations should be made to handle emergencies.

Learning Activities

1. Observe a student in the clinic. Make notes detailing proper and improper ergonomic practices.
2. Observe a student in the clinic. Look for errors in infection control procedures.
3. Make an inventory of the items in a cabinet of clinical supplies. Note which are hazardous materials.
4. Make a list of your daily activities, and note the procedures and equipment that are used to reduce risk.

Review Questions

1. By OSHA mandate, the dental care provider must wear appropriate PPE (glove, mask, eye protection, and clothing) during patient care involving contact with blood and saliva. This PPE should be worn only in the clinical treatment area.
   a) The first statement is true; the second statement is false.
   b) The first statement is false; the second statement is true.
   c) Both statements are true.
   d) Both statements are false.
2. Which type of patient care glove is recommended for noninvasive intraoral procedures?
   a) Sterile surgeon's
   b) Nonsterile exam
   c) Copolymer "overgloves"
   d) Utility gloves
3. Hands should be washed before putting on and after removing gloves. If not visibly soiled and for non-surgical procedures, hands may be cleaned by applying an alcohol-based solution and rubbing the hands for 15 seconds until the agent is dry.
   a) The first statement is true; the second statement is false.
   b) The first statement is false; the second statement is true.
   c) Both statements are true.
   d) Both statements are false.
4. Which type of protective glove should be worn when hand-scrubbing contaminated instruments before sterilization?
   a) Exam gloves
   b) Over gloves
   c) Utility gloves
   d) Sterile surgeon's gloves
5. What type of PPE must be worn while treating a patient with a highly infectious disease, such as tuberculosis, spread by aerosol?
   a) Sterile surgeon's gloves
   b) Full face shield
   c) HEPA mask
   d) Standard face mask
6. Anesthetic needles, orthodontic wire, irrigation needles, and anesthetic cartridges must not be disposed of in the regular trash. These items must be disposed of in appropriately labeled cardboard boxes or plastic bags.
   a) The first statement is true; the second statement is false.
   b) The first statement is false; the second statement is true.
   c) Both statements are true.
   d) Both statements are false.
7. All of the following chemicals are acceptable surface disinfectants except one. Which one is the exception?
   a) Phenols
   b) Iodophors
   c) Chlorine
   d) Quaternaries
   e) Glutaraldehydes
8. An acceptable surface disinfectant must be tuberculocidal and kill both hydrophilic and lipophilic viruses. Hydrophilic viruses are much harder to kill than lipophilic viruses.
   a) The first statement is true; the second statement is false.
   b) The first statement is false; the second statement is true.
   c) Both statements are true.
   d) Both statements are false.
9. According to Spalding's Classification of Inanimate Objects, critical items are those items that may penetrate soft tissue or bone. These items must be sterilized by heat or high-level disinfection.
   a) The first statement is true; the second statement is false.
   b) The first statement is false; the second statement is true.
   c) Both statements are true.
   d) Both statements are false.
10. Surface disinfection occurs after an intermediate-level disinfectant is sprayed onto a surface and allowed to air-dry. Disinfection, however, is not effective unless the surface is first cleaned.
   a) The first statement is true; the second statement is false.
   b) The first statement is false; the second statement is true.
   c) Both statements are true.
   d) Both statements are false.

11. Safety equipment in the dental office should include the following except:
   a) A fire extinguisher
   b) GFI outlets
   c) Steel-toed shoes
   d) Neoprene (rubber) gloves
   e) Eye protection

12. Health care workers have exhibited health problems from exposure to the following except:
   a) Mercury
   b) Disinfectants
   c) Latex gloves
   d) Nitrous oxide
   e) Fluorescent lighting

13. Several chemicals used in the dental office penetrate latex gloves. Information on the proper protective gloves may be found in the MSDS.
   a) The first statement is true; the second statement is false.
   b) The first statement is false; the second statement is true.
   c) Both statements are true.
   d) Both statements are false.

14. Which of the following does not contribute to musculoskeletal problems?
   a) Poor lighting
   b) Poor posture
   c) Indirect vision
   d) Repetitive motions

15. The most hazardous form of mercury encountered in a dental office is:
   a) Mercury vapor
   b) Liquid mercury
   c) Dental amalgam
   d) Amalgam scrap

Supplemental Readings

ADA Council on Scientific Affairs. Dental mercury hygiene recommendations. J Am Dent Assoc 2003;134:1498–1499.

ADA Council on Scientific Affairs. Office emergencies and emergency kits. J Am Dent Assoc 2002;133:364–365.

ADA Council on Scientific Affairs, ADA Council on Dental Practice. Nitrous oxide in the dental office. J Am Dent Assoc 1997;128:364–365.

Alvarez M, Unraveling the Mystery of the Material Safety Data Sheet (MSDS). http://www.osh.net/articles/archive/osh_basics_2000_dec28.htm

Babich S, Burakoff RP. Occupational hazards of dentistry, a review of literature from 1990. N Y State Dent J 1997;63:26–31.

Baratz RS. Minimizing health hazards in the dental workplace, a critical review. Dentistry 1990;10:5–29.

Bednarch H, Eklund K. Management of postexposure prophylaxis. Access 2003;17(2):35–44.

Bednarch H, Eklund K. OSHA compliance directive. Access 2003;17(1):32–34.

Carpal tunnel syndrome: can it be prevented? Dent Hygienist News 1992;Winter:1–3.

Centers for Disease Control and Prevention. Guidelines for Infection Control in Dental Health-Care Settings—2003. MMWR 2003 52(RR-17).

Clark M, Brunick A. Handbook of Nitrous Oxide and Oxygen Sedation. 2nd ed. St. Louis: Mosby, 2003.

Cleveland JL, Barker LK, Cuny EJ, Panlilio AL; National Surveillance System for Health Care Workers (NaSH) Group. Preventing percutaneous injuries among dental health care personnel. J Am Dent Assoc 2007;138:169–178.

Cottone JA, Terezhalmy GT, Molinari JA. Practical Infection Control in Dentistry. 2nd ed. Baltimore: Williams & Wilkins, 1996; Chapters 8–12, 14, 18, and 19.

Graham C. Ergonomics in dentistry, Part 1. Dentistry Today 2002;21(4):98–103.

Graham C. Ergonomics in dentistry, Part 2. Dentistry Today 2002;21(5):106–109.

Hamann CP, DePaola LG, Rodgers PA. Occupation-related allergies in dentistry. J Am Dent Assoc 2005;136:500–510.

Mandel ID. Occupational risks in dentistry: comforts and concerns. J Am Dent Assoc 1993;124(10):40–49.

Michalak-Turcotte C. Controlling dental hygiene work-related musculosketal disorders: the ergonomic process. J Dent Hygiene 2000;74:41–48.

Miller C. Have a written exposure control plan for the office. RDH 2000;20(7)38,50.

Miller C, Palenik CJ. Infection Control and Management of Hazardous Materials for the Dental Team. 2nd ed. St. Louis: Mosby, 1998; Chapters 8 and 10–12.

OSAP. From Policy to Procedure: OSAP's Guide to the Guidelines. Annapolis: OSAP, 2004.

21

Disinfection of Impressions, Dentures, and Other Appliances and Materials

Carol Spear, B.S.D.H., M.S.

Objectives

After studying this chapter, the student will be able to do the following:

1. Describe an effective infection-control protocol for handling impressions and dental appliances that are transferred between the dental operatory and the dental laboratory within the dental office or to an outside commercial laboratory.
2. Discuss and demonstrate the procedure for disinfecting dental impressions.
3. Explain and demonstrate the procedure for disinfecting dentures and other dental appliances after they have been processed or adjusted.
4. Describe and apply the infection-control protocol that must be followed when grinding or polishing dentures and other appliances.
5. Review the preferred method (or methods) of sterilizing or disinfecting instruments or items used during manipulation of dental materials and prostheses.

INTRODUCTION

The primary goal of infection control is to prevent cross-contamination between patients and dental care providers. Because impressions or appliances contaminated by saliva or blood are often transported to and from in-office or remote dental laboratories, the potential for cross-contamination exists. Therefore, when these items are being handled, an infection-control protocol must be explicitly communicated among and observed by the office staff as well as between the office and any remote dental laboratory.

Such an infection-control protocol should include guidelines for the proper handling and disinfection or sterilization of impressions, dentures, appliances, and the equipment or materials used during the processing of these items. Attention must also be given to the personal protective equipment that is worn when handling these items and to the physical layout of the laboratory (see Chapter 20).

Acceptable disinfectants include glutaraldehydes, iodophors, sodium hypochlorite, synthetic phenols, dual or synergized quaternaries, and sodium bromide and chlorine, although all impression materials are not compatible with all disinfectants. Use of quaternaries or sodium bromide and chlorine for disinfecting impressions and prostheses is not found in the literature; however, if you select either of these chemicals for use as such in your dental office or laboratory, test it on samples of materials to check for compatibility. In addition, glutaraldehydes should never be sprayed because they are extremely toxic as aerosols.

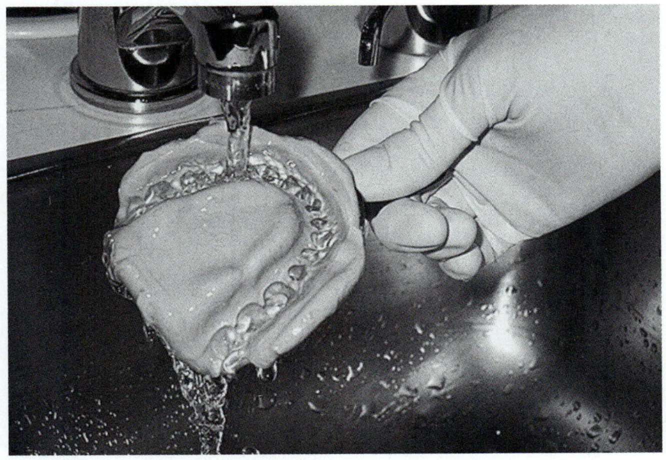

FIGURE 21.1 Rinsing an impression with running water.

I. Disinfection of Impressions

A. Personal Protective Equipment

Wear protective eyewear, an outer cover gown with long sleeves, a mask, and gloves when handling a contaminated impression until it has been disinfected.

B. Rinse the Impression

Immediately after an impression is taken in the dental operatory, rinse it under running water to remove any saliva or blood (Fig. 21.1). This step is essential for optimum disinfection of the impression.

C. Disinfection Techniques

Once the impression has been rinsed and shaken to remove excess water, it must be disinfected. This may be accomplished by immersing the impression in, or spraying it with, an acceptable disinfectant (Table 21.1).

Table 21.1 Recommended Disinfectants for Impression Materials[a]

Impression Material	Glutaraldehydes	Iodophors	Sodium Hypochlorite (1:10 Dilution)	Synthetic Phenols
Alginate	No	Yes	Yes	No
Silicone	Yes	Yes	Yes	Yes
Polyether	No	Yes	Yes	Yes
Polysulfide	Yes	Yes	Yes	Yes
Zinc oxide–eugenol (ZOE) paste	No	Yes	No	?
Compound	No	Yes	Yes	?
Reversible hydrocolloid	No	Yes	Yes	?
Wax bites	No	Yes	No	No

Adapted from Merchant VA. Infection control in the dental laboratory environment. In: Cottone JA, Terezhalmy GT, Molinari JA. Practical Infection Control in Dentistry. 2nd ed. Philadelphia: Lippincott Williams & Wilkins, 1996:240–244; and Miller CH, Palenik CJ. Infection Control and Management of Hazardous Materials for the Dental Team. 2nd ed. St. Louis: Mosby, 1998:213–215.

[a]Bite registrations are made of various materials and should be disinfected with the same chemical that is used on the impression. Incompatibility between materials and disinfectants, as well as between the same material of different companies, may exist.

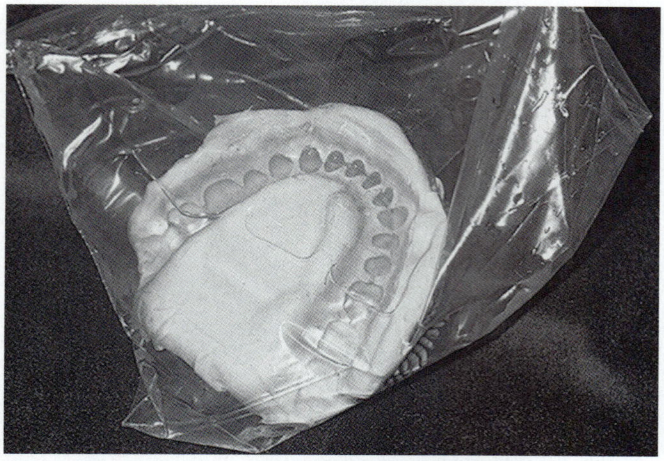

FIGURE 21.2 Impression immersed in disinfectant within a zippered plastic bag.

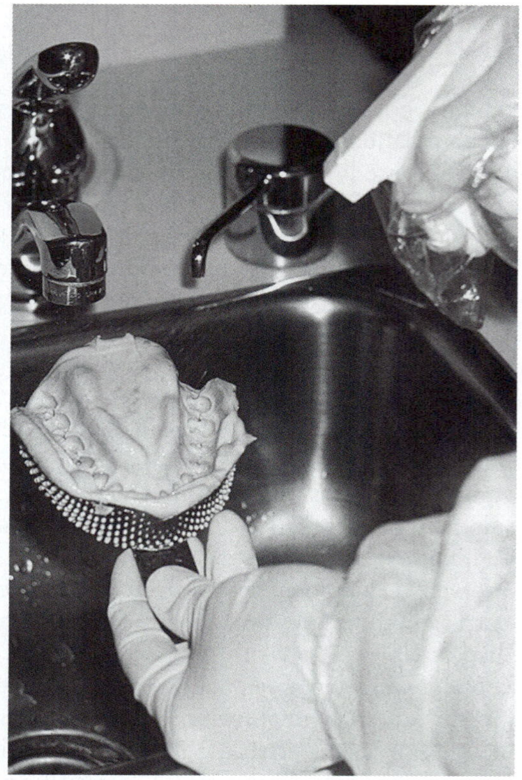

FIGURE 21.3 Disinfection of an impression by spraying and then immediately sealing it in a plastic bag for 15 minutes.

1. Disinfection of an Impression by Immersion

Disinfection by immersion is preferred over disinfection by spraying. Spraying may not be as effective because constant contact of the disinfectant with all surfaces of the impression cannot be assured.

a) Place the rinsed impression into a zippered plastic bag containing appropriate disinfectant (Fig. 21.2).
b) Leave the impression immersed in the disinfectant for 15 minutes. Polyether and hydrocolloid impression materials may be adversely affected by disinfectants; therefore, limit their immersion time to 10 minutes.
c) Remove the impression from the disinfectant.
d) Rinse the impression with running water, and shake to remove excess water.

2. Disinfection of an Impression by Spraying

a) Spray the rinsed impression and impression tray with an acceptable disinfectant (Fig. 21.3).
b) Seal the sprayed impression in a zippered plastic bag for 15 minutes.
c) Remove the impression from the sealed bag.
d) Rinse the impression with running water, and shake to remove excess water.

D. Pour the Impression

Once the impression has been disinfected, it may be poured with the desired gypsum product.

II. Disinfecting Dentures and Other Appliances

Dental prostheses must be cleaned and disinfected in the dental laboratory before they are returned to the dental office for patient try-in. Likewise, dental appliances that have been worn by the patient must be cleaned and disinfected before repairs or adjustments are made in the dental laboratory. Handle contaminated appliances with gloved hands, and return disinfected dental prostheses to the patient with clean, gloved hands.

A. Chairside Adjustments

For chairside adjustments of appliances, use a unit dose of abrasive, a sterile handpiece and burs, and a sterile rag wheel for polishing. This eliminates the need to disinfect the prosthesis during handling.

B. Clean the Prosthesis

Clean the denture or appliance before disinfecting it.

1. Brush the prosthesis with an unused toothbrush or denture brush, or clean it in an ultrasonic unit.
2. To avoid cross-contamination during ultrasonic cleaning, place the appliance in a zippered plastic bag or sterile glass beaker that contains fresh ultrasonic cleaning solution. Then, place the closed bag or beaker into the ultrasonic solution in the unit's holding tank.
3. Rinse the prosthesis after cleaning, and shake to remove excess water.
4. Use air-powered blasters only on cleaned and disinfected prostheses.

Table 21.2 Disinfection of Dentures and Other Appliances[a]

Prosthesis	Glutaraldehydes	Iodophors	Sodium Hypochlorite (1:10 Dilution)	Synthetic Phenols[b]
Complete dentures (acrylic/porcelain)	No	Yes	Yes	Yes
Removable appliances (metal/acrylic)	No	Yes	No	Yes
Fixed prostheses (metal/acrylic/porcelain)	Yes	Yes	No	Yes

Adapted from the American Dental Association (ADA) Council on Scientific Affairs and ADA Council on Dental Practice. Infection control recommendations for the dental office and the dental laboratory. J Am Dent Assoc 1996;127:678; and Miller CH, Palenik CJ. Infection Control and Management of Hazardous Materials for the Dental Team. 2nd ed. St. Louis: Mosby, 1998:210–213.

[a]Routine immersion is 15 minutes. Limit exposure time of metal-containing prostheses to 10 minutes.

[b]Because of their expense, the practical use of phenols is limited to spraying rather than immersion.

C. Disinfect the Prosthesis

Disinfect the cleaned dental prosthesis with the acceptable disinfectant (Table 21.2).

1. Place the prosthesis in a zippered plastic bag containing an acceptable disinfectant for 15 minutes. Immersing a metal prosthesis in a hypochlorite solution may damage the metal; therefore, use one of the other suggested disinfectants.
2. Spraying the prosthesis with a disinfectant and then sealing the sprayed appliance in a zippered plastic bag for 15 minutes is an alternative disinfection method. However, the American Dental Association recommends immersion in disinfectant rather than spraying.

D. Rinse the Prosthesis

Thoroughly rinse the prosthesis as soon as it is removed from the disinfectant. Disinfectant remaining on the appliance may cause tissue irritation.

E. Store the Prosthesis

Store the disinfected prosthesis in a clean, zippered plastic bag containing a mixture of mouthwash and water.

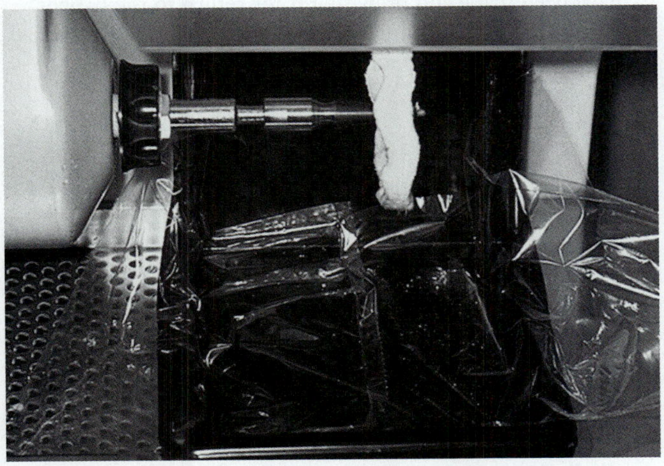

FIGURE 21.4 Dental lathe with sterile rag wheel attached and a single-use liner.

Table 21.3 Recommended Sterilization/ Disinfection Methods for Dental Laboratory tems

Item	Sterilization/Disinfection Method[a]
Impression trays	
Aluminum	AC, CV, EO, DH
Chrome-plated	AC, DH, CV, EO
Custom acrylic resin	EO, Discard
Plastic	EO, Discard
Bowls, water baths	
Stainless steel	DH, CV, AC
Rubber	EO, CV, CDS
Burs	
Carbon steel	DH, CV, EO, Discard
Steel	DH, CV, EO, AC, Discard
Tungsten-carbide	DH, EO, CV, AC, Discard
Polishing wheels and disks	
Garnet and cuttle	DH, CV
Rag	AC, DH
Rubber	DH, CV
Stones	
Diamond	DH, CV, EO, AC
Abrasive (polishing)	AC, CV, EO, DH
Shade guides	CDI, CDS, EO
Spatulas, knives	AC, CV, EO

Adapted from Merchant VA. Infection control in the dental laboratory environment. In: Cottone JA, Terezhalmy GT, Molinari JA. Practical Infection Control in Dentistry. 2nd ed. Philadelphia: Lippincott Williams & Wilkins, 1996:248–250; and the American Dental Association (ADA) Council on Scientific Affairs and ADA Council on Dental Practice. Infection control recommendations for the dental office and the dental laboratory. J Am Dent Assoc 1996;127:676–677.

[a]Preferred method is listed first. AC, autoclave; CDI, chemical disinfect (immersion); CDS, chemical disinfect (spray, wipe, spray); CV, chemical vapor; DH, dry heat; EO, ethylene oxide.

III. Infection-Control Protocol for Grinding or Polishing Dentures or Other Appliances

Laboratory work may be performed on items or materials that have been used or worn by the patient. However, these items or materials must first be disinfected. Manipulation of these materials still requires following an infection-control protocol.

A. Make certain the ventilation system in the room is properly functioning.

B. During operation of the dental lathe (Fig. 21.4), wear protective eyewear and a mask. See Chapter 20 regarding the safe use of a lathe.

C. Clean and disinfect the dental lathe at least once daily.

D. Use sterile rag wheels and stones as well as fresh pumice and pan liners for each prosthesis.

IV. Sterilization/Disinfection of Items Used During Manipulation of Dental Materials and Prostheses

All items that come in contact with oral tissues or touch objects that contact oral tissues must be heat sterilized. These items include metal impression trays, burs, rag wheels and disks, metal spatulas, and glass mixing slabs. Other items that do not come in direct contact with oral tissue may be disinfected or, if disposable, discarded (Table 21.3).

Remember, before an item can be successfully sterilized or disinfected, it must first be cleaned of all bioburden.

SUMMARY

Because many impressions or appliances contaminated with saliva or blood are often transported to and from in-office or remote dental laboratories, the potential for cross-contamination exists. Therefore, an infection-control protocol must be observed by the office staff and between the office and remote dental laboratory.

Personal protective equipment must be worn when handling contaminated impressions and dental prostheses.

Impressions must be rinsed, shaken to remove excess water, and then immersed or sprayed with an acceptable disinfectant.

Dental prostheses must be cleaned and disinfected in the laboratory before they are sent to the office for patient try-in. Likewise, appliances worn by the patient must be cleaned and disinfected before adjustments are made in the dental laboratory.

When grinding or polishing dentures or other appliances on a dental lathe, use sterile rag wheels and stones as well as fresh pumice and pan liners for each prosthesis. Wear protective eyewear and a mask, and make certain that the room is properly ventilated.

Metal impression trays, burs, rag wheels and disks, metal spatulas, and glass mixing slabs must be heat sterilized. Other items should be disinfected or, if disposable, discarded.

Learning Activities

Divide students into pairs, and have each pair observe and critique the infection-control protocol for the situations that follow.

1. Handling an impression before pouring a model. Each student can take an impression of another student's dentition and pour the models.
2. Polishing an appliance in the laboratory after adjustments have been made and preparing it for return to the patient. This can be a mock situation because appliances from actual patients may not be readily available.

Review Questions

1. Immediately after an impression is taken, it must be rinsed under running water to remove saliva or blood. This step is essential before the impression can be disinfected.

   a) The first statement is true; the second statement is false.
   b) The first statement is false; the second statement is true.
   c) Both statements are true.
   d) Both statements are false.

2. It is recommended that all but one of the following types of impression materials be immersed in a disinfectant for 15 minutes. Which one is the EXCEPTION?
a) Alginate
b) Polysulfide
c) Compound
d) Wax bites

3. Chairside adjustments of appliances may be performed with a unit dose of abrasive, a sterile handpiece and bur, and a sterile rag wheel for polishing. This eliminates the need for disinfecting the appliance before handling.
a) The first statement is true; the second statement is false.
b) The first statement is false; the second statement is true.
c) Both statements are true.
d) Both statements are false.

4. What is the routine immersion time for disinfecting a metal dental prosthesis?
a) 5 minutes
b) 10 minutes
c) 15 minutes
d) 20 minutes

5. All but one of the following steps must be performed when disinfecting a removable dental appliance before making laboratory adjustments. Which one is the exception?
a) Handle contaminated appliance with gloved hands
b) Clean ultrasonically by placing the appliance directly into the solution in the ultrasonic unit holding tank
c) Rinse the appliance under running water
d) Shake to remove excess water
e) Disinfect the appliance by spraying it with, or immersing it in, an acceptable disinfect and then allowing contact for the specified time of 10 to 15 minutes

6. In the laboratory, when polishing dentures that have been worn by a patient, it is not necessary to use a sterile rag wheel. This is because the dentures will be disinfected before and after any adjustment is made.
a) Both the statement and the reason are correct
b) Neither the statement nor the reason is correct
c) The statement is correct, but the reason is not

7. After chairside adjustments are made to a dental prosthesis, it is cleaned, disinfected, rinsed, and stored. The recommended storage method is:
a) Placement of the prosthesis back on patient's stone cast
b) An individualized, plastic, closed container for each patient, similar to those used for overnight soaking
c) A zippered plastic bag containing mouthwash and water
d) A zippered plastic bag containing sterile water

8. Which of the following disinfectants are suitable for all impression materials?
a) Glutaraldehydes
b) Synthetic phenols
c) Iodophors
d) Sodium hypochlorite

9. The primary goal of infection control when handling and disinfecting impressions, dentures and appliances is to:
a) Protect the patient from the laboratory personnel
b) Protect the laboratory personnel from the patient
c) Prevent cross-contamination
d) Prevent contamination of equipment in the dental laboratory

10. Disinfection by immersion is preferred over disinfection by spraying. The most important reason is because:
a) Office personnel don't have the necessary time available to spray thoroughly
b) The spraying procedure must be performed twice, with ten minutes in between
c) Constant contact of the spray with all surfaces of the impression cannot be assured
d) The aerosol produced is usually toxic

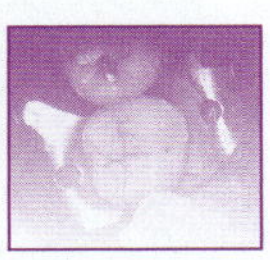

Supplemental Readings

American Dental Association (ADA) Council on Scientific Affairs and ADA Council on Dental Practice. Infection control recommendations for the dental office and the dental laboratory. J Am Dent Assoc 1996;127:672–680.

Cottone JA, Terezhalmy GT, Molinari JA. Practical Infection Control in Dentistry. 2nd ed. Philadelphia: Lippincott Williams & Wilkins, 1996, Chapters 16 and 17.

Miller CH, Palenik CJ. Infection Control and Management of Hazardous Materials for the Dental Team. 2nd ed. St. Louis: Mosby, 1998, Chapter 15.

OSAP. From Policy to Practice: OSAP Guide to the Guidelines. Annapolis: OSAP, 2004, Chapter 18.

22

General Rules for Handling Dental Materials

Objectives

After studying this chapter, the student will be able to do the following:

1. Give reasons why correct dispensing, timing, and mixing of materials are important.
2. Discuss the difference in setting times of dental materials in the oral cavity and on the instrument tray.
3. Summarize the recommended guidelines for light-activated dental materials.

INTRODUCTION

A dental hygienist must understand the composition, use, physical properties, and manipulation techniques for commonly used dental materials. This will promote office efficiency, economy of materials, and quality care for the patient. Based on this understanding, a few general rules should be followed to ensure success in the manipulation and application of these dental materials.

I. Follow the Manufacturer's Directions

A. It is very important to read, understand, and follow the directions that accompany dental materials. One not only should read the directions but also should understand why each step is performed in the manner directed by the instructions.

B. Office personnel should save copies of directions for the materials used in that office. It is recommended that these copies be kept in a file. Thus, if the directions for a kit are lost, a copy will be readily available.

C. When a new material is purchased, practice using the new material at least once before using that material clinically. Check the 'feel' of the new product; how does it compare to other products?

D. Store materials in a cool dry place. The shelf-life of many materials is lengthened by refrigeration. On the other hand, some materials will gel or mixtures separate if they are refrigerated. See manufacturers' directions for proper storage.

II. Mixing and Setting Times

A. Use a clock that has a second hand or displays seconds to time etching, mixing, setting, and other important time spans. This applies to the clinic and to the laboratory.

B. The mouth is a warm environment. Therefore, materials set faster when in the mouth than on the instrument tray or countertop. If a material is set on the instrument tray, it is set in the mouth. Exceptions to this rule are materials that set by cooling, such as impression compound, and light-activated materials.

C. The setting of some materials is also accelerated by the humidity of the mouth.

III. Dispensing Materials

A. Dispense materials properly, as directed by the instructions. Recap tubes and bottles after dispensing materials. Volatile solvents will evaporate from open containers. The chemical composition of the material will then change; performance will suffer.

B. Dispense equal lengths, not equal volumes, of pastes.

C. Dispense consistent drops. Allowing the drop to run onto a mixing pad before it forms into a separate drop and falls from the dispensing tip will result in inconsistent drops. Inconsistent and incorrect powder/liquid ratios result from this type of dispensing method. The powder/liquid ratio is an important determinant of properties.

D. Fluff powders if recommended by the manufacturer. Alginate powder should be tumbled periodically to fluff the powder; it is not necessary to fluff alginate for every impression.

IV. Mixing

A. Mix dental materials aggressively. They are not alive; they cannot be harmed. After mixing alginate, your arm should be tired.

B. The setting rate of some materials is affected by the mixing technique that is used.

C. When mixing cements, force the powder into the liquid.

V. Light-Activated Materials

A. You can undercure, but you cannot overcure, light-activated materials.

B. Maintain a space between the tip of the curing light and the oral tissues. Some light tips become quite warm and may overheat the tooth or soft tissues.

C. Light-activated materials will begin to set in ambient room light. Therefore, light-cure materials need to be covered if not immediately used.

VI. Contamination

Contamination by oral fluids is bad for all materials. This concept applies to adhesive restorative materials as well as nonadhesive restorative materials. It is critical to keep teeth clean and, sometimes, dry when using adhesive materials.

SUMMARY

Following and saving the manufacturer's directions when using any dental material will enhance the quality of patient care. Manipulation factors, such as proper dispensing, correct mixing, adequate curing, and avoiding contamination, will promote successful use and service of the dental material.

Learning Activities

1. Develop a list of dental materials commonly used in your clinic. Which of the general rules presented in this chapter apply to these materials?
2. Can you locate the manufacturer's directions for the materials listed in learning activity #1?

Review Questions

1. When dispensing paste/paste dental materials, equal ______ are usually the proper method for proportioning the two pastes.
   a) Weights
   b) Volumes
   c) Lengths
   d) Loads
2. It is important to read the directions that accompany a dental product. It is more important to understand the dispensing, mixing, and handling of a dental material.
   a) The first statement is true; the second statement is false.
   b) The first statement is false; the second statement is true.
   c) Both statements are true
   d) Both statements are false

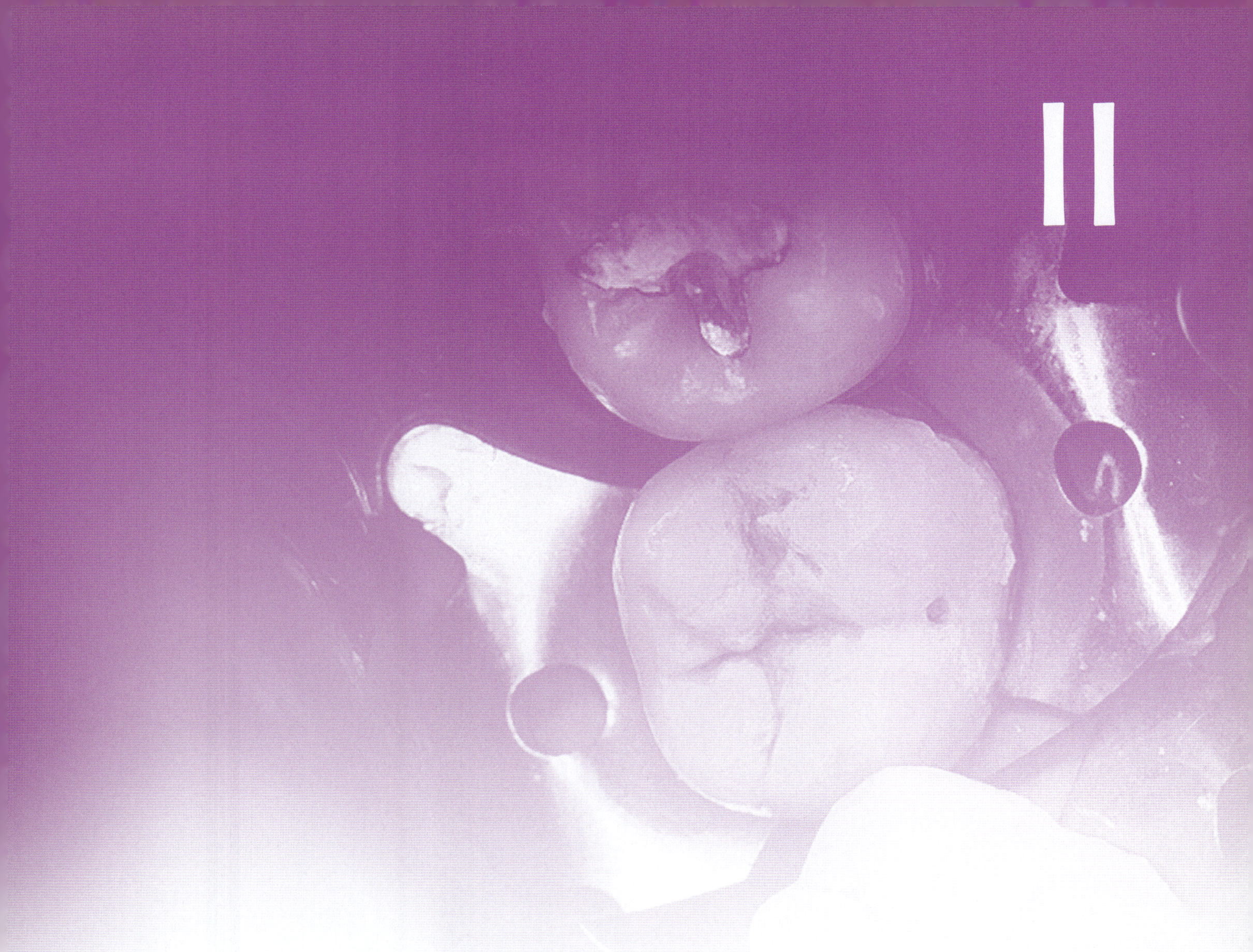

II

Laboratory and Clinical Applications

23

Mixing Liners, Bases, and Cements

Key Words/Phrases

obtundent

exothermic

Objectives

After performing the laboratory/clinical exercises in this chapter, the student will be able to do the following:

1. Describe the use or purpose of the following materials:
   - Calcium hydroxide
   - Zinc phosphate
   - Glass ionomer
   - Zinc oxide–eugenol (ZOE)
   - Temporary cement
2. Demonstrate the proper mixing technique for the materials listed above, and then evaluate the mix according to the criteria stated in this chapter.
3. Recall the approximate mixing and setting times for the liners, bases, and cements discussed in this chapter.
4. Clean the cement spatula or mixing instrument and slab with the appropriate cleaning agent before the material sets.

INTRODUCTION

The various cements, bases, and liners used in restorative dentistry were discussed in detail in Chapter 7. This discussion included the use, composition, and physical as well as chemical properties of each material. As stated earlier, these materials can be used as base or lining agents, cementation materials, or permanent or temporary restorations. This chapter will focus on the manipulation of some of these commonly used materials.

I. Purpose

Mixing of cements, bases, and liners is not a procedure that the dental hygienist typically performs on a routine basis. However, the hygienist may be asked by the dentist to mix these materials if the dental assistant is absent. This situation would include using them as a temporary restoration. Step-by-step instructions for measuring and mixing some of the commonly used cements, bases, and liners serve as the basis for this chapter.

II. Calcium Hydroxide Base/Liner Material

A. Use

Calcium hydroxide may be used in pulp capping and as a base/liner under other dental restorative materials in deep preparations.

B. Protective Properties

Calcium hydroxide serves as a protective barrier between tooth tissues (dentin and pulp) and acid-containing cements and restorative materials.

C. Measuring

1. The items necessary for mixing calcium hydroxide base/liner material are listed in Table 23.1.
2. Dispense small, but equal, amounts on a paper mixing pad, as shown in Figure 23.1.

D. Mixing

1. Mix thoroughly with the crook of a small, ball-pointed instrument until a uniform color is achieved. A completed mix of calcium hydroxide is shown in Figure 23.2.
2. Mixing should be completed within 10 seconds.
3. The criteria for a correct mix of calcium hydroxide are listed in Table 23.2.

Table 23.1 Armamentarium for Mixing Calcium Hydroxide Base/Liner Material

Paper mixing pad
Mixing instrument
Calcium hydroxide base and catalyst
2 × 2 gauze

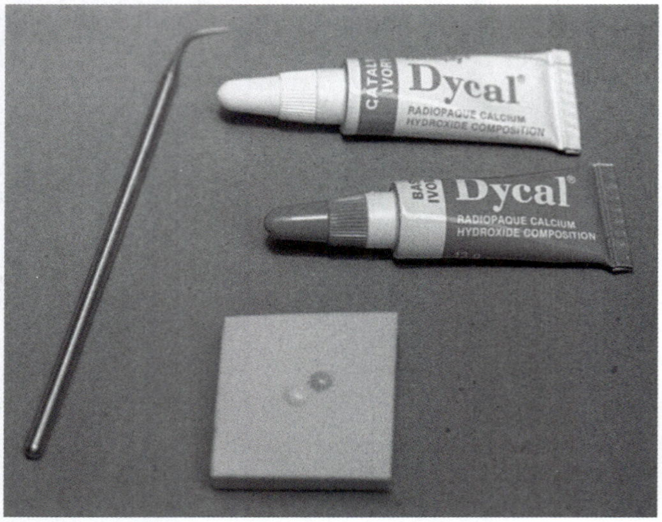

FIGURE 23.1 Calcium hydroxide dispensed on a paper mixing pad.

E. Application

Use the tip of the ball-pointed instrument to place the mixed material on the floor of the cavity preparation. Avoid placing the mixed material on walls and margins, and avoid placing it in large amounts.

F. Setting

1. The setting time of mixed calcium hydroxide is 2 to 3 minutes on the mixing pad at normal room temperature.
2. The setting time for a pulp capping or base/liner will be greatly decreased in the mouth because of the moisture of dentin.

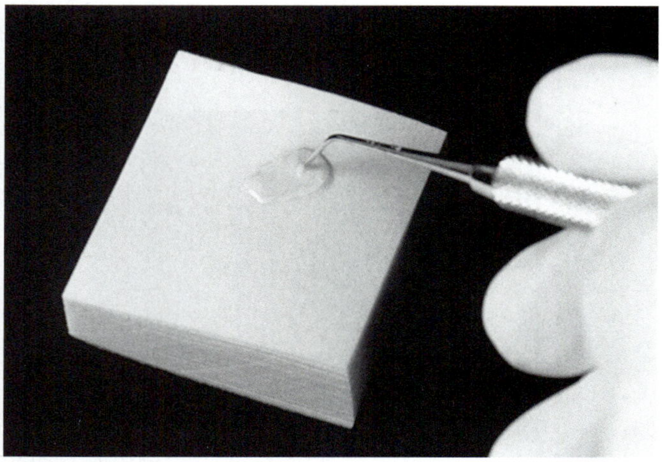

FIGURE 23.2 Completed mix of calcium hydroxide.

Table 23.2 Evaluation Criteria for Mixing Calcium Hydroxide Material

1. An appropriate amount is dispensed.
2. Mixing occurs within 10 seconds.
3. Completed mix is uniform in color.

III. Zinc Phosphate Cement

A. Use

As discussed in Chapter 7, zinc phosphate cement is used to lute inlays, crowns, bridges, orthodontic bands, and other appliances to tooth structure. It can also be used as a base material under restorations.

B. Related Information

Remember that when the powder and liquid are mixed, an **exothermic** (heat-releasing) reaction occurs. Again, this was discussed in Chapter 7. To dissipate the heat of this reaction:

1. A large portion of the glass slab must be used during mixing.
2. The powder must be added in small increments.
3. The mixing time must extend to 1.5 to 2 minutes.

C. Measuring, Mixing, and Application for Luting Consistency

1. The items necessary to mix zinc phosphate cement are listed in Table 23.3.
2. This technique is described in detail, along with illustrations, in Chapter 7.
3. The number of drops of liquid and scoops of powder that are required can be found in the directions provided by the manufacturer.
4. Forcibly mix the powder into the liquid by increments. A figure-8 motion is frequently used, as shown in Figure 23.3. Sometimes, a back-and-forth stropping motion is used.
5. The mixing time is usually 15 seconds for each increment.

Table 23.3 Armamentarium for Mixing Zinc Phosphate Cement

Zinc phosphate powder
Zinc phosphate liquid
Liquid dispenser
Powder scoop
Cement spatula
Glass slab
Solution of bicarbonate of soda (optional)

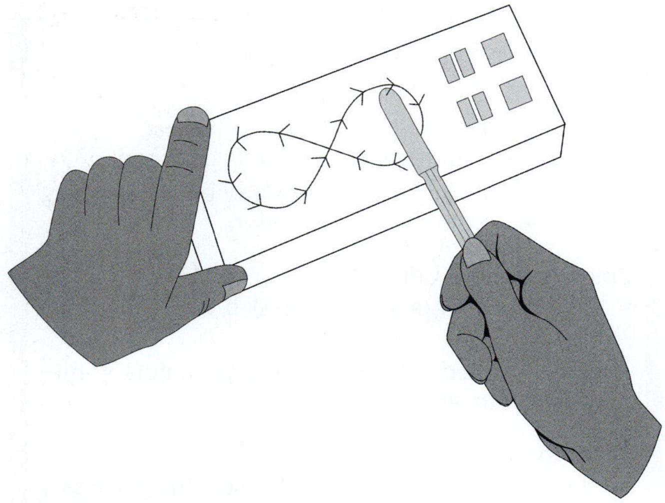

FIGURE 23.3 Figure-8 mixing technique for a dental cement.

6. Remember that for correct luting consistency, the cement should form a "1-inch string" between the spatula and the slab, as shown in Figure 7.6*E*.
7. The Skill Performance Evaluation sheet for mixing zinc phosphate cement to a luting consistency is located in Appendix 2.

D. Measuring, Mixing, and Application for Base Consistency

1. The difference between luting consistency and base consistency is that a higher powder/liquid ratio is used for base consistency. This means that fewer drops of liquid will be needed to mix the cement for a base consistency. The specific amounts to be used are provided by the manufacturer.
2. The powder is also divided into increments for base consistency, but this may include the division of one powder increment into yet smaller increments.
3. The mixing time is approximately the same as that for luting consistency (1.5–2 minutes).
4. The completed mix should be thick, putty-like, and able to be rolled into a ball.
5. The base consistency for zinc phosphate is shown in Figure 7.6*F*.
6. The Skill Performance Evaluation sheet for mixing zinc phosphate cement to a base consistency is located in Appendix 2.

E. Setting

The setting time for both consistencies of zinc phosphate cement is between 5 and 9 minutes.

F. Clean-up

Tap water is used to clean the spatula and glass slab before the cement sets. If the mix has set on the

Tips for the Clinician

Calcium Hydroxide Liner/Base
- Mix until a homogeneous color is obtained.
- Wipe the mixing instrument clean before applying material to the cavity preparation.

Zinc Phosphate Cement
- Mix using a large area of the slab to dissipate the heat.
- When finished, clean the slab and spatula immediately with soap and water.

Glass Ionomer Cement
- When dispensing the liquid, take the necessary time to make precise, uniform drops.
- Mixing time is short, usually 45 seconds or less.

Zinc Oxide–Eugenol (ZOE) Cement
- Use firm pressure with the flat face of the spatula when incorporating powder.
- Enough powder has been incorporated for a base consistency when the mix "flakes" from the spatula pressing on the cement.

Temporary Cement
- Mix until a homogeneous color is obtained.

spatula and slab, the instruments can be cleaned by soaking in a solution of bicarbonate of soda (baking soda) and water.

IV. Glass Ionomer

A. Use

Glass ionomer cement may be used as a base, a luting agent, or a restorative material. As a luting agent, it is used to permanently cement crowns, bridges, and orthodontic bands. As a base, it is used as a thermal insulating material in deep cavity preparations.

B. Related Information

As discussed in Chapter 7, glass ionomer cements are high in strength and low in solubility. Compared to other cements, they are also relatively kind to the pulp. They chemically bond to tooth structure, and they release fluoride ions into enamel and dentin, which is believed to reduce recurrent decay. It is for these reasons this cement has become so popular.

C. Dispensing Systems

Glass ionomer may be dispensed in three ways:

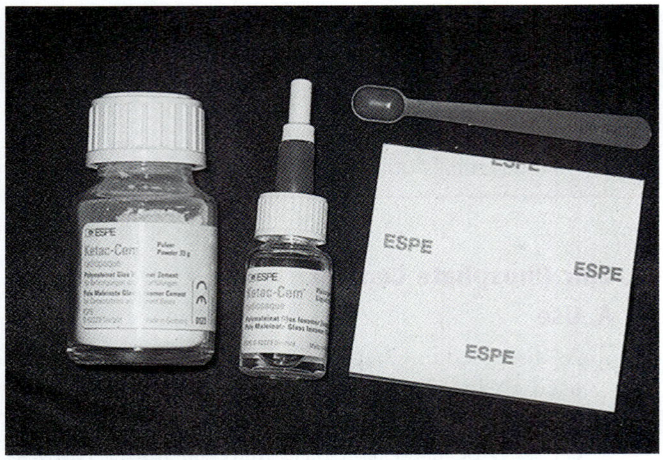

FIGURE 23.4 Glass ionomer cement: powder, liquid, dispensing scoop, and paper pad.

1. Powder/Liquid Systems

Examples of powder and liquid are shown in Figures 7.7*A* and 23.4. This chapter will focus on the powder/liquid systems.

2. Disposable Capsules

The capsule form of glass ionomer cement is illustrated in Figure 7.7*B*. This capsule is mixed in an amalgamator, similar to the way in which an amalgam capsule is mixed. Specific directions for mixing are provided by the manufacturer.

3. Paste/Paste Systems

Paste/paste systems are now being marketed. One such dispensing device is pictured in Figure 23.5. Pressing the lever dispenses the proper ratio of each paste. The material is mixed as in other paste/paste systems until a homogeneous color is obtained.

D. Measuring and Mixing for Luting Consistency

The items necessary to mix a powder/liquid glass ionomer cement are listed in Table 23.4.

1. Measure the Powder

a) Shake the jar of powder to "fluff" the contents.
b) Fill, but not pack, the dispensing scoop.
c) Remove the scoop from bottle by sliding it against the plastic lip in the neck of the bottle, as shown in Figure 23.6. This action will eliminate excess powder.
d) Place one scoop of powder on the paper mixing pad.

2. Measure the Liquid

a) Hold the bottle vertically when dispensing the liquid so that precise and uniform drops will be produced, as shown in Figure 23.7.
b) Dispense appropriate number of drops of liquid.

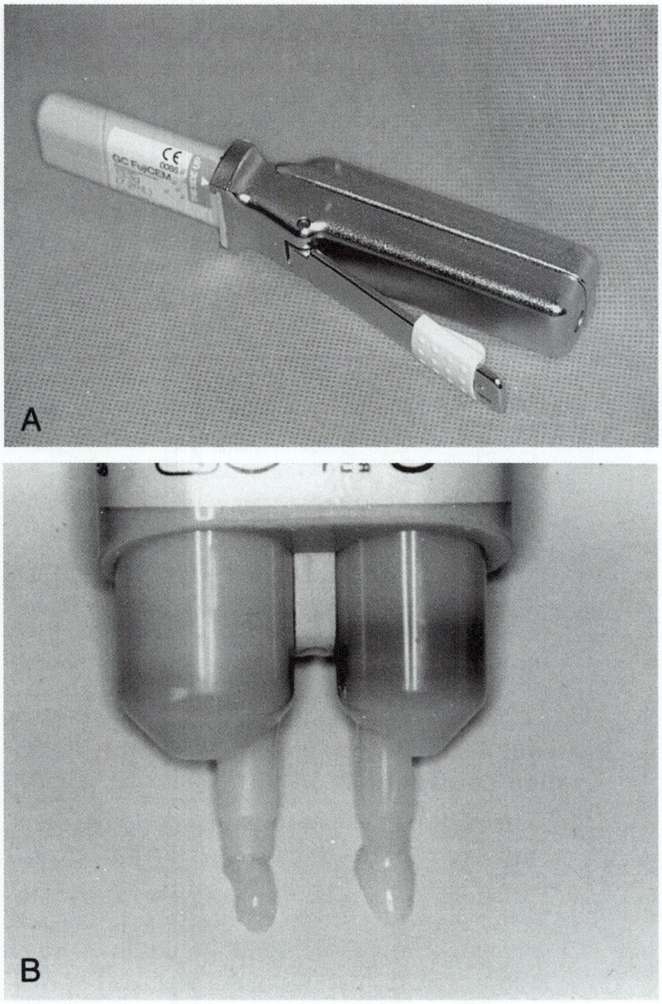

FIGURE 23.5 **A.** Dispenser for a paste/paste glass ionomer material. **B.** Paste materials being dispensed.

3. Mix the Powder and Liquid

To mix, the powder should be added to the liquid in one portion. The typical luting consistency is such that the material stretches 0.5 inch between the spatula and slab, as shown in Figure 23.8.

4. Mixing Time

Mixing time ranges between 15 and 30 seconds. Refer to the manufacturer's instructions.

Table 23.4 Armamentarium for Mixing Glass Ionomer Cement
Glass ionomer powder
Glass ionomer liquid
Dispensing scoop
Liquid dispensing tip
Treated paper pad
Cement spatula

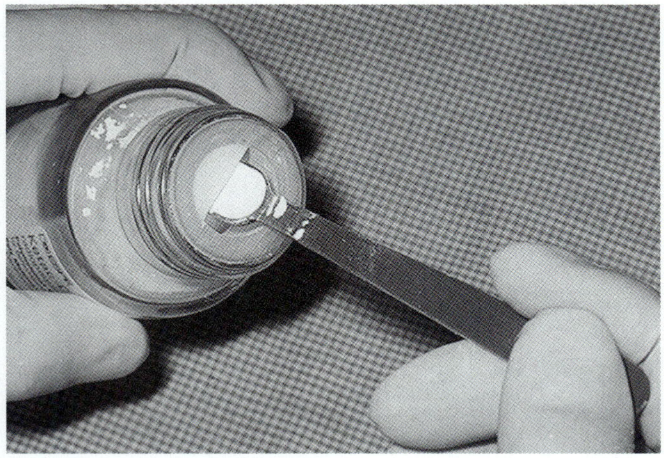

FIGURE 23.6 Eliminating excess glass ionomer powder.

5. Immediate Use

The cement must be used while glossy. When the surface becomes dull, the setting reaction has begun, and the mix should be discarded.

6. Skill Performance Evaluation Sheet

The Skill Performance Evaluation sheet for mixing glass ionomer luting cement is located in Appendix 2.

E. Measuring and Mixing for Base Consistency

1. For bases and liners, a glass ionomer product is employed that differs from the product that is normally used for luting. The product used in this instance has a higher powder/liquid ratio.
2. The powder and liquid are usually measured and mixed in the same manner for base consistency as that described earlier for luting consistency.
3. The mixing time for base consistency ranges between 15 and 30 seconds. Specific directions for mixing are provided by the manufacturer.

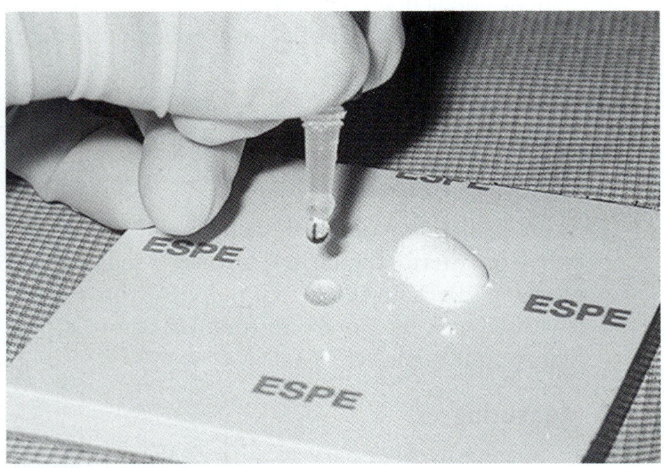

FIGURE 23.7 Measuring glass ionomer liquid.

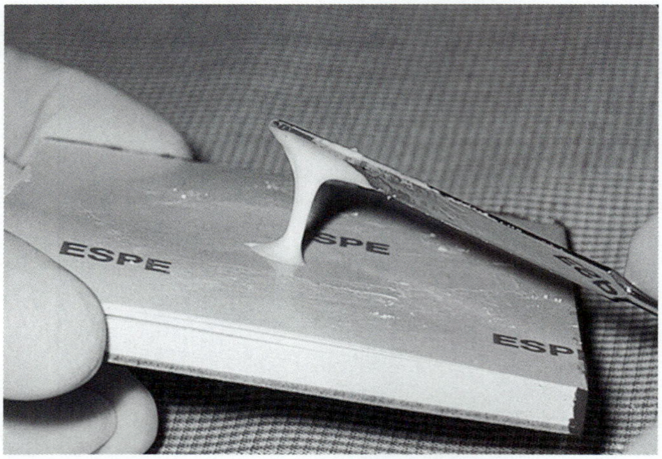

FIGURE 23.8 Proper luting consistency of glass ionomer cement.

F. Setting

The setting time for both consistencies of glass ionomer is usually 7 minutes.

G. Clean-up

The spatula can be cleaned with soap and water before the cement has set.

H. Light-Activated Glass Ionomer Materials

Light-activated glass ionomer materials are typically used as a base or restorative material. They may be a powder/liquid system in bottles or in capsule form. The manufacturer's directions should be followed for mixing.

V. Zinc Oxide–Eugenol (ZOE) Cement

A. Use

Zinc oxide–eugenol (ZOE) cement is one of the least irritating dental materials, and it may be used for several purposes:

1. To cement a temporary crown while a permanent one is being fabricated
2. To create an insulating base under permanent restorations
3. To provide a sedative or **obtundent** (soothing agent) filling for sensitive teeth

B. Protective Properties

As an insulating base, ZOE cement will protect the pulp from thermal trauma. It also has a sedative and soothing effect on the dental pulp; for this reason, it is used as a temporary restoration before a permanent one is placed.

C. Measuring

1. The items necessary to mix ZOE cement are listed in Table 23.5.

Table 23.5 Armamentarium for Zinc Oxide–Eugenol (ZOE) Cement
Zinc oxide powder
Powder scoop
Eugenol
Eye dropper
Glass slab or treated paper pad
Cement spatula
2 × 2 gauze sponges
Isopropyl alcohol

2. Using the measuring scoop provided by the manufacturer, place one scoop of powder on a glass slab or treated paper pad. The product, scoop, and slab are illustrated in Figure 23.9.
3. Dispense two drops of eugenol liquid by holding the dropper perpendicular to the glass slab. The drops should not touch the powder, but they should be placed near it. The measured powder and liquid are shown in Figure 23.10.

D. Mixing Technique for a Base/Temporary Restoration Consistency

1. While holding the spatula in a "flat" position, draw approximately half the powder into the liquid.
2. Using a small portion of the mixing surface, spatulate the powder and liquid in a quick motion with the flat side of the spatula. The mixing technique is illustrated in Figure 23.11.
3. Continue to incorporate small portions of powder by deliberately "pressing" the powder into the mix with the spatula. The mix must be thick, putty-like, and almost "crumbly."
4. The mix should be completed in 1.5 minutes.

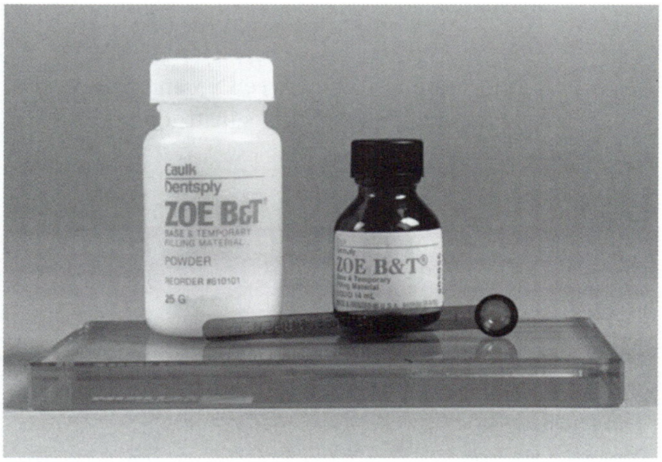

FIGURE 23.9 Zinc oxide and eugenol, measuring scoop, and glass slab.

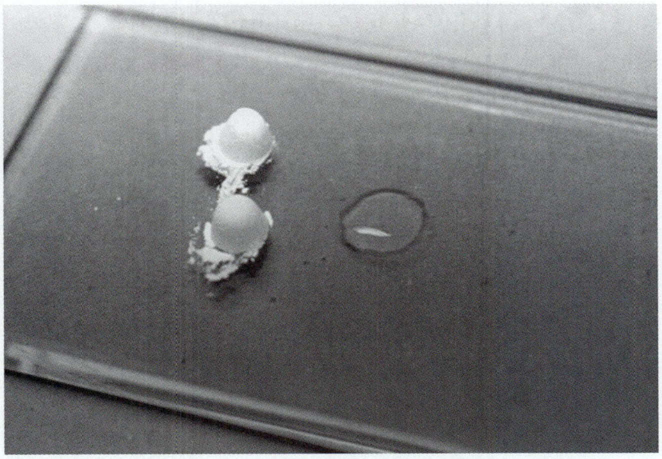

FIGURE 23.10 Zinc oxide and eugenol measured for a base or temporary restoration.

5. The Skill Performance Evaluation sheet for mixing ZOE cement to a base/temporary consistency is located in Appendix 2.

E. Application

1. Gather the cement into one mass on the slab.
2. The cement may be rolled with the fingers to form a ball.
3. Any suitable flat-bladed instrument, such as a plastic filling instrument (PFI), may be used to carry portions of the cement to the cavity preparation. The fingers or instrument may first be dipped into some extra powder to prevent the mixed cement from sticking.

F. Setting

The setting time is between 2.5 and 3.5 minutes in the mouth.

G. Clean-up

The slab and spatula may be cleaned with isopropyl alcohol and 2 × 2 gauze sponges.

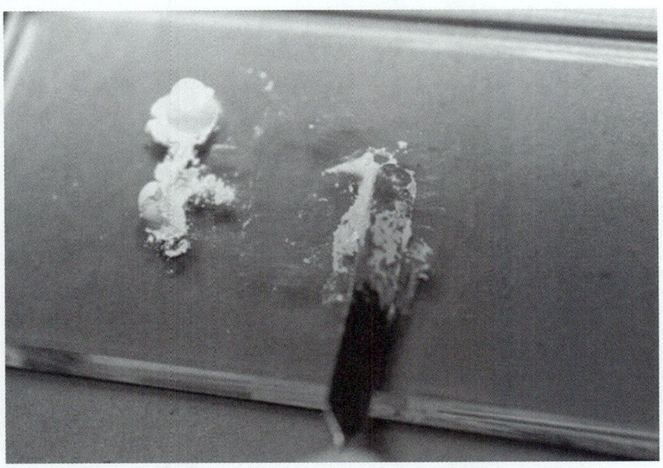

FIGURE 23.11 Mixing of zinc oxide and eugenol for a base or temporary restoration.

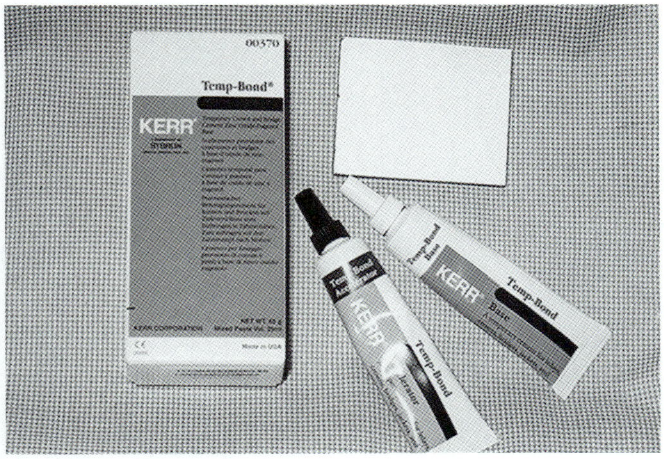

FIGURE 23.12 Base and accelerator of a temporary cement.

VI. Temporary Cement

A. Use

Temporary cement may be used in trial cementing of permanent restorations or in cementing of temporary crowns, bridges, or splints.

B. Properties

Temporary cements have high flow, which permits the restoration to be easily seated. They are strong enough to withstand the stresses of mastication, yet they allow the restoration to be easily removed when desired.

C. Measuring

The components of temporary cement are a base and a catalyst, which are supplied in two tubes. An example of this material is shown in Figure 23.12.

1. The items necessary to mix temporary cement are listed in Table 23.6.
2. Squeeze equal lengths from each tube onto a paper mixing pad, as shown in Figure 23.13.

D. Mixing

1. Thoroughly mix the pastes within 30 seconds.
2. Mix the pastes in a small area until a homogeneous color is obtained.
3. Material should form a string when stretched from the mixing pad. The mixing procedure is illustrated in Figure 23.14.

Table 23.6 Armamentarium for Mixing a Temporary Cement
Cement spatula
Paper mixing pad
Temporary cement base and catalyst

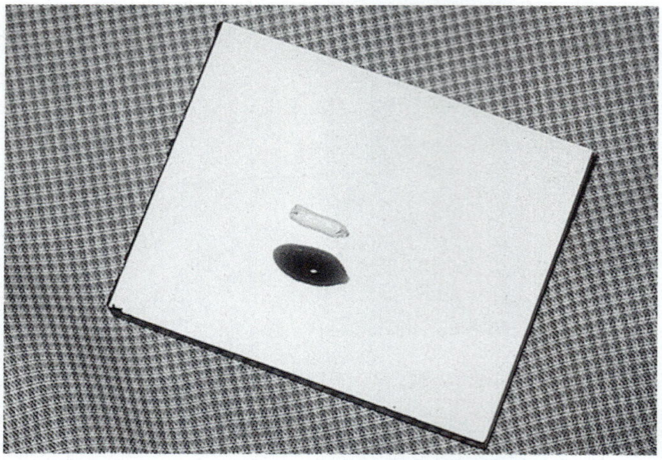

FIGURE 23.13 Equal lengths of temporary cement pastes dispensed on a paper mixing pad.

4. Criteria for the correct mix of a temporary cement are listed in Table 23.7.

E. Application

Spread a thin layer of cement over all areas of the restoration that will contact the preparation.

F. Setting

The setting time is approximately 2 minutes in the mouth.

Precautions

Calcium Hydroxide Liner/Base

- Humid conditions will accelerate the setting reaction.

Zinc Phosphate Cement

- Do not cool the slab beyond the dew point. Condensation will adversely affect the mix and setting time.
- It is critical to mix the cement slowly, in increments, to dissipate heat.
- Make sure the bottles are always properly closed to prevent absorption of moisture.

Glass Ionomer Cement

- The mix must be used while it is glossy.

Zinc Oxide–Eugenol (ZOE) Cement

- For a base consistency, it is important that enough powder is incorporated. Otherwise, the mixture will be "sticky" and difficult to place.

Temporary Cement

- Humidity will accelerate the setting of ZOE-based materials.

Table 23.7 Evaluation Criteria for Mixing Temporary Cement

1. An appropriate amount is dispensed.
2. Mixing occurs within 30 seconds.
3. Completed mix is uniform in color.
4. Cement makes a string between slab and spatula.

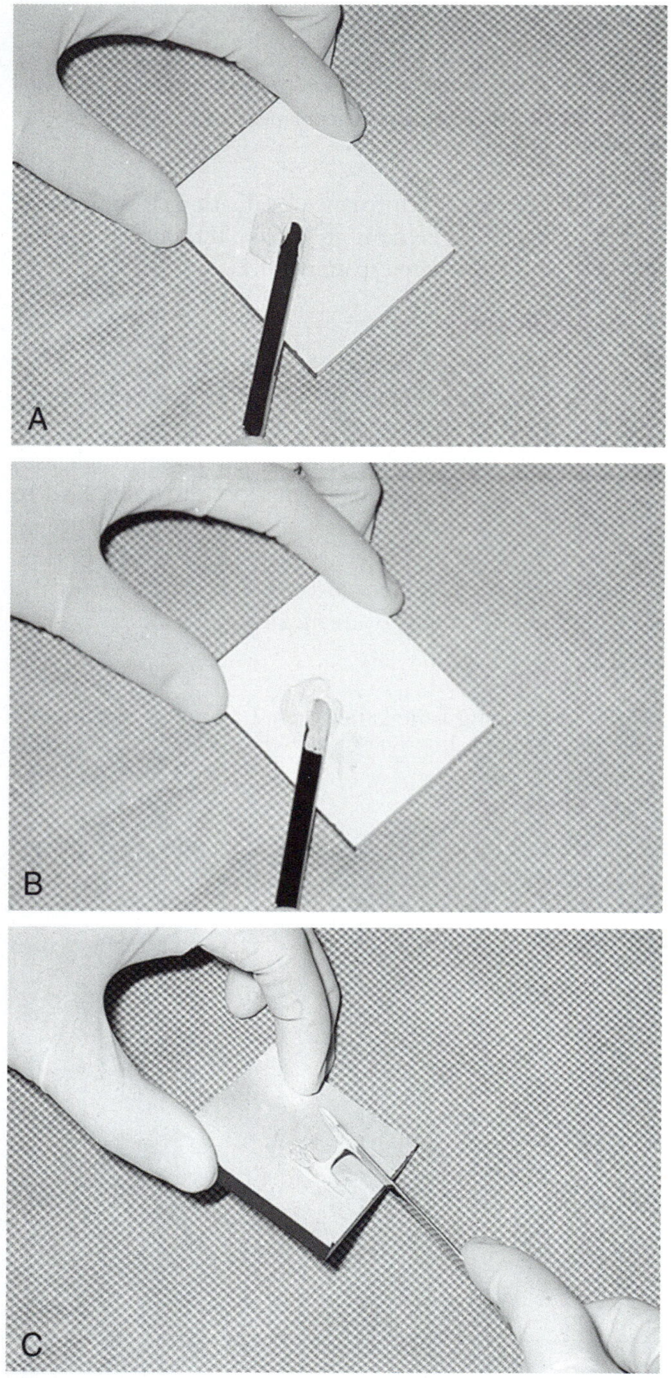

FIGURE 23.14 Mixing procedure for a temporary cement. **A** and **B.** Mixing. **C.** Proper luting consistency.

Summary

Each of the various cements used in dentistry has its own uses, mixing and setting times, mixing techniques, and characteristics of a proper mix. Proper handling will result in the optimum properties for each material.

Calcium Hydroxide Liner/Base

- Dispense small, but equal, amounts on the paper pad.
- Use an appropriate instrument to mix the components in 10 seconds.
- Apply material with a clean instrument. Avoid using large increments.

Zinc Phosphate Cement (Luting and Base Consistencies)

- Dispense the manufacturer's recommended amounts of liquid and powder for the desired consistency.
- Divide into appropriate increments.
- Mix using a large portion of the slab.
- Add powder in small increments.
- Mixing time ranges from 1.5 to 2 minutes (usually 15 seconds per increment).
- Luting consistency: Material forms a 1-inch string between the slab and the spatula.
- Base consistency: Thick, putty-like, and will roll into a ball.

Glass Ionomer Cement

- Measure the powder by "fluffing" the container and then sliding the scoop against the lip of bottle to eliminate excess powder.
- Measure the liquid by holding the bottle vertically to get precise, uniform drops.
- Powder is added to the liquid in one or two portions. Mixing time is usually 30 to 45 seconds.
- Luting consistency: Mix should form a 0.5-inch string between the slab and the spatula.

Zinc Oxide–Eugenol (ZOE) Cement (Base and Temporary Restoration)

- Measure the powder and the liquid according to manufacturer's directions.
- Draw half the powder into the liquid.
- Spatulate using the flat of the spatula and a small portion of the slab surface.
- Continue adding small portions of powder by "pressing" it into the mix.
- Mixing should take approximately 1.5 minutes to complete.
- The finished mix should appear thick, putty-like, and almost "crumbly."

Temporary Cement

- Squeeze equal lengths from each tube onto the paper pad.
- Thoroughly mix to a homogeneous color.
- Material should form a string when stretched from the pad.
- Apply the material to the entire surface to be luted.

Review Questions

1. Which of the following dental cements is significantly accelerated by humidity?
a) Calcium hydroxide
b) ZOE
c) Both
d) Neither

2. Which dental cement is used to calm an irritated dental pulp?
a) Calcium hydroxide
b) ZOE
c) Zinc phosphate
d) Glass ionomer

3. Which dental cement is mixed slowly to dissipate the heat of the setting reaction?
a) Calcium hydroxide
b) ZOE
c) Zinc phosphate
d) Glass ionomer

4. Which dental cement should be used before its glossy appearance becomes dull?
a) Calcium hydroxide
b) ZOE
c) Zinc phosphate
d) Glass ionomer

5. Clean-up of the mixing slab and cement spatula are best accomplished before the material sets. After cement materials set, they are easily cleaned by soap and water.
a) The first statement is true; the second statement is false.
b) The first statement is false; the second statement is true.
c) Both statements are true.
d) Both statements are false.

Supplemental Readings

Anderson PC, Burkard MR. The Dental Assistant. 6th ed. Albany, NY: Delmar, 1987:423–450.

Bird DL, Robinson DS. Modern Dental Assisting. 7th ed. Philadelphia: Saunders, 2002:716–728.

Directions for Dycal. Milford, DE: Dentsply/Caulk, Dentsply International, Inc.

Directions for Temp-Bond Temporary Cement. Romulus, MI: Kerr Corporation.

Directions for ZOE B. & T. Milford, DE: L.D. Caulk Co., Division Dentsply International, Inc.

Ketac-Cem Radio opaque—Information for Use. Norristown, PA: ESPE America.

Application and Removal of the Rubber Dam

Rebecca Thomas, B.S.D.H.

24

Key Words/Phrases

aspirating
isolation
ligature
septum
winged clamps
wingless clamps

Objectives

After performing the laboratory/clinical exercises in this chapter, the student will be able to do the following:

1. List the indications and contraindications for placing the rubber dam.
2. Describe the purpose of the rubber dam armamentarium (rubber dam, rubber dam clamp, punch, etc.).
3. Summarize the steps for placement and removal of the rubber dam.

INTRODUCTION

This chapter will provide basic, step-by-step instructions for application and removal of the rubber dam. In most cases, one of two placement techniques is routinely used: the one-step method, in which the dam and clamp are placed simultaneously or the two-step method, in which the clamp is placed on the anchor tooth and the dam material is then stretched over the clamp. In this chapter, the one-step method will be the technique of choice.

Clinical success of rubber dam **isolation** (exposure of selected teeth) is determined by the placement and retention methods of the clinician. Problems with rubber dam placement are often the result of torn rubber dam material, improper hole size and placement, or inadequate tautness of frame placement.

The rubber dam is usually placed after local anesthesia has been administered and while waiting for that anesthetic to take effect. Proper rubber dam placement can be achieved by a clinician in 3 to 5 minutes or, with a team approach, within 2 minutes.

I. Purpose and Indications

Proper isolation during technique-sensitive dental procedures is important but is also sometimes difficult to achieve. The purpose of rubber dam placement is to improve the overall quality of dental treatment. Indications for rubber dam placement are moisture control, visibility, patient protection, and patient treatment.

Rubber dam placement allows the clinician to achieve a dry field by isolating the tooth (or teeth) indicated for treatment. This prevents the patient from **aspirating** (drawing into the lungs) dental objects that are used during the procedure.

II. Contraindications

Rubber dam placement is contraindicated for patients who are claustrophobic, suffer from severe asthma, or have trouble breathing through their noses. Other contraindications include patients with teeth that are not fully erupted and may not hold the clamp and patients who cannot tolerate the clamp without anesthesia.

III. Procedure

The success of rubber dam placement is dependent on the technique and skill of the clinician. The items needed for rubber dam placement are listed in Table 24.1.

Table 24.1 Armamentarium for Placing the Rubber Dam
Clamps
Floss
Forceps
Frame
Ink pad
Ligatures
Mirror
Plastic filling instrument (PFI)
Punch
Rubber dam material
Scissors
Stamp

A. Choosing the Rubber Dam Material

Selection of the rubber dam material is based on the clinician's preferences regarding size, color, and thickness. Traditional dam material is latex rubber, but nonlatex rubber dams are available for patients or operators with a latex hypersensitivity. The most common size is the precut, 6 × 6-inch square, which is used for isolation of posterior teeth in the permanent dentition. Another common size is the precut, 5 × 5-inch square, which is used for primary dentition or anterior applications. A continuous roll of rubber dam material is available as well, and the choice of colors ranges from pastels to browns and greens. The color is used to contrast the tooth, making the treatment field more visible.

The rubber dam is also available in thicknesses (gauges) of thin, medium, and heavy. The medium rubber dam is widely used because of its ease of handling and resistance to tearing. The armamentarium, less the rubber dam stamp and ink pad, is shown in Figure 24.1.

B. Preparing the Rubber Dam Material

1. Stamp the Material

The rubber dam stamp has markings for the average permanent and primary dentitions. Use of the stamp allows several sheets of dam material to be marked in advance. A rubber dam stamp and stamped dam are shown in Figure 24.2.

2. Punch the Holes

Next, holes are punched into the rubber dam to correspond to the teeth that are to be isolated. The rubber dam punch usually consists of a rotating punch plate that allows holes of five or six different sizes and a metal point (punch) that

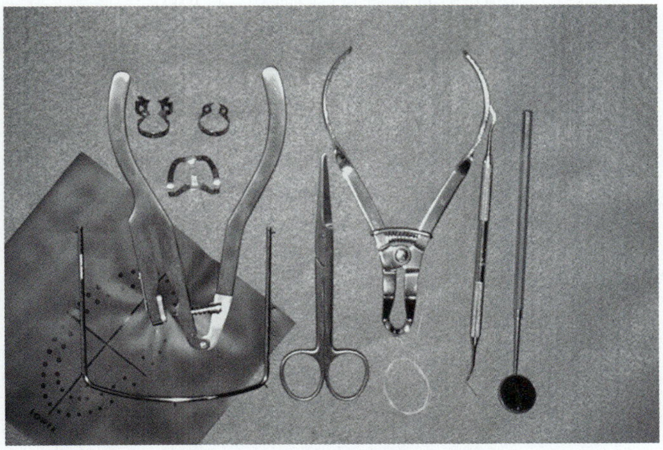

FIGURE 24.1 The basic rubber dam armamentarium.

creates the holes. The larger holes are used for posterior teeth, the smaller holes for premolars and canines, and the smallest holes for incisors. Correct hole size plays a critical role in successful tooth isolation.

3. Prepare the Clamp

The clamp is prepared by threading floss through the facial hole and then tying a knot. This prevents the clamp from being aspirated should it spring free, and allows for quick retrieval. The clamp is used as an anchor for the dam material and to retract the gingiva. Both **winged clamps** (clamps with extra projections) and **wingless clamps** (clamps without projections) are available, as are different shapes and sizes to fit the primary and permanent teeth, as shown in Figure 24.3. The extra projections of winged clamps allow the dam and the clamp to be applied simultaneously, as shown in Figure 24.4. When wingless clamps are used, they are applied first to the tooth, and the rubber dam is then stretched over the clamp and the tooth.

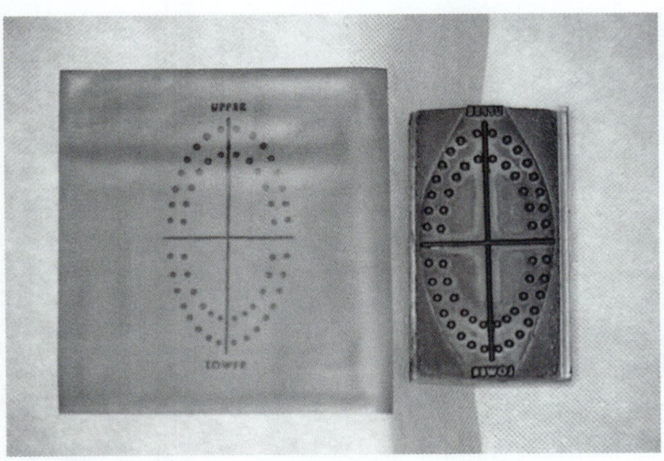

FIGURE 24.2 A rubber dam stamp and a stamped dam.

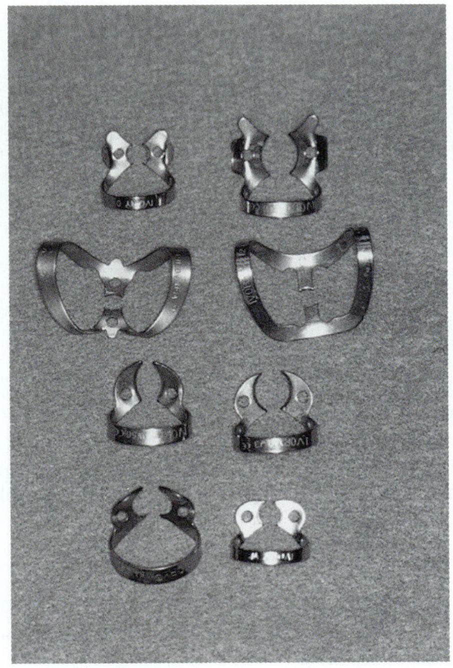

FIGURE 24.3 An assortment of rubber dam clamps: winged clamps (*top*), wingless clamps (*bottom*), and "butterfly-shaped" clamps (*middle*) used to isolate anterior teeth and the buccal of some posterior teeth (see Figure 24.8).

C. Placement of the Rubber Dam

1. Check the patient's record for documentation of the area that needs to be isolated and for potential contraindications. Inform the patient of the procedure and the steps involved in placing the rubber dam.

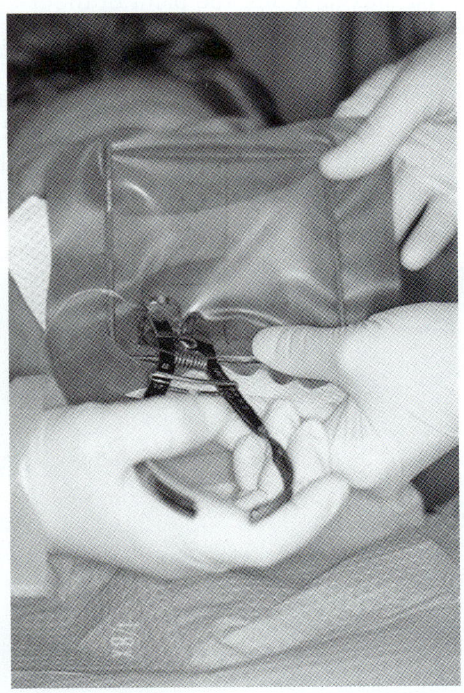

FIGURE 24.4 The transfer of the rubber dam, clamp, and forceps for a mandibular tooth.

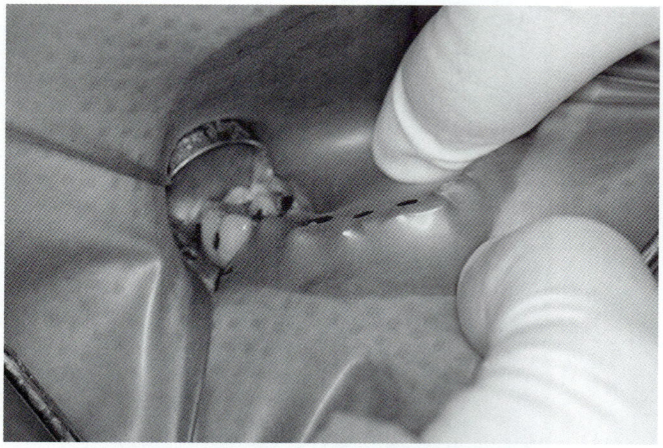

FIGURE 24.5 Once the anchor tooth is clamped, the last-punched hole is placed first for easier orientation when placing rubber dam over the rest of the teeth.

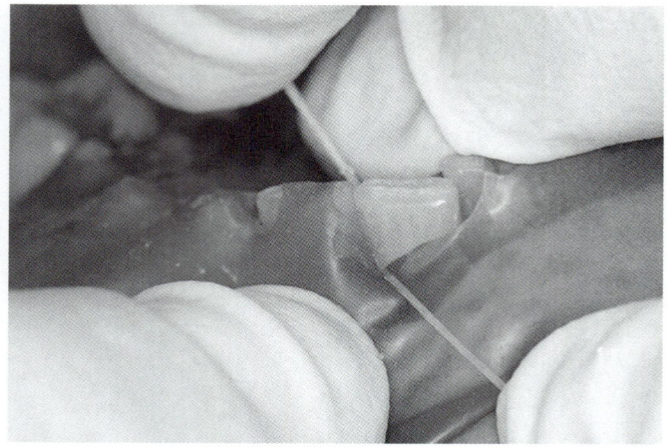

FIGURE 24.6 Flossing of the dam septum past tooth contact areas.

2. Prepare the rubber dam by stamping and punching the correct holes that will be needed for isolation.
3. Stretch the dam material over the bow and wings of the clamp.
4. Place the rubber dam napkin on the patient. This is used to absorb moisture and to reduce latex hypersensitivity.
5. Place the forceps in the clamp, and position it so that the bow of the clamp is at the distal of the anchor tooth. The forceps are held so that the beaks are directed toward the occlusal surface of the tooth (for a maxillary anchor tooth, the palm of the hand will be up; for a mandibular anchor tooth, the palm of the hand will be down). Figure 24.4 illustrates clamp transfer for a mandibular tooth.
6. Place the clamp on the designated anchor tooth. The clamped anchor tooth is distal to the tooth that will be receiving treatment. Check for proper fit when placing the clamp from the lingual to the facial, and keep the clamp stabilized with the index finger while releasing the forceps. Make sure that "all four corners" of the clamp are not seated on the gingiva.
7. Place the frame on the outside of the rubber dam. The dam is stretched and hooked onto the projections of the frame. Make sure the dam is smooth and free of tears.
8. Place the last-punched hole of the dam over the tooth on the opposite side of the anchor tooth, as shown in Figure 24.5. This allows the operator to easily locate the remaining holes for the remaining teeth.
9. Once the punch holes are positioned, floss the dam **septum** (the dam membrane between the punched holes) into the contact areas of the teeth to be isolated, as shown in Figure 24.6.
10. Place a **ligature** (a binding) at the opposite end of the anchor tooth to stabilize the dam. This can be done by using floss or a piece of dam material, as shown in Figure 24.7.

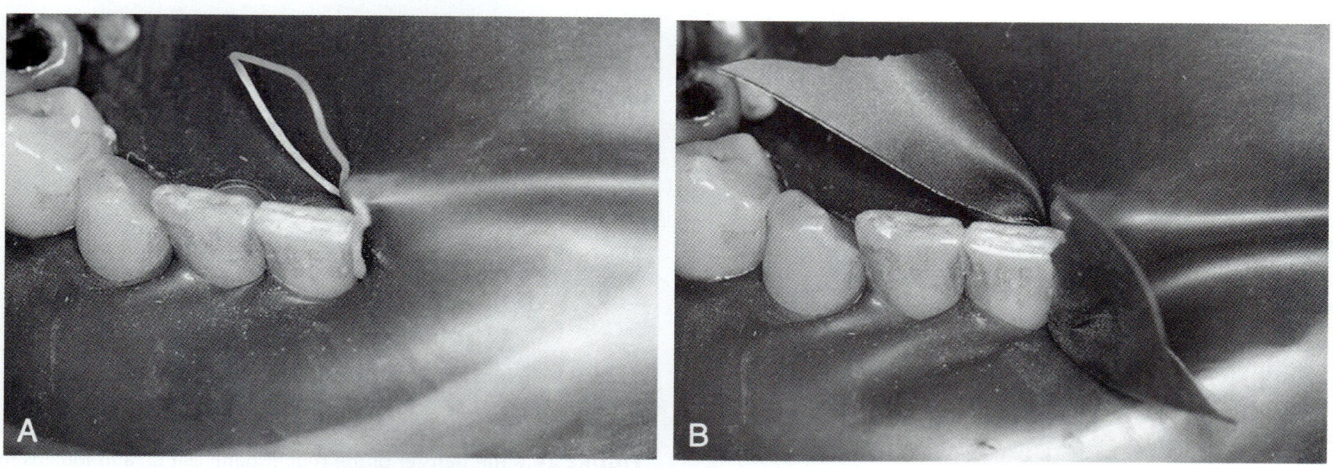

FIGURE 24.7 Two types of ligatures. **A.** Dental floss. **B.** Small corner of the rubber dam.

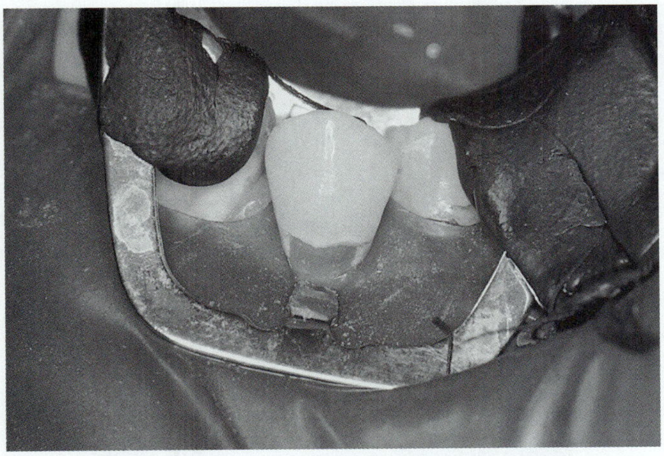

FIGURE 24.8 A "butterfly-shaped" clamp used to isolate the gingiva of the buccal surface of a lower canine.

11. Invert the rubber dam around the necks of the isolated teeth, using the plastic filling instrument (PFI) (beaver tail). Imagine the dam being tucked into the sulci of the isolated teeth. This provides a well-sealed field. If possible, gently use the air syringe to assist with the inversion and to thoroughly dry the area.
12. A variety of special-use rubber dam clamps are available. Use of a "butterfly-shaped" clamp is shown in Figure 24.8. Such clamps are used to retract the gingiva and isolate facial surfaces of the teeth.

D. Removal of the Rubber Dam

The items needed for removal of the rubber dam are listed in Table 24.2. Removal of the dam may be done while the patient is seated in an upright or a supine position.

1. Remove the ligature that is stabilizing the rubber dam.
2. Remove the clamp with the forceps.
3. Before removing the rubber dam, each septum is cut with scissors. The dam is stretched by using a finger rest either under or on top of the dam. This is to protect the gingival tissue and to guide the scissors, as shown in Figure 24.9.
4. Pull the rubber dam occlusally to remove it from the interproximals. Remove the dam and the frame as one unit.
5. Use an explorer in the interproximal areas to inspect and remove any remaining pieces of the rubber dam. Retention of dam fragments will cause gingival irritation.
6. Inspect the removed rubber dam against a contrasting background to make sure that all dam septa are intact (distinct circular openings), as shown in Figure 24.10.
7. Thoroughly rinse and evacuate the treatment area.
8. Massage the gingiva around the clamped tooth to increase circulation.

Tips for the Clinician

- The rubber dam should cover the upper edge of the lip but should not cover the nose.
- All the interproximal gingiva should be covered.
- Make sure the clamp is secure and stable.
- Check for leakage and torn dam material.

Table 24.2 Armamentarium for Removing the Rubber Dam

Scissors
Rubber dam forceps
Explorer
Floss

IV. Other Types of Rubber Dams

Insti-Dam (see Figure 24.11) is a pre-framed rubber dam setup. The flexible frame includes the rubber dam material with a pre-punched hole. The Insti-Dam reduces the number of steps in the application and removal of the rubber dam.

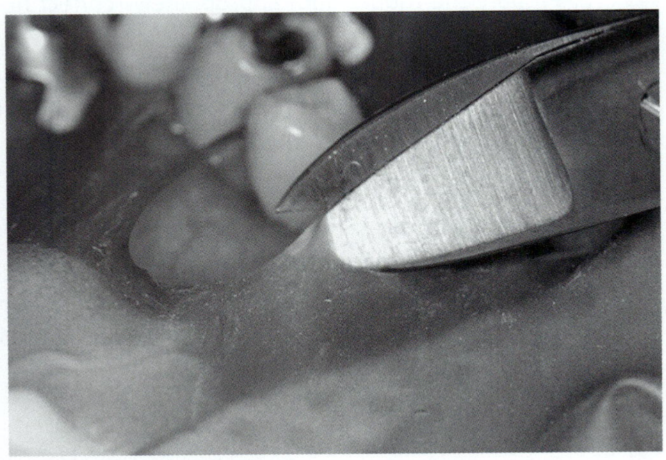

FIGURE 24.9 The rubber dam is stretched, by using a finger rest, when interproximal areas are being cut.

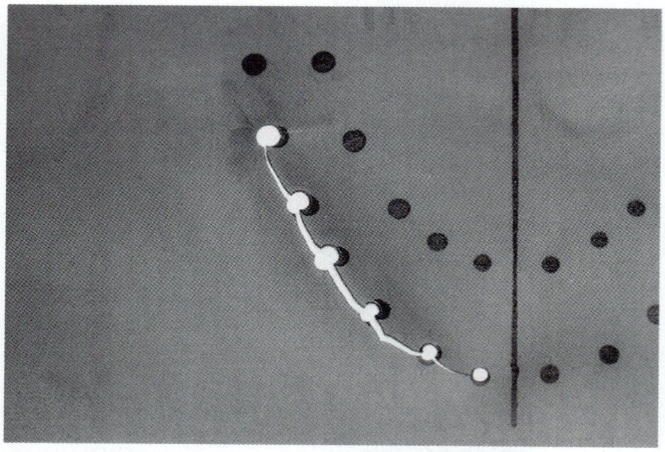

FIGURE 24.10 Inspection of the removed rubber dam against a white background.

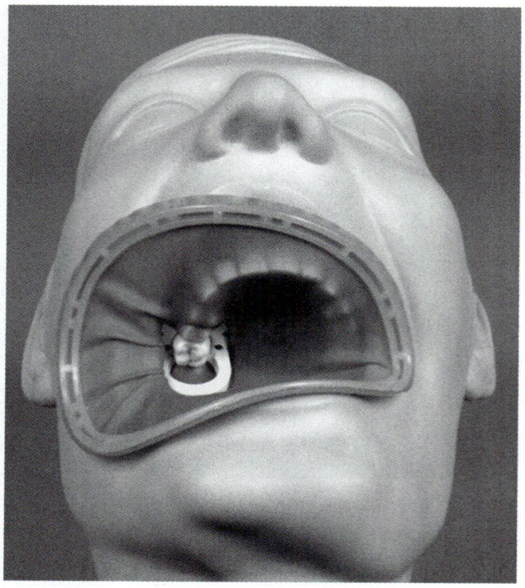

FIGURE 24.11 The Insti-Dam in place on a mannequin to demonstrate the frame's flexibility. (Courtesy of Zirc Company, Buffalo, MN.)

Precautions

- Inadequate stability of the clamp may result in the clamp "springing" off the tooth. Clinicians and patients should wear eye protection during the entire procedure.
- Ligate the clamp with floss so that if the clamp should "spring" free, it can quickly be retrieved.
- During removal of the rubber dam, cut the septa very carefully, using a fulcrum, to avoid injury to the gingival tissue.

Summary

Placement

1. Select appropriate rubber dam material (size, color, etc.).
2. Prepare the rubber dam appropriately (correct hole size, hole distance, clamp ligation).
3. Carefully seat the clamp.
4. Floss the rubber dam between contact areas.
5. Invert the rubber dam around the necks of the teeth.
6. Ligate the last tooth in the exposed sequence.

Removal

1. Remove the clamp from the anchor tooth.
2. Cut the rubber dam septa with scissors.
3. Remove the rubber dam material and the frame as one unit.
4. Inspect the interproximals for rubber dam material.
5. Inspect the removed rubber dam.
6. Rinse and evacuate the oral cavity.
7. Massage the gingiva.

Review Questions

1. The most common size of rubber dam material is:
a) 5 × 5 inch square
b) 6 × 6 inch square
c) 4 × 4.5 inch square
d) None of the above

2. The armamentarium for removing the rubber dam is/are:
a) Scissors
b) Rubber dam forceps
c) Floss
d) Explorer
e) All of the above

3. What is the position of the tooth receiving treatment in relationship to the anchor tooth?
a) The treatment tooth is distal to the anchor tooth
b) The anchor tooth is the same as the treatment tooth
c) The treatment tooth is mesial to the anchor tooth
d) The anchor tooth at the opposite end of the arch of the treatment tooth.

4. Indications for rubber dam placement include all of the following except:
a) Visibility
b) Patient protection
c) Patient with severe asthma
d) Moisture control

5. Which clamp is used for isolation of the facial surfaces of anterior and some posterior teeth?
a) Winged clamps
b) Wingless clamps
c) Butterfly-shaped clamps

Supplemental Readings

Darby ML, Walsh MM. Dental Hygiene Theory and Practice. Philadelphia: Saunders, 1995, Chapter 22.

Sturdevant CM, Roberson TM, Heymann HO, Sturdevant JR. The Art and Science of Operative Dentistry. 3rd ed. St. Louis: Mosby, 1995, Chapter 11.

Torres HO, Ehrlich A, Bird D, Dietz E. Modern Dental Assisting. 5th ed. Philadelphia: Saunders, 1995, Chapter 22.

25

Pit and Fissure Sealants

Key Words/Phrases

air abrasive for polishing
etchant
micropores

Objectives

After performing the laboratory/clinical exercises in this chapter, the student will be able to do the following:

1. Discuss the factors determining the success of a sealant.
2. List the indications and contraindications for applying a sealant.
3. Describe the acceptable, but different, methods for preparing the enamel surface for a sealant.
4. Summarize the steps of applying a sealant.
5. Evaluate a placed sealant regarding proper isolation, coverage, and defects.
6. Explain the importance of recall visits for sealant maintenance.
7. Professionally speak to a parent of a child who is in need of sealants. Include in the discussion the rationale, procedure, time involved, and prognosis.

INTRODUCTION

This chapter will provide the basic steps for pit and fissure sealant application. It is always important to review—and to follow—the manufacturer's directions for the application and storage of a particular sealant material.

Clinical success of sealants is determined by proper placement and retention. The most common reasons for sealant failure are inadequate isolation and subsequent contamination. The dentist must choose a sealant material based on the following properties:

- Autopolymerizing (chemical cure) or visible light cure sealants. Examples of light-activated sealant kits are provided in Figure 25.1
- Fluoride-releasing or nonfluoride-releasing sealants.
- Clear, tinted, or opaque sealants.

The composition, properties, and mechanism for retention of bonding resins were discussed in Chapter 4.

I. Purpose and Indications

Pit and fissure sealant material will literally flow into the deep pit and fissured areas on occlusal surfaces and seal them from bacterial activity. Figure 25.2 illustrates a magnified occlusal surface exhibiting several deep pit and fissure areas. Sometimes, the fissure is shaped in an "I" formation that is very narrow but has a bulbous base. The formation is too narrow to accommodate toothbrush bristles. The "I"-shaped fissure can be seen in Figure 25.3. The American Dental Association Council on Scientific Affairs has determined that sealants are indicated for patients with the following conditions: a moderate or high risk for caries, incipient caries within enamel in pit and fissure areas, or existing pits and fissures anatomically susceptible to decay.

II. Contraindications

Pit and fissure sealants are contraindicated on tooth surfaces having frank caries or on surfaces that have well-coalesced pits and fissures.

III. Procedure

The clinical success of a pit and fissure sealant is dependent on the meticulous technique of the clinician. The items needed to place sealants are listed in Table 25.1.

A. Surface Preparation

The clinician may use one of the following methods to prepare the enamel surface for sealant application. Research has found them all to be acceptable.

1. Bristle brush or rubber cup and low-speed handpiece with plain pumice, then rinse for 10 seconds

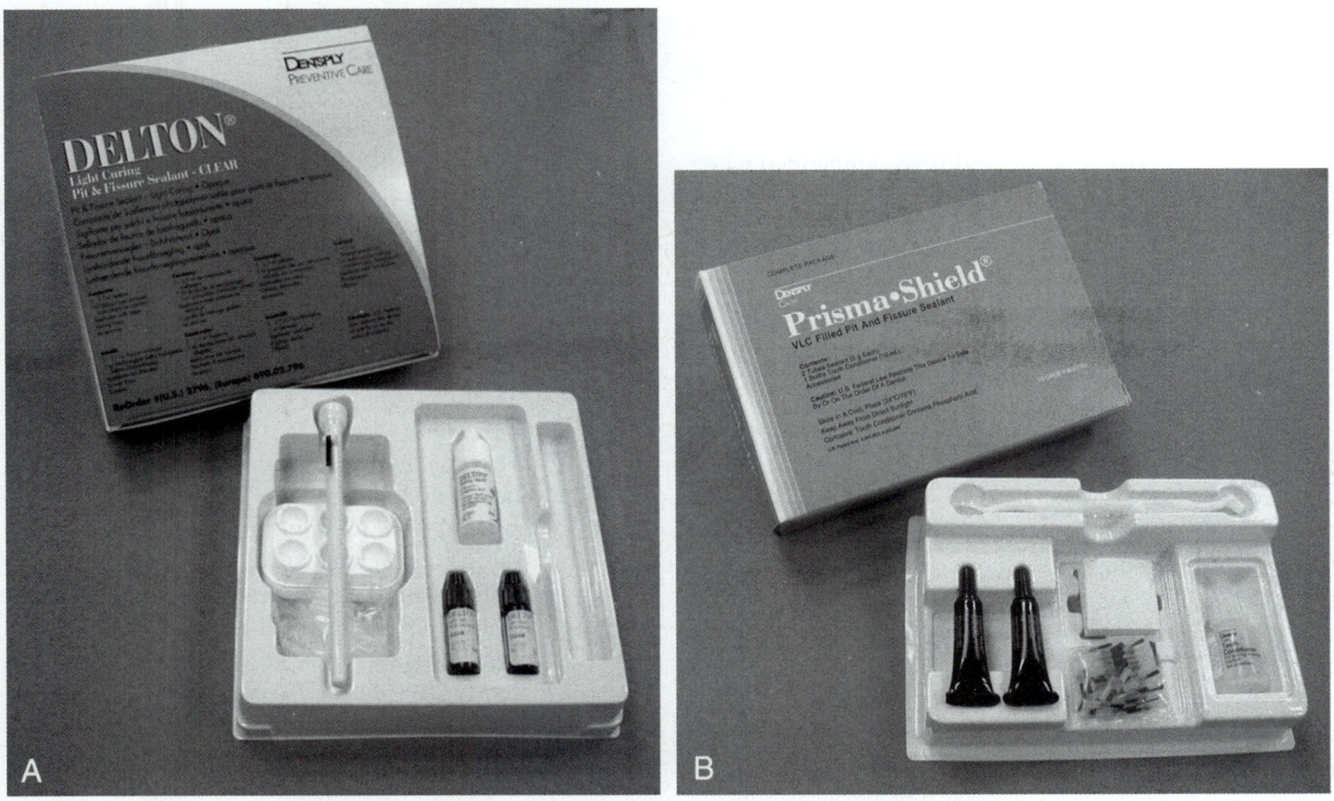

FIGURE 25.1 Examples of light-activated sealant kits. **A.** Clear. **B.** Filled and opaque.

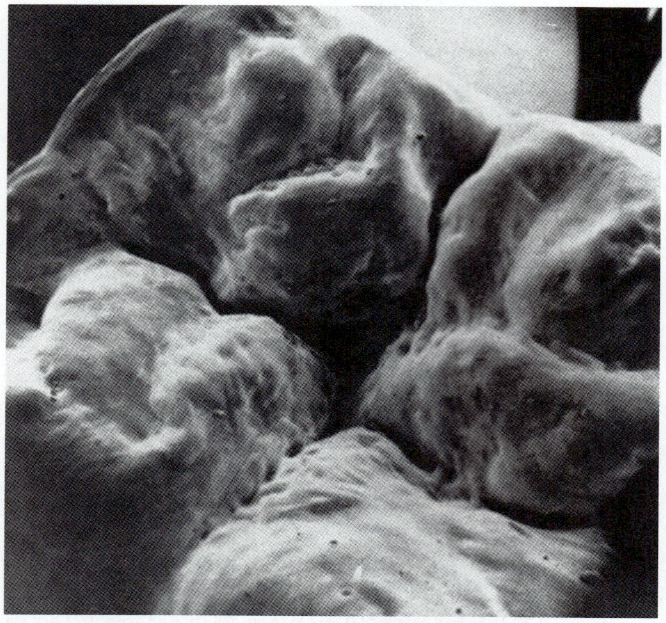

FIGURE 25.2 Magnified occlusal surface showing deep pit and fissure areas. (Reproduced with permission from Gwinnett AJ. The bonding of sealants to enamel. J Am Soc Prevent Dent 1973;3:21.)

Table 25.1 Armamentarium for Placing Sealants

Mirror
Explorer
Cotton pliers
Sealant resin
Etchant (phosphoric acid)
Gauze
Low-speed handpiece
Curing light with shield
No. 6 or 8 round bur or a green or white stone
Triangular saliva absorbers or rubber dam setup
Air/water syringe tip
Saliva ejector
High-speed suction
Bristle polishing brush
Articulating paper
Floss
Pumice
Cotton rolls and Garmer holder
Posterior scaler

2. Bristle brush with water
3. Etchant only (no surface preparation)
4. **Air abrasive polishing** (prophy-jet; sodium bicarbonate particles propelled by compressed air in a water spray) or very light air abrasion with aluminum oxide

B. Isolation

Isolation may be accomplished in two ways.

1. Rubber Dam

The rubber dam method is recommended when more than one tooth in the quadrant is to be sealed.

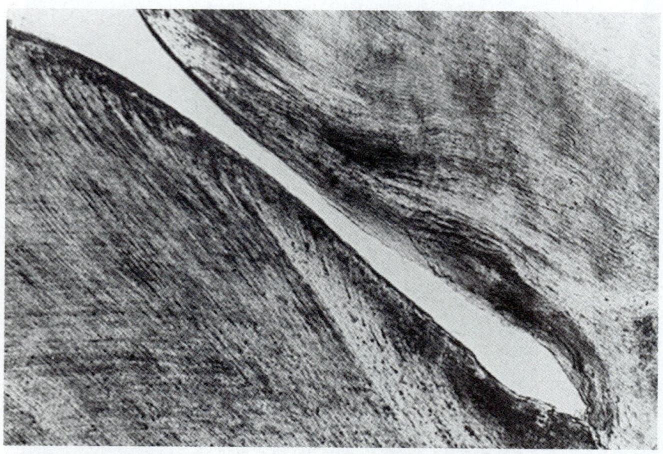

FIGURE 25.3 "I"-shape fissure, very narrow with a bulbous base. (Reproduced with permission from Gwinnett AJ. The bonding of sealants to enamel. J Am Soc Prevent Dent 1973;3:21.)

2. Cotton Roll Application

Use the saliva ejector and Garmer holder for cotton rolls for the mandibular arch (Fig. 25.4, *A* and *B*).

3. Triangular Cotton Isolation

Triangular cotton isolation, as shown in Figure 25.4, *C* and *D*, can also be used in conjunction with either method.

C. Dry the Tooth or Teeth Thoroughly

Make sure the air/water syringe does not leak water or oil because this will interfere with formation of the "enamel tags" or "micropores." These micropores are minute, microscopic openings in the enamel surface, as shown in Figure 4.3. Dry the area for at least 10 seconds and inspect for caries.

D. Apply Etchant

1. Application time is 15 to 20 seconds.
2. If using a liquid etchant, apply with a brush. An enamel **etchant** material is a gel or liquid composed of 37% phosphoric acid.
3. If using a gel etchant, apply and then leave undisturbed. Gel etchants are illustrated in Figure 25.5. Etchant gel clinically applied to a premolar is shown in Figure 25.6.

E. Thoroughly Rinse

1. If using an etching gel, rinse for at least 30 seconds. If using a liquid etchant, rinse for 10 to 15 seconds.

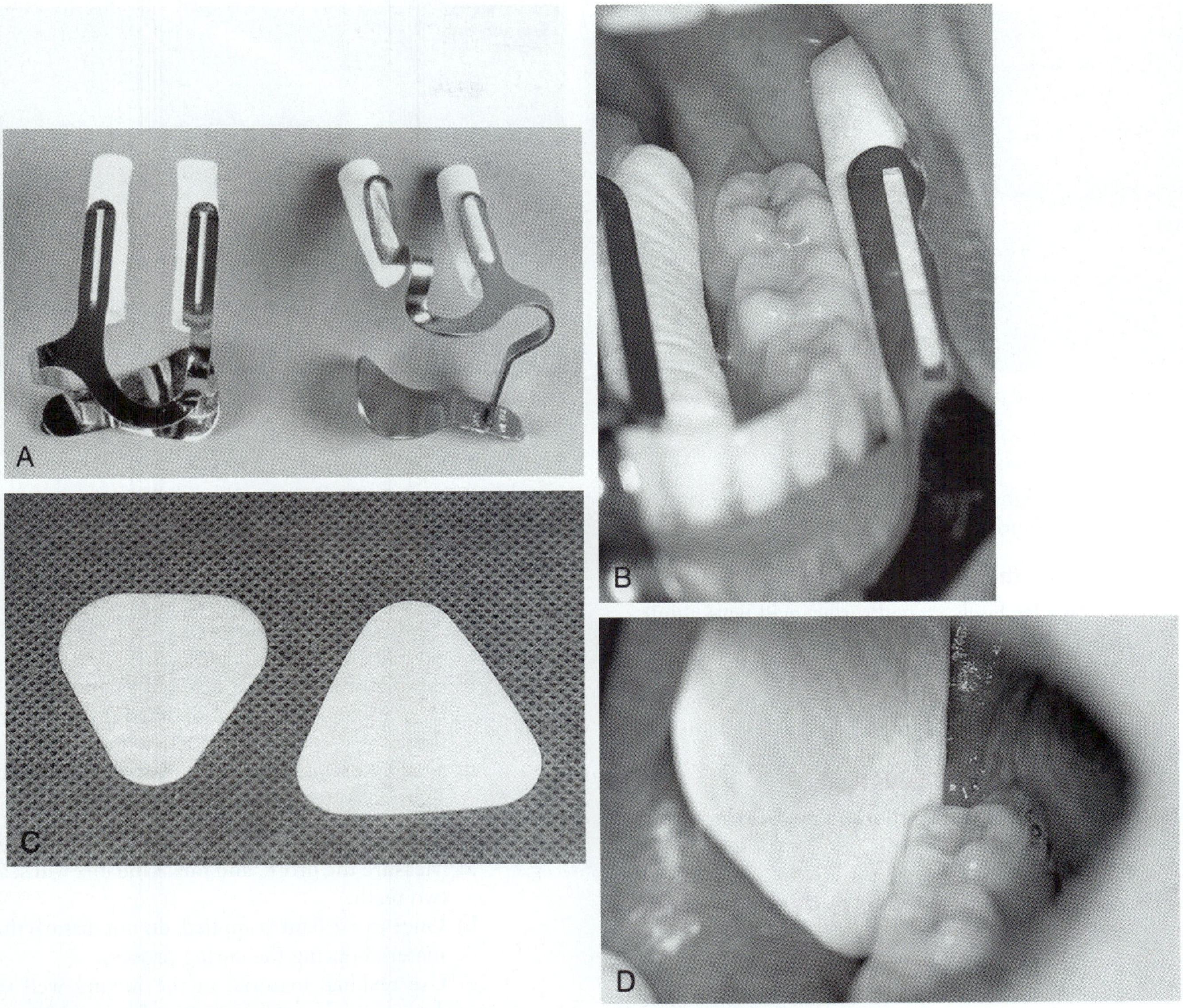

FIGURE 25.4 **A.** Left- and right-side Garmer cotton roll holders. **B.** Cotton roll holder in use. **C.** Triangular cotton substitutes. **D.** Triangular cotton isolation in use.

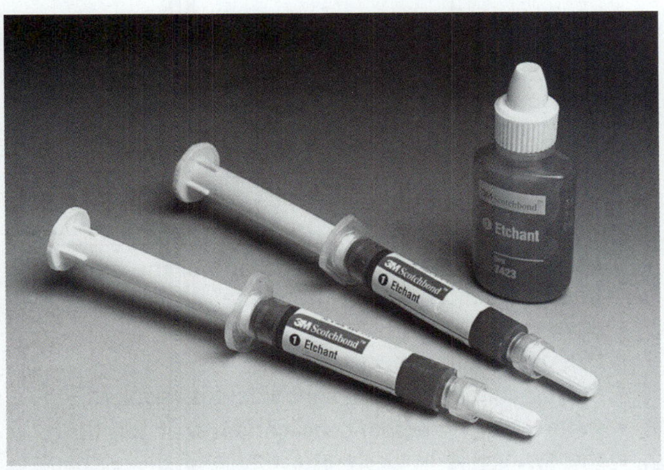

FIGURE 25.5 Gel etchants, syringe delivery, and dispenser bottle for use with a brush/applicator. (Courtesy of 3M Dental Products Division.)

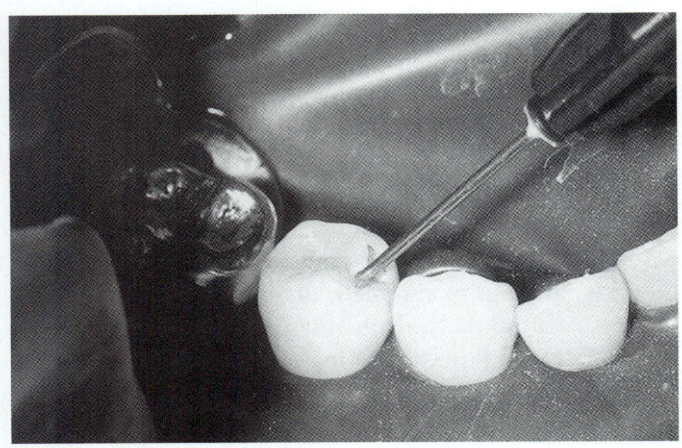

FIGURE 25.6 Clinical application of gel etchant applied to a premolar.

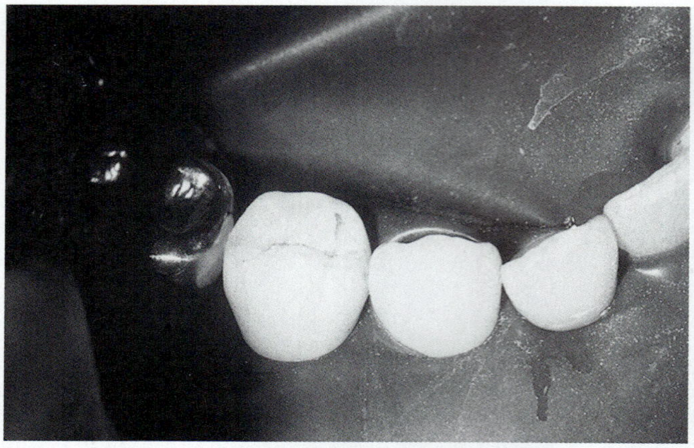

FIGURE 25.7 Etched premolar appearing frosty white.

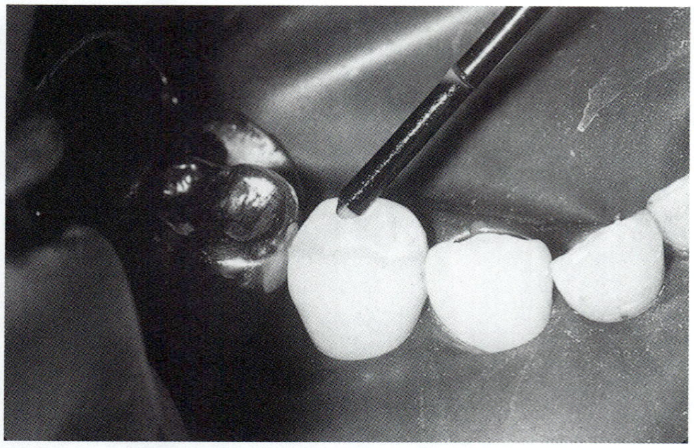

FIGURE 25.8 Sealant material applied to a premolar with an applicator tip.

2. Use high-speed evacuation during the rinse procedure.

F. Evaluate the Etched Surface

1. An adequately etched surface will have a dull, chalky white, opaque appearance.
2. If this appearance is not evident, re-etch the surface by using the same procedure. Figure 25.7 illustrates a properly etched premolar.

G. Dry the Tooth or Teeth Again

Each tooth should be thoroughly dried again for 15 to 30 seconds.

H. Apply a Primer From a Dentinal Bonding System—Optional

Primers from dentinal bonding systems will act as a wetting agent to improve adhesion when contamination of the etched surface occurs. Self-etching primers may also be used; some replace the usual phosphoric acid etching step.

I. Apply the Sealant to the Tooth Surface

1. Sealant may be applied by:
   a) Using the applicator provided by the manufacturer. If applying sealant by this method, allow the material to flow ahead of applicator tip, as shown in Figure 25.8.
   b) Using a small brush.
   c) Using an explorer.
2. Remove excess amounts of material, and attempt to eliminate any bubbles occurring within the sealant.
3. Extend the sealant material along inclined planes of cusps.
4. Don't forget the pits and fissures on the buccal of mandibular and lingual of maxillary molars.

J. Polymerize the Sealant

1. Light-Activated Sealants
   a) Use amber eyewear or light shields during the curing process.
   b) Hold the tip of the curing light as close as possible to the tooth surface.
   c) Curing time is 20 seconds, but an additional 5 to 10 seconds are recommended for each surface.
   d) One new sealant changes color when properly light-activated.
2. Chemically Activated Sealants
   a) Measure the drops, and mix. One mix will seal two teeth.
   b) Once the sealant is applied, do not disturb the material during the curing process.
   c) Use residual material in the mixing well to determine the setting time (~2 minutes).

K. Occlusal Adjustment

1. Unfilled sealants will wear easily, and occlusal adjustment at the time of placement is usually unnecessary.

Precautions

- For sealant retention, it is critical that the area be free of moisture during the entire placement procedure.
- Eye protection is necessary.
- During curing, use of a light shield is required.
- Before placing etchant, be certain that the tip of the syringe is securely attached and the etchant flows freely.

Tips for the Clinician

- Light-cure sealants provide more working time for the clinician than autocure sealants.
- Having additional assistance for this procedure makes placement and retention more effective.
- To avoid the incorporation of bubbles, drag the explorer tip along all pits and fissures before curing.

2. Occlusal adjustment when filled sealants are being used requires articulating paper and either a # 6 or # 8 round bur or a green or white stone.
   a) After using articulating paper, note any markings on the sealants.
   b) Remove any markings with a stone or bur.

L. Evaluate the Sealant

1. Visually and tactilely (with an explorer) inspect the sealant for:
   a) Complete coverage of all etched areas
   b) Absence of voids, bubbles, and defects (overmanipulation of sealant material before curing can incorporate air into the sealant)
2. Attempt to dislodge the sealant with an explorer. If successful, replace the sealant immediately, using a "dry, 10-second re-etch, rinse, dry, seal" sequence.
3. Use floss between the interproximals of all sealed teeth and those adjacent to sealed teeth. If cured sealant material has closed the interproximal space, it can be reopened by removing the material with a scaler and/or floss.

Summary

1. Cleanse the tooth surface(s).
2. Isolate the selected teeth from moisture.
3. Dry teeth for 10 seconds and inspect for caries.
4. Etch for 15 to 20 seconds.
5. Rinse: for liquid etchants, 10 to 15 seconds; for etching gels, 30 seconds.
6. Etched area appears chalky.
7. Apply sealant according to the manufacturer's directions.
8. Polymerize the sealant.
9. Evaluate the sealant for coverage, retention, and absence of voids and bubbles.
10. Check/adjust occlusion and adjacent interproximal spaces.

M. Evaluate the Sealant Placement Procedure

Assess the sealant placement by using the Skill Performance Evaluation sheet in Appendix 2.

N. Follow-up Evaluation

During recall examinations, the dental hygienist will need to re-evaluate sealed tooth surfaces for sealant loss, exposure of voids, and possible caries. This is done both visually and tactilely. If a sealant is partially lost, attempt to dislodge the remaining material with an explorer. If this portion remains intact, simply etch the adjacent enamel and sealant, and then apply additional sealant.

Review Questions

1. Dental sealants are effective in ________ dental caries:
a) Reversing
b) Restoring
c) Preventing
d) Proliferating

2. Properly etched and dried enamel appears:
a) Shiny and pale
b) Chalky white
c) Dull grey
d) Peachy keen

3. After placement, the sealant should be checked for:
a) Hyperocclusion of occlusal contacts
b) Interproximal contacts bonded together
c) Both
d) Neither

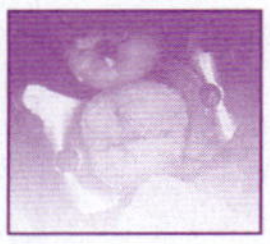

Supplemental Readings

American Dental Association. Dental Sealants, Protecting your teeth. J Am Dent Assoc 2003;134:1018.

American Dental Association. Dental Sealants. J Am Dent Assoc 1997;128:485–488.

Daniel SJ, Harfst SA. Mosby's Dental Hygiene—Concepts, Cases and Competencies. St. Louis: Mosby, 2002, Chapter 26.

Darby ML, Walsh MM. Dental Hygiene Theory and Practice. Philadelphia: Saunders, 1995, Chapter 21.

Waggoner WF, Siegal M. Pit and fissure sealant application: updating the technique. J Am Dent Assoc 1996;127: 351–361.

Wilkins EM. Clinical Practice of the Dental Hygienist. 10th ed. Baltimore: Williams & Wilkins, 2008, Chapter 30.

Woodall I. Comprehensive Dental Hygiene Care. 4th ed. St. Louis: Mosby, 1993, Chapter 22.

Amalgam Finishing and Polishing

Meg Zayan, R.D.H., M.P.H.

26

Key Words/Phrases

amalgam finishing
amalgam polishing
cavosurface margin
flash
open margin
overextension
overhang
premature contacts
submarginal area

Objectives

After studying this chapter, the student will be able to do the following:

1. Explain the rationale for amalgam finishing and polishing.
2. Recall the benefits of properly finished and polished amalgams.
3. List two indications for finishing and polishing amalgams.
4. Discuss the possible results of poor amalgam placement and carving.
5. Assess an amalgam restoration to determine whether it needs replacement or finishing and polishing.
6. Differentiate between the procedures of amalgam finishing and amalgam polishing.
7. Explain the importance of temperature control and related factors during finishing and polishing.
8. Evaluate a well-finished and polished amalgam according to the criteria provided in this chapter.

INTRODUCTION

The procedures discussed in this chapter (or portions thereof) may not be included in the dental hygienist's scope of practice in all states. Procedures that a dental hygienist may legally perform are listed in each state's practice act. Amalgam finishing and polishing is an integral part of the patient's treatment plan in the prevention of periodontal and dental disease, and it should be routinely performed by the dental hygienist. Finished and polished amalgams are less prone to plaque retention and have a greater resistance to tarnish and corrosion than unpolished amalgams. Traditionally, finishing and polishing should be performed at least 24 hours after amalgam placement. This allows the amalgam alloy to set completely before being exposed to abrasives within the oral cavity. Spherical fast-setting amalgams, which could be finished and polished shortly after placing and carving, are the exception. Spherical amalgams were discussed in Chapter 6. For previously placed amalgams, finishing and polishing may be started as soon as the procedure is indicated.

I. Purpose of Finishing and Polishing

The primary purpose of finishing and polishing amalgams is to produce a restoration that can be easily cleaned by the patient, thereby decreasing recurrent decay and increasing the lifetime of the restoration. This allows the surrounding tissues to be healthier, and it provides a more corrosion-resistant surface.

A. Benefits of Finishing and Polishing

The following conditions result from proper finishing and polishing:

1. Smooth and flush cavosurface margins
2. Recreation of defined anatomy
3. Decreased plaque retention
4. Healthier surrounding tissue
5. Higher resistance to tarnish and corrosion
6. Increased longevity of the restoration
7. Improved esthetics

B. Methods by Which These Benefits Are Achieved

These benefits are achieved by properly smoothing the cavosurface margins, reconstructing functional anatomy, and creating an amalgam surface that is both smooth and free of voids. It is necessary to obtain a smooth surface and achieve a high gloss. If only a high gloss is achieved through the polishing sequence, the remaining irregularities will tend to corrode faster than a smooth surface. Ultimately, this will not prolong the life of the restoration.

II. Indications for Finishing and Polishing

Ideally, all amalgam restorations should be finished and polished 24 hours after placement. Realistically, however, this may not happen. Previously existing amalgam restorations, as well as "newer" ones, should be finished and polished to correct various problems or conditions incurred during placement. These problems are often a result of incorrect condensing, poor carving, moisture contamination, natural expansion, or wear. In all these cases, plaque has a greater chance of accumulating on the restoration's surface, which creates a higher risk for recurrent caries.

A. Typical Problems With Amalgam Restorations

1. Overhang at the Cavosurface Gingival Margins

An **overhang** is an excess amount of amalgam that extends beyond the cavosurface margin, and it is caused by improper placement of the matrix band or wedge during amalgam condensation (Fig. 26.1). An overhang increases susceptibility to decay and periodontal disease.

2. Anatomy

Functional anatomy is not created during placement.

3. Contact

Interproximal contact is not created.

4. Tarnish

Tarnish is a removable surface film or discoloration on the amalgam. It does not affect the internal integrity of the restoration.

5. Corrosion

Corrosion is a surface or subsurface chemical deterioration that occurs on or within an amalgam restoration. Corrosion is discussed in detail in Chapter 19.

6. Fracture

A bulk fracture can occur in the amalgam restoration.

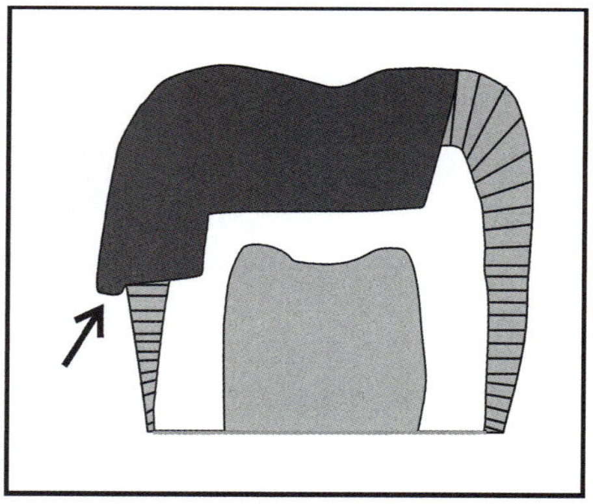

FIGURE 26.1 Amalgam overhang.

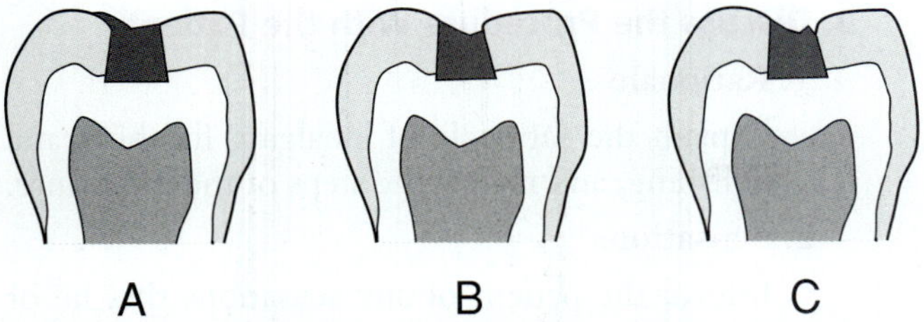

FIGURE 26.2 Results of poor carving. **A.** Overextension or flash. **B.** Submarginal area. **C.** Open margin.

7. Results of Poor Carving

a) Overextension or Flash

Overextension or **flash** are terms used when a thin ledge of amalgam extends beyond the cavosurface margin, as illustrated in Figure 26.2*A*.

b) Submarginal Area (or Deficient Margin)

A **submarginal area** results when the margin is overcarved, creating a deficiency of amalgam, as shown in Figure 26.2*B*. An internal wall of the preparation is exposed.

c) Open Margin

An **open margin** is created as a result of poor condensation or when an opposing cusp fractures an overextended portion of amalgam. An illustration of an open margin is shown in Figure 26.2*C*.

B. Amalgam Restoration Assessment

During patient assessment, all amalgam restorations must be carefully evaluated to determine if amalgam finishing and/or polishing is indicated. As listed in Table 26.1, some amalgam restorations should not be finished and polished but should be replaced instead.

III. Amalgam Finishing and Polishing Considerations

Amalgam finishing and polishing can be considered as two separate procedures or as two steps in a single process. During **amalgam finishing,** marginal irregularities are removed, and all areas of roughness are smoothed. During **amalgam polishing,** the surface is smoothed to a high luster by using a sequence of abrasives (from fine to most fine). Whenever an amalgam restoration is finished, polishing is then performed; for those restorations not indicated for finishing, polishing may be done alone. The abrasives used during finishing are coarser than the milder abrasives that are used during polishing.

During the finishing and polishing procedures, it is essential that the dental hygienist avoid generating any heat within the amalgam restoration. Because of the high thermal conductivity of amalgam, excessive heat could injure the pulp and cause pain to the patient. Also, when heat is generated above 140°F (60°C), mercury from the amalgam restoration may be released to the surface, resulting in a dull, cloudy appearance. Excessive heat generation may also produce increased susceptibility to breakdown and corrosion. Therefore, use of water from a syringe as a coolant during these procedures is recommended. After each step, when burs or abrasives are changed, the area should be thoroughly rinsed, dried, and evaluated. Factors that affect the rate of abrasion must also be considered; these were discussed in Chapter 16.

Table 26.1 Determining Factors for Finishing and Polishing Versus Replacement

Finish and Polish Restoration	Replace Restoration
A. Overhangs	A. Open contact
B. Lack of functional anatomy	B. Excessive corrosion
C. Tarnish	C. Amalgam fracture
D. Overextension	D. Open margin
E. Premature occlusal contacts	E. Recurrent decay

IV. Procedure for Amalgam Finishing

A. Evaluate the Restoration

1. Surfaces

Visually examine the amalgam surfaces for functional anatomy and defects. Functional anatomy includes cusps, cusp ridges, the central groove, and the buccolingual groove. Defects include surface pitting and wear facets.

2. Margins

Using a sharp explorer in a zigzag motion, determine if the cavosurface margins have any excessive discrepancies (Fig. 26.3). The **cavosurface margin** is the area formed by the cavity wall and

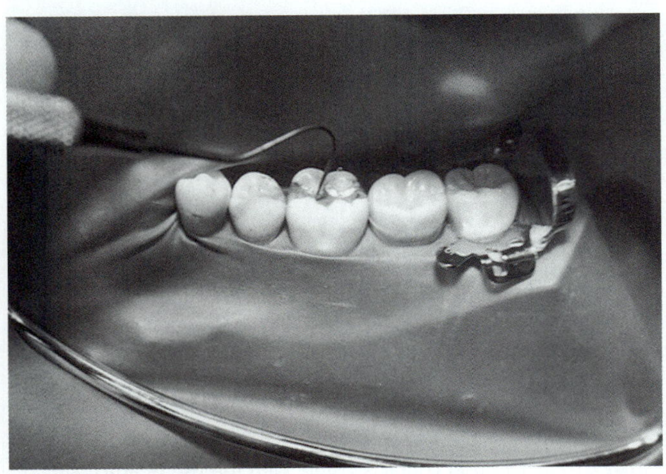

FIGURE 26.3 Examining for marginal discrepancies.

the external tooth surface. Remember that a rough margin is a poor predictor of recurrent decay, as was explained in Chapter 6. Rough surfaces along the margin encourage plaque accumulation, which may result in a greater susceptibility to dental caries. The patient's risk for caries must also be considered.

3. Occlusion

Evaluate the patient's occlusion.

a) **Use Articulating Paper**
Insert articulating paper along the occlusal surface and have the patient tap his or her teeth together.

b) **Determine Intensity**
Observe all markings to determine if they have the same intensity.

c) **Reduce Premature Contacts**
Premature contacts are areas where the amalgam has been undercarved. These will register as darker areas when they are checked with articulating paper. Occlusal contacts, which are registered by using articulating paper, are shown in Figure 26.4.

d) **Check Areas of Equal Intensity**
Check areas of equal intensity throughout the finishing procedure to ensure that occlusal markings of equal intensity are achieved.

4. Proximal Area

a) Check proximal contacts with dental floss. The dental floss should resist passing through the contact. Remember, an open contact serves as a precursor to food impaction.

b) Using dental floss and an explorer, check for overhangs.

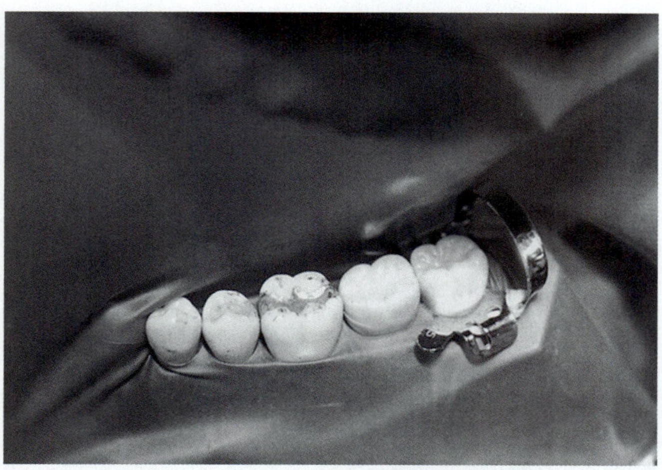

FIGURE 26.4 Occlusal contacts visible with the use of articulating paper.

B. Discuss the Procedure With the Patient

1. Rationale

Explain the rationale of amalgam finishing and polishing, and review the steps of the procedure.

2. Sensations

Inform the patient of any sensations that he or she may experience during the process, especially those of finishing burs with a low-speed handpiece.

C. Gather the Necessary Equipment

Select instruments based on the restoration and the clinician's preference. An example of an equipment listing is shown in Table 26.2.

D. Isolate the Area With Cotton Rolls or a Rubber Dam

Rubber dam isolation is presented in Chapter 24. Cotton roll isolation is described in Chapter 25.

Table 26.2 Armamentarium for Finishing and Polishing Amalgam Restorations

Mouth mirror
Articulating paper
Explorer
Slow-speed handpiece
Contra angle or prophy angle
Air/water syringe
Rubber dam setup or cotton rolls
Finishing burs
Abrasive stones and discs
Green stone (silicone dioxide)
White stone (aluminum oxide)
Finishing discs (zirconium silicate)
Hand instruments
Dental file
Gold knife
Amalgam knife
Dental floss or tape
Finishing strips
Polishing supplies
Rubber points and cups
Brown points or cups
Green points or cups
Yellow-banded green points or cups
OR
Two dappen dishes
Pumice and water
Tin oxide and alcohol/mouthwash
Polishing cups (unwebbed)
Brushes (tapered and wheel)

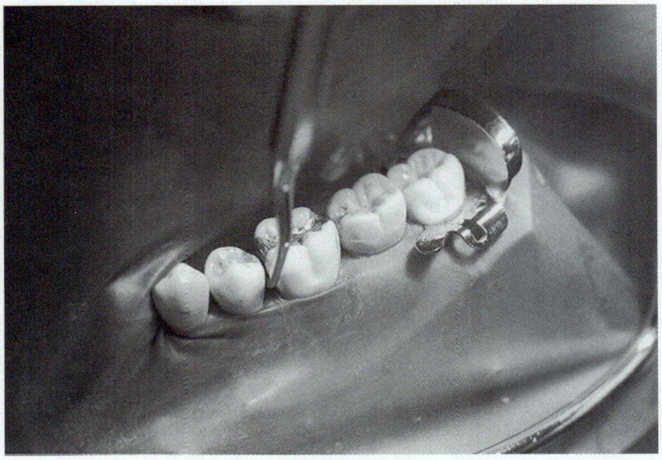

FIGURE 26.5 Hand instrument to smooth amalgam in the proximal area.

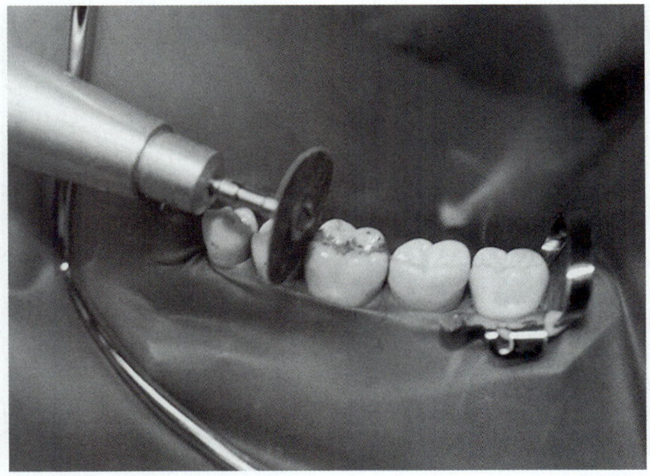

FIGURE 26.7 Disc used to smooth amalgam in the interproximal area.

E. Smooth Proximal Areas if Necessary

This may be done by using hand instruments or finishing burs, discs, and strips.

1. Hand Instruments

a) Use a finishing knife and/or a dental file at the gingival and proximal margins to remove overhangs.

b) Use short, overlapping, shaving strokes to prevent the amalgam from fracturing. This method is illustrated in Figure 26.5.

2. Finishing Burs

a) A flame-shaped bur is recommended when the area is easily accessible.

b) Care must be taken to prevent damage to the contact area or the gingival papilla (Fig. 26.6).

3. Finishing Discs

a) **Selection**
Discs come in varying sizes and grits. Select a size that is easily adaptable to the proximal surface.

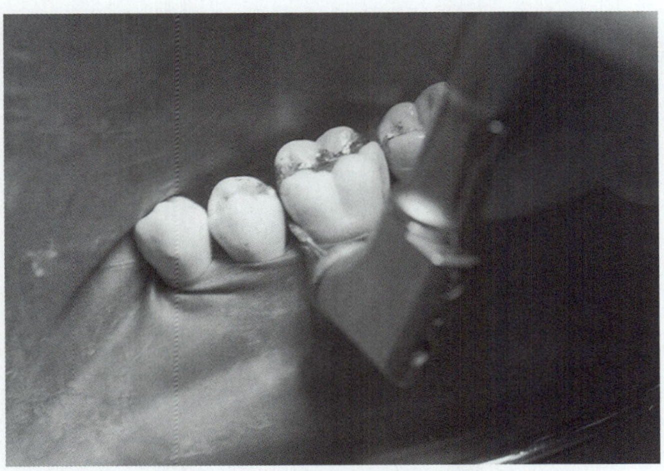

FIGURE 26.6 Finishing bur used to smooth amalgam in the proximal area.

b) **Technique**
Use short, overlapping strokes, and move diagonally across the cavosurface margins.

c) **Sequence**
Discs are used in a sequence of more abrasive to less abrasive grits.

d) **Embrasures**
When you are using discs in embrasure areas, take care not to damage the contact area or papilla. Figure 26.7 illustrates the use of discs for finishing.

4. Finishing Strips

a) Use fine or medium finishing strips after using discs, burs, knives, or files.

b) Position the strip so that it is on both the tooth and the amalgam, and move in a back-and-forth motion.

c) Avoid the contact area when using finishing strips, and use caution in areas of the interdental papilla and surrounding tissue. Wider strips may be cut in half lengthwise to make narrow strips.

F. Remove Occlusal Excess and Eliminate Flash

1. With Burs or Stones

Use a round finishing bur or a green stone to remove excess material and irregularities from the occlusal surface, grooves, and the cavosurface margin (Fig. 26.8).

2. Sequence

Begin with the largest finishing bur that will adapt to the surface, and progress to smaller and less abrasive finishing burs.

3. Technique

Adapt the side of the bur or stone to the margin, contacting both the tooth and the amalgam, as shown in Figure 26.9.

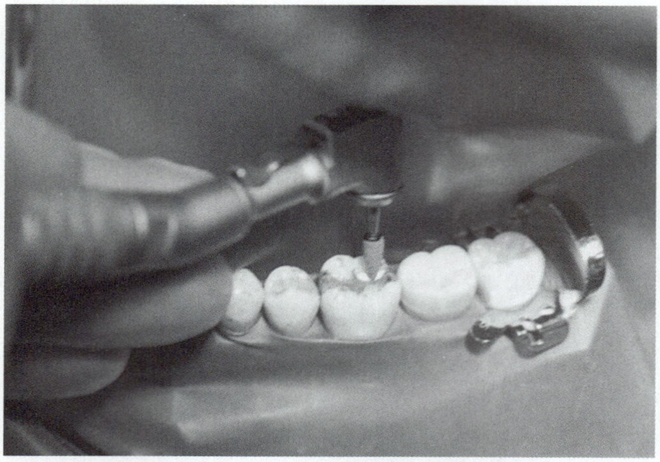

FIGURE 26.8 Green stone used to remove excess material and irregularities.

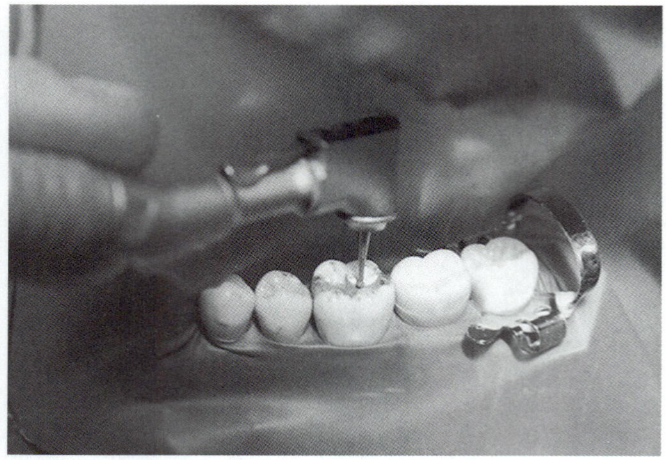

FIGURE 26.10 Defining anatomy by using a small round bur.

4. Direction of Rotating Bur or Stone

Rotate the bur or stone from the amalgam to the tooth to avoid fracturing the amalgam margins.

5. Direction of Stroke

Always begin at the center of the restoration, and work toward the cavosurface margin.

6. Pitted Areas

Use a pointed white stone on tarnished and pitted areas.

G. Define the Occlusal Anatomy

1. With moderate pressure, define the occlusal anatomy by using a steel round bur, green stone, or white stone. Figure 26.10 illustrates this procedure using a small round bur.
2. Refer to existing teeth as a guide for anatomic definition.

H. Smooth Cavosurface Margins and the Occlusal Surface

1. Use a large round or a flame-shaped finishing bur to smooth the occlusal surface and cavosurface margins (Fig. 26.11).
2. Change to a smaller round or a flame-shaped finishing bur to further smooth grooves and cusp slopes.
3. Reduce small areas of enamel (submarginal areas) or amalgam (overextensions) at the cavosurface margin by using a white stone, as shown in Figure 26.12.
4. The restoration should now appear smooth and shiny. Minute scratches may be present but may not be visible to the unaided eye.

I. Smooth Facial and Lingual Surfaces

1. Use a flame-shaped finishing bur or finishing discs, which vary in size and grit, to define and smooth the facial and lingual surfaces.
2. Adapt the bur along the cavosurface margin, contacting both the tooth and the amalgam in the same manner as illustrated in Figure 26.9 but for the facial and lingual surfaces.
3. Use caution when adapting the bur or discs near the gingival margin, especially if near the cementum.

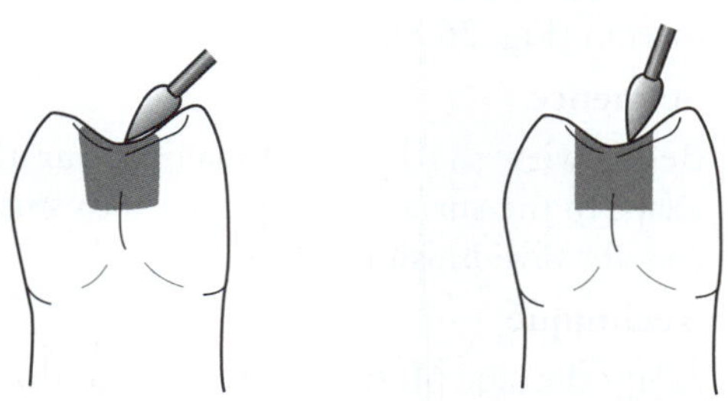

FIGURE 26.9 Adaptation of finishing bur or green stone.

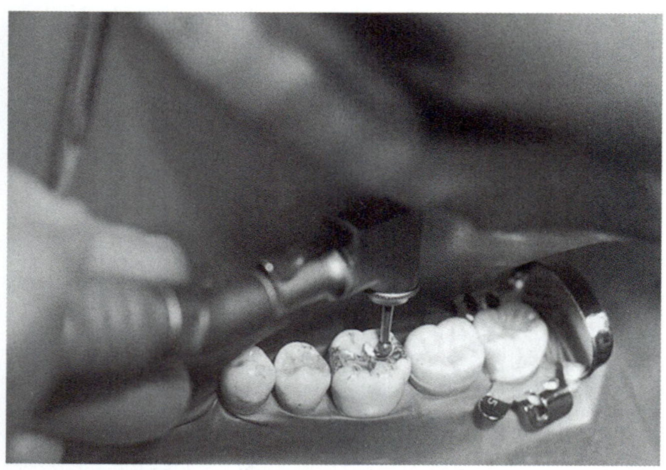

FIGURE 26.11 Smoothing occlusal surface and cavosurface margins by using a large round bur.

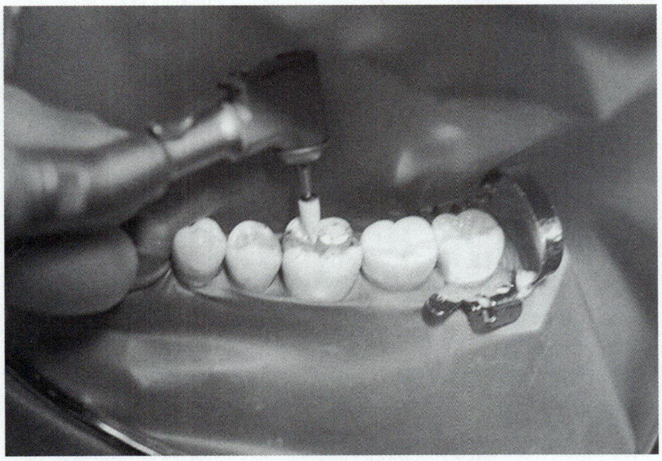

FIGURE 26.12 Reduction of small areas of enamel or amalgam at the cavosurface margin.

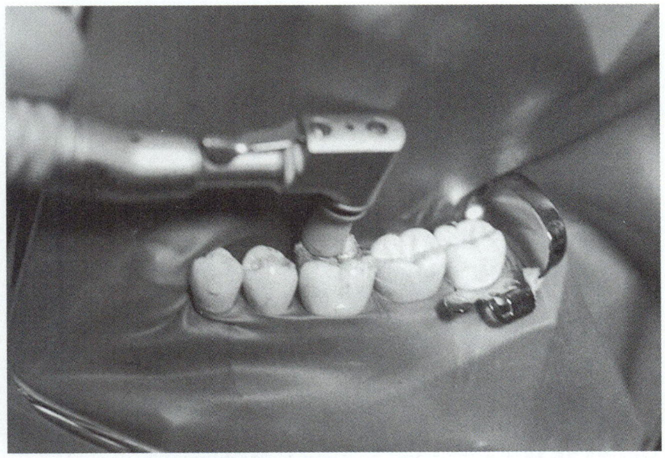

FIGURE 26.13 Polishing with pumice slurry and a rubber cup.

4. When using discs, first use a coarser one, such as garnet, and progress to one having a finer abrasive, such as a cuttle.
5. If developmental grooves are part of the restoration, use a round or flame-shaped bur to define these.

J. Evaluate the Finishing Procedure

Assess the finishing procedure by using the criteria listed in Skill Performance Evaluation sheet in Appendix 2. DO NOT PROCEED TO THE POLISHING PROCEDURE UNTIL THESE CRITERIA HAVE BEEN MET. Polishing will not accomplish a smooth surface unless each step during the finishing process has been successfully accomplished.

V. Procedures for Two Methods of Amalgam Polishing

A. Pumice and Tin Oxide Slurries

This method is accomplished by using a rubber cup, brush, and wheel brush.

1. Prepare a slurry mix of pumice and water in a dappen dish.
2. Polish all surfaces of the restoration with a brush or cup and plentiful pumice slurry (Fig. 26.13). Remember, the pumice does the polishing; the cup only moves the pumice. A smooth satin finish, which will exhibit a dull appearance, is accomplished.
3. Polish the proximal surface with medium and fine polishing strips.
4. Rinse and dry the tooth.
5. Prepare a wet mixture of tin oxide and alcohol in a dappen dish. Water or mouthwash is an acceptable substitute for alcohol.
6. Polish all surfaces of the restoration with a new, clean cup or brush and the tin oxide slurry.
7. An optimal final step may include using a soft wheel brush in a straight handpiece with tin oxide. Continue to polish the amalgam until the tin oxide begins to dry and a high luster is achieved (Fig. 26.14).
8. Rinse and dry the tooth.
9. Assess the polished amalgam by using a mouth mirror, explorer, and the Skill Performance Evaluation sheet in Appendix 2. Figure 26.15

Tips for the Clinician

- Effective lighting allows for ease in evaluating surface irregularities
- The sequence of steps is crucial. Do not proceed to the next step until the previous step is completed.
- The polishing points and cups technique is less messy than the slurry technique

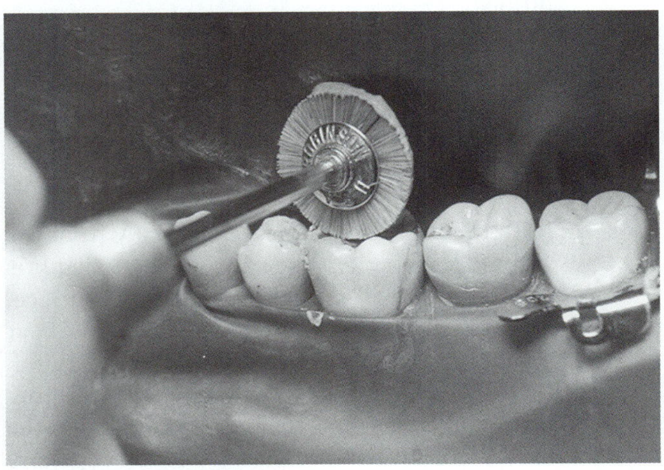

FIGURE 26.14 Polishing with a soft wheel brush.

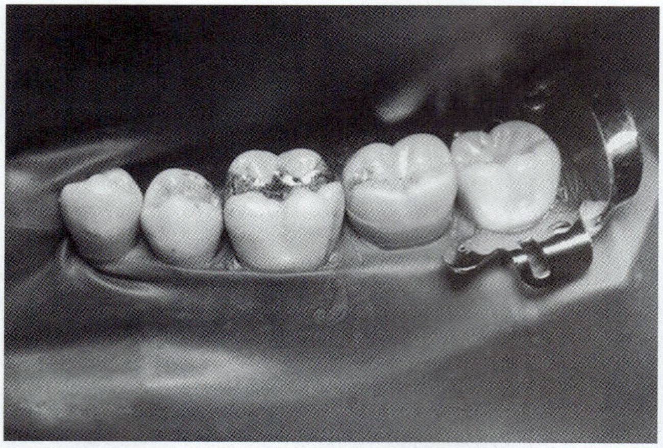

FIGURE 26.15 Finished and polished restoration.

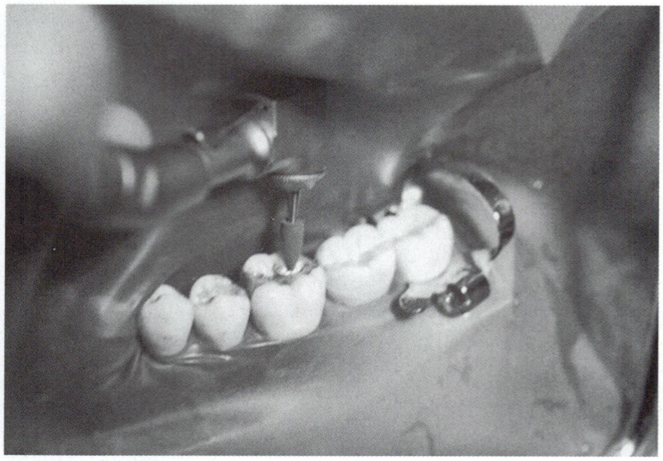

FIGURE 26.16 Brown polishing point adapted to the occlusal surface.

illustrates an amalgam restoration that has been finished and polished.

B. Rubber Cups and Points Impregnated With Abrasive Particles

1. Colors

Abrasive-impregnated rubber cups and points are supplied in three colors: brown, green, and yellow-banded green. Each color denotes a different degree of abrasiveness. In some instances, they are referred to as "brownies," "greenies," and "super greenies."

2. Use

The cups are designed for use on the proximal surfaces, and the points are used on the occlusal surface. Often, they are used interchangeably, providing that the dental hygienist properly adapts them to the amalgam surface. They should be operated at a relatively low speed with light, intermittent strokes under wet conditions.

3. Advantages

The cups and points will polish restorations quickly and tend to be less messy than the use of two slurries of different abrasive agents.

4. Disadvantages

Both the cups and points wear quickly from use and autoclaving. Eventually, a metal shank is exposed that will scratch the amalgam surface. The greatest disadvantage, however, is heat production. The amalgam surface MUST NOT be heated above 140°F by the polishing procedure. Heat is generated rapidly with the use of abrasive-impregnated rubber cups and points.

5. Procedure for Use

a) Brown abrasive cups and points are used first to produce an initial, smooth satin finish. Polish the occlusal, the proximal, and then finally the facial and lingual surfaces. A brown abrasive point polishing the occlusal surface is pictured in Figure 26.16.

b) The green cups and points are used in the same manner as the brown cups and points. After use, examine to determine if a smooth, shiny finish has been achieved.

c) A yellow-banded green cup or point is used as the final step. These cups and points are used in the same manner as the brown and green cups and points. Figure 26.17 illustrates the use of a yellow-banded green point. Examine to determine if a smooth, lustrous polished finish has been achieved.

d) Rinse and evacuate debris.

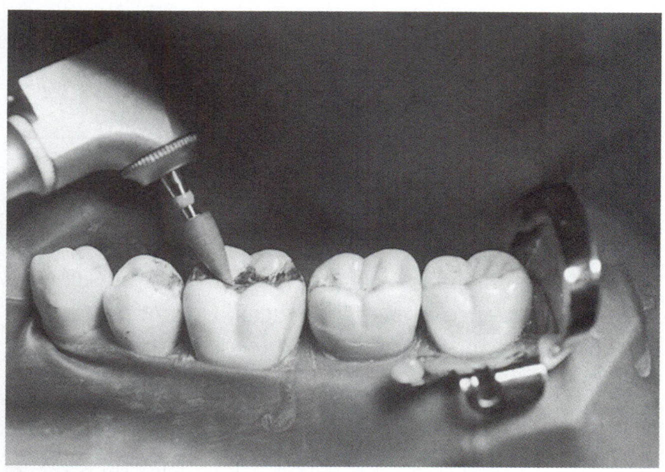

FIGURE 26.17 Yellow-banded green point adapted to the occlusal surface.

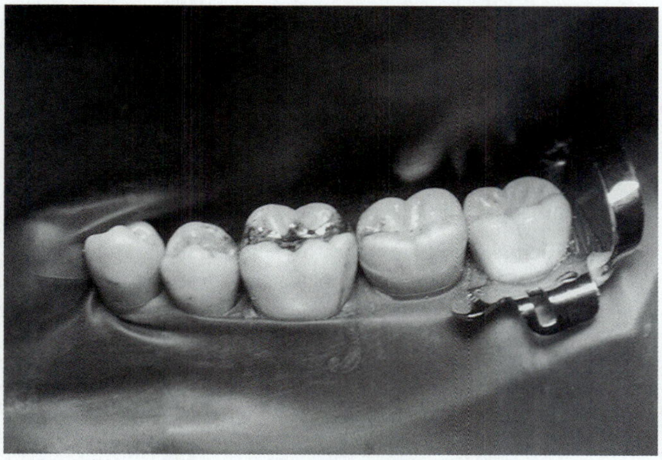

FIGURE 26.18 Final amalgam polish with use of abrasive-impregnated polishing points.

e) Assess the polished amalgam by using a mouth mirror, explorer, and the Skill Performance Evaluation sheet in Appendix 2. The amalgam should appear smooth and highly polished, and it should have a lustrous shine. There should be no damage to the adjacent tooth structure. A final amalgam polish with use of brown, green, and yellow-banded green points can be seen in Figure 26.18.

Precautions

- Heat can be generated rapidly on the tooth during amalgam finishing and polishing.
- Aerosols are frequently created when polishing with pumice and tin oxide.
- Cups and points wear quickly from use and autoclaving. An exposed metal shank will scratch the amalgam surface.

Summary

At each patient recall appointment, amalgam restorations should be evaluated for finishing and polishing. If indicated, this procedure may be performed during the recall visit, or it may be scheduled as a separate appointment. Research has documented the long-term benefits of finishing and polishing amalgam restorations. When an amalgam restoration is properly placed, carved, finished, and polished, the patient will have less plaque retention and, subsequently, a lower incidence of periodontal disease and caries. In addition, finishing and polishing may increase the lifetime of the restoration as well as patient satisfaction.

Finishing

1. Evaluate the restoration (margins, occlusion, proximal areas).
2. Discuss the procedure with the patient.
3. Isolate the area with cotton rolls or a rubber dam.
4. Smooth the proximals if necessary (with files, burs, discs, strips).
5. Remove occlusal excess, and eliminate flash (with burs or stones).
6. Define the occlusal anatomy (with burs or stones).
7. Smooth cavosurface margins and occlusal surface.
8. Smooth facial and lingual surfaces.

Polishing

Slurry Method

1. Prepare slurries of tin oxide and pumice.
2. Polish all surfaces with pumice and cup or brush.
3. Polish proximals with medium and fine polishing strips.
4. Rinse and dry tooth.
5. Polish all surfaces with a clean cup or brush and tin oxide slurry.
6. Rinse and evacuate debris.

Polishing Points and Cups Methods

1. Use brown abrasive cups and points to polish occlusals, proximals, and then facial and lingual surfaces.
2. Use the green cups and points in the same manner.
3. Produce the final polish with a yellow-banded green cup or point.
4. Rinse and evacuate debris.

Learning Activities

1. In the dental materials laboratory, observe existing amalgams on extracted teeth.
2. During patient assessment, evaluate amalgam restorations with an explorer and mouth mirror to determine if the amalgams are indicated for finishing and polishing.
3. Evaluate patient amalgams to determine if any amalgams have already been finished or polished.
4. In the dental materials laboratory and on a typodont tooth with an existing cavity prep, place and carve an amalgam. After 24 hours have elapsed, practice finishing and polishing the restoration.

Review Questions

1. Which of the following polishing agents is used intraorally to give a high luster to amalgam restorations?
   a) Alumina
   b) Tin oxide
   c) Zirconium silicate
   d) Flour of pumice
2. An operator is polishing an amalgam and inadvertently overheats it. The overheating may likely cause the following except one. Which one is the EXCEPTION?
   a) Pulpal injury
   b) Release of mercury
   c) A dull appearance to restoration
   d) Decreased susceptibility to corrosion
3. What occurs when a metal becomes tarnished?
   a) The surface becomes pitted
   b) The surface is discolored
   c) The surface becomes scratched
   d) Mercury has risen to the surface
4. During amalgam finishing and polishing, coarser abrasives should be followed by finer abrasives. This allows for larger scratches in the amalgam surface to be reduced to less defined scratches.
   a) The first statement is true; the second statement is false.
   b) The first statement is false; the second statement is true.
   c) Both statements are true.
   d) Both statement are false.
5. Ideally, amalgam restorations should be finished and polished after:
   a) 1 week
   b) 24 hours
   c) 2 hours
   d) The initial set
6. Polishing amalgam aids in reducing the likelihood that tarnish and corrosion will occur because it:
   a) Helps to create a smooth, homogeneous surface that resists tarnish and corrosion
   b) Brings excess mercury to the surface to aid in preventing tarnish and corrosion
   c) Increases the likelihood for galvanic currents to occur
   d) Forces free mercury to the base of the cavity preparation
7. You are utilizing an explorer in a zigzag motion to examine an amalgam on tooth #18. As you explore the buccal cavosurface, you note a deficient amount of amalgam in several areas. Your explorer catches only as you move from restoration to the tooth. This marginal discrepancy is best described as a (an):
   a) Submarginal area
   b) Open margin
   c) Flash
   d) Overextension
8. When finishing the occlusal surface of an MOD restoration, care must be taken to:
   a) Reduce all occlusal contact with opposing tooth
   b) Reduce both marginal ridges slightly
   c) Maintain the original anatomy of the restoration
   d) Produce a high luster of the amalgam surface
9. Finishing and polishing amalgams improves all of the following except one. Which one is the exception?
   a) Marginal deficiencies
   b) Surface tarnish
   c) Marginal flash
   d) Excessive corrosion
10. When polishing amalgams, green and brown points and cups are utilized to:
    a) Remove gross irregularities from the amalgam surface
    b) Remove bulky contact area
    c) Polish the amalgam to achieve high surface luster
    d) Prepare the surface for finishing burs

Supplemental Readings

Craig RG, Powers JM. Restorative Dental Materials. 11th ed. St. Louis: Mosby, 2002:309–310.

Darby ML, Walsh MM. Dental Hygiene Theory and Practice. Philadelphia: Saunders, 1995:211–212.

Ferracane JL. Materials in Dentistry. 2nd ed. Baltimore: Lippincott Williams & Wilkins, 2001:305–306.

Paarmann C. Finishing, recontouring, and polishing amalgam restorations. J Pract Hyg 1993;Jan/Feb:2,1.

Wilkins EM. Clinical Practice of the Dental Hygienist. 10th ed. Baltimore: Williams & Wilkins, 2008, Chapter 44.

27

Taking Alginate Impressions

Jacqueline Harper, R.D.H., M.S.

Key Words/Phrases

homogeneous
setting time
study models
study casts
working time

Objectives

After studying this chapter, the student will be able to do the following:

1. Select the appropriate tray for the patient by using the criteria listed in this chapter.
2. Prepare the impression trays with rope wax, including the palatal area of the maxillary tray.
3. Discuss the aspects of patient preparation for alginate impressions.
4. Demonstrate proper mixing of the alginate as well as loading, seating, and removal of the tray to obtain acceptable alginate impressions.
5. Evaluate the impression by using the criteria listed in this chapter, and determine if the impression is acceptable.

INTRODUCTION

Use of alginate impression material is the most common method for obtaining diagnostic casts. It is pleasant tasting, inexpensive, and easy to manipulate. It also adequately records details of the patient's oral structures. **Study models** or **study casts** are positive reproductions of the patient's dental arches and surrounding tissues. They are important visual aids in diagnosis and treatment planning for a patient, and they also serve as an important part of the patient's permanent record. In addition, diagnostic study models are useful as pretreatment and posttreatment records for patients who undergo extensive restorative or orthodontic treatment. Taking alginate impressions is a procedure that is included in the scope of practice in most states for both dental hygienists and dental assistants.

I. Purpose

The purpose of taking an alginate impression is to make an accurate reproduction of the maxillary and mandibular arches and adjacent tissues. Study models constructed from alginate impressions can be used for planning patient treatment and can serve as part of the patient's permanent record.

II. Selection and Preparation of the Tray

A. Perforations

Impression trays are usually perforated so that the alginate will flow through the holes when the tray is seated on the dental arch. These perforations act as a retentive mechanism and keep the set alginate from separating from the tray upon removal.

B. Available Varieties

Impression trays are available in a variety of sizes and materials. Disposable (or single-use) trays are usually made of plastic, and autoclavable (permanent) trays are made of stainless steel.

C. Proper Tray Selection

Before taking the impression, the empty tray should be seated in the patient's mouth to determine the correct fit. Each tray should:

1. Extend facially to include all teeth as well as the musculature and vestibule.
2. Extend distally approximately 2 to 3 mm beyond the last tooth in the arch to include the retromolar area.
3. Provide a 2 to 3 mm depth of alginate beyond the occlusal surface and incisal edge.
4. Be comfortable to the patient.

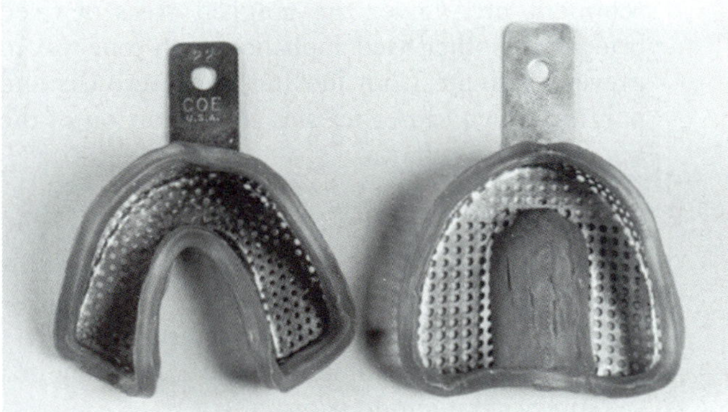

FIGURE 27.1 Beading wax placed around tray peripheries and in the maxillary palatal area.

D. Sterilization

Trays that have been "tried" and those that were "used" for taking the impression should be sterilized before they are returned to storage.

E. Adding Wax to the Tray

After the impression trays have been selected, rope (beading) wax can be molded around the periphery of the tray. This protects the tissues from injury, extends the tray, and may aid in the retention of alginate material within the tray.

F. Adding Wax to the Palatal Area

The maxillary tray may also have rope wax placed in the palatal area of the tray to support the alginate in a high vault and to avoid trapping air. Figure 27.1 illustrates rope wax placed on tray peripheries and the palatal area.

III. Preparation of the Patient

A. Explain the Procedure

Ask the patient if he or she has had impressions taken in the past. If not, explain the procedure. The patient should follow the directions of the clinician during the procedure. Instruct the patient not to talk but, rather, to raise his or her hand to signal any needs or discomfort.

B. Guard Against Spills

Place a napkin on the patient to protect his or her clothing. Give the patient a tissue or paper towel should excessive salivation should occur.

C. Minimize Gagging

Seat the patient in an upright position to minimize the chance of gagging or vomiting.

D. Dental Appliances

Have the patient take out all removable dental appliances, such as full or partial dentures, orthodontic retainers, etc. Cover the gingival areas of fixed bridges and other fixed appliances with rope wax to prevent alginate from locking under crowns and pontics, which causes tearing and distortion of the impression on removal.

E. Rinse

Ask the patient to rinse with mouthwash. This serves two purposes.

1. It will reduce the amount of bacteria.
2. It will reduce the amount of saliva, resulting in a more accurate impression.

F. Sequence

It is recommended that the mandibular impression be taken first to familiarize the patient with the procedure as well as with the taste and consistency of the alginate material.

IV. The Alginate Impression

Alginate material is available in regular-set and fast-set products. The regular-set material has a **setting time** of approximately 3 to 4 minutes, whereas the fast-set material will set (or gel) in approximately 1 to 2 minutes. The **working time,** or the time that it should take to mix the alginate, is 1 minute.

A. Mixing the Alginate

1. You will need the necessary equipment listed in Table 27.1.
2. If the bulk form of alginate is used, shake or "fluff" the can, as discussed in Chapter 8. Both bulk and unit packaging are illustrated in Figure 27.2. Wait 30 seconds to allow the "dust" to settle before opening the lid.
3. Using the calibrated water measure, which is marked and provided by the manufacturer, place one measure of water for each scoop of alginate powder into the flexible rubber bowl. The cooler the water, the more working time you will have; however, the consistency of the mix will be thinner. With warmer water, the working time is decreased.
4. Using the measuring scoop provided, measure the amount of alginate powder needed for the impression as directed by the manufacturer's instructions. Add the alginate to the bowl containing the water.
5. Holding the bowl in one hand and the spatula in the other, gently stir to wet the alginate powder with the water.
6. Once the powder and water have been incorporated, start to rotate the bowl in the palm of one hand, and vigorously press the spatula flat against the bowl with the other. This spatulation method is pictured in Figure 27.3.

   Incorporate the powder and water thoroughly to create a **homogeneous** mix—one that has a smooth consistency. At the completion of spatulation, the alginate will become "creamy," similar to the consistency of peanut butter.
7. With the spatula, gather the alginate material into one mass in the bowl.

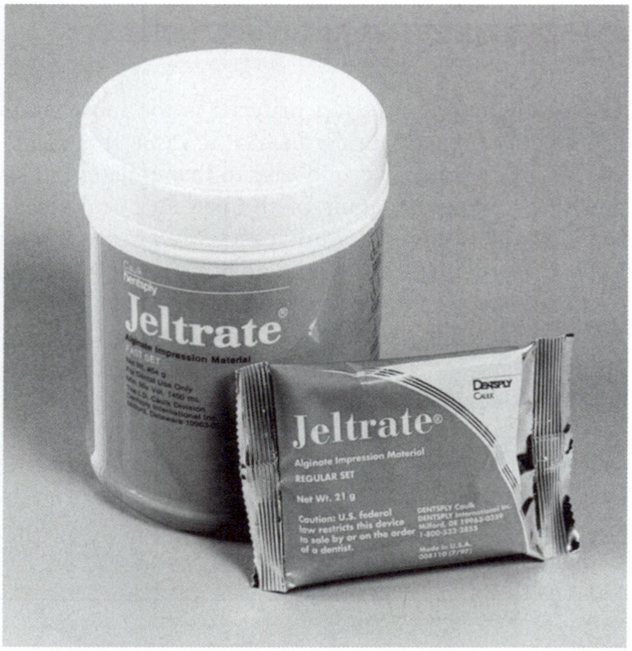

FIGURE 27.2 Alginate in bulk and packet form.

Table 27.1 Armamentarium for Taking Alginate Impressions
Impression trays
Rope (beading) wax
Rubber mixing bowl
Alginate spatula
Alginate powder
Measuring scoop for alginate
Water measurer
Tap water
Disinfecting solution
Mouthwash
Infection control attire

B. Filling the Tray

Load the alginate material onto the spatula. With the spatula in one hand and the tray in the other, begin to place the alginate in the tray.

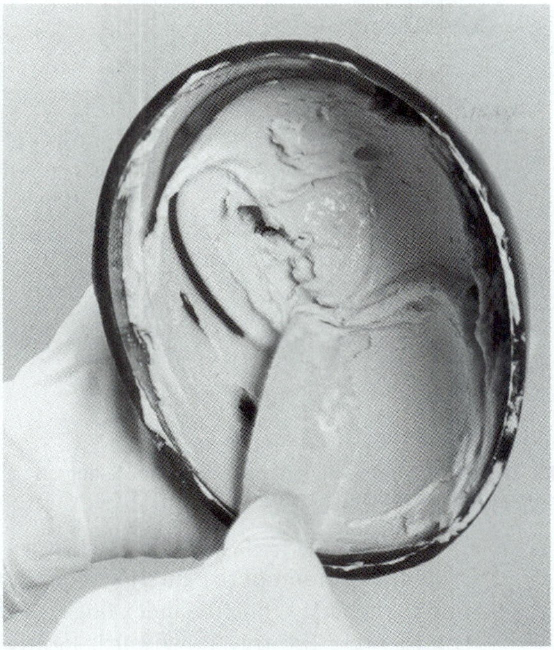

FIGURE 27.3 Spatulation of the alginate impression material.

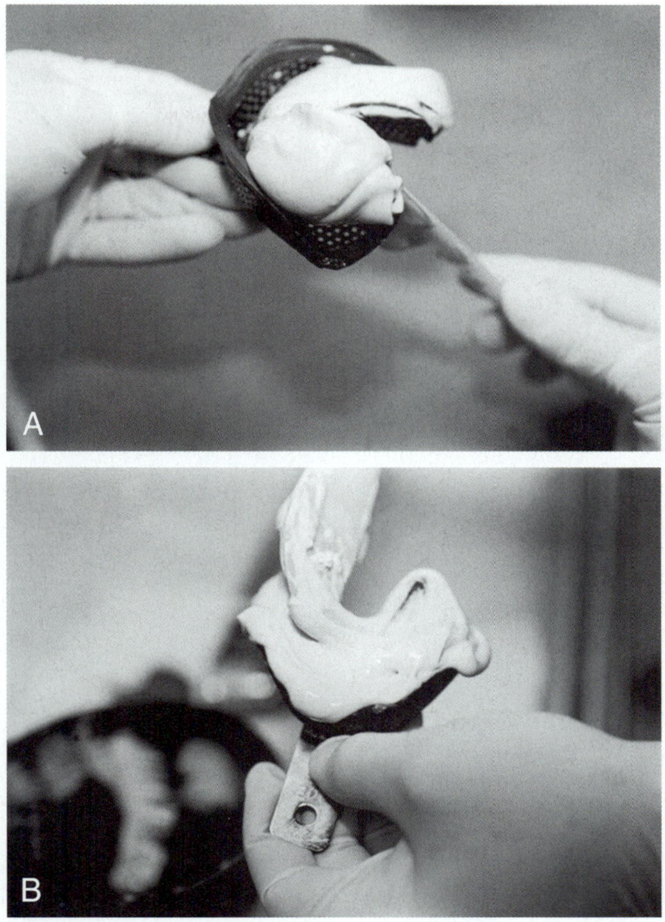

FIGURE 27.4 Loading the mandibular tray with alginate impression material. **A.** Loading from the posterior lingual aspect. **B.** Loading from the anterior aspect.

1. Mandibular Tray

a) Load the Tray

Begin loading the tray from a posterior lingual aspect of the tray, working toward the facial aspect, as shown in Fig. 27.4*A*. Deposit the material into the tray, and fill the tray to its periphery, as shown in Figure 27.4*B*.

b) Eliminate Trapped Air

Using the tip or the end of the spatula, press the material into the tray so that any trapped air in the alginate is released.

2. Maxillary Tray

a) Load the Tray

Begin loading the tray from the posterior aspect of the tray, working anteriorly, as shown in Figure 27.5*A*. With the bulk of the material in the anterior region, fill the tray to its periphery, as shown in Figure 27.5*B*.

b) Eliminate Trapped Air

Using the tip or the end of the spatula, press the material into the tray so that any trapped air between the tray and the alginate is released.

3. Moisten and Smooth the Alginate

Using a fingertip moistened with tap water, smooth the alginate material, and make a slight indentation in the surface, as shown in Figure 27.6. This will help in placing the tray over the teeth correctly and in preventing the formation of air bubbles. Excessive water may prevent bonding of the material in the tray to the material on the occlusal surfaces of the teeth, as will be discussed later.

C. Seating the Impression

1. Mandibular Arch

a) The operator should be in a 7-o'clock position (5 o'clock for left-handed operators) or to the side and in front of the patient.

b) The chair should be raised for easy access to the patient. Adjust the headrest so that the occlusal plane is parallel to the floor. This patient and operator position is illustrated in Figure 27.7.

c) Using a 2 × 2 piece of gauze or the air syringe, dry the patient's teeth as thoroughly as possible to remove excess saliva before seating the impression tray. This will help to increase the accuracy and detail of the impression.

d) Ask the patient to open his or her mouth. Using the index finger and thumb of one hand, retract the patient's cheek. Rub a small amount of alginate material over the occlusal and interproximal surfaces of the mandibular teeth with the index finger of the other hand.

e) Grasp the handle of the impression tray so that the tray and the alginate are facing downward. Rotate the tray into the mouth by using

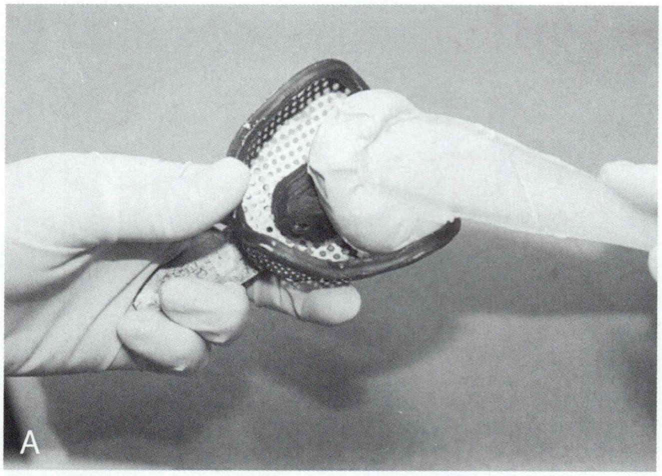

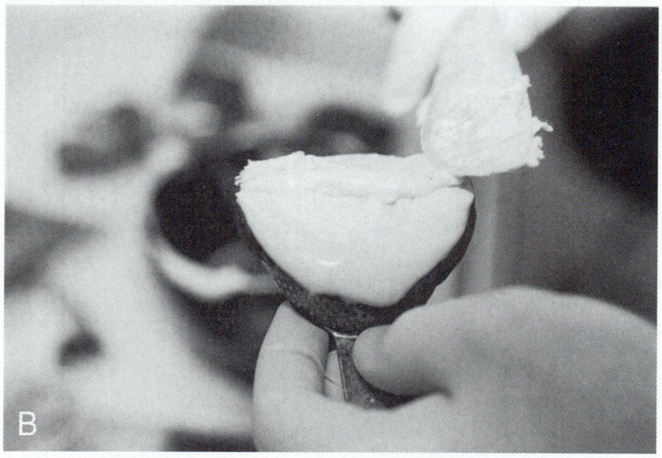

FIGURE 27.5 Loading the maxillary tray with alginate impression material. **A.** Loading from the posterior aspect. **B.** Loading from the anterior aspect.

the front of the tray to retract the near cheek and your free hand to retract the far cheek. Once the tray has been inserted, straighten it so that the tray handle is in line with the patient's midface.

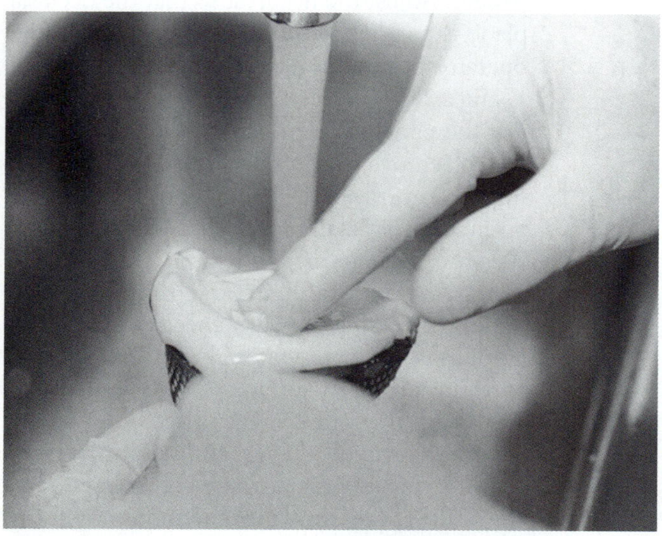

FIGURE 27.6 Moistening and indenting the alginate material.

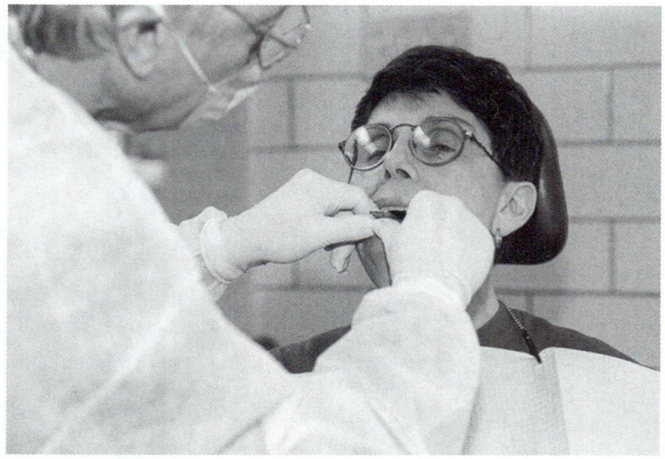

FIGURE 27.7 Operator and patient positioning for taking an impression of the mandibular arch.

f) Note the position of the anterior teeth in relation to the tray. Using the index fingers of both hands, press the tray downward, lightly and evenly, over the mandibular arch until resistance is felt. The lip should lap over the front of the tray, and the alginate should extend into and fill the labial periphery. Excess alginate material will flow out of the perforations as well as into the vestibular and lingual areas. Once the tray has been properly seated, use the index fingers to manipulate the patient's cheeks and release air from the vestibular areas. This will help to create a more detailed anatomy in the facial vestibular area.

g) Ask the patient to raise his or her tongue to the roof of the mouth and move it from side to side. Have the patient close his or her mouth to relax the tongue and cheek muscles, and then carry the tray in a downward direction. This will help to create a more detailed anatomy in the lingual and facial areas.

h) Instruct the patient to breathe normally through his or her nose. If gagging occurs, seat the patient in the most upright position, and ask the patent to lean slightly forward.

i) Keep the tray in place until the alginate is completely set (2–3 minutes after gelation). Alginate material usually sets within 3 to 4 minutes depending on which type of alginate is used (fast or regular set), room temperature, body temperature, water temperature, and consistency of the mix. Because body temperature is higher than room temperature, the alginate material will set faster in the mouth than the remaining alginate will in the bowl.

2. Maxillary Arch

a) Operator position when taking this impression should be from the side and in back of the patient. This patient–operator position is

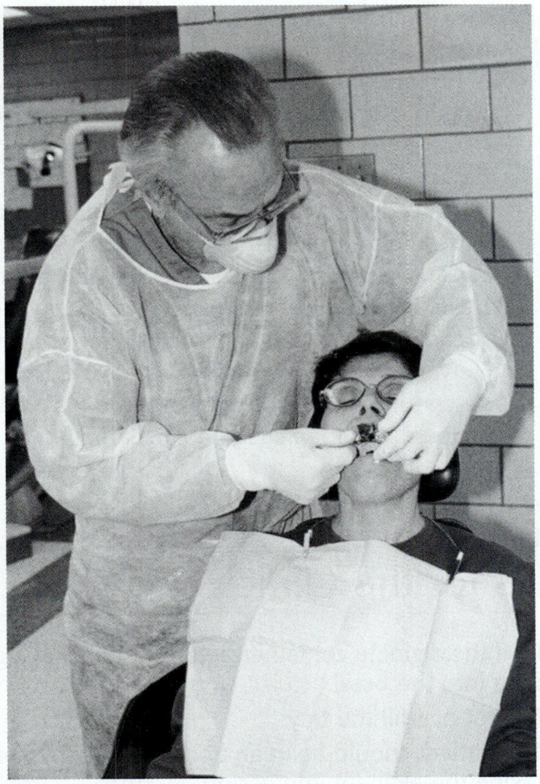

FIGURE 27.8 Operator and patient positioning for taking an impression of the maxillary arch.

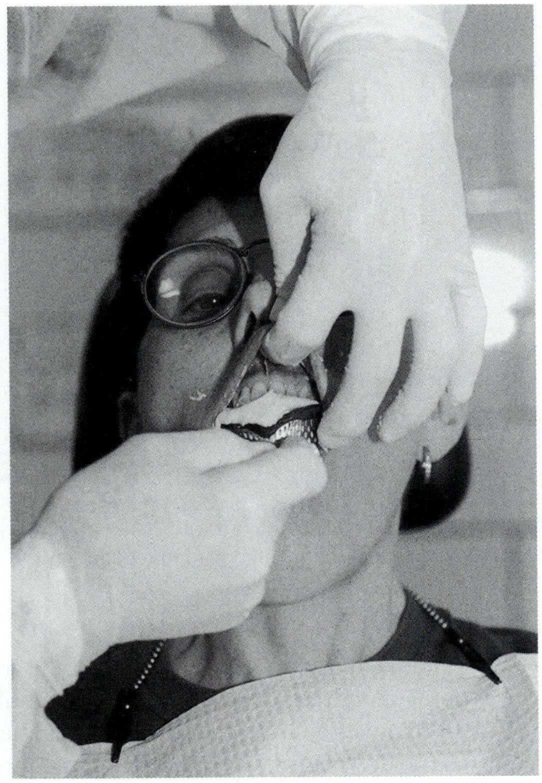

FIGURE 27.9 Seating of the maxillary impression.

frequently referred to as 11 o'clock (1 o'clock for left-handed operators) and is shown in Figure 27.8.

b) As with the mandibular arch, use a 2 × 2 piece of gauze or the air syringe for drying the patient's teeth as thoroughly as possible to remove excess saliva before seating the impression tray.

c) Ask the patient to open his or her mouth. Using the index finger and thumb, again retract the patient's cheek, and rub a small amount of alginate on the occlusal and interproximal surfaces of the maxillary teeth.

d) The impression tray and the alginate material should be facing upward.

e) Turn the tray slightly to one side, placing the tray in the patient's mouth. Insert the tray by rotating it into the mouth as previously described. Once the tray is inserted, straighten it so that the tray handle is in line with the midface of the patient.

f) Begin to apply light and even pressure upward until resistance is felt. Seat the impression tray in the posterior region, and then seat it toward the anterior, allowing the alginate to flow over the molars. Retract the front of the upper lip as the tray is seated, as shown in Figure 27.9. This will allow any excess alginate and air to be expressed through the front of the tray, minimizing the chance of air voids and patient gagging.

g) Instruct the patient to breathe through his or her nose and to lean slightly forward, with the head down toward the chest. This will help to minimize the gagging reflex.

h) Hold the tray in place until the alginate is completely set (2–3 minutes after gelation).

D. Removing the Impression Tray

1. Mandibular Tray

a) Use the fingers of one hand to retract the corner of the mouth and allow air to enter the vestibule.

b) To remove the tray, place the thumb and index finger on the tray handle and use a firm, sideways lifting motion, as shown in Figure 27.10. The impression tray should flip free, with the alginate material held securely in the impression tray. The free hand should be used to stabilize the mandibular arch during tray removal to decrease injury to the temporomandibular joint and the teeth in the opposing arch.

c) If the tray does not release, a suction seal has been created. To break this seal, place the index finger of one hand under the periphery of the posterior portion of the tray on either the right or left side. The tray should now be easy to remove.

d) Assess the impression by using the Skill Performance Evaluation sheet in Appendix 2.

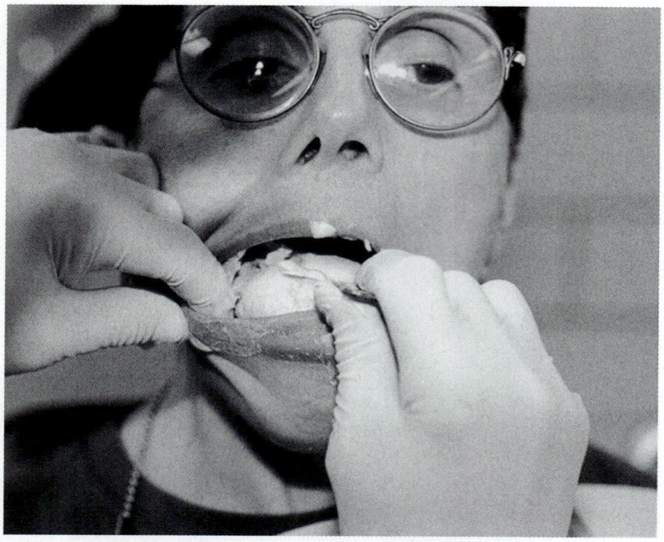

FIGURE 27.10 Removal of the mandibular impression tray.

2. Maxillary Tray

a) With the fingers of one hand, retract the corner of the mouth to allow air to enter the vestibule.

b) To remove the tray, grasp the tray handle and use a downward, sideways flipping motion with the thumb and forefinger. The tray should remove easily, with the set alginate secured in the impression tray. The fingers of the free hand should protect the teeth in the opposing arch during tray removal.

3. Postremoval Procedures

a) After an impression procedure, ask the patient to rinse with water or mouthwash to remove any excess alginate.

b) Remove any alginate that may be remaining on the teeth or in the interproximal spaces by using an explorer or floss.

c) Before dismissing the patient, have the patient rinse again. Use a moistened towel to remove any alginate on the face or lips.

d) Be sure to return any removable dental appliances to the patient.

E. Disinfecting the Impression

1. Gently rinse the alginate impression under cool tap water to remove any debris that may be remaining in the impression.
2. Gently shake off any excess water.
3. Spray the entire impression (top and bottom) with an Occupational Safety and Health Administration–approved disinfecting solution.
4. Place the impression in a headrest cover or plastic bag.
5. Disinfection is usually complete in 10 minutes depending on the disinfectant used.
6. Rinse again with water, shake dry, and place in a clean headrest cover or plastic bag.
7. If the impression(s) cannot be poured immediately, store them in an area with 100% humidity.
8. Assess the impression by using the Skill Performance Evaluation sheet in Appendix 2.

Precautions

- Wear a mask when fluffing the alginate.
- Remember that the impression is contaminated with saliva and should be properly handled and disinfected.

Tips for the Clinician

- Fluff the alginate container before dispensing alginate into the bowl.
- Do not overfill the tray.
- The patient should be in an upright position when taking the alginate impression.
- Do not clean the mixing bowl immediately. Use the alginate remaining in the bowl as an indicator for setting time. If the alginate in the bowl is set, then the material in the mouth is also set.
- If taking impressions for both arches, take the mandibular impression first to get the patient accustomed to the procedure.

SUMMARY

1. Discuss the procedure with the patient.
2. Select the proper tray by inserting an empty tray in the patient's mouth.
3. Prepare the trays by adding wax to the periphery and palatal areas if needed.
4. Have the patient rinse with mouthwash.
5. Mix the alginate following the manufacturer's directions, and fill the tray.
6. Smooth the alginate with a moistened finger.
7. Take a mandibular impression from the 7-o'clock position.
8. Take a maxillary impression from the 11-o'clock position.
9. With a quick motion, remove the impressions 2 to 3 minutes after gelation.
10. Properly disinfect the impression.
11. Pour the impression as early as convenient.

Review Questions

1. When preparing the patient for an impression the operator should:
a) Explain the procedure to the patient
b) Place a napkin on the patient to protect his/her clothing
c) Place the patient in the upright position
d) Have the patient remove all removable appliances
e) Have the patient rinse with antibacterial mouthwash
f) All of the above
g) a, b, and d only

2. When taking a maxillary impression, a right handed operator should be standing in which position?
a) 12:00
b) 7:00
c) 11:00
d) 9:00

3. When mixing alginate impression material:
a) Add the water to the powder
b) Add the powder to the water
c) Add the powder and water together, at the same time
d) Either water or powder can be added in any sequence

4. All of the following statements are true about the "working time" of alginate material except one. Which one is the EXCEPTION ?
a) Working time begins when water and powder come together
b) Cooler water increases working time
c) Warmer water decreases working time
d) Working time begins when the impression is seated.

5. The typical mixing time for alginate is _______ and the setting time for regular-set material is _______.
a) 1 min; 1–2 min
b) 1 min; 3–4 min
c) 3–4 min; 1 min
d) 1–2 min; 1 min

Supplemental Readings

Ehrlich A, Torres HO. Essentials of Dental Assisting. 3rd ed. Philadelphia: Saunders, 2001, Chapter 22.

Medcom-Trainex. The New Dental Assistant—Impressions and Models. Cypress, CA: Medcom, Inc., 1992.

Wilkins EM. Clinical Practice of the Dental Hygienist. 10th ed. Baltimore: Lippincott Williams & Wilkins, 2008, Chapter 11.

28

Key Words/Phrases

diagnostic model
study model

Fabrication and Trimming of Study Models

Joan Gibson-Howell, R.D.H., Ed.D

Objectives

After studying this chapter, the student will be able to do the following:

1. Demonstrate the following laboratory procedures:
   - Use a gypsum product to pour a study model from an impression.
   - Trim the study model on the model trimmer.
2. Differentiate between the two methods of diagnostic cast/study model fabrication.
3. Describe and demonstrate the cast cuts that are used to trim a study model for patient consultation and dental treatment planning.
4. Explain the laboratory safety procedures and necessary equipment for use in the laboratory mandated by the Occupational Safety and Health Administration.
5. Critique the completed study model for acceptable cuts.

INTRODUCTION

The composition, properties, and uses of gypsum materials were discussed in Chapter 9. **Study models** (or **diagnostic models**) are defined as "a positive replica of the dentition and surrounding structures used as a diagnostic aid and/or base for construction of orthodontic appliances or prosthetic devices."

Because a dental hygienist is legally permitted to perform these procedures, competency is expected in the associated knowledge and skills. These procedures are commonly performed in the practice of dentistry to gather information concerning the patient's dentition and to establish an accurate diagnosis. As with all skills, however, "practice makes perfect." Most people must continue to practice to be consistently competent. Therefore, do not feel bad if your first attempt is not exact.

During any process, each step is important to the quality of the final outcome. If a flaw is present in step one, that flaw will be reproduced throughout the entire procedure and be present in the final product. The ability to self-critique to make adjustments or repeat the step is critical for obtaining satisfactory results. The procedural steps for these techniques will be detailed in this chapter.

Table 28.1 Armamentarium for Constructing Study Models

Equipment and Supplies
Plaster bowl
Plaster spatula
Gypsum material
Vibrator
Ruler
Lab knife
Protractor (optional)
Boxing wax (optional)
Beading wax (optional)
Wet/dry sandpaper (optional)
Maxillary and mandibular impressions
Scale
Graduated cylinder
Pencil
Pink baseplate wax
Model trimmer
Glass or acrylic slab
Infection Control and Safety
Protective eyewear
Lab jacket or clinic gown
Gloves

I. Purpose/Indications

The purpose of this chapter is to apply previously learned information and acquire the necessary skills to prepare esthetically pleasing and useful study models. The process of pouring an alginate impression, preparing a base for the model, separating the model from the impression, and trimming the model, is described in the following pages. It is also important that these skills are practiced both safely and effectively; therefore, compliance with Occupational Safety and Health Administration (OSHA) guidelines is mandatory.

II. Construction of a Study Model

Several laboratory techniques for fabricating study models are acceptable. The armamentarium is listed in Table 28.1. This chapter will present two of these techniques: one using a "double-pour" and another using boxing wax around the impression.

A. Using a Double-Pour Technique

A two-stage pour will prevent distortion and provide an adequate base for reproduction of the oral structures. The double-pour technique involves two separate mixes and, thus, two separate setting times.

1. First-Stage Pour

a) Measure 100 g of the dental stone or other gypsum. Regardless of the material, follow the manufacturer's directions.

b) Measure the correct quantity of the corresponding water (25–30 mL), and pour it into your plaster mixing bowl. Pour the powder into the liquid.

c) Spatulate (stir) the mixture for 30 seconds with a stropping motion. Pressing the spatula against the side of the bowl helps to remove air bubbles from the mixture.

d) Place the mixing bowl on the vibrator, and compress the sides of the bowl. Bubbles should rise to the surface and break. Remove the mixing bowl from vibrator.

e) Place the impression on the vibrator. Starting at one corner and using a wax spatula, "deliver" a small amount (pea size) of the mix into the mold distal to the last molar (Fig. 28.1*A*). Allow this material to flow into the impression under vibration, filling the impression of the last tooth in the opposite quadrant.

f) Repeat the previous step until the impression is filled, adding the new material at the same location as the initial increment. The material

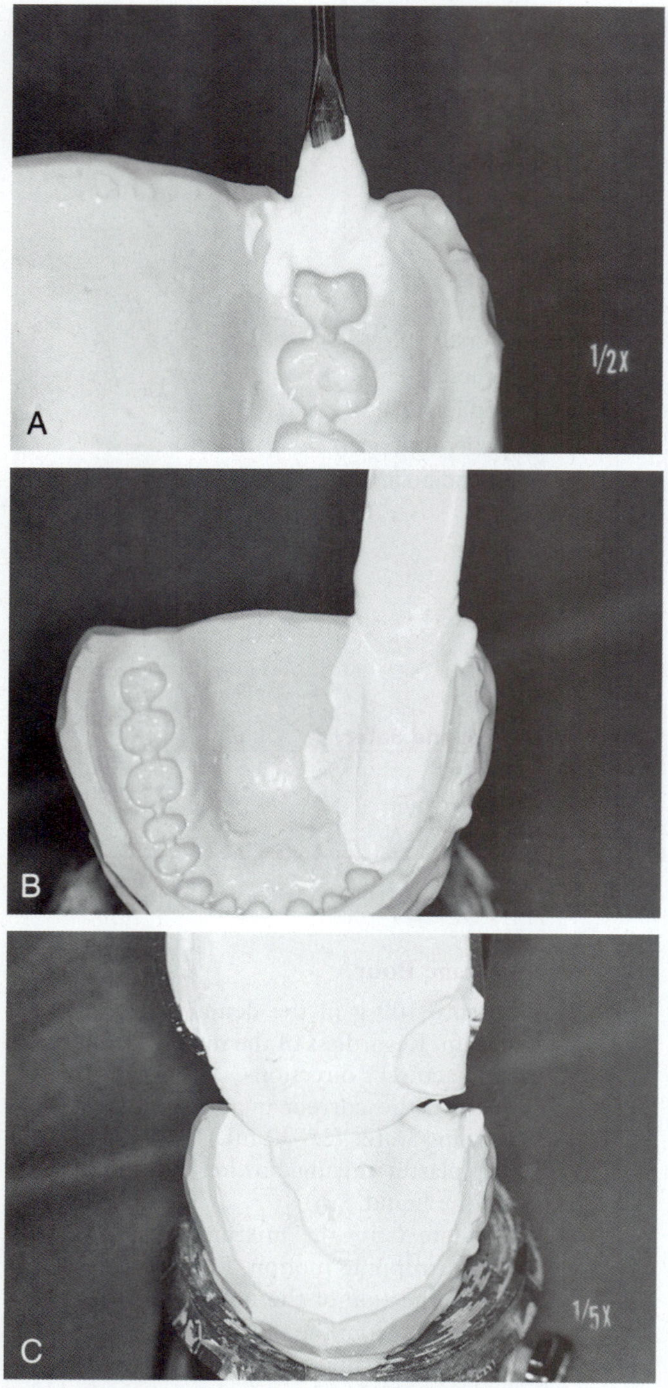

FIGURE 28.1 Pouring an impression. **A.** A small amount of gypsum material is added distal to the most posterior molar. **B.** Larger increments are added with the plaster spatula. **C.** After the teeth are filled, the remaining gypsum material is poured to fill the impression.

should flow around the arch, filling one tooth at a time. You may increase the size of the increment when the material has a greater distance to flow around the arch. You may use the plaster spatula to add larger amounts of material for these final additions (Fig. 28.1*B*).

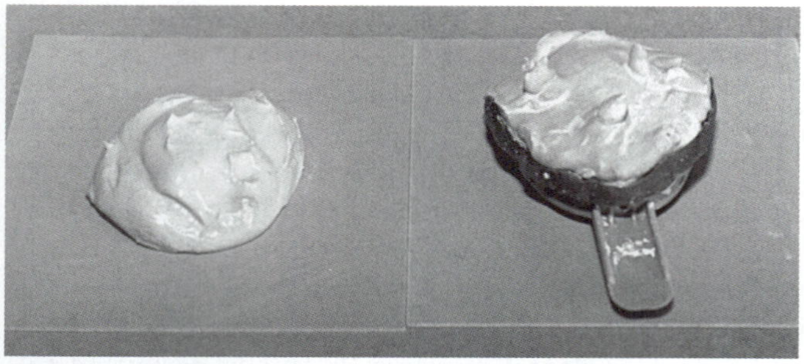

FIGURE 28.2 Alginate impression poured with gypsum. The gypsum paddy serves as a base for the alginate impression.

g) After all the teeth are filled, pour the remainder of the mix from the bowl into the impression (Fig. 28.1*C*). Overfill the impression with gypsum material sufficiently to cover all areas by approximately 0.25 inch.

h) Add small amounts of the gypsum material to the surface of the pour to assist in retention of the second pour (Fig. 28.2). Allow the impression to set facing up.

i) Allow the mix to reach the initial set (see the manufacturer's instructions). This will be several minutes after the "loss of gloss," or approximately 10 minutes after the initial pour.

2. Second-Stage Pour

a) Make a thicker mix of gypsum product (100 g of gypsum to 25–30 mL of water) to serve as a base to support the first pour.

b) Make a paddy of gypsum material approximately 1 inch thick in a shape resembling the size of the impression tray, and place it on a glass or acrylic slab or a surface that will not absorb water or stick to the mix (Fig. 28.2).

c) Invert the poured impression onto the paddy. Do not apply pressure to the inverted impression tray. Do not allow the impression to sink closer than 0.5 inch to the surface. Do not allow the gypsum material to overlap outside the tray (Fig. 28.3).

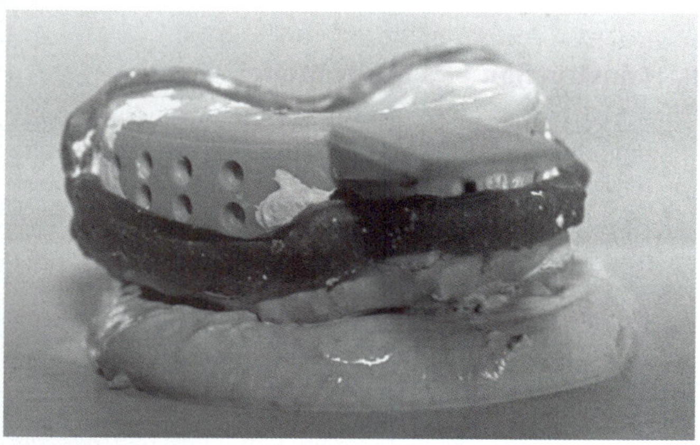

FIGURE 28.3 Inverted set impression on the gypsum paddy.

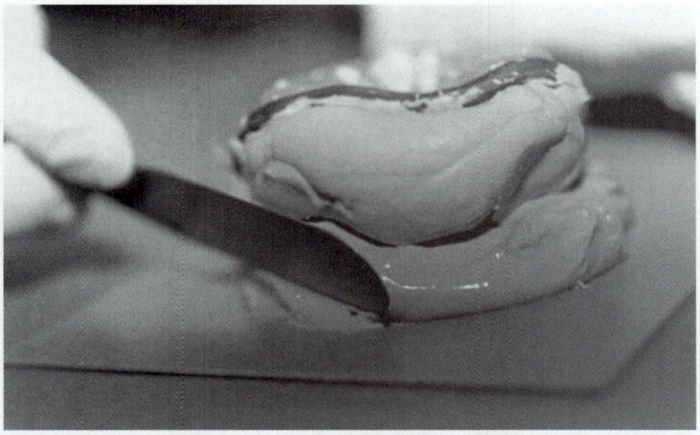

FIGURE 28.4 Adapting the gypsum base material to the set gypsum in the impression tray.

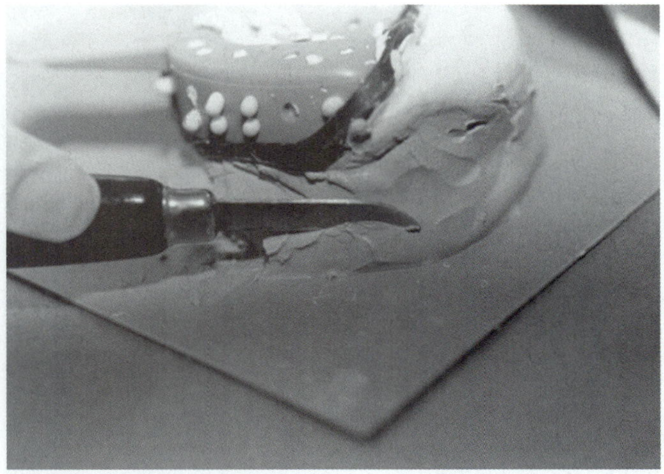

FIGURE 28.6 Trimming the excess gypsum with a laboratory knife after loss of gloss.

d) Blend the two gypsum mixes together with the plaster spatula to create a continuous connection of the two mixes (Fig. 28.4). While holding the handle of the impression tray, use the spatula to shape the sides of the stone around the first pour. Avoid placing the wet gypsum material from the base onto the impression tray because this would create a mechanical lock that is difficult to separate when set. Be certain that the handle of the impression tray and the occlusal surface of the teeth are parallel with the slab to promote a base of uniform thickness. A cross section of the base and impression is illustrated in Figure 28.5. Note how the additional small mounds of gypsum added to the first pour "interlock" into the base to provide a stronger finished product.

e) After loss of gloss, trim the excess stone base with a laboratory knife to approximately 1/4 inch from the outer border of the impression (Fig. 28.6). This will develop the sides and base area of the cast, thus requiring minimal use of the model trimmer.

f) Separate the cast from the impression 45 to 60 minutes after the beginning of the second pour.

g) To begin tray removal from the cast, place the laboratory knife on the edges of the periphery of the tray, and slightly twist the knife to release the adhering alginate and gypsum materials (Fig. 28.7). Repeat this procedure around the periphery of the tray.

h) When the margins of the tray are free of the cast, use an upward, pulling motion to facilitate the separation (Fig. 28.8).

i) If the tray does not freely separate from the cast, determine the location of the obstruction on the periphery, and carefully remove it with a laboratory knife.

j) Avoid rocking the impression tray back and forth or side to side. This may cause the teeth to fracture.

k) Trim the base and sides of the cast on the model trimmer. Use of the model trimmer will be discussed later in this chapter.

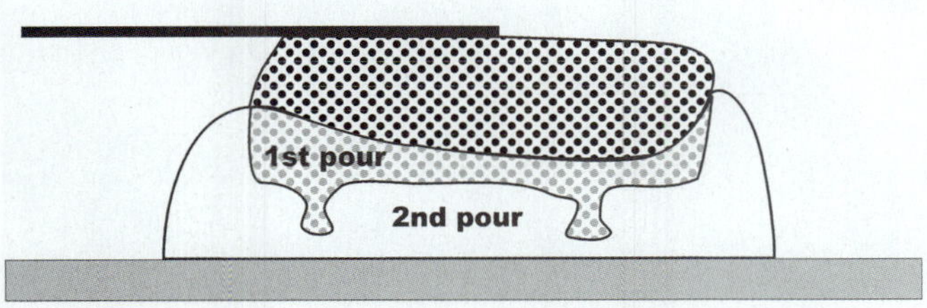

FIGURE 28.5 Cross section of the poured alginate impression inverted onto the gypsum paddy (base).

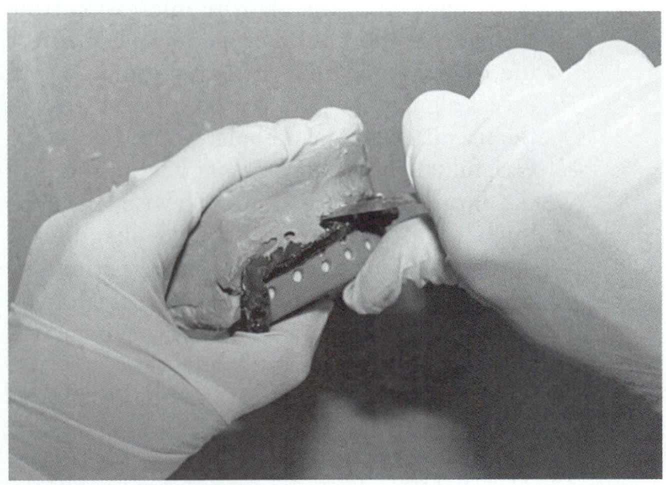

FIGURE 28.7 Removing the cast from the impression tray with the laboratory knife.

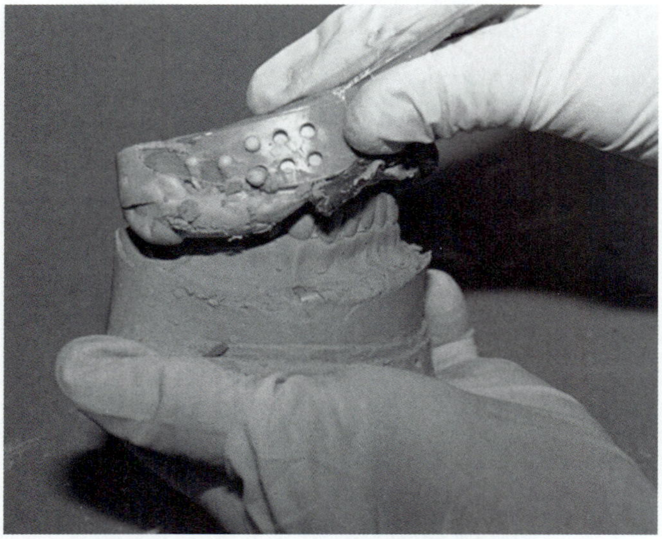

FIGURE 28.8 Using an upward, pulling motion to separate the cast from the impression.

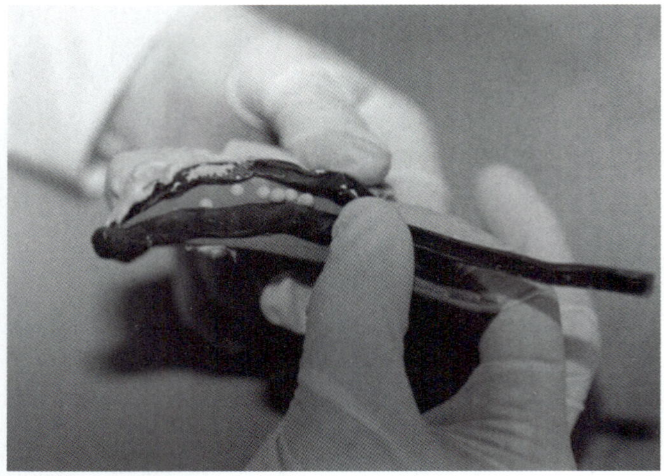

FIGURE 28.9 Application of the beading (rope) wax to the periphery of the impression.

B. Using a Single-Pour Technique

After developing skill with the double-pour technique, a single-pour technique may be used for some models or casts. In the single-pour technique, a larger amount of material is initially mixed. The impression is filled and the paddy prepared as described above. The filled impression is inverted and placed on the paddy before the material sets. Greater care is needed to prevent the impression tray from being locked into the setting gypsum material.

C. Using Boxing Wax

Boxing wax completely encircles the impression tray and creates a temporary mold to contain the plaster or stone. A base is formed for the study model when the gypsum material has set inside the boxing wax.

1. After removal of the alginate impression from the patient's mouth and proper disinfection, use the laboratory knife to carefully trim away the excess alginate beyond the posterior border of the maxillary and mandibular impression.
2. Carefully trim the palatal and heel portions of the maxillary impression. Likewise, trim the lingual and heel portions of the mandibular impression. Be conservative with the trimming procedure. Removal of this excess alginate helps to box the impression and to maintain the anatomic landmarks on the final cast.
3. Apply and attach a piece of beading (rope) wax to the periphery of the impression above the handle so that the entire impression tray is encircled (Fig. 28.9). Use a warm wax spatula to affix the wax approximately 2 to 3 mm down from the peripheral roll of the impression to the impression tray. To avoid distortion, do not overheat the spatula, beading wax, or alginate.
4. Add the boxing wax around the entire impression, and have it extend and overlap 0.5 inch beyond the vestibular edge of the tray (Fig. 28.10).
5. Set the vibrator on a slow setting, and slowly fill the tooth impressions as previously described. Tilt the impression to encourage thorough wetting and movement of gypsum throughout the dentition (Fig. 28.11).
6. Continue adding larger increments until the impression is filled to half the boxing wax height, then set the impression on a flat surface.
7. Completely fill the boxed impression with the remainder of the gypsum product (Fig. 28.12).
8. Allow the material to set for 45 to 60 minutes.

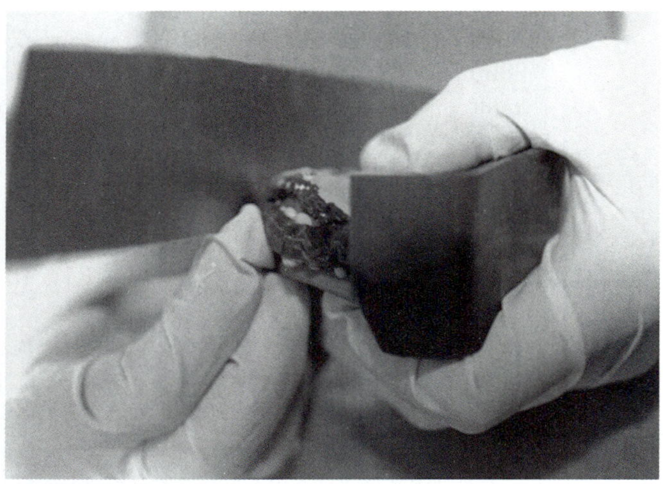

FIGURE 28.10 Boxing and beading (rope) wax attached to the impression.

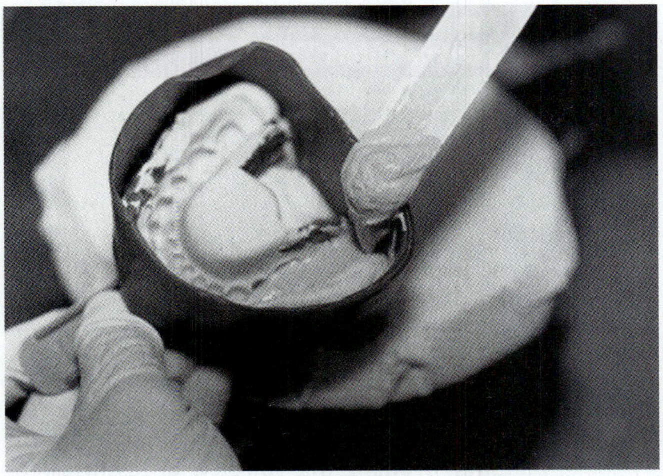

FIGURE 28.11 Initial fill of a boxed alginate impression.

9. Remove the beading and boxing wax (Fig. 28.13).
10. Carefully separate the gypsum cast from the alginate impression.
11. Trim the base and sides as described in the next section.

Tips for the Clinician—Pouring An Impression

- Properly proportion and mix the gypsum product.
- Fill one tooth at a time.
- Do not lock the impression tray into the cast.
- Do not allow the material to vibrate out of the impression at the opposite end of the arch.

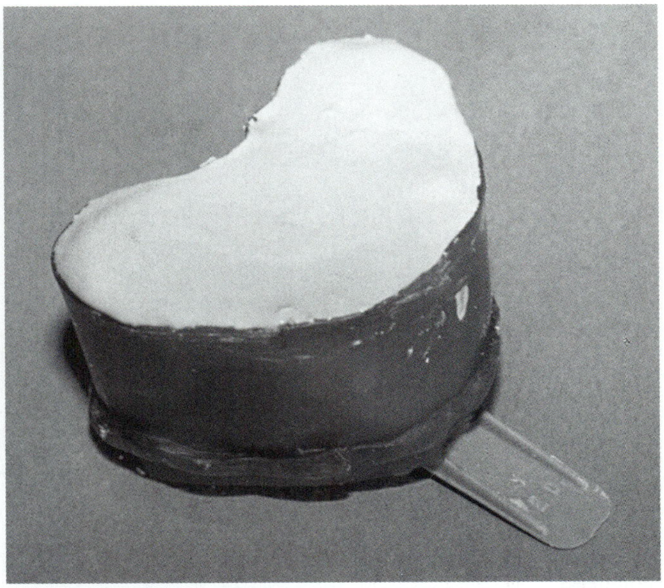

FIGURE 28.12 Boxed impression filled with gypsum.

Precautions—Pouring An Impression

- Disinfect the impression before pouring.

III. Trimming Diagnostic Casts or Study Models

A nicely trimmed cast or study model gives the patient a professional and esthetic-looking representation of their oral tissues. It can be used during a consultation appointment to inform the patient about his or her

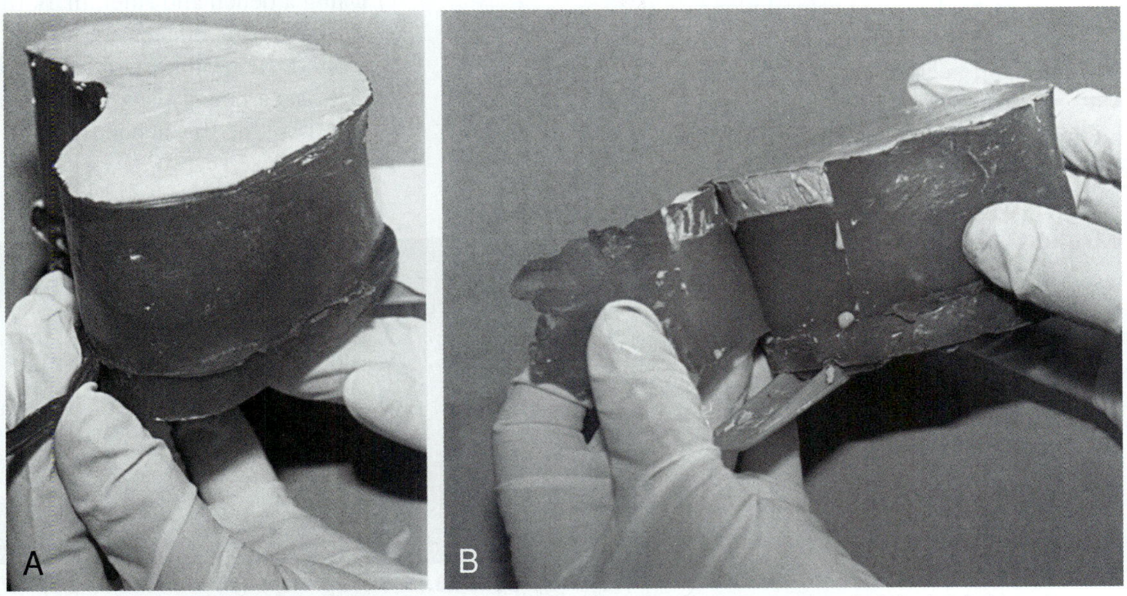

FIGURE 28.13 Wax removal. **A.** Removal of the beading (rope) wax. **B.** Removal of the boxing wax.

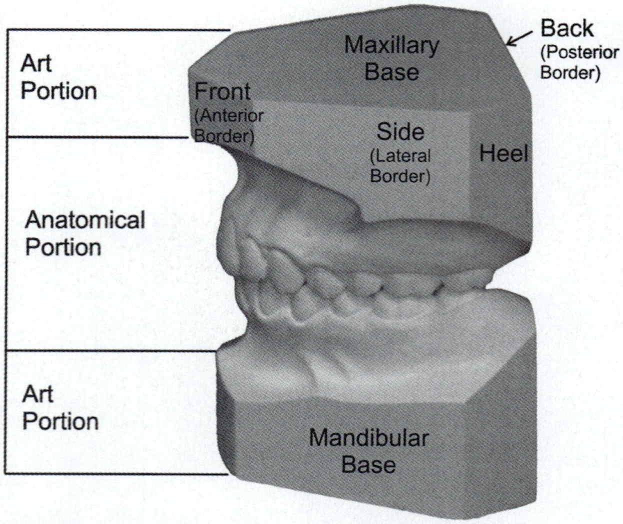

FIGURE 28.14 Cast terminology and identification of cast landmarks.

existing oral status and the proposed plans for dental treatment. A prepared study model that is neat and accurate adds to the precise, professional content of the presentation. Study models may also serve as part of the patient's record.

The following general directions are intended for a wide variety of clinical needs. Specific needs may require the trimming technique to be modified.

A. Cast Design and Terminology

Note the cast's appearance and terminology in Figure 28.14. Note the similarities and differences in the cuts and shapes between the maxillary and mandibular casts.

1. Bases are parallel to the occlusal plane.
2. The backs are perpendicular to the bases.
3. The sides and heels are trimmed even.
4. The anterior of the upper cast has a point at the midline, but the anterior of the mandibular cast is rounded.

B. Preparation for Trimming

1. Assemble the necessary materials and equipment, which are listed in Table 28.2.
2. Don appropriate personal protective equipment.
3. Make sure the casts have set for a minimum of 30 minutes, and then separate the casts from the impressions. If the casts are dry, thoroughly wet them.
4. Remove small nodules of stone on the casts and/or residual bits of alginate with a wax spatula, particularly on the occlusal surfaces of the teeth (Fig. 28.15).

Table 28.2 Armamentarium for Trimming Study Models

Models or casts
Model trimmer
Pencil and ruler
Wax spatula and laboratory knife
Eye protection
Handpiece and burs
Lathe and attachments

5. Secure hair away from your face. Remove any hanging or dangling jewelry, accessories, or clothing. Removal of rings is recommended.
6. Turn on the model trimmer. Establish a steady flow of water over the grinding wheel of the model trimmer so that it does not become clogged and will function smoothly.
7. Trim excess stone that grossly extends beyond the anatomy of interest. At this and all other steps, DO NOT TRIM AWAY CRITICAL ANATOMY!

C. Trimming Models

1. Maxillary Base

a) Establish a Plane for the Maxillary Model Base

To make the base of the maxillary model parallel to the occlusal plane, place the model occlusal surface down on a cushioned (several layers of paper towels), flat surface. If the cast is not stable when resting on the occlusal surface, rock it onto the anterior teeth and do one of the following:

1) Using a pencil and ruler, mark the model in at least four places at an equal height around the periphery of the model.
2) OR, use a pencil placed between the pages of a book at the needed height. Mark the

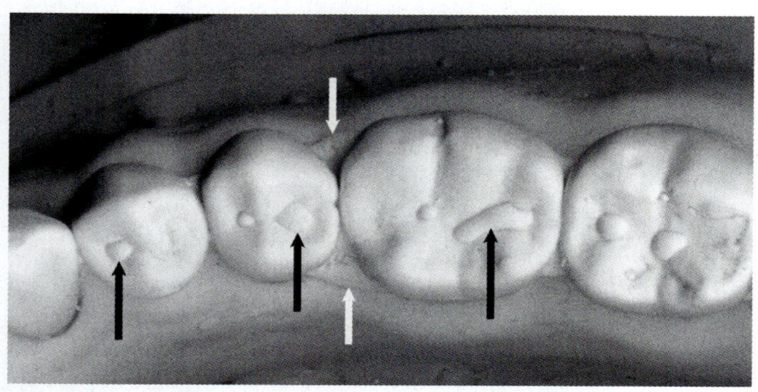

FIGURE 28.15 Blebs of stone (*black arrows*) and bits of alginate (*white arrows*) to be removed from the model.

Step-By-Step Checklist for Trimming Models

1. The Maxillary Base

   ______ A. To make the maxillary arch parallel to the bench top, do one of the following after you have rocked the arch forward onto the anterior teeth:

   1. Use a pencil and ruler to mark the model in 4 places at an equal height around the periphery
   2. Use a pencil between the pages of a book to the required height. Turn the model to mark it in at least 4 places (Fig 28.16)

   The base should be approximately one third of the total model height in the anterior region.

   ______ B. Trim the base of the maxillary model (Fig. 28.17)

   Place on grinding wheel and trim the base parallel to the pencil marks. The trimming goal is one flat surface. Rinse clean. Check periodically by laying trimmed surface on counter and attempt to "rock" the base from side to side. It should not have any bevels or exhibit a rocking motion.

2. Maxillary Posterior Border (Fig. 28.18)

   ______ Put both arches in occlusion and mark with a pencil the location on the maxillary cast of the most posterior anatomy that is present on either cast (so you know "how far in" to grind) (Fig. 28.18A).

   ______ Also mark the median raphae (midline of palate) with a pencil (Fig. 28.18B).

   ______ Now trim the maxillary model at a right angle to the penciled midline. Grind to the marked area identifying the most posterior anatomy (Fig. 28.18).

3. Mandibular Posterior Border (Fig. 28.19)

   Place the base of the maxillary model on the stage of the model trimmer. Occlude the mandibular model with the maxillary (mandibular model will be on top–look closely at Figure 28.18A).

   ______ Trim the back of the mandibular model until it is even with the back of the maxillary model but do not trim away any anatomy.

   ______ Both posterior sides (backs) should be flat and the occluded models should not open when set "on end" (on posterior sides).

4. Mandibular Base

   ______ Keep both models in occlusion with the backs on the trimmer stage. Trim the base of the mandibular model so that it is parallel with the maxillary model (Fig. 28.20A and B). The combined height should be 2 to 2¾ inches.

   ______ The bases of the models and the occlusal plane should be parallel to the bench top.

5. Lateral Borders (Fig. 28.21)

   ______ Trim the sides of the widest cast first from canine to the last molar (Fig. 28.21A). Trim parallel to the central grooves (Fig. 28.21B).

   ______ Next, put teeth in occlusion and trim the other arch to match (Fig. 28.21C).

6. Anterior Borders (Fig. 28.22)

   A. Maxillary Cast

   ______ Mark the canine eminence and the midline <u>on the base</u> portion of the model with a pencil.

   ______ Trim the anterior portion from the canine eminence to anterior midline on both sides (Fig. 28.22 A and B). These cuts will form a point with each other, and with each lateral border.

   B. Mandibular Cast

   ______ Trim the anterior portion from canine to canine following the form of the arch (Fig. 28.22A and C). It will be rounded in appearance.

7. Posterior Angles

   ______ Place the teeth in occlusion and trim the posterior angles (heels) (Fig. 28.23) of both casts to be even and symmetrical with the lateral and posterior sides of the casts.

8. Finishing the Casts

   ______ A. Trim and smooth the tongue area of the mandibular cast with a lab knife or large acrylic bur and lab handpiece

   ______ B. Trim the excess "lip" (land area) of lateral and posterior borders of both casts (Fig. 28.24). Do not remove mucobuccal fold unless instructed to do so.

   ______ C. Fill in voids with a putty of matching gypsum product in the base portion of casts. Use waterproofs and paper to smooth the base; do not round or sand the edges.

   ______ D. Remove any remaining nodules or blebs of gypsum from the cast with a lab knife.

   ______ E. Check casts for symmetry.

   ______ F. Label both casts with your name (for laboratory exercises) or the patient's name (for the clinical setting) and the date.

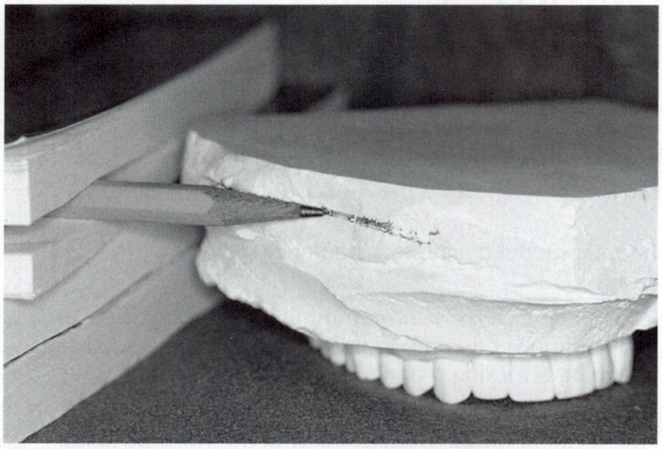

FIGURE 28.16 The base of the maxillary cast is marked parallel to the occlusal plane.

model in at least four places around the periphery, as shown in Figure 28.16.

3) Connect the pencil marks with a solid line as shown in Figure 28.17*A*.

4) The base should be approximately one third of the total model height in the anterior region.

b) Trim the Base of the Maxillary Model (Fig. 28.17)

Gently feed the maxillary cast into the grinding wheel of the model trimmer with a steady pressure to trim the base and leave a smooth, flat cut. Cut parallel to the penciled line (and the occlusal plane). Trim until the model base is approximately 0.5 to 1 inch in height at the maxillary anterior region and the base is flat. It is not necessary to trim to the pencil marks, only to trim parallel to them. Evaluate the cuts by periodically placing the cast on the countertop to assess the overall cast appearance. The base should be parallel to the occlusal plane in both the anteroposterior and the lateral directions. When using the model trimmer, immediately rinse away any gypsum debris on the model.

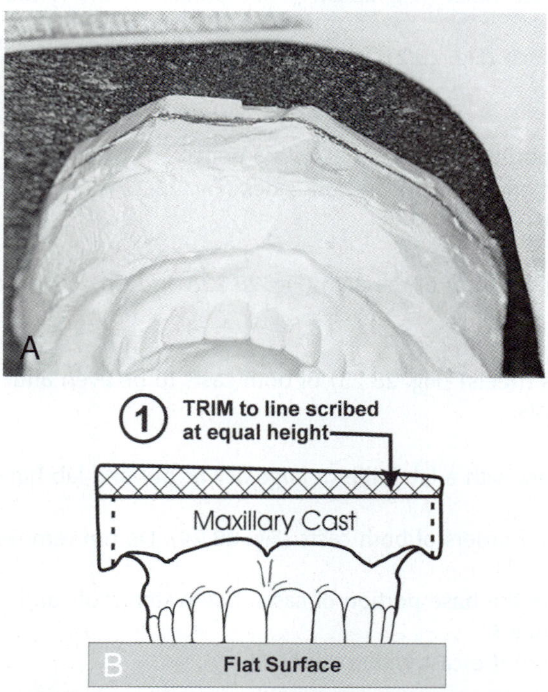

FIGURE 28.17 A. The base of the maxillary cast is trimmed parallel to the pencil line. **B.** Drawing showing the portion of the cast to be removed. The *cross-hatched area* indicates the material to be trimmed in this step. The *dashed lines* indicate areas to be trimmed in subsequent steps.

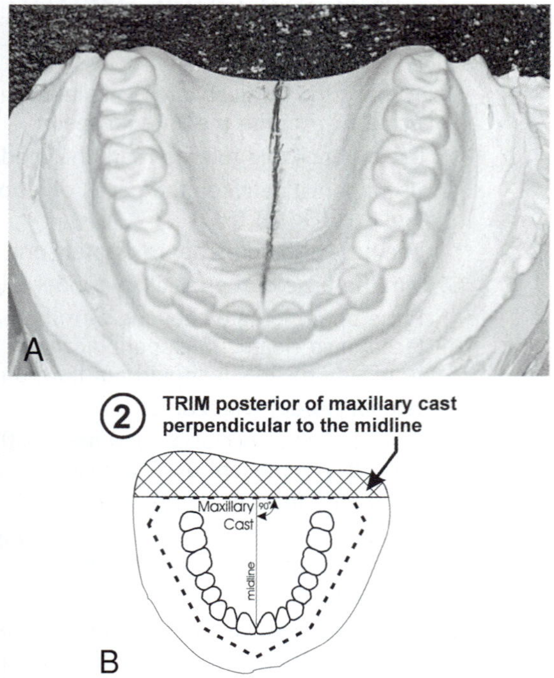

FIGURE 28.18 A. The posterior of the maxillary cast is trimmed perpendicular to the midline. **B.** Drawing showing the portion of the cast to be removed. The *cross-hatched area* indicates the material to be trimmed in this step. The *dashed lines* indicate areas to be trimmed in subsequent steps.

2. Maxillary Posterior Border (Fig. 28.18)

a) Occlude models with or without a wax bite. If the models will not completely occlude, trim the interfering base material. Do not trim away any anatomy of interest.

b) With a pencil, mark the location on the maxillary cast of the most posterior anatomy of either cast: retromolar pad, hamular notch, or maxillary tuberosity. Also, on the maxillary cast, mark the midline and the median raphe with a pencil.

c) Trim the posterior surface of the maxillary model at a right angle to this line, as shown in

Figure 28.18. Trim to the most posterior anatomy of either cast.

3. **Mandibular Posterior Border (Fig. 28.19)**

Place the base of the maxillary model on the model trimmer table. Articulate the mandibular model with the maxillary having the interocclusal bite registration wax between the teeth if available to avoid fracture. In other words, place the maxillary and mandibular model in occlusion and turn them upside down (maxillary now on bottom) on the trimmer table. Trim the back of the mandibular model until it is even with the back of the upper model, but do not trim away any anatomy. The backs (posterior borders) should be flat and the models should not open when they are placed "on end" (posterior borders), see Figure 28.19.

4. **Mandibular Base (Fig. 28.20)**

Keep the upper and lower casts in occlusion with their backs resting on the trimmer table. Trim the base of the lower cast so that it is perpendicular to the backs of both casts and parallel to the base of the upper cast and occlusal plane. The combined height of both models should be approximately 2 to 2.5 inches. When finished,

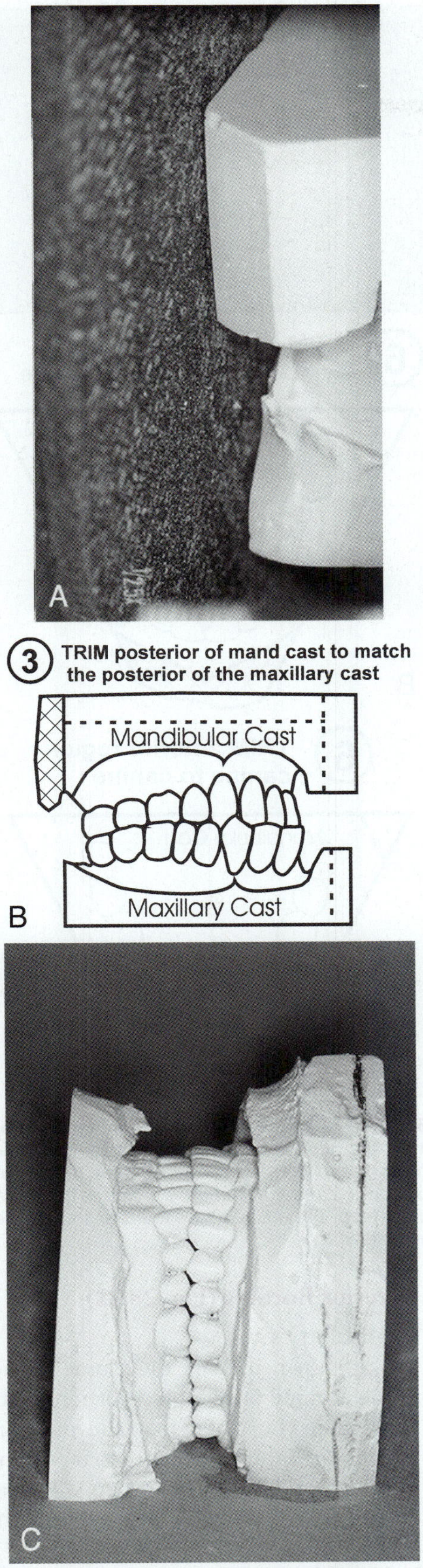

FIGURE 28.19 A. The posterior of the mandibular cast is trimmed to match the posterior of the maxillary cast. **B.** Drawing showing the portion of the cast removed. The *cross-hatched area* indicates the material to be trimmed in this step. The *dashed lines* indicate areas to be trimmed in subsequent steps. **C.** The models sit on their posterior borders with the teeth in occlusion.

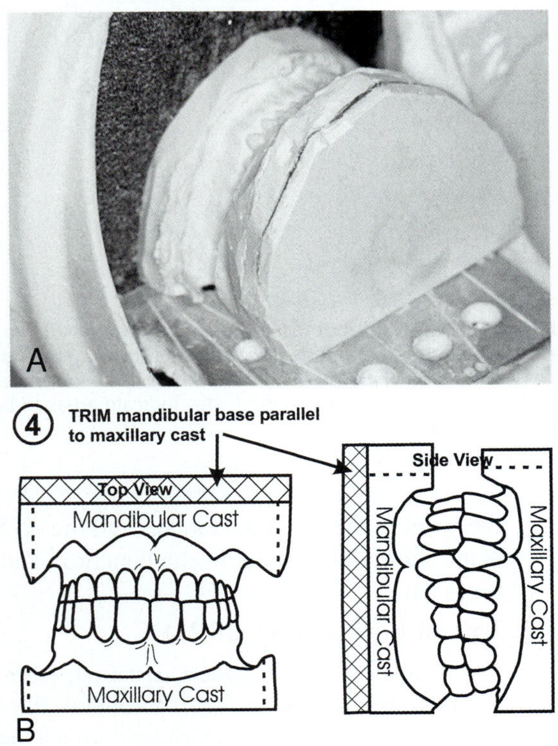

FIGURE 28.20 A. The posterior of the mandibular cast is trimmed perpendicular to posterior of the maxillary and mandibular casts. **B.** Drawing showing the portion of the cast to be removed. The *cross-hatched area* indicates the material to be trimmed in this step. The *dashed lines* indicate areas to be trimmed in subsequent steps.

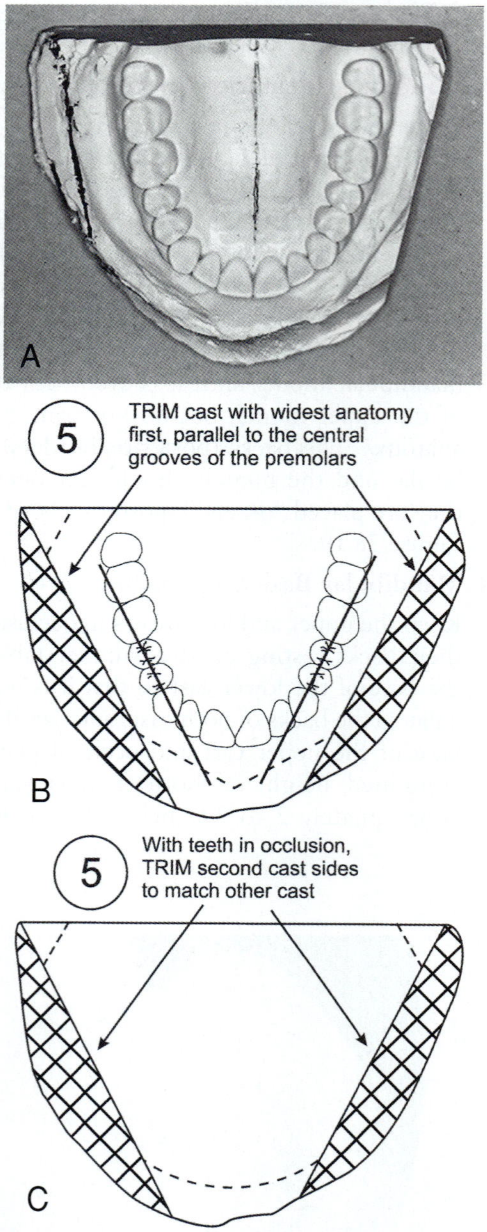

FIGURE 28.21 **A.** The sides of the casts are trimmed parallel to the central grooves of the teeth. **B** and **C.** Drawings showing the portion of the cast removed. The *cross-hatched area* indicates the material to be trimmed in this step. The *dashed lines* indicate areas to be trimmed in subsequent steps.

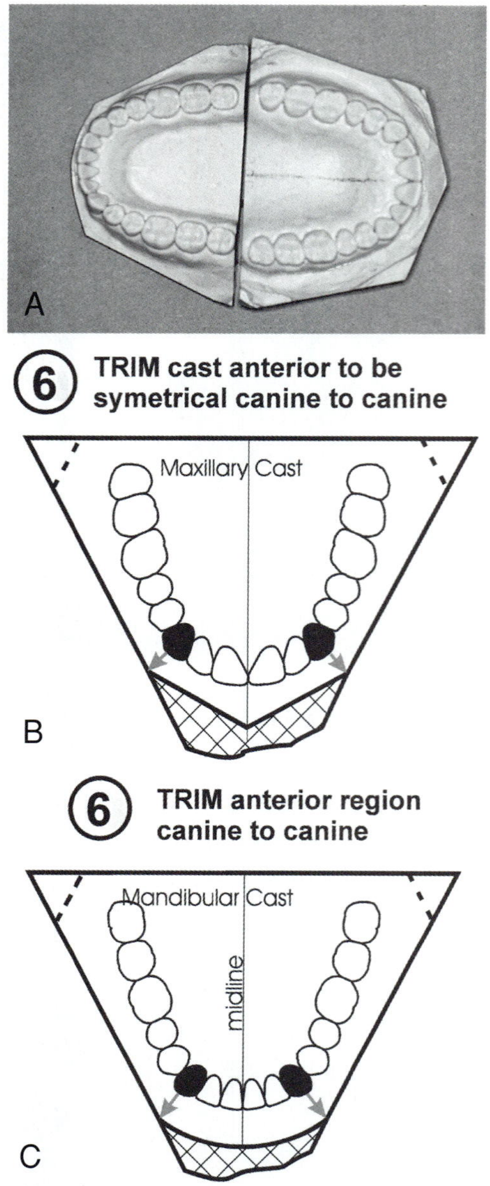

FIGURE 28.22 **A.** The anterior of the maxillary cast is trimmed to form a point at the midline, while the anterior of the mandibular cast is rounded. **B** and **C.** Drawings showing the portion of the cast to be removed. The *cross-hatched area* indicates the material to be trimmed in this step. The *dashed lines* indicate areas to be trimmed in subsequent steps.

the bases of the occluded models and the occlusal plane should be parallel to the benchtop and the bases flat.

5. Lateral Borders (Fig. 28.21)

Trim the sides of the widest cast first, from the canine to the last molar. Trim parallel to the central grooves of the teeth. With teeth in occlusion, trim the lateral borders of the opposing cast to match those of the first cast trimmed. When finished, the lateral borders of both casts should be flat and flush with each other.

6. Anterior Borders (Fig. 28.22)

a) Maxillary Cast

With a pencil, mark the canine eminence and the midline on the base portion of the model to guide your cuts. Trim the anterior portion from the canine eminence to the anterior midline on both sides. These cuts will form a point with each other and with each of the lateral borders.

b) Mandibular Cast

Trim the anterior portion from canine to canine following the form of the arch. The result is a rounded cut.

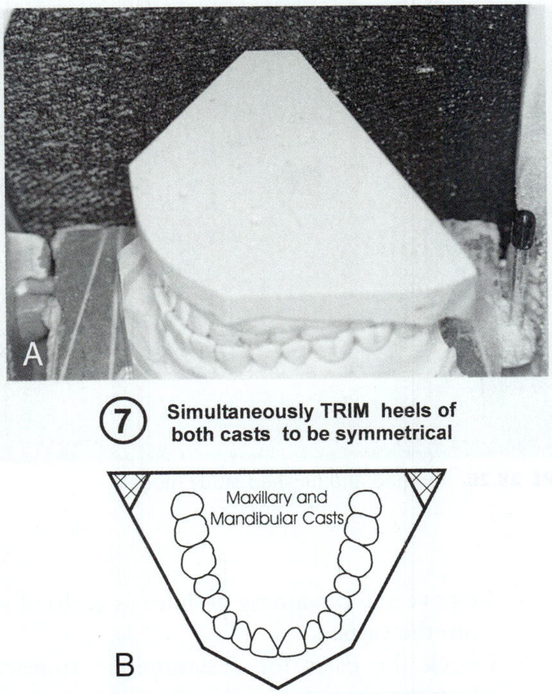

FIGURE 28.23 **A.** The heels of both casts are trimmed to form equal angles with the posterior and the sides. **B.** Drawing showing the portion of the casts to be removed (*cross-hatched areas*).

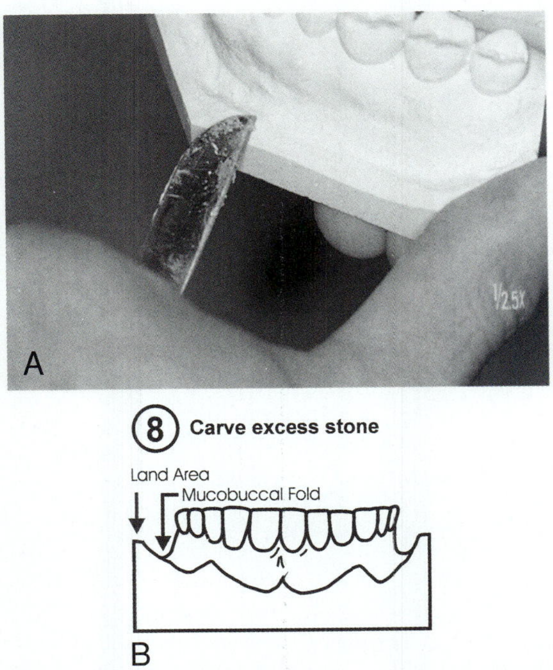

FIGURE 28.24 **A.** The land area is created by trimming the excess material above the mucobuccal fold. **B.** Drawing showing the portion of the cast to be removed.

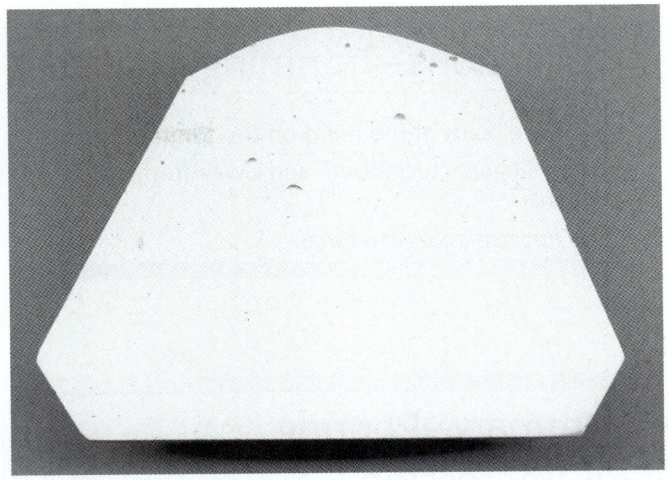

FIGURE 28.25 Pores and voids are present in the upper half of the base of this cast. In the lower half, the pores and voids have been filled and sanded for final finishing.

7. **Posterior Angles (Fig. 28.23)**

   With the casts in occlusion, trim the posterior angles (heels) of both casts to be even and symmetric with the lateral and posterior sides of the casts.

D. Finishing the Casts

1. Use a lab knife, handpiece, or lathe and accessories to trim and smooth the tongue area of mandibular cast. Do not remove any anatomy (lingual frenum). Preserve the lingual alveolar sulcus.
2. Trim the excess "lip" (land area) of the lateral and posterior borders of both casts, as shown in Figure 28.24. Do not remove the mucobuccal fold unless directed to do so.
3. Fill voids in the base portion with the proper gypsum material. Use waterproof sandpaper to smooth the base portion of the casts (Fig. 28.25). Do not round or sand the edges.

Tips for the Clinician—Trimming Models

- Make sure that adequate water is flowing through the model trimmer to prevent clogging.
- Rinse the trimming debris from the model immediately after using the model trimmer.
- Take care not to trim away teeth and other oral anatomy.

Precautions—Trimming Models

- Rest the palm of the hand on the trimmer's table.
- Keep fingers "tucked in" and away from rotating wheel.
- Do not use excessive force.

Summary—Pouring An Impression

1. Mix the gypsum material.
2. Fill the impressions of the teeth.
3. Fill the rest of the impression.
4. Construct a base.
5. Wait 30 to 45 minutes for the gypsum material to set.
6. Separate the model from the impression by lifting the impression upward (do not use a tipping motion).

Summary—Trimming Models

1. Trim the maxillary base parallel to the plane of occlusion.
2. Trim the posterior of the maxillary model perpendicular to its base.
3. Trim the posterior of the mandibular model even with that of the maxillary model.
4. Trim the base of the mandibular model perpendicular to the backs of both models.
5. Trim the sides parallel to the central grooves of the posterior teeth with the models in occlusion.
6. Trim the anterior of the models.
7. Trim the heels of the models while they are in occlusion.
8. Remove blebs of excess stone or plaster.
9. Fill in pores, and sand smooth.

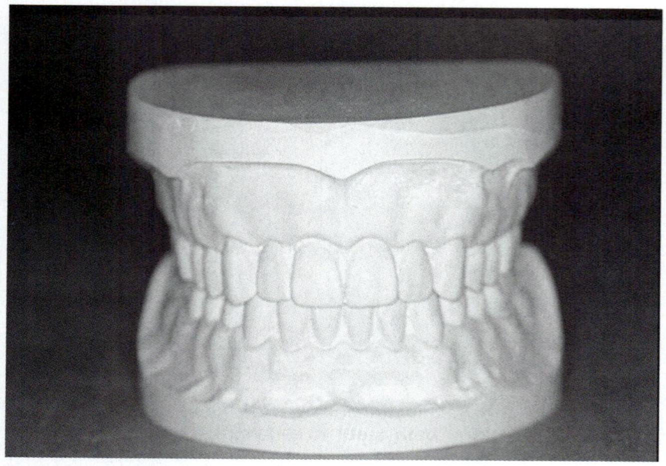

FIGURE 28.26 Trimmed and finished study models.

4. Remove any remaining nodules or blebs of stone from the casts.
5. Check the casts for a symmetric appearance where appropriate.
6. Label both casts with your name (for laboratory exercise) or the patient's name (for clinical setting) and date.
7. Assess your casts by using the Skill Performance Evaluation sheet in Appendix 2. Completed study models are shown in Figure 28.26.

Review Questions

1. Why would the double-pour technique be a preferred method of fabricating a cast/study model?
a) It is the quicker method of the two
b) Prevents distortion of oral structures
c) Produces a better reproduction of oral structures
d) It is a safer technique

2. Which is the best indicator of the initial set of gypsum products?
a) Loss of gloss
b) Loss of resilience
c) Decreased compressive strength
d) Decreased elasticity

3. The overall, combined height of both maxillary and mandibular models should be ______ inches.
a) 1.5–2.0
b) 2.0–2.5
c) 2.5–3.0
d) 3.0–3.5

4. Listed below are the basic steps in model trimming. Starting with #1 as the first step, identify the steps in the proper sequence using #'s 1 through 7.

_____ Trim the posterior surface of the maxillary model perpendicular to the marked midline

_____ Trim the base of the lower cast so it is perpendicular to the backs of both casts and parallel to the base of the maxillary cast

_____ Remove small nodules on the casts with a wax spatula

_____ Trim the lateral borders

_____ Trim the anterior borders

_____ Trim the base of the maxillary model parallel to the established plane (pencil line)

_____ Trim the back of the mandibular model until it is even with the back of the maxillary model

Supplemental Readings

Bird DL, Robinson DS. Modern Dental Assisting. 7th ed. Philadelphia: Saunders, 2002, Chapter 47.

Dofka CM. Competency Skills for the Dental Assistant. Albany, NY: Delmar, 1996, Chapter 9.

Wilkins EM. Clinical Practice of the Dental Hygienist. 8th ed. Baltimore: Lippincott Williams & Wilkins, 1999, Chapter 10.

Woodall IR. Comprehensive Dental Hygiene Care. 4th ed. St Louis: Mosby, 1993, Chapter 15.

29

Fabrication of a Custom Impression Tray

A. Todd Walls, D.D.S.*

Key Words/Phrases

arbor band
burley arbor
exothermic reaction
occlusal stops
visible light–cure (VLC) resins

Objectives

After studying this chapter, the student will be able to do the following:

1. List the differences between the acrylic resin and visible light–cured (VLC) tray fabrication techniques.
2. Briefly describe the characteristics of an exothermic reaction.
3. Name the three purposes of an impression tray.
4. Recall the four reasons why a dentist may choose to fabricate a custom tray for a patient rather than use a stock tray.
5. Explain the purpose of the occlusal stops that are designed in a custom impression tray.
6. Discuss two methods of trimming a custom tray.

*The original chapter contributor for the 1st and 2nd editions was Norton P. Smith, D.D.S., M.A., West Virginia University.

INTRODUCTION

Custom impression trays can be constructed of several types of resins. Autopolymerizing acrylic resins and **visible light–cured (VLC) resins** are two types of useful materials for the production of custom impression trays, orthodontic appliances, temporary restorations, and denture fabrication. These materials were discussed in detail in Chapter 5.

Autopolymerizing resins (Fig. 29.1) may be formed by adding measured amounts of the monomer liquid to the polymer powder, then mixing and molding the resin into the desired shape before the initial set. When the material cools from the exothermic phase (material gives off heat) of the setting reaction, it may be removed from the die, cast, or model and then trimmed and/or polished.

The VLC resins are supplied in lightproof plastic packages. After the package is opened, the material is molded to the desired shape and then made rigid by exposure to high-intensity visible light in a light-curing unit.

I. Purpose

The purpose of an impression tray can be remembered by using "the 3 Cs"—to carry, control, and confine the impression material. Custom-made impression trays produced from either acrylic or VLC resins are used in final impressions for crown and bridge restorations and for denture construction.

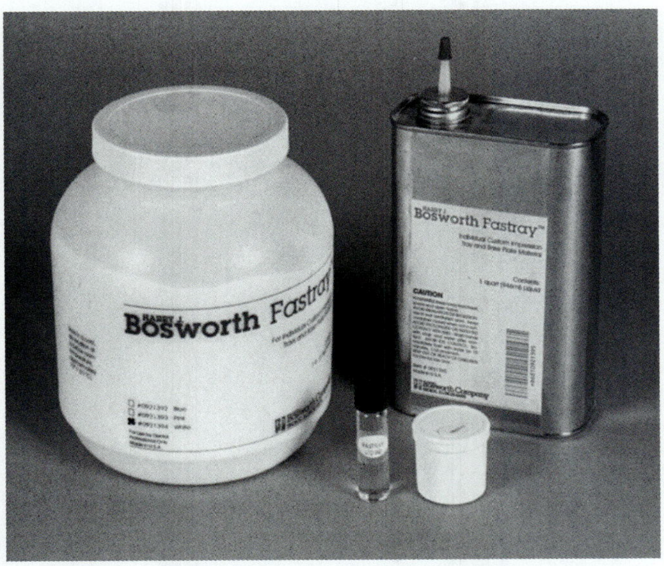

FIGURE 29.1 Tray resin powder and liquid supplied in bulk form and in single-use packaging.

Tips for the Clinician

- If adding a handle to an autopolymerized resin tray, wet the tray in the area of intended handle placement with monomer. This will enhance the bond.
- Make sure the resin is a doughy consistency before manipulating it. If the resin is a viscous consistency, it will be difficult to adapt into the shape of a tray.

Custom rather than stock trays are used for the following reasons:

- The operator can better control the thickness of the material.
- Custom trays can accommodate any anatomic anomaly, such as large lingual tori.
- Custom trays are more stable than stock trays.
- Custom trays can be used again for the same patient.

These are accomplished best with custom impression trays. Use of custom trays was described in Chapter 8. A custom tray requires a preliminary impression to produce a preliminary cast.

II. Tray Spacing Procedure (for a Dentulous Custom Tray)

For this discussion, we will assume that fabrication of a custom tray will be a laboratory exercise, with the impression being taken on a dentoform rather than on an actual patient. For this reason, fabrication of a quadrant tray will be presented so that the subsequent impression can be easily removed from the dentoform. In clinical practice, however, custom impression trays are usually made as a full maxillary or mandibular arch tray rather than as a quadrant tray for greater stability and ease of articulation. The VLC tray will be illustrated with this technique.

Precautions

- The monomer liquid and vapors are flammable.
- The monomer liquid will dissolve many plastic materials and penetrate some gloves.
- Frequent contact with autopolymerizing resin monomer liquid will cause skin irritation. Use of Vaseline or butyl rubber gloves will prevent this.
- Wear eye protection during the entire procedure. Monomer may splash, especially when rotary equipment is used.
- Hold the tray firmly while trimming with a dental lathe.

Table 29.1 Armamentarium for Custom Tray Blockout

Stone cast of patient	Aluminum or tin foil
Laboratory knife	Foilcote
Baseplate wax	Small paint brush
Bunsen burner	

Impression materials need a uniform thickness to produce the most accurate casts. The construction of a custom tray uses a blockout procedure and "stops" to accomplish this uniform thickness. These procedures are the same for both autopolymerizing and VLC resin trays. The blockout procedure adds wax to eliminate or "block out" any cast undercuts that would lock the set custom tray to the cast. The same wax provides an even space for impression material. Stops are holes in the blockout wax that result in a precise seating of the custom tray. The exact location of stops, thickness of wax and extent of the wax and impression tray depend on the patient, impression material, and clinician's personal preferences. The following is a general technique useful for most patients. The items necessary to prepare a cast for custom tray construction are listed in Table 29.1.

A. Coat the preliminary cast with Foilcote (Whip Mix Corp., Louisville, KY) or a similar separator material, see Figure 29.2.

B. Using a Bunsen burner or hot water, soften a piece of baseplate wax that is approximately 2 × 3 inches in size for the quadrant tray. Be careful not to overheat the wax, as this could result in unwanted thin areas.

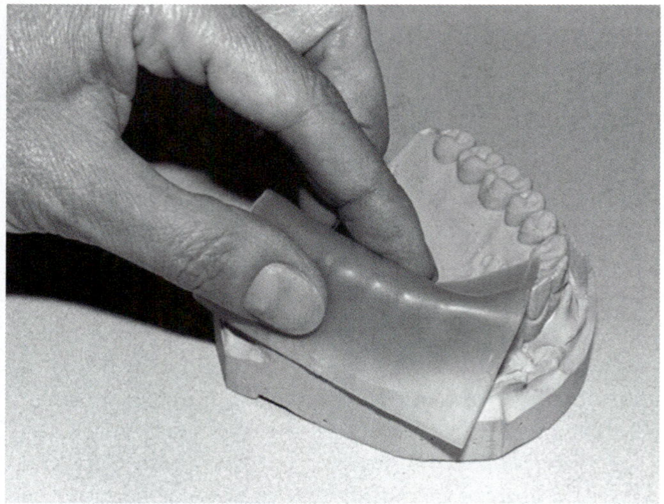

FIGURE 29.3 Adapting baseplate wax over patient's cast.

C. Loosely adapt the warm wax over the tooth to be restored and adjacent teeth, see Figure 29.3. Extend the wax onto the buccal and lingual tissues 3–4 mm beyond the gingival margin of the teeth. Adapt a second layer of wax on top of the first. This will give a space of about 2–3 mm for the impression material. Trim the excess wax with a warm dental lab knife.

D. Provide occlusal stops by cutting three 1 to 2 mm openings in the wax on the occlusal portion of three teeth, not teeth to be prepared for restoration. When preparing a full arch custom tray, three occlusal stops should be cut in a tripodal configuration: two posterior stops and one anterior stop. The cut openings in the wax for occlusal stops are shown in Figure 29.4. They allow the tray material

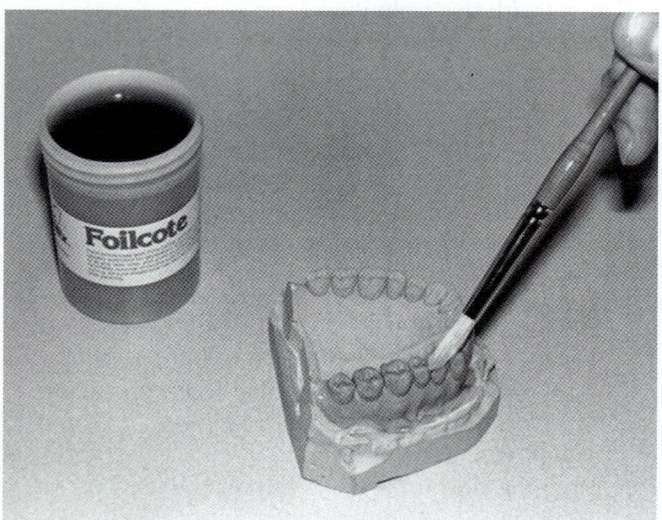

FIGURE 29.2 Stone cast coated with a separating medium.

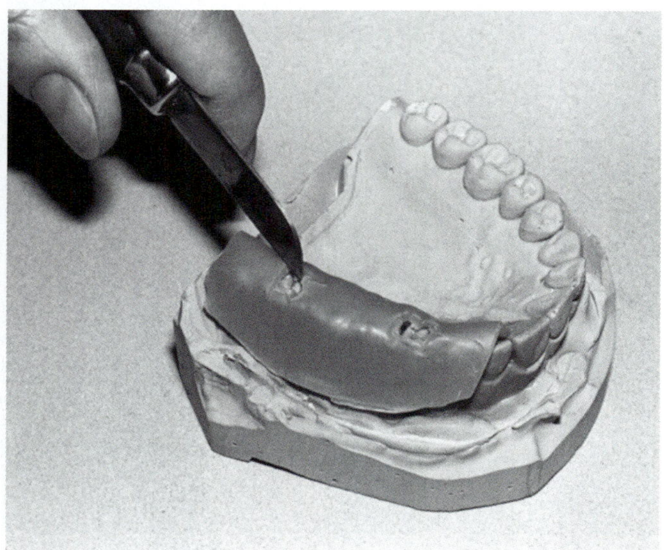

FIGURE 29.4 Adapted wax cut with openings for occlusal stops.

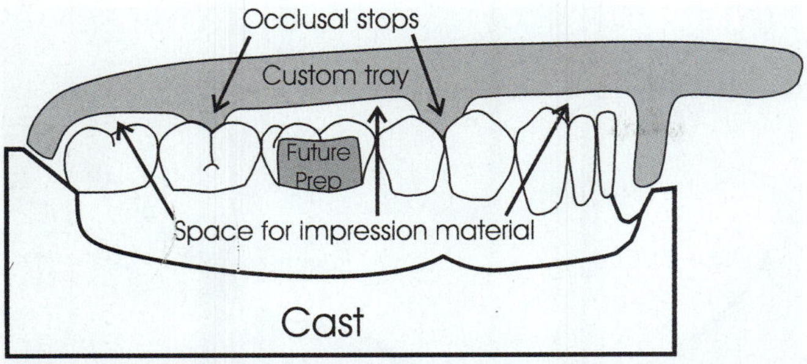

FIGURE 29.5 Cross section of tray, impression material, occlusal stops, and prepared tooth.

to flow into these openings and create a "bump" or a protuberance on the tissue side of the tray. When the tray is made, the tray will seat until these occlusal stops or bumps fit onto their mating surfaces of the teeth in a stable and predictable manner. Precise seating of the tray will provide space for a uniform layer of impression material. Figure 29.5 illustrates this result in cross section. Occlusal stops are pictured on the inside of a tray in Figure 29.6.

E. Place a layer of aluminum or tin foil over the wax to ensure the tray material separates from the blockout after fabrication and the inside surface of the tray is not contaminated with wax (Fig. 29.7). Your instructor (or future employer) will select which separating material to use.

III. Construction Procedure for Autopolymerizing Resin Trays

The armamentarium necessary to fabricate a traditional custom tray is listed in Table 29.2.

A. Mix one unit of tray resin, or measure the powder and liquid of the bulk material with the measuring devices supplied by the manufacturer. Use a waxed paper cup as a mixing bowl. Remember that acrylic monomer is a powerful solvent and will dissolve certain plastics.

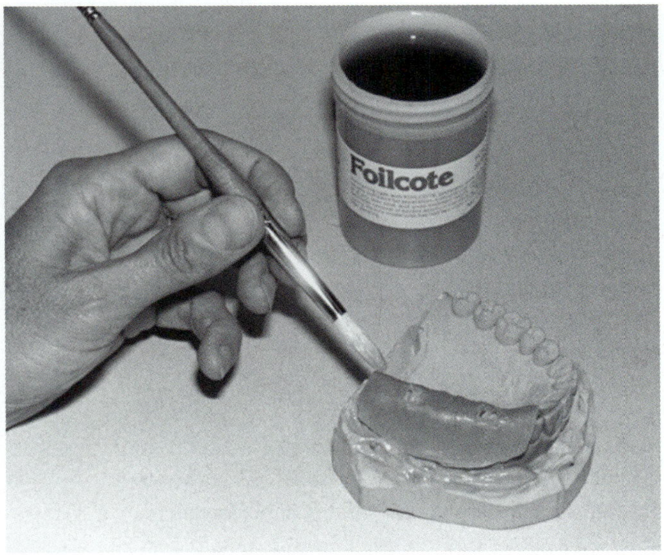

FIGURE 29.7 Painting baseplate wax with a separating medium.

B. Stir thoroughly with a wooden tongue depressor. All liquid and powder must be homogeneously incorporated into the resin mass.

C. When the mixture reaches a doughy consistency, lightly coat your hands with petroleum jelly or wear gloves so that the tray resin will not stick to them while you are working.

D. Once the doughy mixture no longer sticks to the fingers when touched, remove it from the paper cup, create a short "sausage" shape with your hands, and lay it on the blocked out area of the cast (Fig. 29.8).

E. Adapt the mixture over the blockout and cast while keeping a uniform thickness, and extend the tray borders to the edge of the blockout, as illustrated in Figure 29.9. Push the resin into the occlusal stop areas so that it contacts the cast.

F. Form a handle in the anterior portion of the tray by pressing some of the material between your thumb

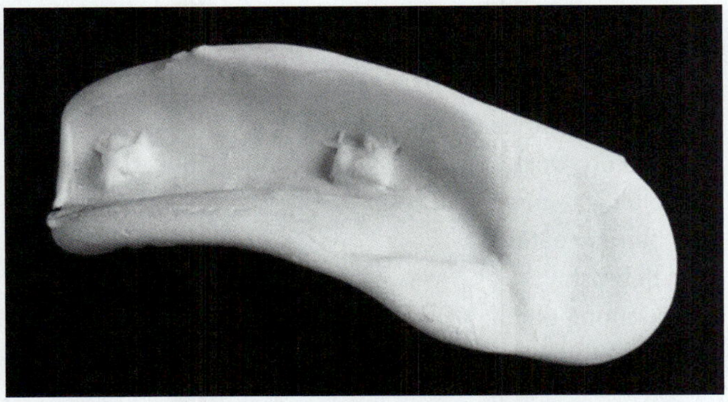

FIGURE 29.6 Untrimmed custom tray showing "stops" on the inside surface.

Table 29.2 Armamentarium for Acrylic Custom Tray Construction

Blocked-out stone cast of patient
Waxed paper cup
Laboratory knife
Tray resin powder
Tray resin liquid
Wooden tongue depressor
Petroleum jelly or butyl rubber gloves
Dental lathe, burley arbor, and arbor band
OR
Barrel-shaped acrylic bur and laboratory handpiece

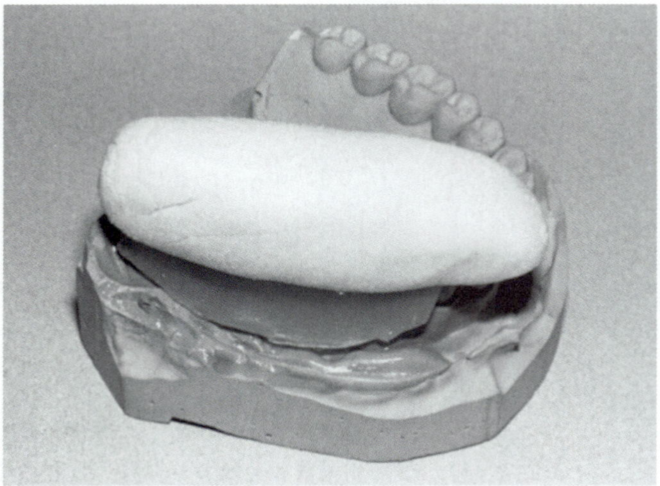

FIGURE 29.8 Initial shape of resin before adaptation.

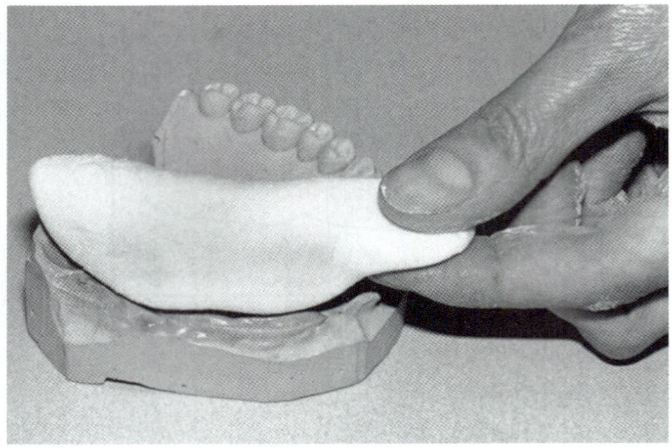

FIGURE 29.10 Handle formation on the custom tray.

and forefinger. The handle must not set in a drooped position. A functional handle is shown in Figure 29.10.

G. Note the temperature of the tray as it sets (**exothermic reaction**). After the tray is almost cool, remove it from the cast. If wax sticks to either the tray or the cast, soak the wax-covered object in hot water for a few minutes, and then gently pull the wax away.

H. Tray trimming will be discussed later in this chapter.

IV. Construction Procedure for VLC Resin Trays

The armamentarium necessary to fabricate a full arch VLC resin tray is listed in Table 29.3.

A. Follow the tray spacing procedures described earlier in this chapter to block-out the cast.

B. Remove the VLC resin from its package (Figure 29.11)

C. Next, adapt the resin over the blocked-out cast keeping a uniform thickness, and extend the tray borders to the edge of the blockout as illustrated in Figure 29.12. Push the resin into the occlusal stop areas of the cast.

D. Mold an unused piece of VLC resin into a handle shape and adapt it to the anterior of the tray as illustrated in Figure 29.13.

E. Paint the tray with Triad air barrier (Dentsply International, York, PA) as illustrated in Figure 29.14.

F. Place the cast and tray into a Triad light curing unit and cure for 2 minutes, see Figure 18.6.

G. Remove the tray from the cast and remove all blockout materials inside the tray.

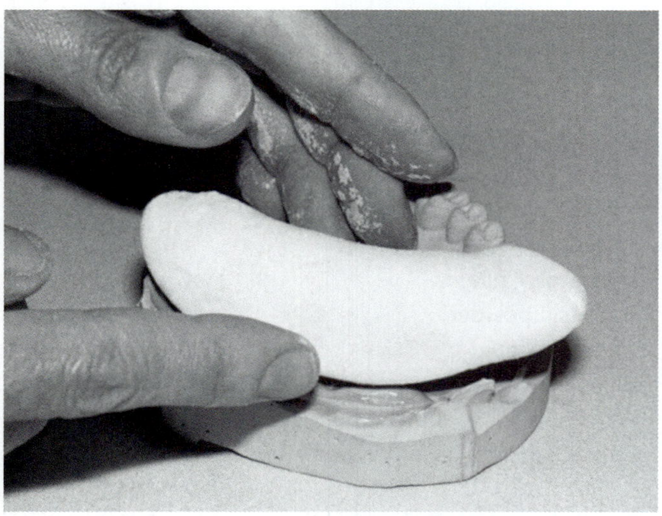

FIGURE 29.9 Tray resin adapted over wax and cast.

Table 29.3 Armamentarium for Visible Light–Cure Custom Tray Construction

Blocked-out stone cast of patient
Laboratory knife
Visible light–cure (VLC) resin
Air barrier coating
Small brush
Light-curing unit
Dental lathe, burley arbor, and arbor band
OR
Barrel-shaped acrylic bur and laboratory handpiece

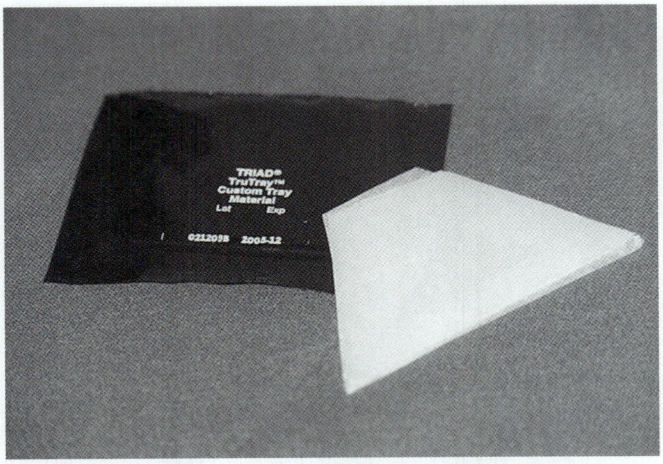

FIGURE 29.11 Visible light–cure (VLC) tray material removed from package.

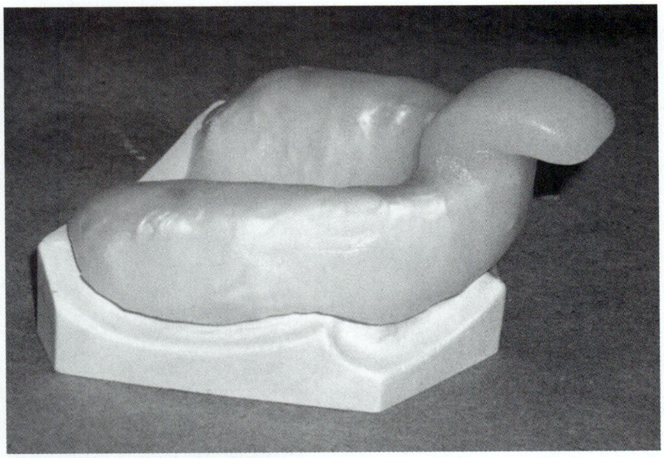

FIGURE 29.13 VLC material added to form the tray handle.

H. Paint the tissue side of the tray with Triad air barrier coating.

I. Place the tray in the curing unit tissue side up and cure for an additional 2 minutes.

J. Remove the air barrier coating by washing with soap and water.

K. Check that tray properly seats on the cast. It should be stable and all stops should seat accurately.

L. Proceed to the next section to trim the tray.

V. Trimming the Tray

A. Trim the tray to eliminate excess material and rough edges in all areas. Do this by using the dental lathe, burley arbor, and arbor band. The **burley arbor** attaches to the lathe and holds the arbor band. The **arbor band** is a 0.75-inch-wide, coarse sandpaper ring. The lathe, burley arbor, and arbor band are pictured in Figure 29.15.

B. During trimming, check for smoothness by gently pushing on all edges with your finger. If the edge hurts your finger, it will hurt the patient. Trim sharp edges so that they are smooth and rounded.

C. An alternative method of finishing the tray is to trim it with a laboratory handpiece and barrel-shaped acrylic bur. Use a palm grasp for this procedure, as illustrated in Figure 29.16.

D. Evaluate the custom tray by using the Skill Performance Evaluation sheet in Appendix 2.

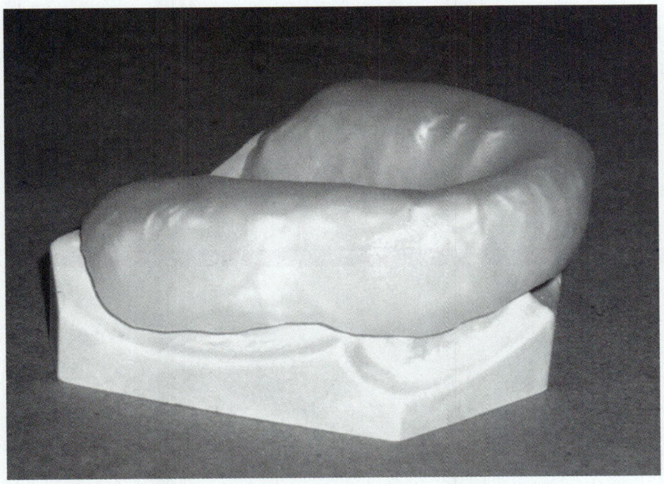

FIGURE 29.12 Visible light-cure (VLC) tray material, molded onto the cast and trimmed.

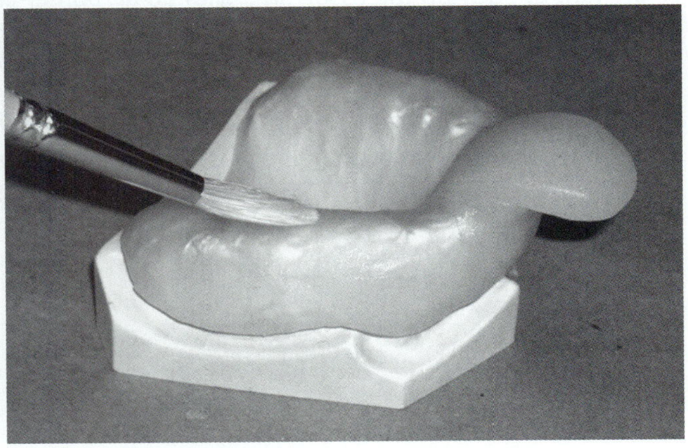

FIGURE 29.14 Painting the tray with air barrier coating.

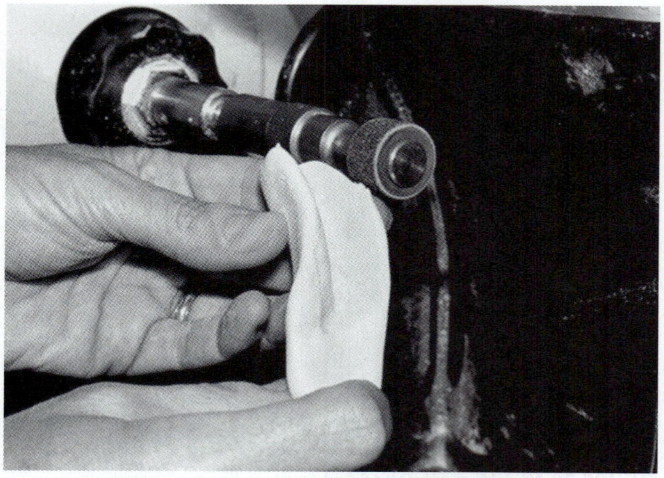

FIGURE 29.15 Trimming the tray with the dental lathe.

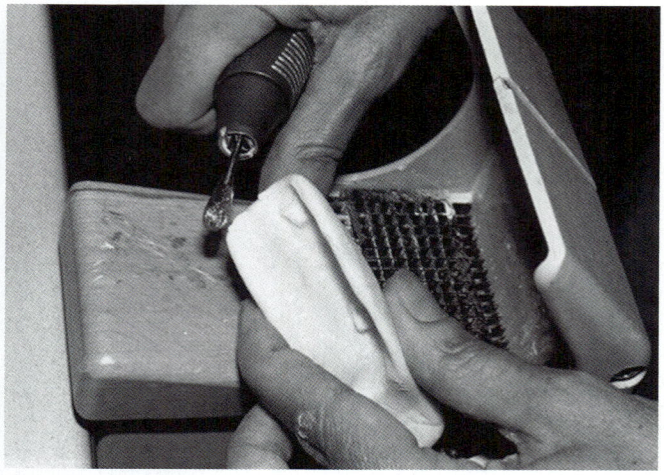

FIGURE 29.16 Trimming the tray with a handpiece and bur.

Summary

Application of Wax Spacer

1. Coat the cast with a separating material.
2. Apply softened wax, and cut stops.
3. Reapply separating media or foil.

Tray Construction Procedure

Autopolymerizing Resin

4. Mix the resin to a homogeneous consistency.
5. Coat your hands with petroleum jelly or wear gloves.
6. When the mix reaches a doughy consistency, adapt over the blockout and form a handle.
7. When the resin begins to heat, remove the tray from the cast.
8. Remove the blockout, and reseat the tray on the cast.

Visible Light–Cure (VLC) Resin

1. Remove VLC resin from the package, and adapt it over the blockout.
2. Add the handle.
3. Paint the tray with an air barrier coating.
4. Place the resin in a curing unit for 2 minutes.
5. Remove the tray from the cast, and remove the blockout.
6. Paint the tray on the tissue side with an air barrier coating, and cure again for 2 minutes.
7. Remove barrier with soap and water.

Tray Trimming

1. Smooth the surfaces and edges with a bur or other abrasive.
2. Check the entire tray and all edges by rubbing with a finger.

Review Questions

1. All of the following are true regarding custom trays except one. Which one is the exception?
   a) There is better control of the thickness of impression material with the use of a custom tray
   b) Custom trays cannot accommodate anatomic features such as tori
   c) A custom made impression tray can be used again for the same patient
   d) There is more stability when using a custom tray as compared to a stock tray

2. The tray spacing (blockout) procedure during custom tray fabrication should provide _____ mm of space between the cast and the tray.
   a) .5–1
   b) 1
   c) 2–3
   d) 4–6

3. What is important to do when adapting resin on the blocked-out cast?
   a) Always extend the resin over the land area
   b) Extend the resin onto the tissues 3–4 mm beyond the gingival margin
   c) Press out the resin to make it as thin as possible
   d) Ensure the final thickness of the resin is at least 6–7 mm for rigidity

4. Which of the following is true about occlusal stops?
   a) Are needed to ensure proper seating of the custom tray
   b) Should be placed on centric cusps
   c) Are only needed on the maxillary arch
   d) Are placed on the buccal gingiva

5. Trimming the tray can be accomplished with a dental lathe or a laboratory handpiece with a barrel-shaped acrylic bur. The tray borders should have sharp edges to ensure patient comfort.
   a) The first statement is true; the second statement is false.
   b) The first statement is false; the second statement is true.
   c) Both statements are true.
   d) Both statements are false.

Supplemental Readings

Rosenstiel SF, Land MF, Fugimoto J. Contemporary Fixed Prosthodontics. 3rd ed. St. Louis: Mosby, 2000:364–368.

Shillingburg HT, Hobo S, Whitsett LD, Jacobi R, Bracket SE. Fundamentals of Fixed Prosthodontics, 3rd ed. Chicago: Quintessence Publishing, 1997:290–293.

30 Elastomeric Impressions

Key Words/Phrases

addition silicone impression material
automix gun
retraction cord
tray adhesive

Objectives

After studying this chapter, the student will be able to do the following:

1. Briefly discuss the rationale for dental hygienists to learn the preparation and technique of addition silicone impression material.
2. Recall the reasons for using addition silicone impression material.
3. Explain the tray preparation that is necessary for use of addition silicone impression material.
4. Summarize the steps involved in:
   - Preparing the putty (tray) material
   - Preparing the wash (syringe) material

INTRODUCTION

This chapter will address the manipulation of **addition silicone** (polyvinylsiloxanes or polysiloxanes) **impression material.** This is one of the four types of impression materials discussed in Chapter 8. This material commonly involves the use of an automix gun, as shown in Figure 8.14. Use of the **automix gun** eliminates hand mixing with a spatula and paper mixing pad.

I. Purpose

Addition silicone impression material is generally used as a "final impression material" for the fabrication of crowns and bridges. Dental hygienists may (or may not) take this type of impression depending on their state practice act. From time to time, however, even those who do not take this type of impression may find themselves assisting with this procedure. An advantage of this material is that it does not need to be poured soon after the impression is taken. Its stability and accuracy make it a very popular material.

II. Procedure for the Double-Mix Putty-Wash Technique

The double-mix impression technique uses two different viscosities of impression material. One is very thick and is used in the tray. The second has a low viscosity. It is syringed on and around the tissues of interest. The tray is seated immediately after the syringe material is injected into place. Typically, the tray and syringe materials are prepared simultaneously by two people.

A. Tray Preparation (Table 30.1)

1. A plastic stock tray is selected and painted with a **tray adhesive.** This adhesive aids in retention of the impression material in the tray. Use an adhesive from the same manufacturer as the impression material.

Table 30.1 Armamentarium for Addition Silicones

Stock tray
Tray adhesive
Impression material (putty)
Cartridge gun
Impression syringe
Syringe tips
Impression cartridges (wash or light body)

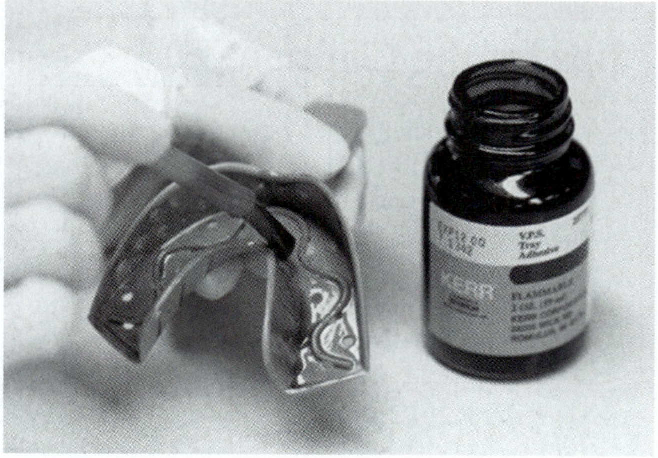

FIGURE 30.1 Stock impression tray coated with adhesive.

2. Be sure to coat the facial, lingual, and occlusal surfaces of the inside of the tray, as shown in Figure 30.1.
3. Allow approximately 10 minutes to air-dry so that the adhesive becomes tacky.

B. Preparing the Automix Gun

Two types of automix guns are on the market at this time. The guns, cartridges, and mixing tips are not interchangeable. When the older system is used, the tip is left on the cartridge after each use. The newer system has a cap, which is replaced after each use.

1. Older Automix System

a) Load the cartridge into the gun.
b) Twist off and dispose of the sealing cap. If cartridge has been used for a previous impression, remove the previous self-mixing tip.
c) Dispense a pea-sized amount of material onto a paper towel by squeezing the trigger. This ensures that the base and catalyst materials have not set and clogged either opening of the cartridge. Wipe the end of the cartridge.
d) Install a new mixing tip, and twist it into the locked position.
e) After use of the automix system, leave the used mixing tip in place until the material is needed again. This serves as a self-sealing device and keeps base and catalyst material from setting at the cartridge opening.

2. Newer Automix System

a) Load the cartridge into the gun.
b) Twist off the sealing cap.
c) Dispense a pea-sized amount of material onto a paper towel by squeezing the trigger. This ensures that the base and catalyst materials have not set and clogged either opening of the cartridge. Wipe the end of the cartridge.

Tips for the Clinician

- Avoid wearing latex gloves when mixing the putty.
- For best results, tray and syringe materials are prepared simultaneously by two people.
- Moisture control is critical.
- It is much easier to wait and remove set material from a patient's face (or other places) than it is to remove unset material.

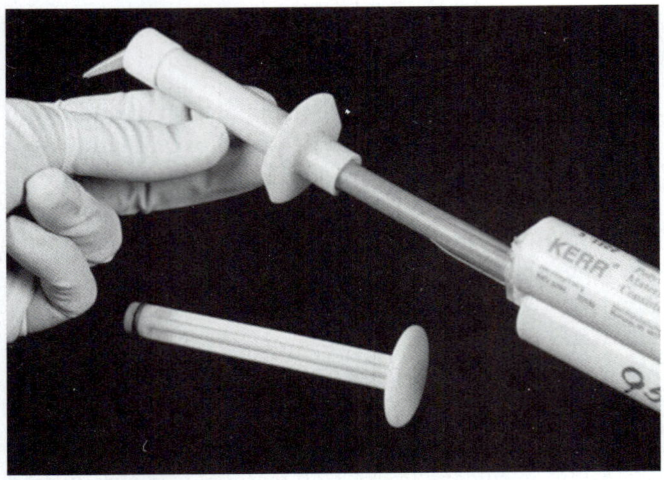

FIGURE 30.3 Filling the impression syringe from the cartridge gun.

d) Install a new mixing tip, and twist it into the locked position.

e) After use of the automix system, remove the used mixing tip, and replace the cap.

C. Preparing the Putty Material

1. Don plastic overgloves. Latex gloves are not used because they may inhibit the setting of the material.
2. Dispense equal volumes of the putty base and catalyst materials, using the appropriate scoops. Using the same scoop in both jars will contaminate the remaining material.
3. Knead the material with your fingertips rather than in the palm of the hand. Kneading with your palms will warm and accelerate the set of this material. A homogeneous color should be obtained in 30 seconds.
4. Roll the mix into a 3 to 4-inch-long cylinder, and place this into the tray, as shown in Figure 30.2.

D. Preparing the Wash Material

1. Squeeze the trigger of the automix gun to dispense an appropriate amount into the back end of the barrel of an impression syringe, as shown in Figure 30.3. Backfill by withdrawing the tip of the automix gun from the syringe barrel.
2. Place the plunger into the impression syringe. It is important to do this in a way that does not trap air.

E. The Impression

1. Most impressions for crown and bridge restorations use retraction cord. **Retraction cord** is a fine string that is placed in the gingival sulcus of the prepared teeth below the margins, as shown in Figure 8.6. Retraction cord pushes the gingiva away from the teeth. Many times retraction cord is treated with a hemostatic or vasoconstrictive agent to reduce bleeding and temporarily shrink the gingival tissues. Depending on the dentist's preference, the retraction cord may or may not be removed before the impression is taken. When the retraction cord is removed, the syringe material will flow into the space that the

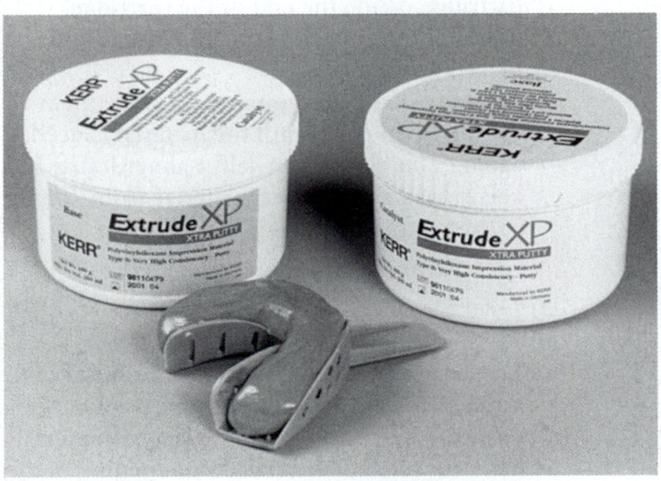

FIGURE 30.2 Putty material placed in tray.

Precautions

- To avoid an accelerated set, mix the putty material with your fingertips.
- Follow the manufacturer's directions regarding used tips and cartridge caps.
- For putty material, use the designated scoops for each jar to avoid cross-contamination.
- Protect the patient's clothing when using impression materials to prevent staining.

retraction cord created. This captures the fine details of the preparation's margins.

2. The syringe material is placed in the interproximal areas and over the margins and occlusal surfaces of the prepared teeth, as shown in Figure 30.4.
3. The previously prepared tray material is immediately placed directly over the syringe material. It is then held without motion for approximately 5 to 7 minutes (or the appropriate amount of time as specified by the manufacturer).
4. The tray is removed with a quick snap motion, rinsed, and disinfected. It is then poured or sent to a dental laboratory.
5. Assess the impression by using the Skill Performance Evaluation sheet in Appendix 2.

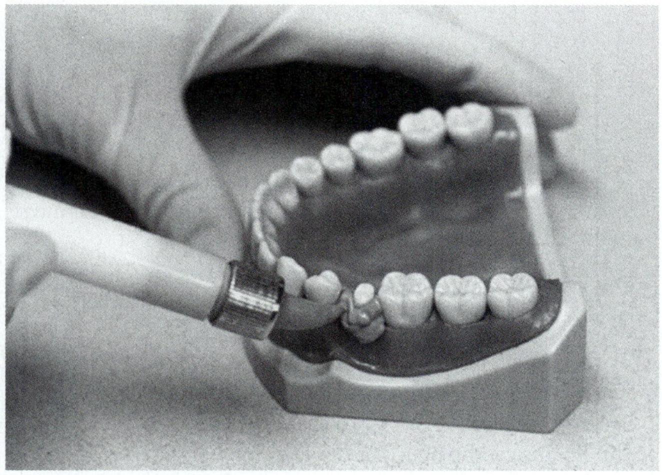

FIGURE 30.4 Application of syringe material around the preparation.

Summary

Tray Preparation

1. Coat the impression tray with adhesive.
2. Wait 10 minutes.

Automix Gun

3. Load the cartridge into the gun, and squeeze out material to ensure its free flow.
4. Install a mixing tip.
5. After use, follow the manufacturer's directions regarding the used tip and cartridge cap.

Putty Material

6. Don nonlatex overgloves.
7. Dispense equal volumes of putty base and catalyst.
8. Knead the material with your fingertips for 30 seconds (until a homogeneous color occurs).
9. Roll mix into a 3- to 4-inch-long cylinder, and place this into tray.

The Impression

10. Remove the retraction cord if desired, and control moisture.
11. Place the syringe material over the margins and in the interproximal areas, and then cover the entire preparation.
12. Seat the tray directly over the syringe material.
13. Hold the tray without motion for 5 to 7 minutes.
14. Remove the tray with a quick snap motion, rinse, and disinfect.

Review Questions

1. The addition silicone tray material is placed over the syringe material and held in place for approximately _____ minutes.
a) 1–3
b) 3–5
c) 5–7
d) 6–8

2. An advantage of addition silicone impression material is:
a) Stability
b) That it can be poured at a later time
c) Accuracy
d) All are advantages

3. Addition silicone material is best prepared:
a) By a single operator
b) With two people
c) Using latex gloves
d) In a moist environment

4. The putty material of addition silicone should be kneaded in the preparer's fingertips rather than in the palm of the hand because of:
a) Staining from the material
b) Difficulty in removing from hands
c) Accelerating the set of the material
d) Increasing the setting time

5. The tray adhesive used in the double-mix putty-wash technique should dry in the impression tray for approximately ______ minutes.
a) 3
b) 5
c) 7
d) 10

Supplemental Readings

Bird DL, Robinson DS. Modern Dental Assisting. 7th ed. Philadelphia: Saunders, 2002, Chapter 46.

31

Vital Tooth Whitening: Patient-Applied, Professionally Supervised Clinical and Laboratory Procedures

Michele R. Sweeney, R.D.H., M.S.D.H.*

Key Words/Phrases

block-out resin
custom whitening tray
informed consent
paint-on resin dam
reservoir
shade guide tab
sheet resin
spectrophotometer
white swabs

Objectives

After studying this chapter, the student will be able to do the following:

1. List the indications and contraindications for use of patient-applied, professionally supervised whitening technique.
2. List the indications and contraindications for professionally applied power whitening techniques.
3. Outline the steps in the clinical phase of patient-applied, professionally supervised vital whitening technique.
4. Identify the essential elements of home care instruction for the patient using the professionally supervised, self-applied technique.
5. Outline the steps in construction of the whitening tray, and identify the equipment and materials used.
6. Outline the steps in the professionally applied power whitening technique. Identify the equipment and materials used.

*The original chapter contributor for the 1st and 2nd editions was William R. Howard, D.D.S., M.P.H., Western Kentucky University, Bowling Green, Kentucky.

INTRODUCTION

Delivery of the patient-applied and professionally applied power (light- or heat-activated) whitening technique may be shared between the dentist and the dental hygienist. The critical elements of both techniques include the patient's medical history, intraoral examination, discussion of benefits and risks, informed consent, collection of data, record maintenance, detailed patient instruction, and follow-up evaluation. The hygienist may assume many of these responsibilities.

I. Purpose/Indications

Patient-applied whitening or professionally applied power whitening is generally effective on vital teeth that are affected by slight to moderate intrinsic staining. Yellow, orange, and light brown intrinsic stains are more susceptible to whitening than are dark blue-gray and dark brown stains. White spots can be difficult to mask with whitening. Tetracycline staining becomes more difficult to treat as the degree of staining intensifies. Extrinsic stains are more easily whitened than intrinsic stains; however, a prophylaxis may be all that is necessary to obtain the desired esthetic result.

II. Contraindications

Teeth that have been stained as a result of caries, pulpal necrosis, or endodontic therapy are not good candidates for patient-applied whitening. Stains caused by amalgam restorations also resist whitening. Teeth with sensitive root surfaces should not be whitened aggressively because of the potential for increased tooth sensitivity. A small minority of patients may be sensitive or allergic to a component in the whitening agent, and occasionally, a patient may not exhibit the degree of motivation and/or cooperation that is necessary for successful treatment. Table 31.1 lists the indications and contraindications for use of patient-applied, professionally supervised vital whitening.

Professionally applied power whitening should not be used on patients with photosensitivity due to drugs or herbal supplements. Patients undergoing chemotherapy or radiation therapy must not be bleached with the power technique. Patients with a history of melanoma should avoid the power bleaching systems because of the potential exposure to harmful light sources. Severe intrinsic stains, cervical erosion/sensitivity, cracks in the enamel, caries, and anterior restorations not scheduled for replacement are also contraindications for power whitening procedures. Nonvital teeth may undergo professionally applied power bleaching systems. Table 31.2 lists indications and contraindications for the Professionally Applied Power Bleaching Whitening.

Before whitening treatments are prescribed, the patient's medical history should be thoroughly reviewed. The procedure is contraindicated in the following patients:

- Pregnant or lactating women
- Children under the age of 18 years
- Heavy smokers
- Patients who are sensitive to any ingredient in the whitening agent
- Anterior restorations that will not be replaced

III. Clinical Procedure—Three Patient Appointments for Professionally Monitored Patient-Applied Whitening

Professionally prescribed whitening agents for patient application are available in the popular kit form, which contains all the necessary supplies for an average treatment sequence. The following is a brief description of the recommended clinical procedure for vital tooth bleaching using carbamide peroxide agents. Necessary items for this procedure are listed in Table 31.3.

Table 31.1 Patient-Applied, Professionally Supervised Whitening

Indications	Contraindications
Vital teeth	Nonvital teeth
Extrinsic stain	Severe intrinsic stain
Light to moderate intrinsic stain	Sensitive root/dentin
Cooperative/compliant patient	Sensitivity to components of whitening agent
	Unreasonable expectations

Table 31.2 Professionally Applied Power (Light/Heat Activated) Whitening

Indications	Contraindications
Vital teeth, endo treated nonvital teeth	Untreated nonvital tooth
Extrinsic stain	Severe intrinsic stain
Light-to-moderate intrinsic stain	Sensitive root/dentin
Cooperative/compliant patient	Sensitivity to whitening components
	Unreasonable expectations
	Use of photosensitive drugs/herbs
	Hx of melanoma
	Hx of chemo/radiation therapy

Table 31.3 Armamentarium for the Clinical Procedure

Forms: medical history, informed consent, clinical examination, and treatment
Prophylaxis instruments
Camera: video, film, or digital
Shade guide or spectrophotometer
Written instructions

A. First Appointment

A summary of the clinical procedures in this section can be found at the end of the chapter.

1. Medical History

Obtain a complete medical history from the patient. Other than conditions listed above or a sensitivity or allergy to carbamide peroxide or other ingredients contained in the bleaching agent, there are no medical contraindications.

2. Informed Consent

An **informed consent** should be read and signed by the patient at this time. The consent form should briefly describe the bleaching procedure as well as the possible benefits and side effects. The informed consent should become a part of the patient's record. A sample consent form is illustrated in Figure 31.1.

3. Intraoral Examination

Perform a complete intraoral examination. Examine the soft tissues for lesions, which would be irritated by the tray or the bleaching agent. Examine the teeth for caries, exposed root surfaces, exposed dentin, and broken or cracked restorations as well as teeth. Any findings from this exam should be documented in the patient's record.

4. Prophylaxis

Perform a prophylaxis. Scale and polish the teeth to remove plaque, calculus, and stain.

5. White Swabs

White Stain Remover Swabs with Aqueous Cleaning Technology™ from GRINrx may also be used to enhance bleaching. The tabs are swabbed gently over all surfaces to be whitened.

6. Intraoral Photograph

Take an intraoral photograph showing both the upper and lower teeth. In this photograph, include a **shade guide tab** that is matched to the shade of the anterior teeth. The tab may be positioned adjacent to the incisal edge of a central incisor. Figure 3.4 shows a Vita shade guide. Intraoral color-measuring devices, such as the **spectrophotometer** shown in Figure 31.2, may also be used to document the initial tooth color.

7. Full-Arch Impression

Take a full-arch alginate impression of the teeth that are to be whitened. Carefully pour the impression in dental stone. The whitening tray is fabricated on the stone model before the next appointment.

B. Second Appointment

1. Test Fit

Try the custom tray in the patient's mouth, and make any necessary adjustments. Figure 31.3

Informed Consent for Patient-Applied, Professionally Supervised, Tooth Whitening Treatment

The product you will apply to your teeth contains the active whitening ingredient, ***Carbamide Peroxide.*** The most frequently reported side effects of peroxide tooth whitening are tooth sensitivity and irritation of the gums. Sore throat and nausea may occur if you accidentally swallow some of the product.

Patient Consent: I ______________________________ (full name), hereby consent to treatment using a patient-applied, professionally supervised tooth whitening agent. I have been informed of the potential benefits and side effects of the treatment, and affirm that I have read and understand the instructions below.

Signed: ______________________________

Witness: ______________________________

Date: ______________________________

One copy for the patient.

One copy for the patient's record.

FIGURE 31.1 Patient informed consent form.

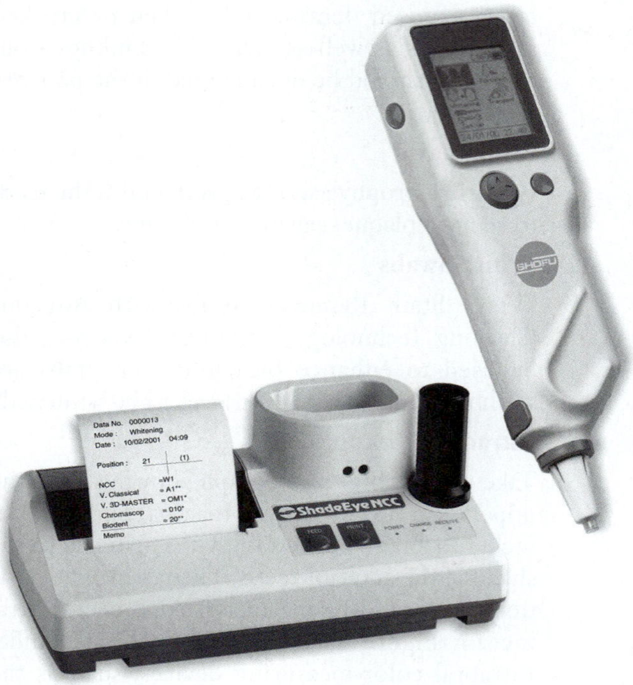

FIGURE 31.2 Photograph of a intraoral spectrophotometer, a clinical color-measuring device. (Courtesy of Shofu Dental Corp.)

shows a custom tray in place over the maxillary teeth. The tray should not impinge on frenal attachments.

2. Patient Instruction

Instruct the patient regarding use of the tray. The patient may wear the tray at night or during the day. When used at night, the tray is worn over the teeth while the patient sleeps. When used during the day, the tray is worn twice daily for 1 hour each. On average, initial results are achieved in 2 weeks; however, longer treatment may be required to achieve the desired result.

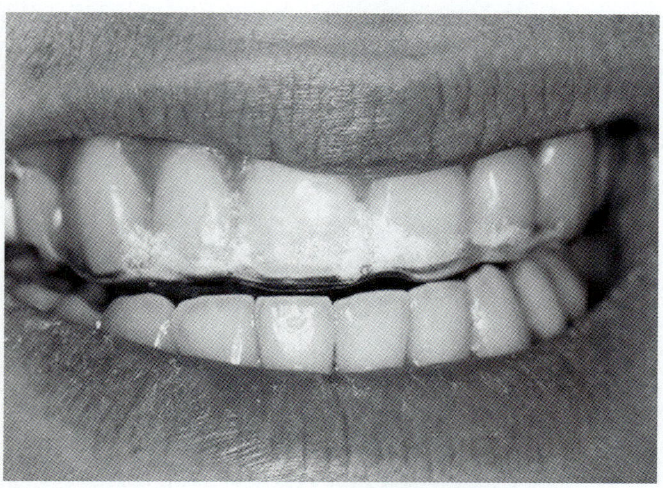

FIGURE 31.3 Custom resin whitening tray in place over the maxillary teeth.

a) Load the tray with fresh whitening agent before each treatment. Do not fill the tray completely. Fill only the space that is created by the reservoirs in the tray; use only one dot of material per facial surface.
b) Place the tray firmly over the teeth. Wipe any excess whitening agent from outside the tray with fingers or a piece of gauze.
c) Do not swallow the excess whitening agent.
d) Remove the tray at the end of each treatment period, and rinse it with cold water.
e) Brush the teeth and rinse the mouth at the end of each treatment.
f) Store the tray in the storage box between treatments. Do not expose the tray or box to heat.
g) Record each whitening treatment with the date and the hours treated.

3. Side Effects

Describe the possible side effects, such as tooth sensitivity or soft-tissue irritation (gums, lips, or cheeks), to the patient. Instruct the patient to call the office should any side effects occur. If the teeth become sensitive, the patient should discontinue treatment until the sensitivity disappears and then begin treatment again with a reduction in the daily treatment time. Tooth sensitivity can be effectively treated with application of neutral sodium fluoride or potassium nitrate in the whitening tray twice daily for 1 hour each.

4. Written Instructions

Give the patient written instructions. These instructions should include space to record the date and length of treatment (Fig. 31.4).

5. Follow-up Appointment

Schedule an appointment for the patient to return when the treatment is completed. The duration of treatment may vary but usually requires 2 to 6 weeks.

Whitening one arch at a time will allow the patient to better visualize the results of treatment by allowing comparison between treated and untreated teeth.

C. Third Appointment

1. Examination

Examine the patient for results of the whitening treatment. Record the total amount of treatment in hours, and note any negative side effects.

2. Additional Whitening

If additional whitening is desired, dispense more whitening agent to the patient, and schedule an appointment for a follow-up examination at the

Instructions for Patient-Applied, Professionally Supervised Tooth Whitening

You should expect a gradual improvement in the whiteness of your teeth with repeated applications of the whitening product. Apply the whitening product to your teeth twice daily for one hour each application, following these directions:

- Brush and floss your teeth in the usual manner.
- Place one dot of the whitening gel on each facial surface in the custom tray.
- Place the tray securely over your teeth.
- Remove any excess gel with your toothbrush.
- Do not swallow the gel.
- After one hour, remove the tray from your teeth and rinse your mouth with plain water.
- Rinse the tray in cool water and store it in the storage box away from heat.
- Repeat the application twice daily.
- If you experience any negative side effect, discontinue use and call the office for instructions. (Telephone: ______________)
- Return to the office for re-examination and evaluation at the appointed time.
- Store the whitening gel safely out of reach of small children.

Record of Treatment (patient name ______________________________)

Make an entry each time you apply the whitening agent to your teeth. Record the date of treatment and the length of time of each treatment in hours or fraction of an hour.

Date of Treatment	Length of Treatment

FIGURE 31.4 Patient instruction form.

end of a sufficient treatment sequence (usually 2–4 weeks).

3. Intraoral Photograph

When the desired result has been achieved, take a posttreatment intraoral photograph of the treated teeth, including a matching shade guide tab (as in the first photograph). Together with the pretreatment photograph, this photograph becomes part of the patient's record to document the results of the bleaching treatment. Alternatively, a new color measurement with an intraoral color-measuring device can be used to document the color change.

The Skill Performance Evaluation sheet for patient protocol and bleaching tray fabrication as a clinical procedure is located in Appendix 2.

IV. Laboratory Procedure–Constructing the Custom Tray

The **custom whitening tray** is made of clear vinyl resin. A stone model is produced from an alginate impression, and the custom tray is fabricated on the model. Many of the oral appliances discussed in Chapter 18 are constructed in a similar way. Necessary items for the laboratory procedure are listed in Table 31.4.

A. Make a Stone Working Model

1. Mix the dental stone and pour into the alginate impression. The impression need not be boxed, but should be poured into a horseshoe-shape to avoid additional trimming.
2. Remove the model from the impression after the stone has completely set, and trim on a model

Table 31.4 Armamentarium for the Laboratory Procedure

Vacuum former
Resin-curing light
Light-cure block-out resin
Small, curved scissors
Microtorch
Sheet vinyl (thickness, 0.040 inch)
Dental laboratory stone
Storage container for tray(s)

trimmer. Keep the base small, thin, and horseshoe-shaped.

B. Create a Reservoir for the Whitening Agent

1. After the model has completely dried, create a reservoir on the facial surface of the teeth to be bleached. The **reservoir** is a space created between the tray and the teeth to hold the bleaching material. It should be no more than 1 mm thick. Carefully place light-cure **block-out resin** on the facial surface of each tooth to be whitened. Stop the material 1 mm short of the gingiva. Do not cover the incisal or occlusal surfaces, and do not fill the interproximal spaces.
2. Cure the resin on each tooth by exposing the resin to a curing light for 10 seconds (Fig. 31.5).

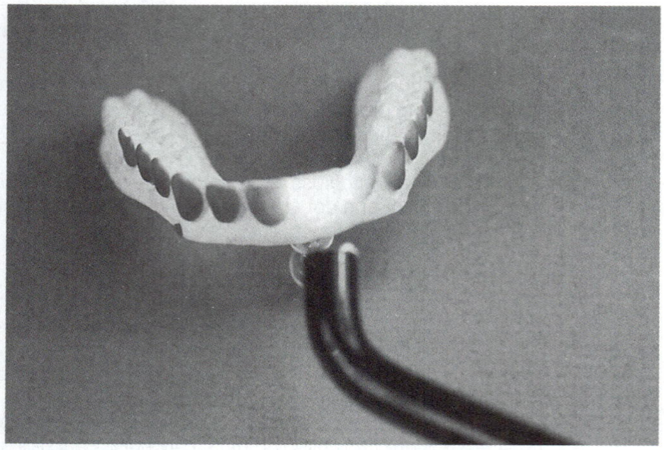

FIGURE 31.5 Block-out resin exposed to curing light (10 seconds for each tooth).

C. Vacuum Sheet Resin Over the Working Model

1. Place a 6 × 6-inch piece of **sheet resin** material in the frame of the vacuum former. Vinyl resin with a thickness of 0.040 inch makes an adequate tray.
2. Place the thoroughly dry model in the center of the vacuum former platform.
3. Heat the resin material until it sags downward approximately 1 inch below the frame. Figure 31.6 shows the heated resin in the vacuum former frame over the stone model.
4. Turn on the vacuum, and immediately pull the frame down over the model. Vacuum for 30 seconds.

Tips for the Clinician

Patient Instructions

- For best results, encourage patients not to smoke, eat food, or drink beverages that stain.
- Emphasize that "more is not better." Stress that the patient should follow instructions given by dental professional.

Tray Construction

- Trim the base of the stone model as thin as possible.
- Allow the stone model to dry completely before performing the vacuum procedure.
- Allow the resin to cool completely before attempting to trim or remove it from the model.
- A thin layer of Silly Putty (available in toy stores) can be substituted for the block-out resin. Cover all but the gingival third of the facial surfaces of the teeth to be whitened.

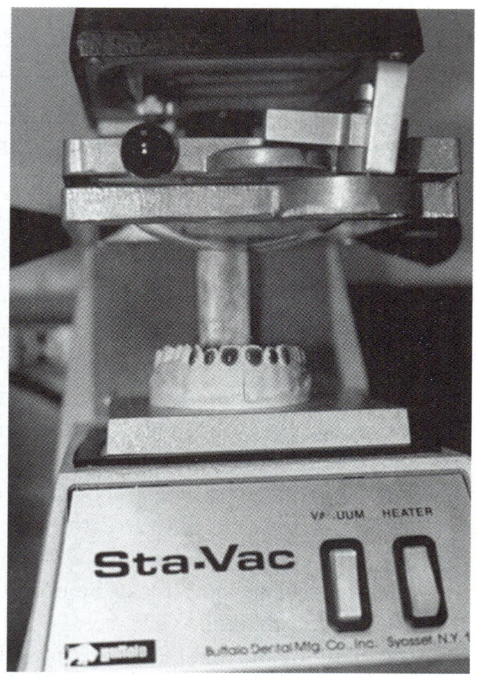

FIGURE 31.6 Stone model with facial reservoirs centered on the vacuum former. Warm resin is sagging below the frame.

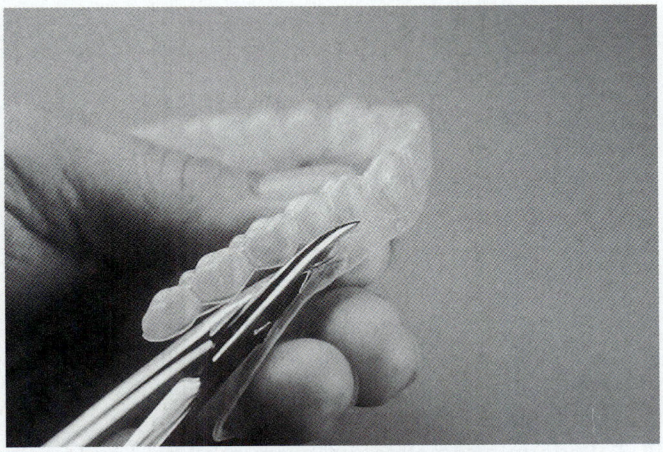

FIGURE 31.7 Trimming of the whitening tray with curved scissors.

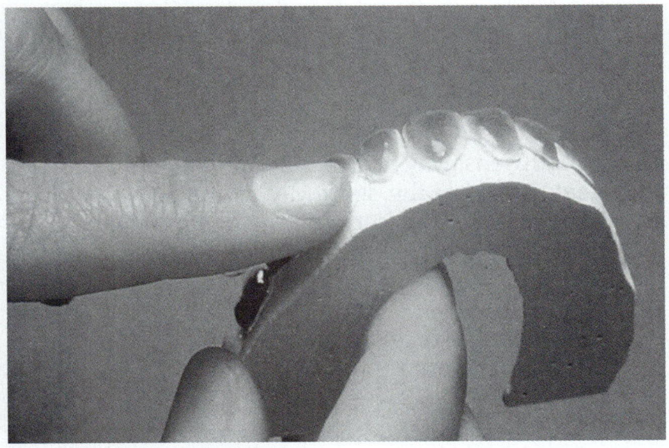

FIGURE 31.9 Warmed edges of the tray being readapted to the model with a wet finger. (Courtesy of Ultradent Products, Inc.)

5. Allow the resin to cool, and then remove the resin-covered model from the frame.

D. Trim the Whitening Tray

1. Trim the vinyl material with scissors, and carefully separate the tray from the model. Trim the tray again, creating a scalloped border following the gingival margins of the teeth. The tray border should end on the teeth, just gingival to the reservoir spaces. A tray being trimmed is shown in Figure 31.7.
2. Gently heat the cut edges of the tray with a microtorch or warm instrument (Fig. 31.8).
3. Immediately return the tray to the model, and with a wet finger, readapt the edges to the model (Fig. 31.9). Readapting with dry fingers could leave fingerprints on the tray material.
4. Keep the tray on the model until it is delivered to the patient. Instruct the patient to keep the tray in the storage box and away from heat. Figure 31.10 shows a trimmed custom bleaching tray inside its storage box.

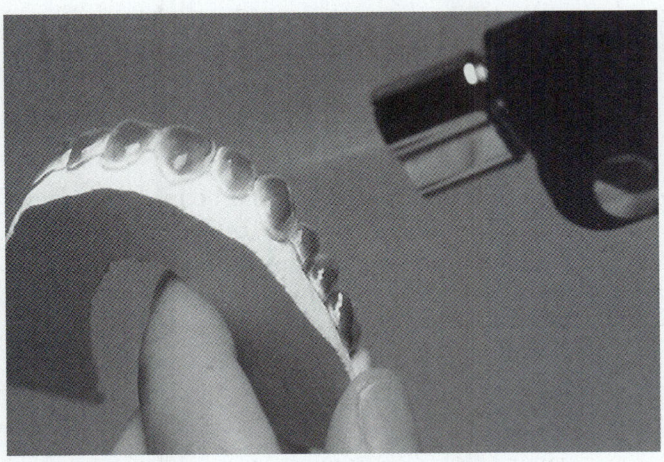

FIGURE 31.8 Edges of the trimmed tray softened with a microtorch. (Courtesy of Ultradent Products, Inc.)

5. Assess the tray by using the Skill Performance Evaluation sheet in Appendix 2.

V. Clinical Procedure Professionally Applied Power Whitening (Light-/Heat-Activated Chairside): Two Appointments

Increasing patient demands for faster methods of whitening has created a need for clinical competence in chairside power whitening. Armed with higher percentages of peroxide whiteners enhanced with activators and light equipment, the dental team may now offer those near immediate results. Clinically the patient may be seen only once for the procedure and once for a follow up evaluation. Now higher concentrations of hydrogen peroxide formulas enhanced with activators are available in power bleaching systems. These systems activate the whitening agent with heat or light. Some agents require no light. Those using

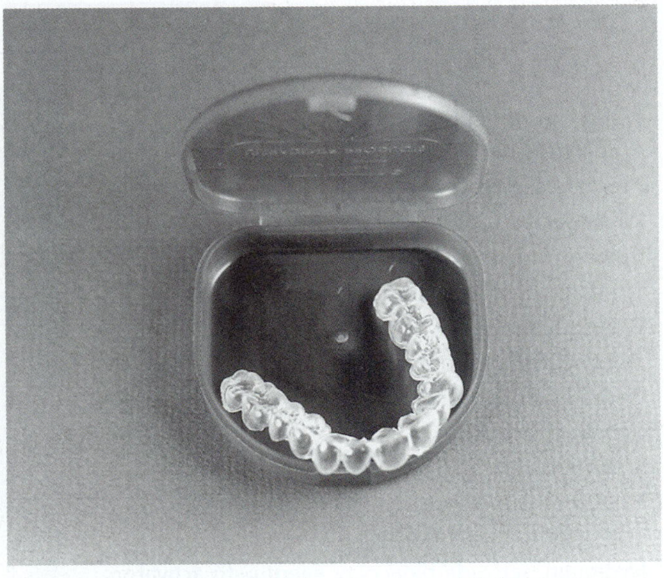

FIGURE 31.10 Custom whitening tray, trimmed, in its storage box.

Precautions

Patient Instructions

- If tooth sensitivity occurs, stop treatment. Resume treatment after the sensitivity disappears (usually in a few days), but decrease the treatment time by half.

Tray Construction

- Do not look directly at the curing light when curing the block-out resin.
- The heating element and the frame that holds the resin remain hot after the vacuum has been turned off.

lights require resin curing lights, violet wavelength lights, gas plasma lights or LED lights. The following describes the clinical methods for applying those higher percentage (15%–35%) hydrogen peroxide whitening agents. Necessary items for this procedure are listed in Table 31.5. A summary of this section's clinical procedures can be found at the end of this chapter.

A. Whitening Appointment

1. Medical History

Obtain a complete medical history from the patient. Carefully evaluate that there are no contraindications such as sensitivity to whitening agent, use of photosensitive drugs or herbs, radiation or chemotherapy, history of melanoma, caries, cracked enamel, or root sensitivity, as in Table 31.2. The dental professional should determine if the patient is overusing whitening procedures. Review the number of times a patient has undergone whitening procedures. Proceed once medical history is cleared.

2. Informed Consent

An informed consent should be read and signed by the patient prior to the procedure. The bleaching consent should briefly describe the treatment, the benefits, and the possible side effects. Informed consent should be kept with the patient's records. A sample consent is found in Figure 31.11.

3. Intraoral Examination

Patient is given a thorough intraoral exam. Soft tissues must be free of lesions or potential areas

Table 31.5 Armamentarium for Professionally Applied Light/Heat Activated Whitening Agents

Forms: medical history, informed consent, clinical exam, and treatment
Prophylaxis instruments
White swabs (optional)
Camera: video, film, digital
Shade guide or spectrophotometer
Written instructions
Safety glasses for operator and patient
Gauze and cotton rolls
Cheek retractors
Sunscreen
Paint on resin dam
Curing light, bleaching light
Hydrogen peroxide bleaching agent with activators

Summary—Clinical Procedures For Patient-Applied Professionally Supervised Whitening

First Appointment

1. Obtain a complete medical history for the patient.
2. Obtain the patient's signed informed consent after a full explanation.
3. Perform a complete oral exam of all hard and soft tissues.
4. Perform a scale and polish procedure.
5. Obtain intraoral photographs, including a shade guide tab, of the maxillary and mandibular teeth.
6. Take impression for model and tray construction.

Second Appointment

1. Try the custom tray in the patient's mouth; make any adjustments.
2. Provide the patient with instructions for using the tray.
3. Provide the patient with written instructions, and schedule a follow-up appointment.

Third Appointment

1. Examine the teeth for results; record the hours of treatment and any side effects.
2. Provide more whitening if desired. Schedule another appointment.
3. Take a posttreatment intraoral photograph, again including a shade guide tab.

Summary—Laboratory Procedures

1. Construct a stone model, then trim the model, making the base small and thin.
2. Place block-out resin (and cure) on the desired teeth in the proper location and thickness.
3. Heat the resin material until it sags 1 inch below the frame.
4. Turn on the vacuum, and immediately pull down the frame. Vacuum for 1 minute.
5. Trim any excess vinyl from the model with scissors.
6. Trim the tray again, up to gingival margins.
7. Heat the cut edges of the tray with a microtorch or warm instrument.
8. Replace the tray on the model, and readapt the edges to the model.

of irritation. Caries, root sensitivity, cracks, or broken restorations must not be present. Any anterior restorations that are not being replaced would negate the procedure. At this time evaluate the need for whitening. Check for already whitened teeth with chalky appearance. Patients with body dysmorphic disorder (BDD), may insist on a procedure that is highly unnecessary.

4. **Prophylaxis**

   Complete a prophylaxis that includes scaling and polishing to remove plaque, calculus, and stain. Remove extrinsic stains and floss.

5. **White Swabs with Aqueous Cleaning Technology™ from GRINrx**

   Optionally, you may swab the surfaces to be whitened with white swabs. The swabs will remove stain and hydrate teeth before the whitening procedure.

6. **Intraoral Photograph**

   Photograph both the upper and lower teeth. This front view will show the teeth in the smile line. The photography must include a shade guide tab that is matched to the tooth shade of the anterior teeth. Tabs may be positioned to the incisal edge of a central incisor, see Figures 31.12 and 31.13. A spectrophotometer could also be used, see Figure 31.2. The photo will document the initial tooth color for the patient record.

7. **Isolate and Condition Patient's Soft Tissue**

   If lights are used, apply sunscreen to patient's lips and nose if they are possibly in the area to be exposed, see Figure 31.14. Retract lips and cheeks and isolate tissues with gauze and cotton rolls as in Figure 31.15.

Informed Consent for Professionally Applied Power Whitening (Light/Heat Activated) Chairside Treatment

The product our dentist/dental hygienist will be applying to your teeth is **Hydrogen Peroxide** ________(Percentage) with an activator. Your tissues will be isolated and the material will be applied to the tooth surfaces requiring whitening. A light/heat source will be activated to initiate the whitening. A series of three applications of the hydrogen peroxide material with light/heat activation will occur. Immediate whitening results should occur.

The most frequently reported side effects of peroxide tooth whitening are sensitivity and irritation to the gums. Sore throat and nausea may occur if product is accidentally swallowed. In rare cases pulpal necrosis (tooth death) could occur.

Patient Consent: I________________________________
(Full name), hereby give consent to treatment allowing the dentist/dental hygienist to apply a whitening agent to my teeth. I have been informed of the potential benefits and side effects of the treatment, and affirm that I have read and understand the instructions below.

Signed:____

Witness:____

Date:____

One Copy for Patient
One Copy for Patient's Record

FIGURE 31.11 Sample of bleaching consent form.

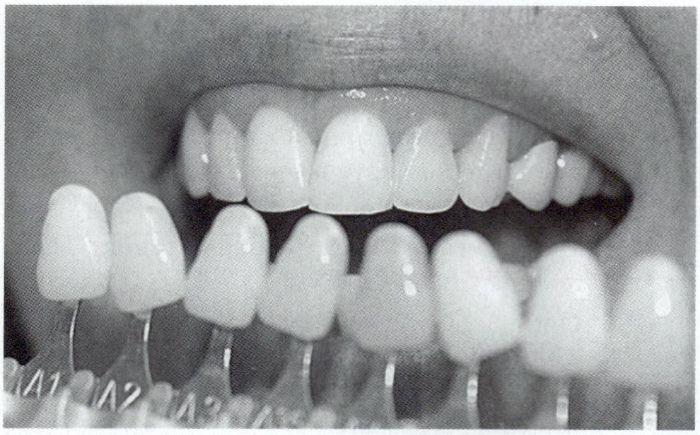

FIGURE 31.12 Shade guide for evaluation of original color.

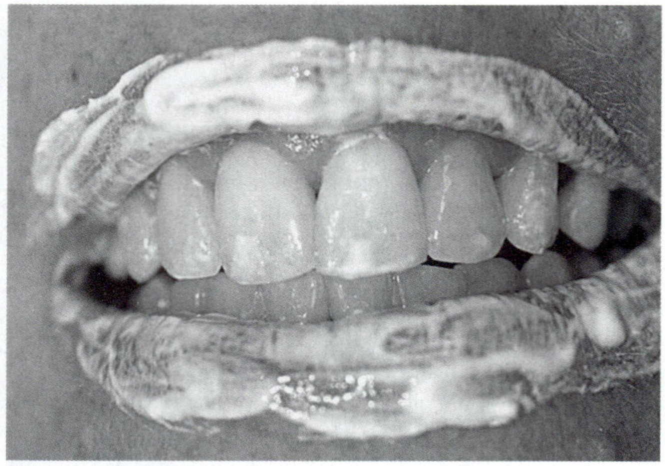

FIGURE 31.14 Patient's lips with applied sunscreen.

8. Paint on Resin Dam

Carefully apply **paint-on resin dam** to all exposed gingival tissues. Light cure material. Reapply to any gingival areas still exposed, see Figure 31.16.

9. Protective Eyewear

To avoid exposure to damaging light, both operator and patient must be wearing eyewear as shown in Figure 31.17. Although splatter does not usually occur, the eyewear can protect from potential splash hazards. Protective eyewear can also filter the activation light.

10. Application of Whitening Agent

Whitening agent is applied to all facial surfaces in the smile line. The agent is syringed to the surface and then spread evenly over the tooth as shown in Figure 31.18.

11. Light Activation of Whitener

If the whitener requires light activation, place light evenly over smile line as shown in Figure 31.19. Activate for 20 minutes. Rinse, evacuate whitener, and reapply whitener. Repeat sequence two more times, totaling 3 applications and 3 light activations for the entire procedure. If a curing light is used, the light must be placed individually for 30 seconds for each tooth whitened. Between each application give the patient the chance to rest or opt to discontinue if uncomfortable. At the end of the procedure, rinse, evacuate the whitener, and remove the paint-on dam and isolation materials.

12. Second Intraoral Photograph

A second intraoral photograph should be taken at the completion of procedure to document final

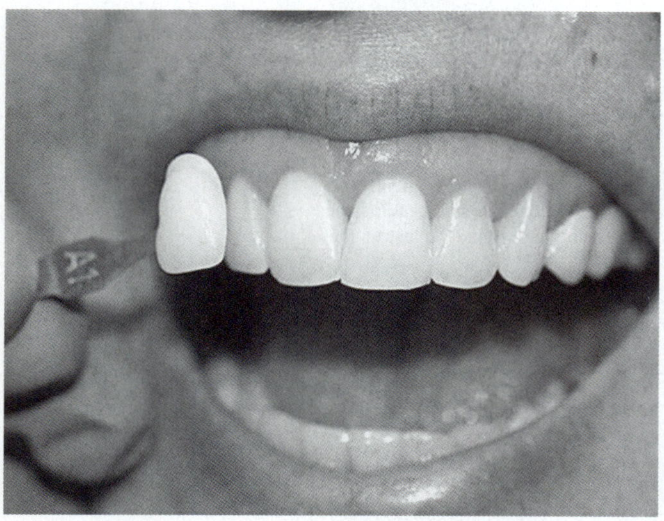

FIGURE 31.13 Aligning matched shade guide with anterior tooth.

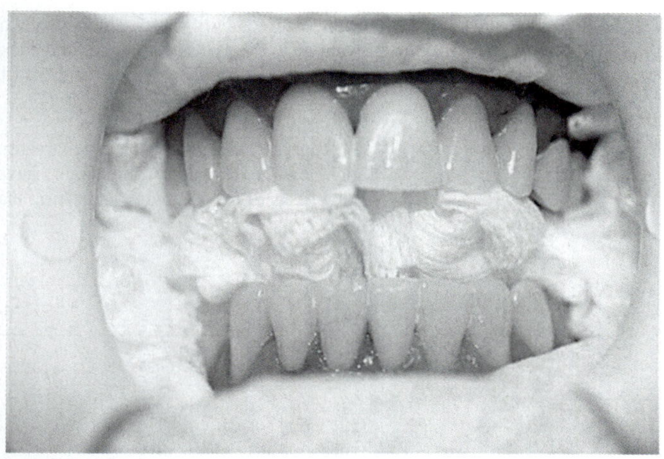

FIGURE 31.15 Retraction and isolation in place prior to placement of resin dam.

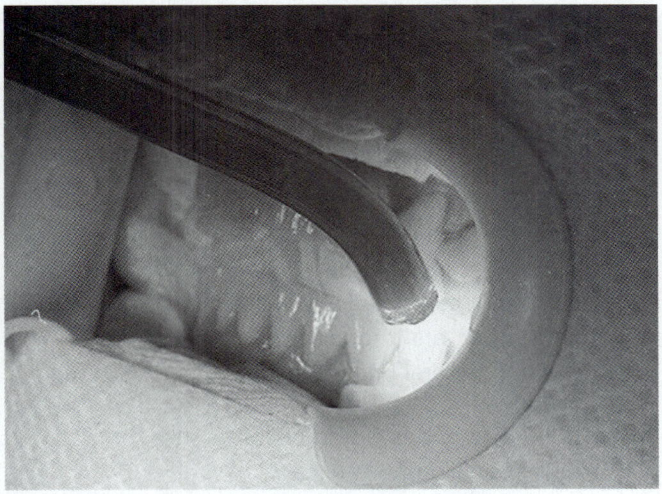

FIGURE 31.16 Light curing paint on resin dam.

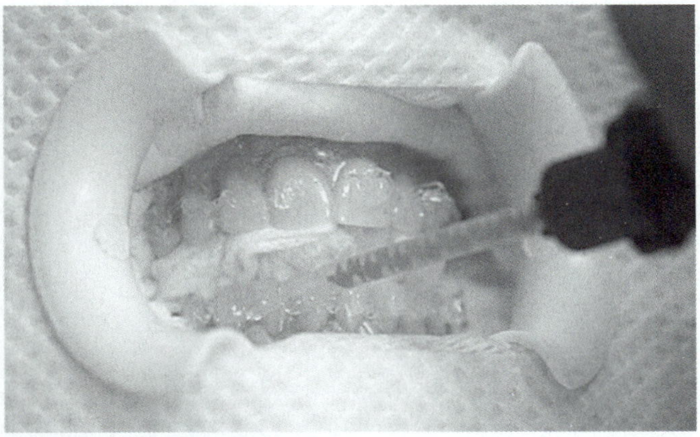

FIGURE 31.18 Hydrogen peroxide gel with activator syringed onto facial surfaces.

results. Again, the shade guide should be used to determine whitening effects, Figure 31.20.

13. Patient Instructions

At this time patient must be informed of side effects. An instruction sheet should be given to the patient. An example is included as Figure 31.21. Patient must realize that tooth sensitivity and gingival irritation could occur. Examine tissue for any gingival irritation. Instruct patient on the use of Vitamin E oil for gingival irritation. A nonsteroidal anti-inflammatory drug (NSAID) may be recommended for tooth sensitivity. NSAIDs are often recommended prior to the procedure also. Advise patient to avoid eating colored foods/drinks that may stain the dentition (e.g., tea, coffee, mustard, red sauces). No smoking should occur. Neutral sodium fluoride gel or potassium nitrate can be used in bleaching trays for 30 minutes twice/day. Additional bleaching enhancement may take place with the use of night guard bleaching trays often created prior to the power whitening procedure. Allowing for no sensitivity, the patient may choose to further enhance the whitening by using the trays for a few nights after the power procedure. Any pain lasting more than 24–48 hours should be reported immediately to the dental office.

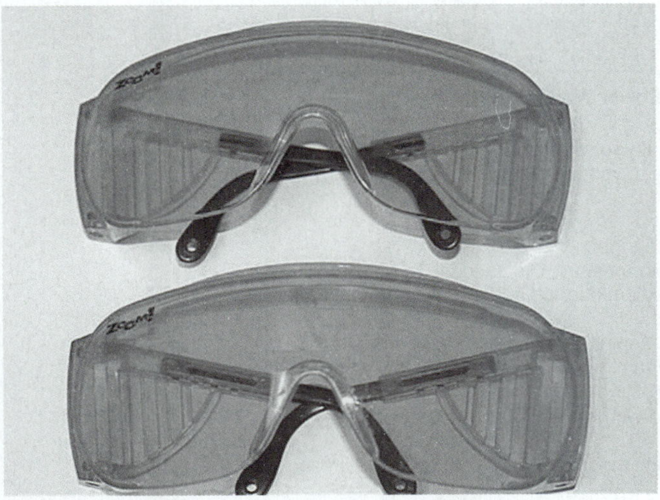

FIGURE 31.17 Eyewear must be provided for both patient and operator.

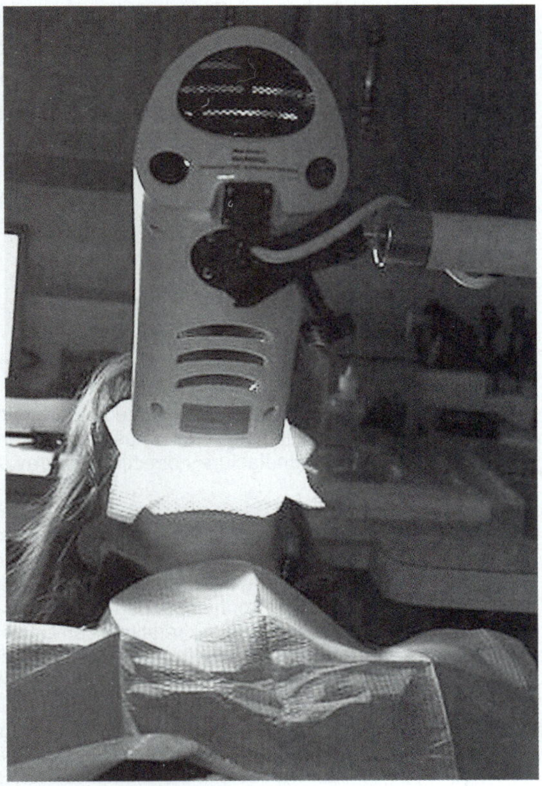

FIGURE 31.19 Activation light in use.

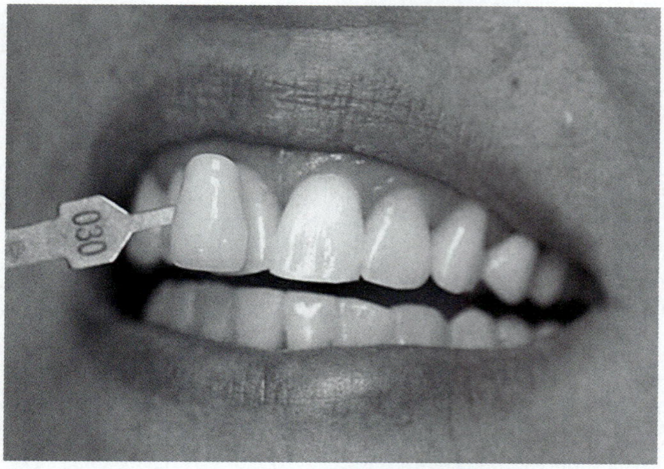

FIGURE 31.20 Second photograph documenting results of whitening procedure.

14. Documentation

Document the procedure in the patient records. Include medical history, intraoral evaluation, informed consent, photograph, material used, the amount of time light activated, and the beginning and ending shade guide results.

15. Evaluation Appointment

Before the evaluation, a telephone call could be made to the patient to confirm patient's comfort with the procedure. The patient then may return within 1 week for a follow-up appointment. At this time the gingival tissues and the whitening results could be evaluated. Anterior restorations in need of replacement can be scheduled one week later allowing for the two weeks post whitening. Any lingering sensitivities should be addressed at this time.

Summary Clinical Procedures for Professionally Applied Power Whitening

1. Obtain a complete medical history.
2. Obtain the patient's signed informed consent.
3. Perform a complete intraoral evaluation.
4. Perform an oral prophylaxis.
5. Obtain intraoral photographs with shade guide included.
5. Retraction and isolation of soft tissues.
6. Apply paint-on resin dam.
7. Apply whitening agent.
8. Activate with light for 20 minutes.
9. Rinse and evacuate whitening agent.
10. Apply whitening agent for the second time.
11. Activate with light a second time for 20 minutes.
12. Rinse and evacuate whitening agent.
13. Apply whitening agent for the third time.
14. Activate with light for the third time for 20 minutes.
15. Rinse and evacuate whitening agent.
16. Remove retractors, isolation gauze, cotton rolls, and paint-on dam.
17. Obtain second intraoral photograph with shade guide.
18. Document procedure in the patient's record.
19. Explain and give written instructions to patient.
20. Reevaluate results at second appointment.

Instructions for Post Power Whitening

You should see immediate whitening results. If you wish to further enhance the whitening you may use night guard bleaching trays for 2-3 days. Follow the manufacture's directions for tray use.

- Brush and floss your teeth in the usual manner.
- Avoid foods that stain such as tea, coffee, mustard, red sauces.
- If tooth sensitivity occurs, use neutral sodium fluoride gel or potassium nitrate in trays twice/day for 30 minutes.
- Prophylactic use of NSAIDS (Ibuprofen, aspirin) may be used for sensitivity.
- Gingival irritations can be treated with Vitamin E oil.
- Night guard whitening may be undertaken to enhance results.
- Whitening maintenance can be achieved with whitening mouthrinses and dentifrices.
- Touch up maintenance can be achieved in the future with night guard whitening trays.

FIGURE 31.21 Patient instructions to be given after power whitening.

Review Questions

1. Which of the following is the professionally applied whitening material?
   a) Whitening dentifrice
   b) Night guard whitening agents
   c) Power (light/heat activated) whitening agent
   d) Whitening mouthrinse
2. Which of the following would be used for night guard tooth whitening?
   a) Boil and bite mouth guard
   b) Fluoride tray
   c) Custom vinyl tray
   d) Athletic custom mouth guard
3. Which of the following helps prevent gingival irritation while night guard whitening?
   a) Using a scalloped tray
   b) Using a small dot of whitening in facial surfaces of tray
   c) Using a mouthrinse prior to whitening
   d) Both a and b
4. Why is the intraoral photograph with the shade guide necessary?
   a) To document the initial tooth color
   b) To document the final tooth color
   c) To document for patient records
   d) All of the above
5. Application of a paint-on resin dam prior to power whitening helps
   a) Isolate teeth and protect gingival tissue
   b) Activate the whitening agent
   c) Hydrate the teeth and tissue
   d) Nourish the teeth and tissue

Supplemental Readings

Aqueous Cleaning Technology™ A disruptive new technology promoting oral health and smile aesthetics. GRINrx Corporation, NY, NY; 2006.

Buchalla W, Attin T. External bleaching therapy with activation by heat, light or laser – A systematic review. DentMat 2006;23:586–596.

"Dam that's Kool" Tech Specifications from the Manufacturer Contemporary Esthetics and Restorative Practice. January 2004. retrieved March 14, 2007 from http://www.pulpdent.com/studies/Kool_Dam_Glazer.pdf

Goldstein RE, Garber DA. Complete Dental Bleaching. Chicago: Quintessence, 1995:71–100.

Haywood V, Cordero R, Wright K, et al. Brushing with a potassium nitrate dentifrice to reduce bleaching sensitivity. J Clin Dent 2005;16:17–22.

Turkin M, Turkin L. Effect of nonvital bleaching with 10% carbamide peroxide on sealing ability of resin composite restorations. Int Endo J 2004;37:52–60.

What takes place when your dentist performs professional teeth whitening treatments? Retrieved March 1, 2007 from www.animated-teeth.com

Ziempa S, Felix H, Ginger M, Ward M. Randomized Prospective Effectiveness of Zoom2™ Dental Whitening Lamp and Light-catalyzed peroxide gel. Clinical White Paper. Discus Dental Inc. Feb 2005.

32

Debonding Orthodontic Resins

Marylou Gutmann, R.D.H., M.A.

Key Words/Phrases

debonding

Objectives

After studying this chapter, the student will be able to do the following:

1. Explain the rationale for removing composite adhesive resin from the teeth following orthodontic treatment.
2. Discuss the clinical objectives for debonding.
3. Describe the effects of using improper debonding techniques or materials on enamel.
4. Demonstrate each step in the debonding procedure.
5. Self-evaluate the effectiveness of the debonding procedure.
6. Explain three follow-up considerations to be discussed with the newly debonded orthodontic patient.

INTRODUCTION

Adhesive composite materials are commonly used to attach **orthodontic brackets** to enamel surfaces. These brackets hold the arch wire in place by means of elastics or ligature wires, as illustrated in Figure 13.1. Common orthodontic materials are discussed in Chapter 13. The orthodontist generally removes the fixed appliances and the adhesive resin at the end of therapy (debonding). **Debonding** is the complete removal of composite material from enamel surfaces after orthodontic treatment. Generally the orthodontist performs this procedure. However, if the orthodontic practice employs a dental hygienist, then he or she usually debonds the patient. Patients are generally referred to their general dentist for a complete dental examination, radiographs, and prophylaxis after the debonding appointment. The dental hygienist in the general practice is often the first person to see the patient after the active phase of orthodontic treatment is completed. Occasionally fine remnants of adhesive resin remain on the facial surfaces of the patient's anterior and premolar teeth where the orthodontic brackets had been attached. The task of eliminating the residual composite material is then the responsibility of the general practice dental hygienist. It is important to completely remove all composite resin material to avoid:

- Plaque accumulation
- Stain
- Poor esthetics
- Demineralization and/or caries formation
- Gingival inflammation
- Mucosal response from rough resin

All debonding methods remove some enamel. The dental hygienist must select the least traumatic instruments and methods to accomplish the resin removal.

I. Objective of Debonding

The primary objective of debonding is to return the enamel surface to its natural, pretreatment appearance. A secondary objective is to return the enamel surface to its pretreatment texture or feel.

II. Problems With Improper Debonding Techniques and Materials

A number of hand and rotary instruments as well as a variety of abrasives have been investigated for use in debonding. Most studies indicate that some enamel alteration results from the debonding process. In addition, decalcified enamel surfaces (white spots) are much more likely to exhibit enamel loss than intact enamel. Faster techniques and coarser abrasives cause more damage to the enamel surfaces. Researchers generally agree that diamond burs, rubber wheels, green stones, white stones, sandpaper discs, manual or ultrasonic scalers, pliers, and band removers should not be used to remove the composite adhesive resin that remains after bracket removal.

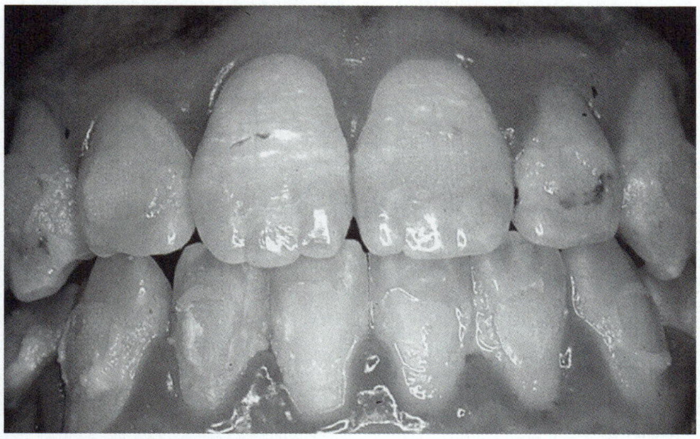

FIGURE 32.1 Facial view of anterior teeth with adhesive resin still remaining after removal of orthodontic brackets. (See color insert.) (Reprinted with permission from Gutmann ME. Composite adhesive resin removal following active orthodontic treatment. J Pract Hyg 1996;5(3): 16–19; (c)1996, Montage Media Corporation; see the color insert for a color version of this image.)

III. Debonding Procedure

Enamel surfaces that are gouged or scratched as a result of improper debonding methods or materials may cause the same problems that would result from leaving remnants of adhesive resin on the tooth. It is critical for the dental hygienist to follow the steps in the debonding procedure in sequential order to provide a smooth enamel surface. The materials needed for debonding are listed in Table 32.1.

A. Identification of the Resin

Identification of the remaining composite adhesive resin is necessary to avoid causing inadvertent damage to the enamel surface during resin removal. The resin that remains immediately after bracket and band removal (Fig. 32.1) is easier to see than the residual remnants that are frequently seen in general practice settings. The clinician may use one of the following methods to identify the location and amount of remaining resin:

1. Dry the tooth with air to see the resin. The resin appears as a square, opaque substance on the tooth surface.
2. Apply disclosing solution to the tooth with a cotton-tipped applicator. The composite material may stain the same as plaque.
3. Examine the tooth surface with an explorer. Resin will feel rough compared to smooth

Table 32.1 Armamentarium for Debonding Orthodontic Adhesive Resin

Mirror
Explorer
Low-speed handpiece
Tapered, plain-cut, tungsten carbide finishing bur
Aluminum oxide composite polishing cups and points
Rubber cup
Wet slurry of fine flour of pumice
Brown polishing cup
Green polishing cup
Gauze
Disclosing solution
Two dappen dishes
Cotton-tipped applicator
Prophy angle
Contra angle
Safety glasses (for patient and clinician)
Personal protective equipment
Floss
Air/water syringe tip
Saliva ejector

enamel. Some composite materials may also abrade the metal explorer, leaving a gray line on the surface.

4. Ask the patient to rub his or her tongue over the tooth surface to identify the exact location of the resin.

B. Removal of the Resin Bulk

Removal of the resin bulk requires use of a slow-speed handpiece and a tapered, plain-cut, tungsten carbide finishing bur. A slow-speed handpiece is preferred for better access and control.

Avoid decalcified areas that frequently surround the adhesive resin due to inadequate plaque/biofilm removal by the patient during active orthodontic treatment. Use the bur on the adhesive resin only and avoid the decalcified enamel as much as possible. In cases of significant decalcification, complete removal of bonding material may exacerbate the problem. An alternative procedure is: 1) gross removal of bonding material, 2) followed by remineralization via fluoride treatments, and 3) three months later, complete bonding material removal and enamel polishing. This alternative should reduce loss of tooth structure.

1. Use a brush-like stroke in one direction only.
2. Begin at the cervical aspect of the resin, and move to the incisal (Fig. 32.2).
3. As the resin is removed with the bur, it will resemble fine white shavings.

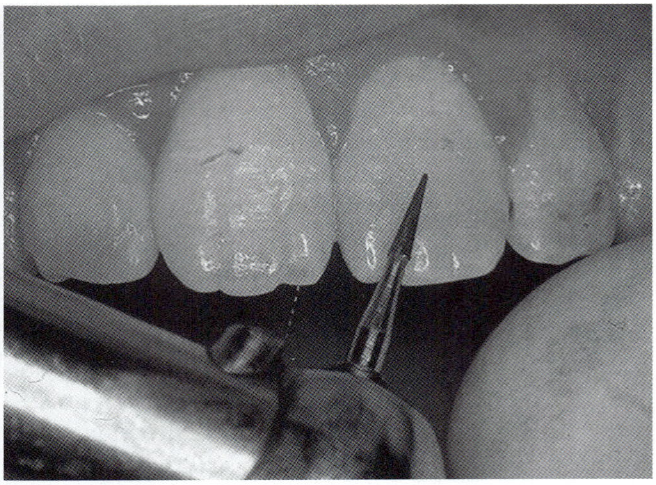

FIGURE 32.2 Use of finishing bur on a low-speed handpiece to remove the bulk of adhesive resin. (Reprinted with permission from Gutmann ME. Composite adhesive resin removal following active orthodontic treatment. J Pract Hyg 1996;5(3):16–19; (c)1996, Montage Media Corporation.)

4. Rinse the tooth with water frequently, and then dry the surface to evaluate progress and to avoid using the bur on intact enamel. The resin remnant appears opaque and dull next to the glossy enamel surface.
5. The dental hygienist should strive to reach a balance between smoothness of the enamel surface and enamel removal. More enamel is removed as the surfaces become smoother. It is critical to frequently evaluate the tooth surface for remaining resin deposits. When none are visible, you are ready to proceed to the final finishing of the enamel surface.
6. During the procedure, ask the patient for feedback regarding smoothness.

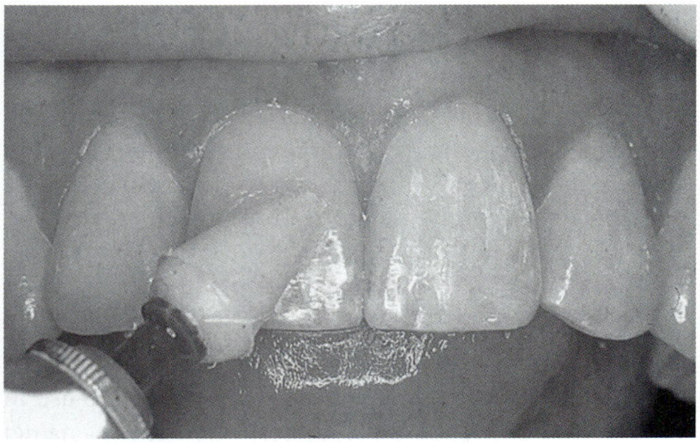

FIGURE 32.3 Aluminum oxide finishing point used to remove any enamel scarring resulting from burs. (Reprinted with permission from Gutmann ME. Composite adhesive resin removal following active orthodontic treatment. J Pract Hyg 1996;5(3):16–19; (c)1996, Montage Media Corporation.)

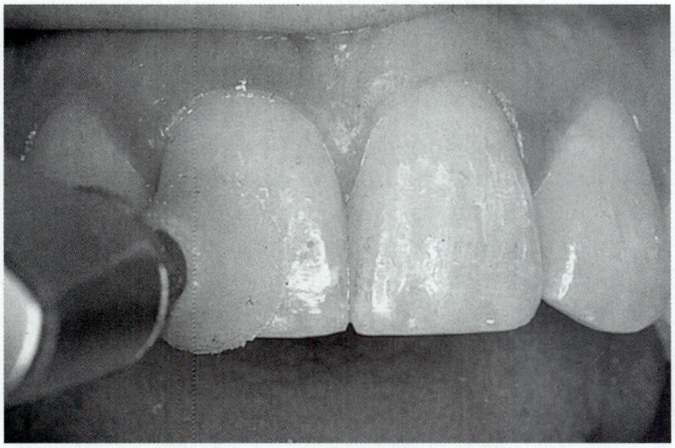

FIGURE 32.4 Aluminum oxide finishing cup used to remove any enamel scarring resulting from burs. (Reprinted with permission from Gutmann ME. Composite adhesive resin removal following active orthodontic treatment. J Pract Hyg 1996;5(3):16–19; (c)1996, Montage Media Corporation.)

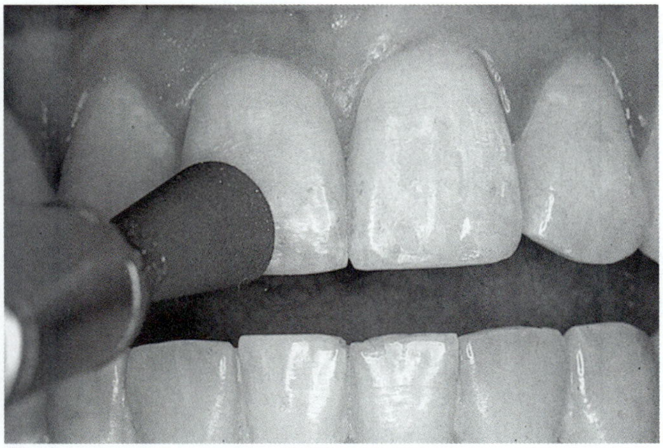

FIGURE 32.6 Brown polishing cup used for maximum gloss to enamel surface. (Reprinted with permission from Gutmann ME. Composite adhesive resin removal following active orthodontic treatment. J Pract Hyg 1996;5(3):16–19; (c)1996, Montage Media Corporation.)

7. A final check with the explorer and disclosing solution will confirm if all the resin has been removed.

C. Final Finishing

When no visible resin remains, the enamel surface is then finished and polished to restore its pretreatment appearance:

1. Use aluminum oxide composite finishing cups and points (Enhance Caulk/Dentsply, Milford, DE) at low speed over the resin-free enamel surface (Figs. 32.3, 32.4).
2. Polish each tooth with a fine pumice slurry and a rubber prophylaxis cup (Fig. 32.5).
3. To produce a natural-appearing, glossy enamel surface, two additional steps are recommended: final polish with brown followed by green (Figs. 32.6 and 32.7) polishing cups (Brasseler, Savannah, GA).

Tips for the Clinician

- During use of the bur, apply air frequently to dry the tooth and examine the surface; do not keep using the bur unnecessarily.
- Make sure that the patient moves his or her tongue over each tooth surface slowly to detect any residual resin.
- Emphasize the importance of office and home fluoride to remineralize enamel after debonding.

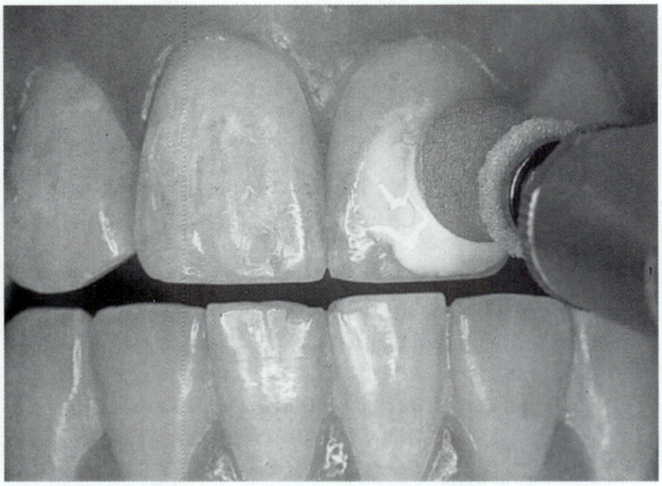

FIGURE 32.5 Polishing with fine pumice slurry and rubber cup. (Reprinted with permission from Gutmann ME. Composite adhesive resin removal following active orthodontic treatment. J Pract Hyg 1996;5(3):16–19; (c)1996, Montage Media Corporation.)

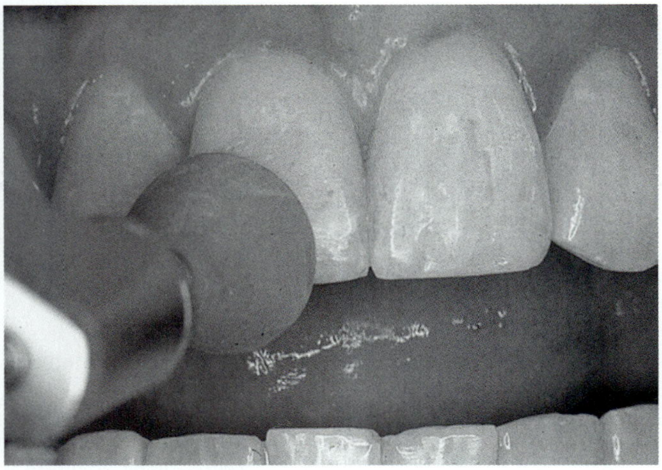

FIGURE 32.7 Final polishing with a green polishing cup. (Reprinted with permission from Gutmann ME. Composite adhesive resin removal following active orthodontic treatment. J Pract Hyg 1996;5(3):16–19; (c)1996, Montage Media Corporation.)

Precautions

- Begin the stroke with the bur at the cervical portion of the resin, and move toward the incisal or occlusal surface to avoid accidental trauma to the gingiva.
- To avoid enamel damage, do not try to remove composite adhesive resin with curets, scalers, diamond burs, high-speed handpieces, sandpaper discs, rubber wheels, green stones, white stones, orthodontic pliers and band removers, or ultrasonic instruments.
- Because aerosols are produced during debonding, it is important to wear a face mask.
- During use of the bur, flying particles of resin may cause injury to the eyes, so safety glasses for the patient and the clinician are essential.

D. Evaluation

Use the Skill Performance Evaluation sheet in Appendix 2 to assess the effectiveness of the debonding procedure. Provide the patient with a hand mirror to view the results.

IV. Postdebonding Considerations

As with other dental hygiene care, educating the patient is important and should be included as part of the procedure. Include the following in your instructions:

A. Recommend a topical fluoride treatment or application of fluoride varnish to replenish the lost fluoride in the outermost layer of enamel.

B. Reinforce use of a fluoride dentifrice. Recommend use of a fluoride rinse on a daily basis.

C. Schedule a maintenance appointment for a complete examination, radiographs, prophylaxis, and other preventive services as indicated by the patient's oral conditions (if the debonding procedure is performed in the orthodontic office). If residual composite material is found during the maintenance appointment in the general practice, it can be removed during the course of the maintenance visit.

Summary

1. Use air, an explorer, disclosing solution, and patient feedback to identify the resin.
2. Use a tapered, tungsten carbide finishing bur in a low-speed handpiece.
3. Move the bur from the cervical to the incisal surface of the resin in a light, brush-like stroke.
4. Evaluate resin reduction frequently by rinsing and drying, exploring, disclosing, and asking the patient to evaluate smoothness with his or her tongue.
5. After the resin is removed, polish the enamel with aluminum oxide polishing points.
6. Follow step 5 with aluminum oxide polishing cups.
7. Polish each surface with a fine pumice slurry, using a rubber cup and a slow-speed handpiece.
8. Use intermittent strokes to avoid heat generation.
9. Polish the enamel with a brown polishing cup.
10. Polish the enamel with a green polishing cup.
11. Provide the patient with appropriate self-care instructions.

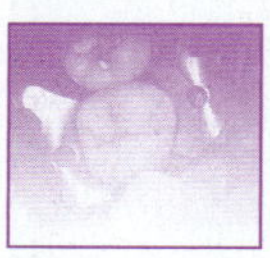

Review Questions

1. Which of the following should be used to correctly debond?
   a) Tapered plain-cut finishing bur and a high speed handpiece
   b) Tapered plain-cut finishing bur and a low speed handpiece
   c) Tapered cross-cut finishing bur and a low speed handpiece
   d) Straight fissure, plain-cut bur and a high speed handpiece
   e) Straight fissure, crosscut bur and a low speed handpiece

2. All debonding methods remove some enamel. It is the responsibility of the hygienist to select the least traumatic method for resin removal.
   a) The first statement is true; the second statement is false.
   b) The first statement is false; the second statement is true.
   c) Both statements are true.
   d) Both statements are false.

3. The direction of the stroke of the bur during debonding should be toward the:
a) Gingival margin
b) Proximal surface
c) Embrasure spaces
d) Incisal or occlusal

4. It is important to remove all composite resin material during debonding to avoid all of the following *except* one. Which one is the EXCEPTION?
a) Changes in occlusion
b) Gingival inflammation
c) Stain
d) Plaque accumulation

5. During the debonding procedure, which of the following should be done to avoid unnecessary use of the bur?
a) Change to a new bur after the resin is removed on 2 teeth
b) Apply air frequently and examine the surface
c) Polish with the pumice slurry after 5 seconds of bur use
d) Use a constant circular motion with the bur

Supplemental Readings

Brown CRL, Way DC. Enamel loss during orthodontic bonding and subsequent loss during removal of filled and unfilled adhesives. Am J Orthod 1978;74:663–671.

Campbell PM. Enamel surfaces after orthodontic bracket debonding. Angle Orthod 1995;65:103–110.

Diedrich P. Enamel alterations from bracket bonding and debonding: a study with the scanning electron microscope. Am J Orthod 1981;79:500–522.

Eminkahyagil N, Arman A, Cetinahin A, Karabulut E. Effect of resin-removal methods on enamel and shear bond strength of rebounded brackets. Angle Orthod 2006;76: 314–321.

Everett MS. Debonding orthodontic adhesives. Dent Hyg 1985;59:364–370.

Fitzpatrick DA, Way DC. The effects of wear, acid etching, and bond removal on human enamel. Am J Orthod 1977;72: 671–681.

Gutmann ME. Composite adhesive resin removal following orthodontic treatment. J Pract Hyg 1996;5(3):16–19.

Pus MD, Way DC. Enamel loss due to orthodontic bonding with filled and unfilled resins using various clean-up techniques. Am J Orthod 1980;77:269–283.

Retief DH, Denys FR. Finishing of enamel surfaces after debonding of orthodontic attachments. Angle Orthod 1979;49:1–10.

Thompson RE, Way DC. Enamel loss due to prophylaxis and multiple bonding/debonding of orthodontic attachments. Am J Orthod 1981;79:282–295.

Tufekci E, Merrill TE, Pintado MR, Beyer JP, Brantley WA. Enamel loss associated with orthodontic adhesive removal on teeth with white spot lesions: an in vitro study. Am J Orthod Dentofacial Orthop 2004;125:733–739.

Zachrisson BU. Bonding in orthodontics. In: Graber TM, Vanarsdall RL, eds. Orthodontics, Current Principles and Techniques. 3rd ed. St. Louis: Mosby, 2000:557–639.

33

Placement of the Periodontal Dressing

Cathryn Frere, B.S.D.H., M.S.Ed.

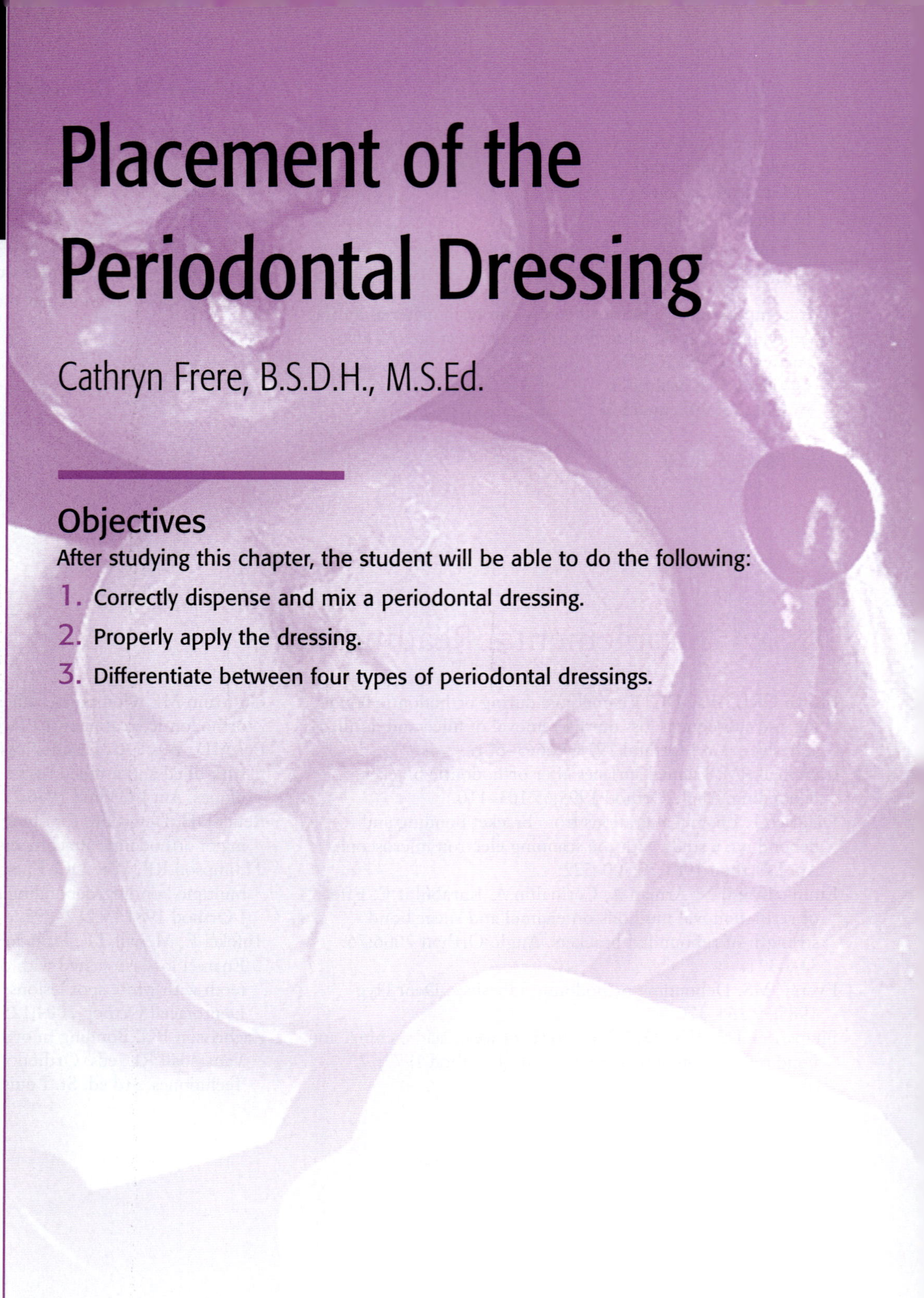

Key Words/Phrases

periodontal dressing
adhesive foil

Objectives

After studying this chapter, the student will be able to do the following:

1. Correctly dispense and mix a periodontal dressing.
2. Properly apply the dressing.
3. Differentiate between four types of periodontal dressings.

INTRODUCTION

The **periodontal dressing** is a physical barrier that is placed on surgical sites to protect the healing tissues from the forces produced during mastication, thereby providing patient comfort. These dressings also provide some splinting of mobile teeth during healing and they help shape newly forming tissues by maintaining close adaptation of mucosal flaps and gingival grafts to the underlying tissues after periodontal surgery. Periodontal dressings help prevent post surgical bleeding by keeping the initial blood clot in place. At present, no periodontal dressings are manufactured that contain therapeutic agents to aid in healing.

I. Purpose

The dental hygienist may be given the responsibility of placing a periodontal dressing when assisting the dentist during surgery, when performing postoperative care, or when a patient returns to the practice with a postsurgical emergency. Necessary items for a periodontal dressing are listed in Table 33.1.

II. Dressing Types

A. Zinc Oxide-Eugenol (ZOE) Dressing

Early periodontal dressings were made by mixing zinc oxide with eugenol. These were described in Chapter 7. Because some patients experience adverse reactions to the eugenol, these packs are seldom used today.

B. Noneugenol Zinc Oxide Packs

Coe-Pak (G.C. America, Inc.) is the most commonly placed, American Dental Association-accepted noneugenol periodontal dressing in the United States. Its clinical preparation and application will be discussed in this chapter, and postoperative instructions for patients with a noneugenol zinc oxide dressing are listed in Table 33.2. Compared to the ZOE dressing, this is a more pliable and smoother dressing. However, it must be prepared at the time it is used.

Table 33.1 Armamentarium for Placement of a Periodontal Dressing

Plastic-coated mixing pad
Wooden tongue depressor or broad, flexible, stainless-steel spatula
Tube of Coe-Pak accelerator
Tube of Coe-Pak base
Petroleum jelly
Plastic instrument
Curet
Gauze squares
Dentoform (for laboratory exercises)

Table 33.2 Postoperative Instructions for Patients with a Noneugenol Zinc Oxide Dressing

1. To prevent disturbance of the dressing while it is setting, avoid the following for 2 hours after the surgery:
   - Smoking, excessive talking, eating warm foodstuffs, or drinking warm beverages
   - Rubbing or applying pressure to the face in the area of surgery
   - Pushing on the dressing with the tongue
2. If a small piece of the dressing crumbles off, simply discard it.
3. If a piece of dressing breaks off, creating a sharp edge or exposing a sensitive area of the surgical site, call the treating dentist.

C. Visible Light–Activated Surgical Packs

A urethane dimethacrylate resin-based material (e.g., Barricaid; Dentsply International, Inc.) is available in a syringe carrier for direct placement. There is no mixing of pastes or powder required. The material is activated by a visible light, giving the operator control over manipulation and setting time. On activation, a nonbrittle, protective, tasteless, translucent, elastic covering is formed. This dressing is especially useful in the anterior region, where esthetics are a concern.

D. Cyanoacrylate Dressing

N-Butyl cyanoacrylate is a liquid that polymerizes shortly after contact with the moisture of the oral tissues. An example of this dressing is PeriAcryl (Glustitch, Inc.), which is available in single-dose applicators (Fig. 33.1) or multiuse kits with a dispensing tray and applicator pipettes. This clear dressing adheres to the tissues, and it is hemostatic, bacteriostatic, and biodegradable. It does not need to be removed at a post-surgical follow-up. It is useful for securing the gingival margin after placement of intrasulcular local delivery antimicrobials and as a dressing for postbiopsy sites. Although it has many applications in periodontal surgery, it is not widely used at present.

III. Preparation of the Noneugenol Zinc Oxide Pack

A. Dispensing

1. Coe-Pak is supplied as two pastes, which are mixed immediately before placement.

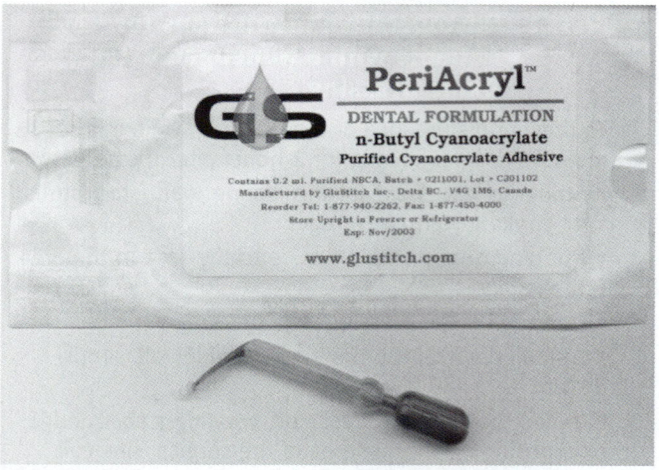

FIGURE 33.1 Single-dose applicator of PeriAcryl (Glustitch, Inc.), a cyanoacrylate dressing.

2. The larger tube, containing the base paste, is composed primarily of petrolatum, rosin, and fatty acids.
3. The smaller tube, containing the accelerator, is a mixture of zinc and magnesium oxides and vegetable oils.
4. Equal lengths of base and accelerator are expressed onto the mixing pad, as shown in Figure 33.2*A*. The diameters of the expressed pastes (but not the lengths) will differ, corresponding to the size of the tube orifice. Usually, strips equal in length to the span of the surgical site are adequate to provide coverage.

B. Mixing

1. Using a small area of the mixing pad, mix the base and accelerator with a tongue depressor (Fig. 33.2, *B* and *C*) or metal spatula until the mixture is uniform in color, such as that illustrated in Figure 33.2*D*. Spatulation should take from 30 to 45 seconds. A capsule of tetracycline may be added during mixing to give antimicrobial properties to the dressing.
2. Gather the mixture into a compact mass (Fig.33.2*E*), and let it rest for 2 to 3 minutes.
3. Lightly lubricate your fingers with petroleum jelly or sterile saline, and test the dressing. When the dressing is no longer tacky but is still soft and pliable, it is ready to apply.

IV. Placement

A. Hemostasis should be achieved before a dressing is placed. Blot-dry the surgical site and the teeth in the area with sterile gauze. There should not be excessive bleeding. A dry application site will help with dressing retention.

B. If the surgical site is in the posterior region of the mouth, roll the dressing with lightly lubricated fingers into a rope about the diameter of a pencil. The rolled dressing is shown in Figure 33.2*F*.

C. Starting in the anterior facial area, place the roll on the cervical area of the teeth. Flatten the pack against the involved soft tissues and the cervical third of the teeth. Loop it around the distal of the terminal tooth, and continue covering the involved lingual tissues, pressing the lingual and facial interproximal segments firmly together.

D. If the surgical site is in the anterior portion of the mouth, divide the pack material into two equal portions, and place the strips on the facial and lingual sites.

E. Adapt the interproximal areas with a plastic instrument or the back of a curet, as shown in Figure 33.3*A*. These interproximal projections create mechanical retention for the dressing. The dressing should be only thick enough to give strength to the material and should cover only the surgical wound.

F. To help with retention in areas with open embrasures, small pieces of the dressing material can be shaped to wedge into the interproximal spaces before the dressing is applied.

G. When the surgical site includes a small edentulous area, the dressing is continued over that space, with the facial and lingual portions joining at the alveolar crest.

H. To aid in retention, include at least four or five teeth in the dressed area.

I. In certain cases, adhesive foil may be placed between the surgical site and the dressing to prevent the inadvertent introduction of the dressing under the tissue margins or the incorporation of sutures into the dressing. **Adhesive foil** is a tinfoil coated with a pharmaceutical adhesive (Fig. 33.4).

J. The final placement is shown in Figure 33.3*B*. The dressing should be only 2 to 3 mm in thickness at the area of greatest depth and only 8 to 10 mm in total width.

K. Working time for Coe-Pak dressing is 10 to 15 minutes for the regular set and 5 to 8 minutes for the fast set.

L. Assess placement of periodontal dressings by using the Skill Performance Evaluation sheet in Appendix 2.

V. Characteristics of a Well-Placed Dressing

A. The dressing should be non-mobile and rigid. A pack that moves is irritating to the tissues and may cause prolonged bleeding.

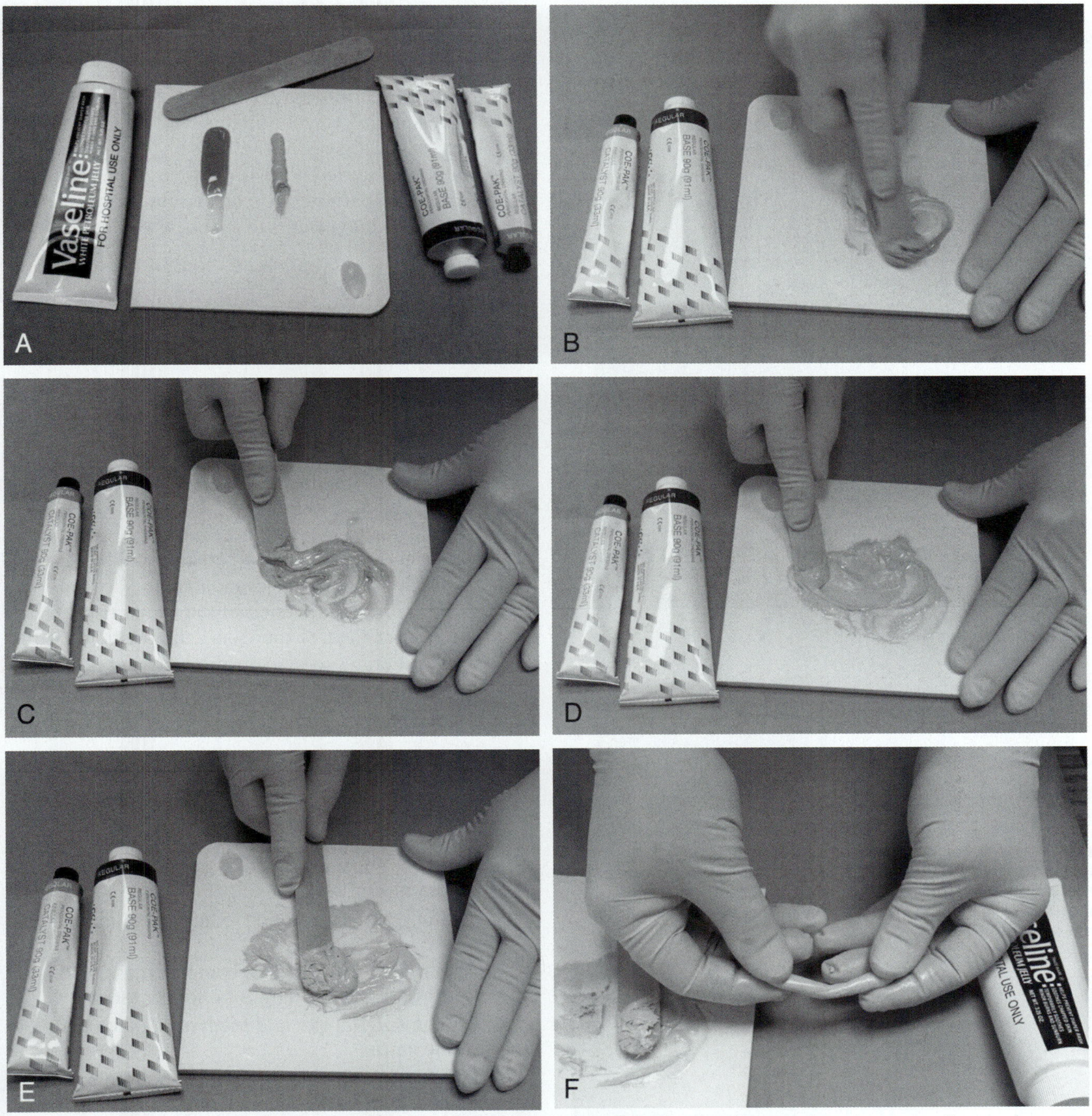

FIGURE 33.2 Mixing and placement of the periodontal dressing. **A.** Equal lengths of base and accelerator are dispensed on the mixing pad. **B–D.** The base and accelerator are mixed on the mixing pad until uniform in color. **E.** The mixture is gathered into a compact mass. **F.** When the dressing is no longer tacky, it is rolled into a "rope."

B. The pack should not extend coronally from the cervical third of the teeth. There should be no occlusal contact with the pack during mastication.

C. The wound should be covered without unnecessary overextension. The dressing should not extend more than two millimeters apical to the surgical site.

D. Dressing material should not extend into the vestibule or impinge on frenum attachments. Trim excess material that interferes with muscle movement.

E. There should be as little bulk as necessary to give rigidity.

F. The surface should be smooth and edges tapered to provide patient comfort and to discourage plaque retention.

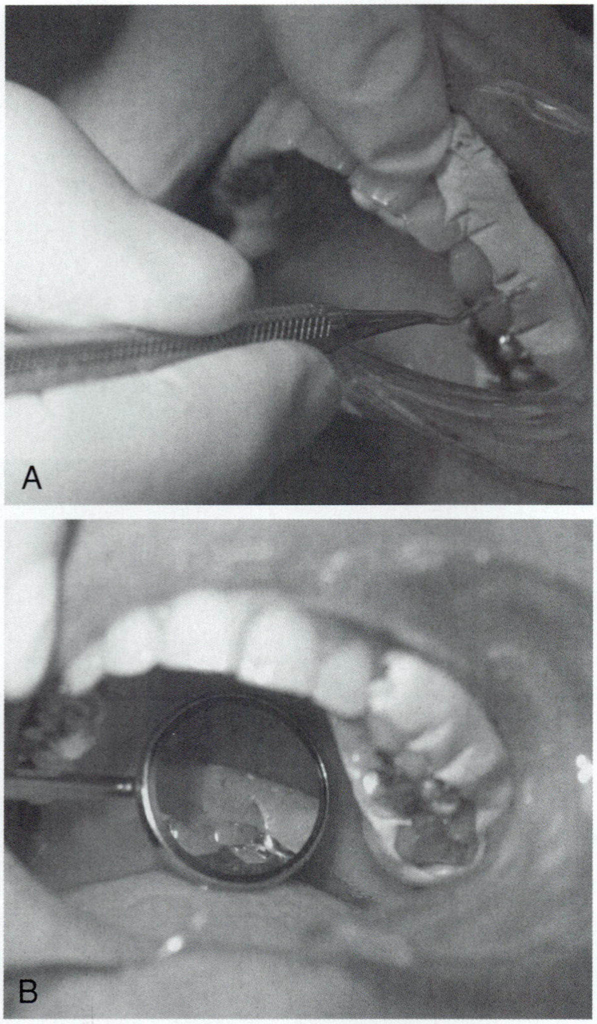

FIGURE 33.3 A. The dressing is pressed onto the surgical site and necks of the teeth. The dressing is pressed into the interproximal areas with the back of a curet or plastic instrument to create mechanical retention. **B.** Final placement. The dressing is removed from occlusal surfaces.

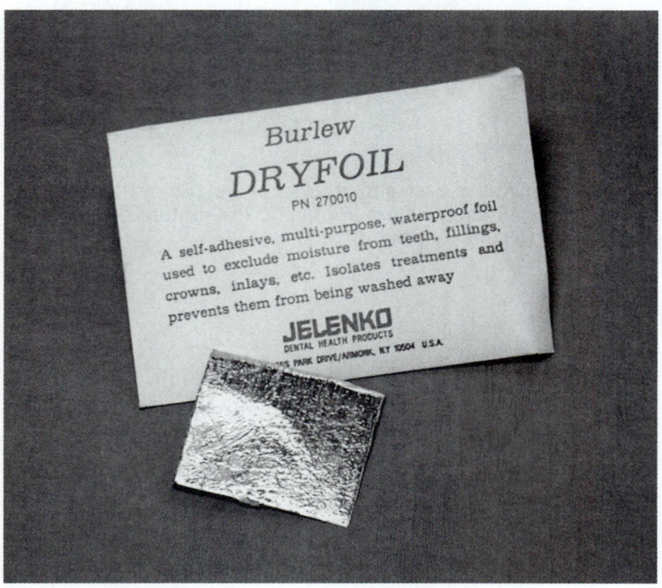

FIGURE 33.4 Adhesive foil.

Tips for the Clinician

- Keep gloves moistened to prevent the dressing from adhering to your fingers.
- Retract the tissues in the area of the dressing to check for interference with muscle attachments.
- Have the patient try retraction, protraction, and lateral movements to check for occlusal interference.

Precautions

- Avoid using cyanoacrylate dressings for patients reporting sensitivity to cyanoacrylate and formaldehyde.
- Both the clinician and the patient should wear eye protection when the cyanoacrylate dressing is used, to prevent adhesion of the ocular tissues.
- Avoid placement of the Coe-Pak in patients with known allergies to pine tar products and peanuts.

Summary

1. Dispense equal lengths of base and accelerator onto a mixing pad.
2. Mix for 30 to 45 seconds to achieve a uniform color.
3. Gather the mixture into a compact mass, and let it rest until the dressing is no longer tacky.
4. Dry the surgical site and teeth in the area with sterile gauze.
5. Roll the dressing into a "rope" about the diameter of a pencil and equal in length to the span of the surgical site.
6. Starting at the anterior facial area of the surgical site, flatten the pack against the involved soft tissues and the cervical third of the teeth. Include at least four or five teeth in the dressing.
7. Apply the dressing to the lingual surface of the surgical site, pressing the lingual and facial interproximal segments together.
8. Adapt the interproximal areas with a smooth instrument surface to create retention.
9. Trim any excess dressing away from muscle attachments and occlusal surfaces, and smooth the edges.

Review Questions

1. Which of the following would be a purpose for using the noneugenol mineral oxide surgical dressing?
   a) To decrease healing time
   b) To stop post-surgical bleeding
   c) To help hold the healing tissues in place
   d) To keep bacteria away from the healing tissues
2. The noneugenol zinc oxide dressing is held in place by:
   a) Physical retention
   b) Adhesion to the tissues
   c) Sutures
   d) Adhesive foil
3. The finished noneugenol zinc oxide dressing placed after flap surgery should be:
   a) Extended to the occlusal surface.
   b) Extended to the depth of the vestibule.
   c) Lightly pressed into the interdental space to allow for easy removal.
   d) Rigid with tapered edges.
4. A patient is in the office to have a five millimeter, deep growth excised from the attached gingiva between the maxillary left lateral and central incisors. The patient is concerned about the subsequent esthetics. He is a consultant with many companies and will be out of town with work for the next 2 months. Which of the following would be the best choice of surgical site care for this patient?
   a) Recommending warm saltwater rinses TID
   b) Placement of a noneugenol zinc oxide surgical dressing
   c) Placement of a visible light-activated surgical dressing
   d) Placement of a cyanoacrylate dressing
5. Which of the following statements regarding the noneugenol zinc oxide dressing would <u>NOT</u> be included in post-surgical instructions following periodontal flap surgery?
   a) Do not consume warm foodstuffs for 2 hours following surgery
   b) If a piece of the dressing breaks off, return to the office immediately for emergency care
   c) If a small piece of dressing crumbles off, simply discard it
   d) Do not smoke for 2 hours following the surgery.

Supplemental Readings

Lindhe J, Karring T, Lang NP, eds. Clinical Periodontology and Implant Dentistry. 3rd ed. Copenhagen: Munksgaard, 1997, Chapter 18.

Newman MG, Takei HH, Klokkevold PR, Carranza FA. Carranza's Clinical Periodontology. 10th ed. Philadelphia: WB Saunders, 2006, Chapters 64, 66.

Wilkins EM. Clinical Practice of the Dental Hygienist. 10th ed. Baltimore: Lippincott Williams & Wilkins, 2008, Chapter 40.

34

Removal of the Periodontal Dressing and Sutures

Cathryn Frere, B.S.D.H., M.S.Ed

Key Words/Phrases

chromic gut
continuous suture
interrupted sutures
surgical gut
suture abscess
sutures
swaged

Objectives

After studying this chapter, the student will be able to do the following:

1. Remove a surgical dressing without damage to the oral tissues.
2. Debride both hard and soft tissues after dressing removal.
3. Remove all placed sutures without contamination of or damage to the tissues.
4. List the items to record in the patient's chart.
5. Identify and name common suture patterns used in dentistry, and give an example of their application.
6. Describe the classification of suture materials.

INTRODUCTION

Following periodontal surgery, the patient is frequently scheduled with the dental hygienist for a "post-op" appointment. Collagen deposition and primitive epithelium have usually repaired a surgical site by the end of the first postsurgical week. This provides enough strength to the wound to allow for dressing and suture removal. Therefore, the patient returns for a follow-up evaluation 7 to 10 days after the surgery. If the dressing has not been lost, the hygienist will remove the periodontal pack followed by suture removal and documentation of healing state.

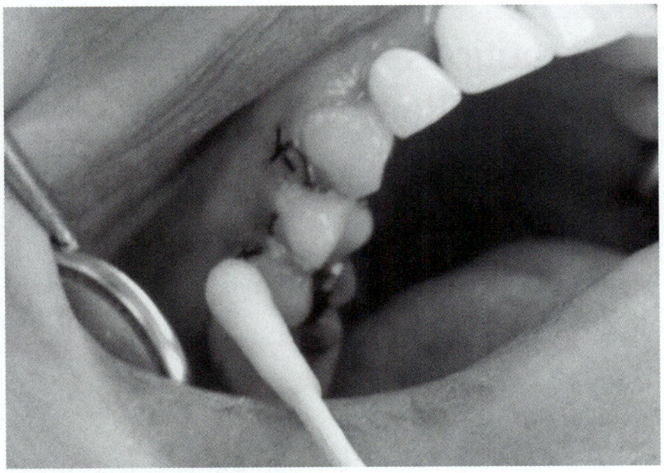

FIGURE 34.1 Teeth and tissues are swabbed with a disinfectant.

I. Removal of the Periodontal Dressing

A. A sturdy, blunt instrument, such as a surgical hoe, plastic instrument, or curet, is inserted under the edge of the dressing with a smooth surface against the tissue. Gentle lateral pressure is applied, and the pack is carefully loosened. Sutures that may have become incorporated into the dressing material must be detected and cut before each piece of pack can be removed. Remove dressing pieces with the forceps, being careful not to scratch the sensitive tissues. Suture removal is discussed later in this chapter, and the necessary items for removal of the periodontal dressing are listed in Table 34.1.

B. After the dressing has been removed, the teeth and tissues are swabbed gently with diluted disinfectant mouthwash or hydrogen peroxide on a cotton-tipped applicator to loosen food and bacterial debris, as shown in Figure 34.1. The area is then rinsed with warm water. This may need to be repeated to débride the area.

C. Inspect the surgical site for approximation of incision edges and absence of drainage, inflammation, and edema. The healing state is evaluated and noted in the patient's chart. The tissues that had been surgically manipulated should be epithelialized (covered with epithelium); however, the epithelium will be friable at this early stage of healing. These tissues may appear more red than the surrounding tissues due to the greater vascularity and lesser degree of keratinization. Red, head-like projections of granulation tissue are an indication of residual calculus. If healing is delayed and the tissues are sensitive, another periodontal dressing may be placed for a second week.

D. Residual dressing material and any visible calculus are removed, taking care not to disturb the fragile epithelium.

E. Assess periodontal pack removal by using the Skill Performance Evaluation sheet in Appendix 2.

II. Suture Removal

Sutures are stitches that are used to control bleeding and to hold body tissues in a desired position until healing has progressed to the point at which sutures are no

Table 34.1 Armamentarium for Removal of the Periodontal Dressing and Sutures

Gauze squares
Cotton-tipped applicators
1:1 dilution of chlorhexidine gluconate mouthwash or hydrogen peroxide
Forceps
Scaling instruments
Suture scissors or Dean scissors
Orange solvent (for laboratory exercises)
Skinless chicken breast with interrupted sutures (for laboratory exercises)

Tips for Periodontal Dressing Removal (Laboratory Exercise)

- If the dressing is placed on a dentoform for a laboratory exercise, prompt removal of the pack will facilitate cleaning of the dentoform.
- Large pieces of retained material can be removed with a scaling instrument.
- The last traces of pack on the dentoform can then be dissolved with orange solvent on a gauze square.

Precautions—Periodontal Dressing Removal

- Remove the surgical dressing with controlled force, checking for and cutting imbedded sutures.
- Loosened pieces of dressing are better removed with forceps to prevent scratching of the primitive epithelium.

longer needed. This healing normally takes place in 5 to 7 days for oral tissues. Removal of the sutures is usually performed at the 7- to 10-day postsurgical follow-up visit. All sutures that are not removed at this time act as a foreign body and promote inflammation to varying degrees. An infection at the sight of a suture is called a **suture abscess** or a stitch abscess.

A. Classifications of Suture Materials

Suture materials were introduced in Chapter 13. A typical suture package is shown in Figure 34.2*A*.

1. Suture materials can be monofilaments (one strand of material) or multifilaments (multiple threads twisted or braided together in a strand). Greater capillary action, or "wicking effect," is created by the multifilaments, which draw more bacteria into the tissues and create a greater inflammatory reaction than the monofilaments. Multifilament sutures are often coated and elicit less tissue response. Sutures may also be dyed to make them easier to see.
2. Suture materials can be natural or synthetic. Natural suture materials elicit a strong inflammatory response because of the presence of foreign proteins.
3. Suture materials can be divided into two broad categories: absorbable and nonabsorbable. Absorbable sutures are broken down and absorbed by the body. Those that have not been completely absorbed before the postsurgical evaluation visit must be removed. Natural suture materials are absorbed by the process of phagocytosis and enzymatic resorption. Some synthetic materials are resorbed by hydrolysis, causing less inflammatory response.
4. **Surgical gut** or "gut" is a monofilament made from the connective tissue of sheep or cattle intestinal mucosa.
5. **Chromic gut** is surgical gut that has been treated with chromic salts to inhibit enzymatic resorption. These sutures stay in place for 14 days or longer.
6. Synthetic, biodegradable sutures are commonly being used in dentistry today. These may be braided polymer fibers of polylactic acid or polyglycolic acid. Monofilaments of other polymers having more flexibility are also available.
7. Nonabsorbable sutures can also be of natural or man-made materials. These materials cannot be absorbed; they must be removed at the postsurgical visit.
   a) Silk sutures are braided fibers of protein excreted by the silkworm. Although made of a natural, biodegradable protein, the absorption of silk progresses much more slowly than the healing process. Therefore, silk sutures are classified as nonabsorbable because they must be removed.
   b) Synthetic, nonabsorbable sutures may be made of polypropylene, polyester, nylon, or Gortex.
8. In the United States, sutures are sized according to diameter and are labeled numerically. As the number of zeros increases, the diameter decreases. For example, a "000" suture is larger in diameter than a "0000" suture. The "000" suture can also be expressed as "3-0" suture and is pronounced as "three ought" or "three zero." The suture sizes used most commonly in dentistry are 3-0 to 5-0.
9. The European system of sizing simply states the metric diameter of the suture.

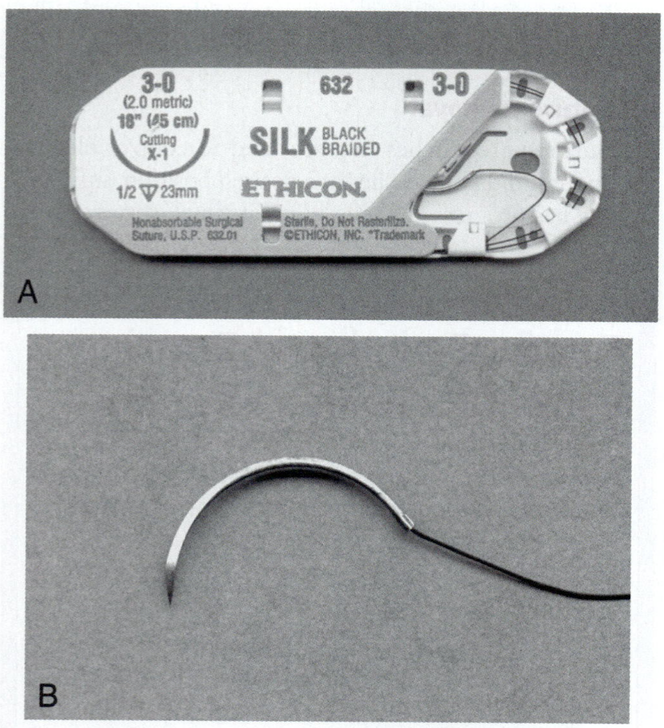

FIGURE 34.2 A. Silk suture material. **B.** Swaged suture needle.

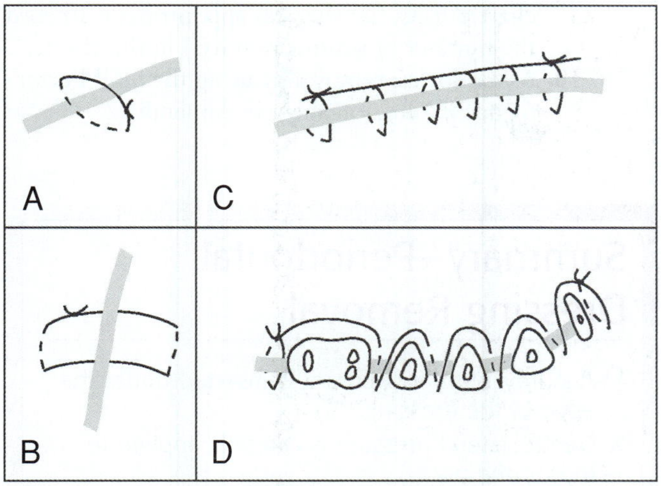

FIGURE 34.3 A. Single interrupted suture. **B.** Mattress interrupted suture. **C.** Continuous blanket suture. **D.** Simple continuous suture. The *wide gray lines* represent the incision. The *solid line* represents the suture above the tissues. The *dashed lines* represent the suture below the tissues.

10. The suture material can be supplied separate from the suture needles, or it can be manufactured attached to the needle, creating a continuous unit of suture and needle. The latter option is termed **swaged.** A swaged needle with silk suture material is shown in Figure 34.2*B*.

B. Suturing Techniques

1. Sutures that are placed in such a way that each stitch is tied and knotted separately are termed **interrupted sutures.** Examples are the single interrupted suture (Fig. 34.3*A*) and the mattress interrupted suture (Fig. 34.3*B*).
2. The uninterrupted or **continuous suture** is a series of stitches made with one thread, and it is tied at the beginning and at the end of the run. Examples of continuous sutures are the continuous blanket (Fig. 34.3*C*) and the simple continuous suture (Fig. 34.3*D*).

Tips for the Clinician—Suture Removal

- Know how many sutures are to be removed by checking the patient's chart for the number of sutures that were placed.
- A topical anesthetic can be used to provide patient comfort during suture removal.
- If scissors cannot get under the loop, a # 11 scalpel blade may be used.
- For the laboratory simulation exercise, keeping the sutures placed in the chicken breast moist will better simulate the oral cavity and facilitate removal.

Precautions—Suture Removal

- Use an intraoral or an extraoral rest when cutting sutures.
- Know the placement pattern that was used when removing sutures, taking care not to leave residual material submerged in the tissues.

C. Procedure for Removing the Single Interrupted Suture

The single interrupted suture is the most versatile suture. It can be used in most flap and graft surgeries.

1. The periodontal dressing is removed, and the surgical area is cleaned as discussed earlier in the chapter (Fig. 34.1).
2. Holding the forceps in the nondominant hand, the suture knot is grasped with the forceps, taking care not to pinch the tissues.
3. The knot is lifted away from the tissues, to create an opening to insert a scissors blade. This also exposes a portion of previously submerged suture material. Suture material that has been beneath the surface is considered to be free of bacteria.
4. With the dominant hand, insert one cutting tip of the suture scissors into the opening of the suture loop (Fig. 34.4*A*). Dean scissors are also commonly used for suture removal. Maintaining an intraoral or extraoral rest will provide stability and control of the hand holding the scissors.
5. In the section of suture material that was previously submerged, snip only one thread close to the tissue. Cutting both "ends" of the suture may result in suture material being left in the tissues and, possibly, causing a suture abscess. Take care not to cut the soft tissues. If scissors are used with blades that are curved, the blade is inserted in the loop with the tip curved away from the tissues.
6. In a continuous, smooth action, pull the suture out in one piece (Fig. 34.4*B*), and place the suture on a gauze square.
7. Do not pass the knot (ouch) or suture material, previously exposed in the oral cavity, through the tissue. The knot or suture material will contaminate subepithelial tissues with bacteria.

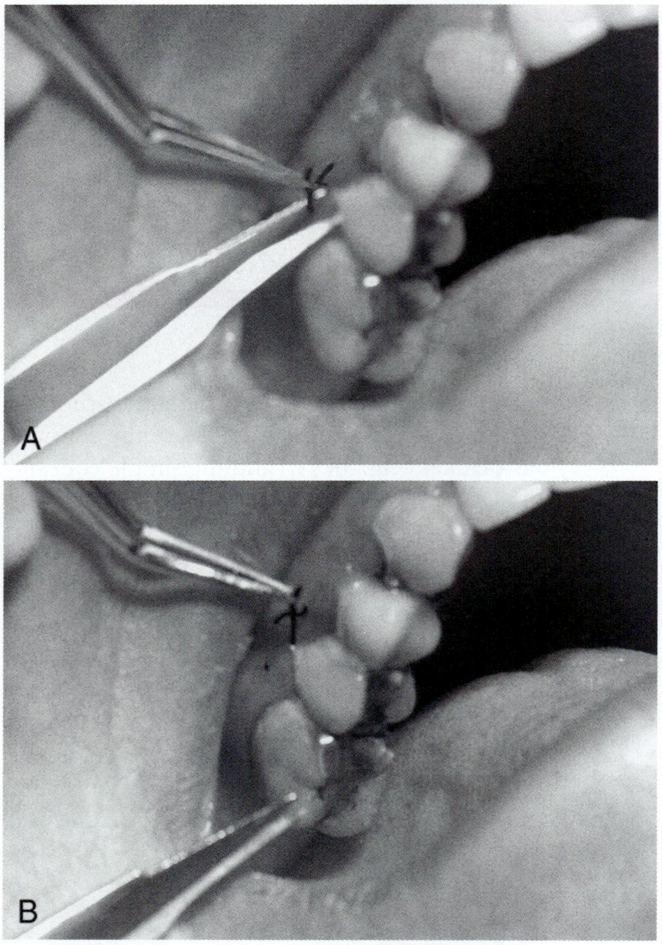

FIGURE 34.4 Suture removal. **A.** The suture knot is gently pulled away from the tissues, and the scissors tip is inserted into the suture loop. **B.** One thread is cut, and the suture is pulled out in one piece.

8. Continue removing all visible sutures and placing them on the gauze square. Bleeding of the suture sites can be controlled by gauze applied with moderate pressure.
9. When finished, count the removed sutures. This count should equal the number of sutures that were placed and recorded in the patient's chart during the surgical appointment. Record the number of sutures removed in the chart.
10. Assess suture removal by using the Skill Performance Evaluation sheet in Appendix 2.

Summary—Periodontal Dressing Removal

1. A sturdy, blunt instrument is inserted under the edge of the dressing.
2. Gentle, lateral pressure is carefully applied to loosen the pack.
3. Check for and cut sutures that have become incorporated into the dressing.
4. Remove dressing pieces with forceps.
5. Swab teeth and tissues with a disinfectant mouthwash and rinse.
6. Evaluate and record the healing state of the tissues.
7. Scale residual dressing material and residual calculus.

Summary—Suture Removal

1. The suture knot is grasped with forceps (held in the nondominant hand) and lifted.
2. Insert one blade of the scissors (held in the dominant hand) into the opening of the suture loop, and cut the suture in the section that was previously submerged.
3. Pull the suture out in a continuous, smooth action.
4. Count the number of removed sutures, and record this in the patient's chart.

Review Questions

1. Which of the following methods is the best way to loosen and remove a periodontal dressing?
a) Using a rigid curette with slow, controlled movement
b) Using a sickle scaler with slow, controlled movement
c) Using a periodontal probe with quick lateral movement
d) Using a surgical hoe with quick lateral movement

2. Seventy-eight-year-old Mrs. Wilson has come to the dental office as an emergency appointment with discomfort in a recent surgical site. Two weeks previously she was in for a post-surgical appointment at which the dressing and sutures were removed. Reviewing the chart, you notice that Mrs. Wilson is a controlled diabetic and has hypertension controlled with medication. She had reported a portion of the pack had been lost a few days after placement. Eight sutures were placed, however, only seven sutures were able to be found and were removed. Clinically, you find a localized red and edematous area distal to the maxillary second molar. Pus exudes from the area when pressure is applied. What is most likely the cause of the inflamed area?
a) She is healing poorly due to her age
b) She is healing poorly due to her diabetes
c) There is a retained suture
d) There is retained calculus in the area

3. All of the following are procedures that correctly follow removal of the periodontal dressing *except* one. Which one is the EXCEPTION?
a) The area is swabbed with a disinfectant and rinsed to remove food and bacterial debris.
b) The tissues are checked for the healing response and noted in the chart.
c) Residual pieces of dressing in and around the tissues are removed.
d) Areas of residual calculus are charted for removal at the next scale and polish appointment.

4. To remove a single interrupted suture the suture knot is grasped with forceps and gently lifted away from the tissues before being cut for all of the following reasons *except* one. Which one is the EXCEPTION?
a) To create an opening in which to insert the scissors blade
b) To keep the introduction of bacteria into the tissues to a minimum
c) To allow the clinician to cut the knot away from the rest of the suture material
d) To prevent passing the knot through the tissues

5. You are preparing a surgical tray for the dentist who has asked for "Four-ought" or smaller size non-absorbable suture material. You find the following suture materials in the supply cabinet. Which one do you choose?
a) 00000 chromic gut
b) 000 polylactic acid
c) 5-0 silk
d) 3-0 polytetrafluoroethylene

Supplemental Readings

Fedi PF, Vernino AR, Gray JL, eds. The Periodontic Syllabus. 4th ed. Philadelphia: Williams & Wilkins, 2000, Chapter 11.

Kozier B, Berman AJ, Erb G, Snyder S. Techniques in Clinical Nursing. 5th ed. Redwood City, CA: Addison-Wesley, 2003, Chapter 32.

Nevins M, Mellonig JT, eds. Periodontal Therapy: Clinical Approaches and Evidence of Success. Chicago: Quintessence, 1998, Chapter 12.

Newman MG, Takei HH, Klokkevold PR, Carranza FA. Carranza's Clinical Periodontology. 10th ed. Philadelphia: WB Saunders, 2006.

United States Pharmacopeial Convention, Inc. The United States Pharmacopeia/The National Formulary. 26th ed. Easton, PA: Mack, 2003.

35

Temporary Crowns

Key Words/Phrases

preformed shell crown
provisional
temporary crowns

Objectives

After studying this chapter, the student will be able to do the following:

1. Describe the reasons for placing a temporary crown.
2. Describe the materials used to construct temporary crowns.
3. Describe a method to make a temporary crown with acrylic resin.

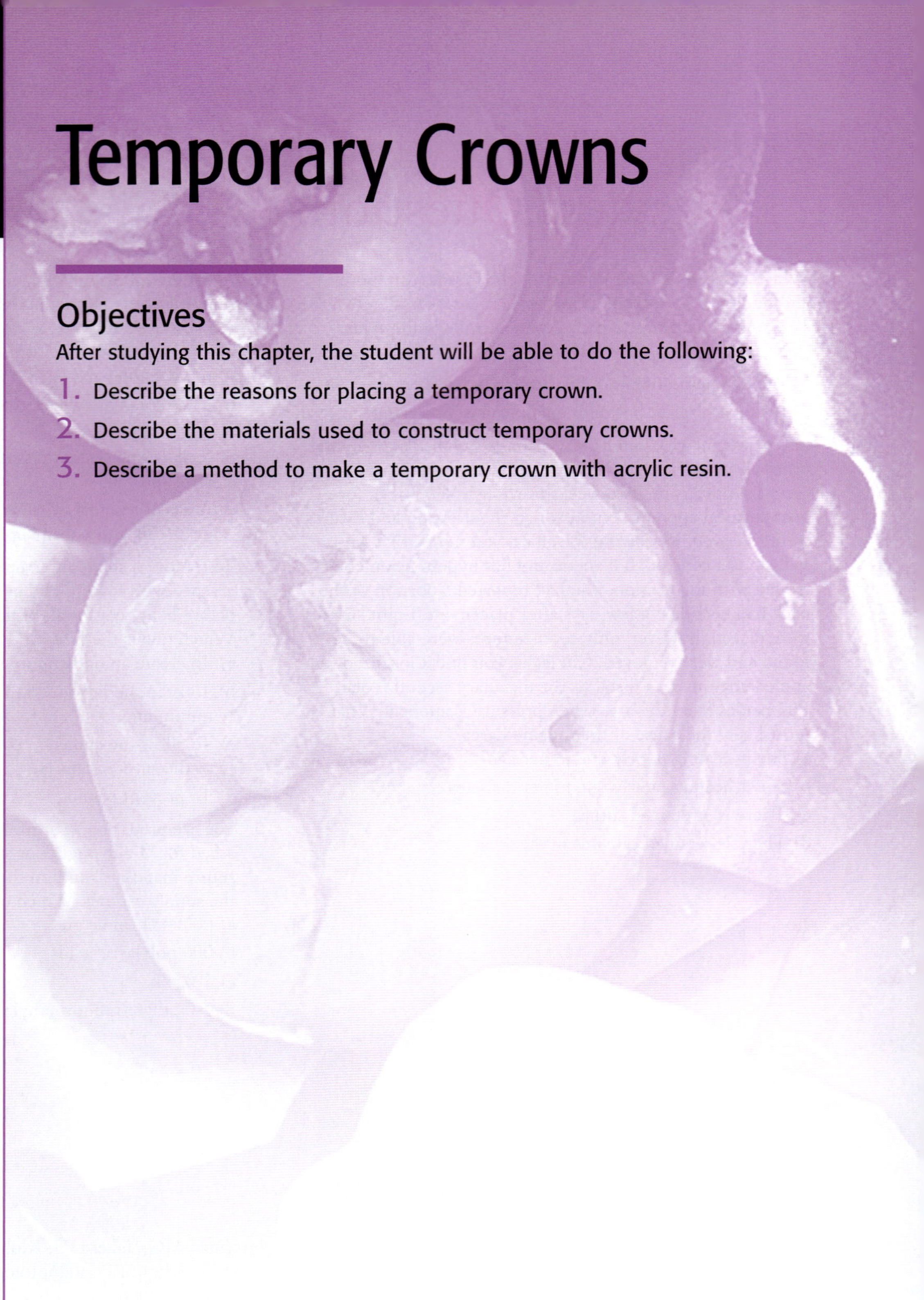

INTRODUCTION

A crown is a restoration that provides complete coverage of the coronal portion of a tooth. It may be composed of a variety of materials. Steps in the construction of a crown are shown in Figure 1.10. After diagnosis and treatment planning, the tooth is prepared. A temporary crown is made and then "worn" between the preparation appointment and the cementation appointment. **Temporary crowns** are made for patient comfort and esthetics. The temporary crown will protect the pulp from temperature extremes and other irritants. Temporary crowns are cemented on with temporary cement and are removed when the permanent crown is ready to be placed. Temporary restorations are also used while making other indirect restorations, such as an inlay or bridge. The terms "interim" or "**provisional**" are replacing the term "temporary" in some dental circles; however, they basically mean the same thing. Necessary items for constructing a temporary crown are listed in Table 35.1.

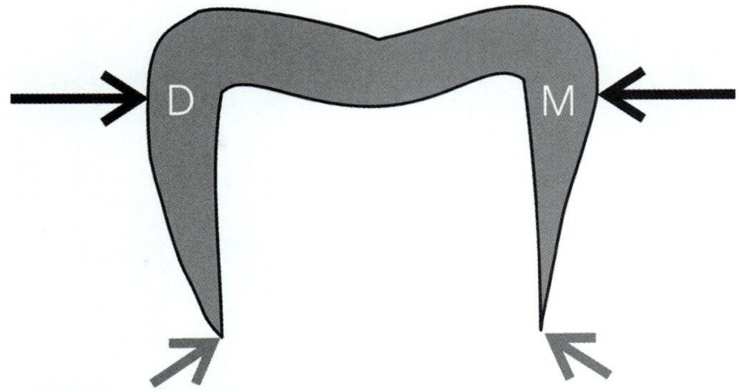

FIGURE 35.1 Cross section of a crown. *Dark arrows* point toward the mesial (*M*) and distal (*D*) contacts. *Light arrows* point toward the margins.

I. Methods

A. Three aspects must be considered when making a temporary crown (Fig. 35.1).

1. The outer surface of the crown should reproduce the anatomy of the tooth that is being restored. The shape of the crown includes occlusal contacts, proximal contacts, and side contours. The occlusal contacts must not be heavy (high), or the tooth will become sore from excessive biting forces. However, if the temporary crown has no occlusal contact, the tooth may drift occlusally or "super-erupt." Super-eruption of the tooth will require excess occlusal adjustment of the permanent crown. Proximal contacts (dark arrows in Fig. 35.1) are also important. If the proximal contacts are too tight, the excessive force may push (orthodontically move) the adjacent teeth in a mesial or distal direction. The permanent crown will not have good contact, and food will impact between the teeth, causing periodontal problems. If the interproximal contacts of the temporary crown are open, food will again impact and cause periodontal problems. Proper interproximal contacts and side contours will facilitate periodontal health.
2. The inner surface of the temporary crown must closely follow the shape of the prepared tooth for retention. As with a permanent crown, the preparation should be covered by the temporary crown to prevent postoperative sensitivity. The margins of the temporary crown (light arrows in Fig. 35.1) should be smooth and properly contoured to promote periodontal health and esthetics.
3. The temporary crown material must be thick enough and strong enough to withstand occlusal forces for several weeks.

B. The outer surface of a temporary crown can be made in several ways. It is either part of a **preformed shell crown,** as shown in Figure 35.2, or it is constructed with use of a "mold" (negative shape). The mold can be made in the mouth before the tooth is prepared, or it can be made on a cast. The inner surface of the temporary crown conforms to the preparation because the temporary crown is typically made in the mouth, directly on the prepared tooth. Chemically activated acrylic resins were the most popular material for the construction of temporary crowns, but have been replaced by resin systems called "bis-acryl" materials; see Figure 35.3*A*. Bis-acryl materials can be

Table 33.1 Armamentarium for Constructing a Temporary Crown
Dentoform with a prepared tooth (a cast may be substituted)
Cast of the dentoform with an unprepared tooth
Vacuum form material (0.020 inch in thickness)
Scissors
Wax spatula
Sharp knife or scalpel
Petroleum jelly
Acrylic powder and liquid
Lab handpiece
Pumice, miscellaneous discs, stones, and polishing devices
Articulating paper (optional)

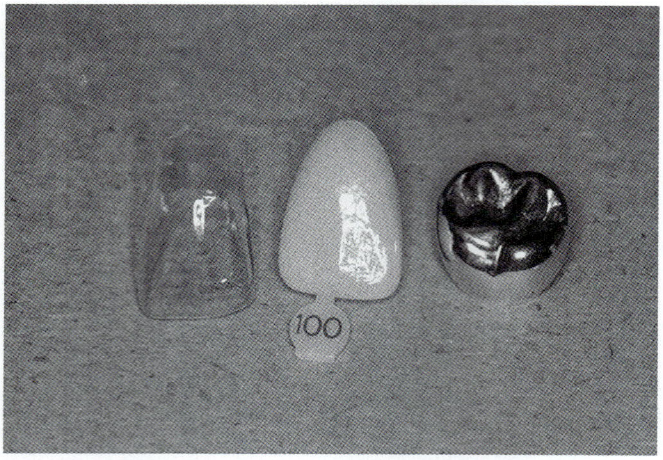

FIGURE 35.2 A celluloid crown form (*left*), a polycarbonate shell crown (*middle*), and an aluminum shell crown (*right*).

described as having a chemical structure that is intermediate between that of acrylic resin and those of dental composite materials. They often contain some filler. Both acrylic resin and bis-acryl resins are available in a variety of shades; see Figure 35.3*B*.

C. The various techniques for construction of a temporary crown use a variety of materials and products. Each patient is unique, and he or she presents specific challenges to the dentist. Each clinician also has favorite materials and techniques, several of which are presented in this chapter.

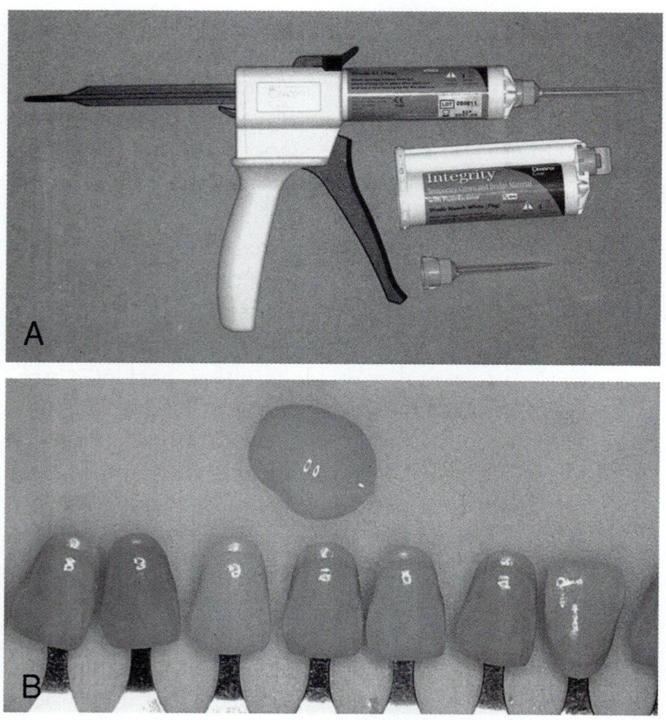

FIGURE 35.3 **A.** A bis-acryl resin automix product. **B.** Shade A3 and a shade guide.

One popular technique uses a disposable triple tray impression (Fig. 8.5*B*). The impression is taken before preparing the tooth. After preparing the tooth, the impression of the unprepared tooth of interest is filled with the temporary material in a doughy state. The impression is replaced in the patient's mouth. The patient closes into their normal bite, seating the impression (the form for the temporary) into place. The material sets. The patient opens and the impression is removed. The temporary crown is removed from the impression or tooth and trimmed. Because the form is precisely seated by the opposing arch, the occlusion of the temporary crown is nearly perfect.

Tips for The Clinician

- Mix the acrylic material, and wait for the doughy stage before seating the material on the prepared tooth. If the material is too runny, it will flow excessively.
- Remove and replace the temporary crown several times during the setting process to prevent the material from becoming locked in the interproximal undercuts.

Precautions

- Methyl methacrylate is irritating to the skin. Coat your hands with petroleum jelly.
- Methyl methacrylate is highly flammable. Do not use this material around a flame.

II. Preformed Temporary Crowns

Preformed crowns are shown in Figure 35.2. The preformed crown becomes the outer surface of the temporary crown.

A. Use

1. Some preformed crowns can be directly luted with a "stronger" temporary cement, such as reinforced zinc oxide–eugenol (ZOE). The cement forms the inner surface.
2. Alternatively, the preformed crown can be first lined with a chemically activated polymer system. First, the resin system is mixed and placed inside the preformed crown. Next, the filled crown form is seated on the prepared tooth. The

resin lining sets and forms the inner surface of the temporary crown. The lined crown is trimmed and then luted with temporary cement.

B. Materials

1. Polycarbonate Crowns

Polycarbonate crowns are supplied as maxillary and mandibular incisors, canines, and premolars. Each crown comes in a variety of widths, but only one shade is usually available. They are usually lined with acrylic resin, which will bond to the polycarbonate material. If polycarboxylate crowns are not lined with a resin, the color of the cement may show through.

2. Metal Shell Crowns

At one time, aluminum shell crowns were popular, but other soft metals, such as tin, have now replaced aluminum. Soft metal shell crowns are similar in shape to, but are much easier to adapt than, stainless-steel crowns. Stainless-steel crowns were discussed in Chapter 13. Metal shell crowns are typically used for molars and premolars because these crowns are not considered to be esthetic. Typically, they are lined with a polymer material before cementing. At times, however, they are not lined and are cemented with a thick mix of reinforced ZOE.

III. Constructed Temporary Crowns

A. The "constructed" temporary crown is made in the mouth on the prepared tooth by using a mold to form the outer surface. The mold can be made on a cast or in the mouth before the tooth is prepared. The mold should have an "ideal" shape.

B. The mold may be made from wax, elastic impression material, or a thermoplastic polymer, as shown in Figure 35.4. The material must first be soft so that it can be adapted to the "ideal" form. The material then sets or cools and becomes semisolid, forming a negative of the ideally shaped tooth, as shown in Figure 35.5*A*. When the temporary crown is made, the mold forms the outer surface.

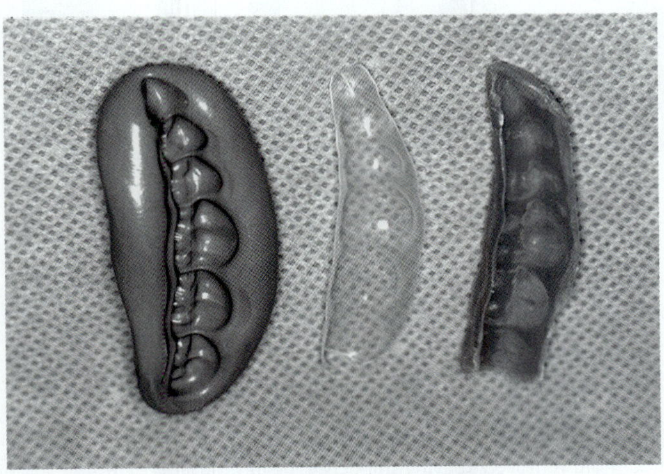

FIGURE 35.4 Molds (negative shapes) made of impression putty (*left*), a thermoplastic resin (*middle*), and wax (*right*).

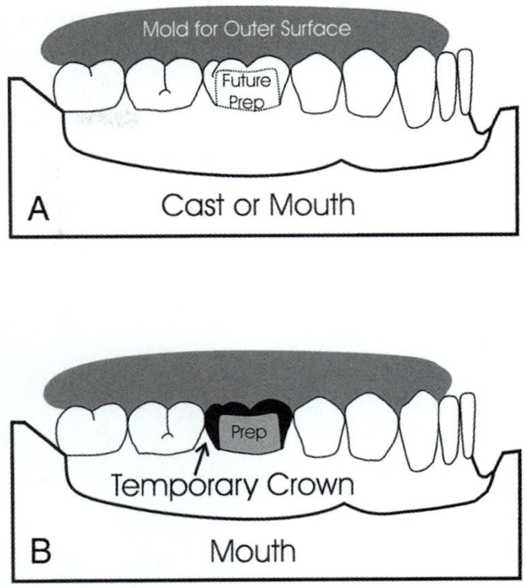

FIGURE 35.5 Side views of a mold made before the tooth is prepared (**A**) and use of the mold to construct the temporary crown (**B**).

C. Next, a resin system is mixed and placed in the mold. The mold is seated in the mouth over the prepared tooth, matching the positive surfaces of adjacent unprepared teeth with the negative surfaces of the mold, as illustrated in Figure 35.5*B*. The material then sets. The mold is removed, and the set material is removed. Excess set material is trimmed to form the temporary crown.

IV. Celluloid Crown Forms

A clear, thin, preformed celluloid crown, as shown on the left in Figure 35.2, can be used as a mold. The mold is filled with acrylic or other resin material, as done with other types of molds. Celluloid is not affected by, and does not bond to, acrylic materials. Celluloid is thermoplastic; it can be warmed and stretched to enlarge the opening. Celluloid crown forms can be made smaller by cutting a slit, overlapping the edges, and then joining the overlap with a drop of acetone. They are filled with an acrylic material, as previously discussed. The thin celluloid material is stripped off (removed) before trimming and cementing of the temporary crown.

V. Laboratory-Constructed Temporary Crowns

A dental laboratory may make a temporary crown or bridge for a complex case. Casts of the teeth to be restored are sent to the lab. The teeth on the cast are minimally prepared at the lab, and a temporary "shell" crown is made. In the mouth, after the teeth are prepared, the temporary shell crown is lined with acrylic resin. The crown is trimmed and cemented as done with other techniques.

VI. Constructing a Temporary Crown

A temporary crown can be constructed on a dentoform by using a "vacuum-formed" mold and chemically activated acrylic resin. Necessary items are listed in Table 35.1. Both an unprepared and a prepared tooth for the dentoform are used. Techniques for taking an

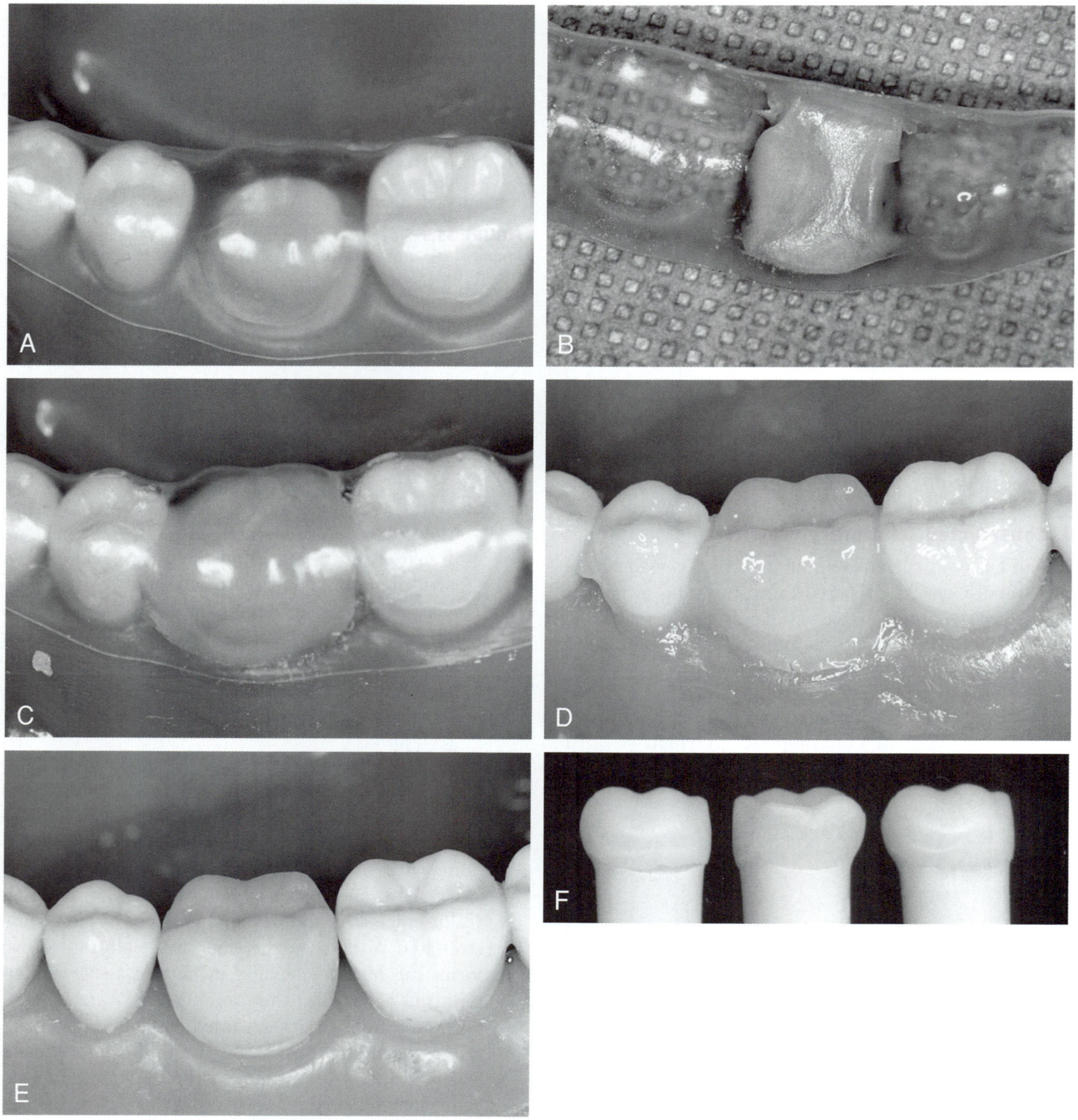

FIGURE 35.6 Steps in the construction of a temporary crown. **A.** Vacuum-formed mold on the dentoform with crown prep in place. **B.** Vacuum-formed mold filled with freshly mixed acrylic resin in the area of the prepared tooth. **C.** Mold and acrylic resin seated on the prepared tooth. **D.** Vacuum-formed mold removed, leaving the acrylic resin on the prepared tooth. **E.** The trimmed and polished temporary crown. **F.** Margins of a temporary crown (from *left* to *right*): open buccal margin, acceptable lingual margin, and the same buccal margin now repaired.

alginate impression, pouring and trimming the model, and use of the vacuum former are presented in other chapters.

A. Making the Thermoplastic Vacuum-Formed Mold

1. Make a cast of the dentoform, using the original, unprepared tooth.
2. Heat the plastic sheet, and apply it to the cast as presented in Chapter 31. While the plastic is still hot, use an instrument such as a wax spatula to force the plastic into the four interproximal areas of the tooth of interest.
3. Trim the mold to include several teeth mesial and distal to the tooth of interest. Trim to the gingival extent of the crown of interest. A vacuum-formed mold on the dentoform is shown in Figure 35.6*A*.

B. Constructing the Temporary Crown

1. Insert the "crown prep" tooth into your dentoform.
2. Lubricate the dentoform with the prepared tooth (including the teeth) with petroleum jelly.
3. Mix the powder and liquid of the acrylic resin system to a thick consistency.
4. Fill the mold in the area of the prepared tooth (Fig. 35.6*B*). Wait until the acrylic material has reached a doughy consistency.
5. Seat the material on the prepared tooth on the dentoform (Fig. 35.6*C*). The material may ooze over the gingiva, but do not try to remove it at this time.
6. Allow the material to set to a semirigid state. Remove the vacuum-formed mold and acrylic material from the dentoform (Fig. 35.6*D*).
7. Trim any gross excess with scissors. Trim any excess in the interproximal areas with a sharp-bladed instrument or the curved scissors. Reseat the temporary crown on the dentoform, and wait until the acrylic resin has become hard and rigid.

C. Trimming Excess Flash With a Handpiece, Burs, and Discs

1. Trim any excess flash, creating proper interproximal contacts (Fig. 35.6*E*).
2. Trim any excess flash at the margins. The temporary crown should end at the margin of the preparation. The contour of the crown at the margin should be in line with that of the remaining tooth structure.
3. If the temporary crown has a short margin, add more material to "repair" the temporary crown (Fig. 35.6*F*).
4. If desired, adjust the occlusion by using articulating paper and the opposing dentoform arch.
5. Polish the temporary crown with pumice or other materials. It is now ready to be cemented.
6. Assess the temporary crown by using the Skill Performance Evaluation sheet in Appendix 2.

SUMMARY

1. Assemble the necessary materials.
2. Coat the dentoform with petroleum jelly.
3. Mix the acrylic material.
4. Place the material in the previously made tooth-form mold.
5. Seat the filled mold on the dentoform.
6. Remove the mold and acrylic resin, and trim any gross excess.
7. Allow the acrylic resin to set.
8. Trim any excess.
9. Adjust the occlusion.
10. Finish and polish.

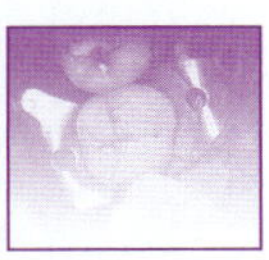

Review Questions

1. Another name for a temporary crown is a(n):
a) "One size fits all" crown
b) Provisional restoration
c) Suck-down crown
d) Resin crown

2. Important contacts of a temporary crown include:
a) Occlusal
b) Interproximal
c) Both
d) Neither

3. Temporary crowns are placed for:
a) Patient comfort
b) Esthetics
c) Function
d) All of the above
e) None of the above

Supplemental Readings

Burke FJ, Murray MC, Shortall AC. Trends in indirect dentistry: 6. Provisional restorations, more than just a temporary. Dent Update. 2005;32:443–444, 447–448, 450–452.

Christensen GJ. The fastest and best provisional restorations. J Am Dent Assoc 2003;134:637–639.

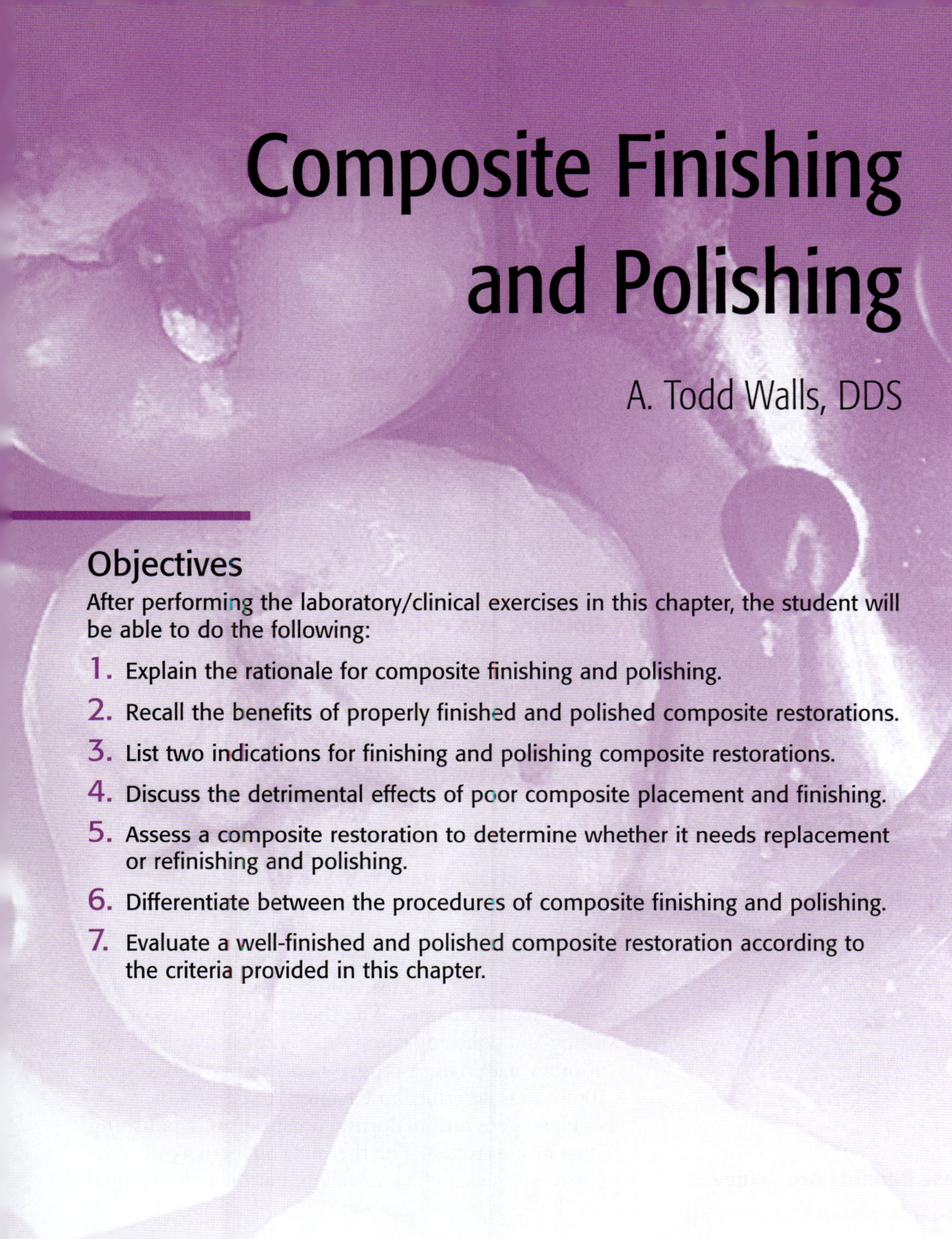

36

Composite Finishing and Polishing

A. Todd Walls, DDS

Objectives

After performing the laboratory/clinical exercises in this chapter, the student will be able to do the following:

1. Explain the rationale for composite finishing and polishing.
2. Recall the benefits of properly finished and polished composite restorations.
3. List two indications for finishing and polishing composite restorations.
4. Discuss the detrimental effects of poor composite placement and finishing.
5. Assess a composite restoration to determine whether it needs replacement or refinishing and polishing.
6. Differentiate between the procedures of composite finishing and polishing.
7. Evaluate a well-finished and polished composite restoration according to the criteria provided in this chapter.

Key Words/Phrases

finishing
flash
polishing

INTRODUCTION

The use of composite resin as a restorative material has been on the rise for the past several years and its popularity will only increase as manufacturers introduce stronger composite materials. Once relegated to primarily anterior regions of the dentition where esthetics is a chief concern, composites are now being used to restore the entire dentition in a variety of situations. With this in mind, it is imperative that the dental hygienist be aware of the proper maintenance of composite materials to ensure periodontal health and prevent dental disease.

I. Purpose of Finishing and Polishing

The primary purpose of finishing and polishing composite restorations is to create a restoration that is smooth, uniform, and easily cleaned by the patient. This, in turn, can increase the longevity of the restoration, decrease the incidence of recurrent caries, and promote the health of surrounding tissues. Occasionally patients will need to have their composite restorations polished, and less often refinished.

A. Advantages of Finishing and Polishing

The following conditions result from proper finishing and polishing:

- Smooth, undetectable margins
- Plaque-resistant surface
- Healthier gingival tissues
- Increased longevity
- Enhanced esthetics
- Proper contours

B. Methods by Which These Benefits Are Achieved

These benefits are achieved by properly smoothing the cavosurface margins, reconstructing functional anatomy, and creating a surface that is smooth and free of voids. A smooth surface is necessary to simulate the high gloss of enamel.

II. Evaluation of Composite Restorations

Unlike amalgam restorations, composites can be completely finished and polished immediately after they are placed. Improper placement, incomplete finishing and polishing, or normal wear and tear, increase the risk of recurrent caries, plaque retention, periodontal disease, and restoration failure. Composite restorations are evaluated as part of the dental exam. Some restorations may need to be finished and polished. In other instances, the restoration will need to be repaired or replaced.

A. Indications for Finishing and Polishing

1. Overextension or **flash**
2. Premature occlusal contact
3. Overhang
4. Limited stain
5. Limited re-contouring of anatomy
6. Small chips or defects

B. Indications for Repair or Replacement

1. Gross overextension or overhang
2. Open margin
3. Fracture
4. Extensive stain
5. Recurrent caries
6. Open proximal contact
7. Larger defects

III. Finishing and Polishing Considerations

Similar to amalgam finishing and polishing discussed in Chapter 26, the process of finishing and polishing composite restorations can be considered two different procedures or two steps of a single procedure. During the **finishing** procedure, contours are corrected while margins and irregularities are smoothed. The **polishing** procedure should produce a smooth lustrous finish.

A variety of products are available ranging from burs, finishing strips, finishing disks, points, cups, pastes, and brushes, as pictured in Figure 36.1. Many manufacturers even market their own polishing systems. Some of the most common products are discussed in this chapter. The theory and process of finishing and polishing composites is consistent with that of other materials; a progression from coarse to finer abrasives is described in Chapter 16.

Heat generation during finishing and polishing must be controlled. The thermal conductivity of composite is not as high as amalgam, but the risk of pulpal

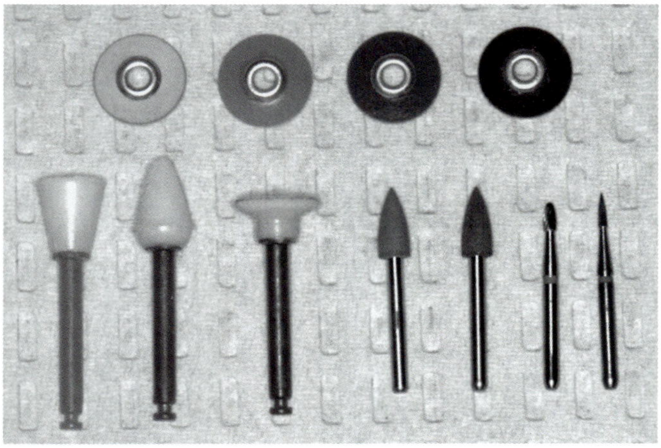

FIGURE 36.1 Abrasive disks, points, a cup and burs used to finish and polish composite restorations.

irritation or injury from increased temperatures must be considered. The use of a slow-speed handpiece, water as a coolant, and intermittent strokes is recommended to avoid heat build-up and transmission.

Finally, care must be taken not to damage adjacent teeth or soft tissues. Isolate the tooth or teeth with cotton rolls, dry angles, or a rubber dam to prevent iatrogenic injury to surrounding tissues.

IV. Procedure for Composite Finishing and Polishing

A. Evaluate Restoration

Because dental composites are tooth-colored and often difficult to see, it is useful to thoroughly dry the restored tooth with a light stream of air from the air-water syringe. With the restoration dry, visually inspect the contours to detect proper anatomical form, chips, voids, stains, or defects. Occlusal contacts can be evaluated using articulating paper. Use an explorer to gently examine all of the margins of the restoration. Proximal surfaces can also be evaluated with an explorer. Proper contacts and gingival margins can be confirmed with dental floss.

B. Discuss Procedure With Patient

Explain the rationale of composite finishing and polishing and review the steps of the procedure with the patient. Inform the patient of sensations he or she may experience during the process, especially those of finishing burs with a low-speed handpiece.

C. Gather Necessary Equipment

Select instruments based on the restoration and the clinician's preference. A list of equipment is included as Table 36.1.

D. Isolate the Area with Cotton Rolls or a Rubber Dam

TABLE 36.1 Armamentarium for Finishing and Polishing Composite Restorations

Mouth mirror
Articulating paper
Explorer
Slow-speed handpiece
Air-water syringe
Cotton rolls, dry angles, or rubber dam
Finishing burs
Finishing strips
Finishing and polishing disks, cups, and points
Dental floss

Tips for the Clinician

- Effective lighting and dried surfaces allow for improved evaluation of surface irregularities.
- The sequence of steps is crucial. Do not proceed to the next step until the previous step is completed.

Precautions

- Heat can be generated rapidly on the tooth during composite finishing and polishing.
- Aerosols are created frequently when polishing with disks.
- An exposed metal shank or center of a disk will scratch and discolor the composite surface. Use care in positioning the disk.

E. Finish, Evaluate, Polish and Reevaluate Restoration

V. Finish the Composite Restoration

A. Proximal Surfaces

Overhangs are most frequently encountered in proximal areas. Access to proximal surfaces can be challenging and often dictate which finishing and polishing procedures can be incorporated.

1. Scalpel Blade

A curved scalpel blade is the most effective instrument to remove interproximal overhangs and flash. Use of a scalpel blade is shown in Figure 36.2. It is

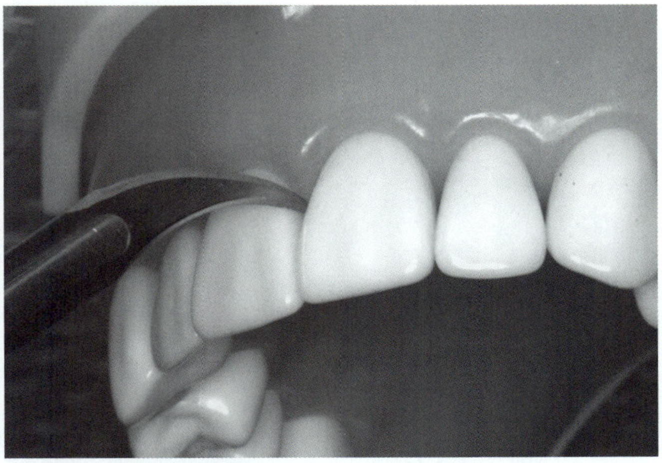

FIGURE 36.2 Removal of an interproximal overhang with a curved scalpel blade.

important the operator uses a curved blade with a single cutting edge on the inside curve. The outer edge of the blade that contacts the gingiva lacks a cutting edge; therefore, the outer edge is not likely to traumatize the soft tissues. The blade is carefully held at a slight acute angle with the cutting edge in contact with the tooth surface. The blade is guided by tooth contours and shaves rather than carves the excess composite material. If the hygienist is not comfortable or this in not in the scope of the state's practice act, the hygienist should use an alternative technique or ask for assistance from the dentist. Use of a scalpel blade to remove a composite overhang is quite similar to debridement of a root surface with a curette.

2. **Flame-shaped Finishing Burs**

Flame-shaped finishing burs can be used to smooth contours and margins, and remove overhangs, as shown in Figure 36.3. As with disks, move from tooth structure to restoration using smooth, deliberate, intermittent brush strokes. Stay in constant motion while engaging the surface to prevent gouging the restoration or tooth surfaces.

3. **Finishing Disks**

Finishing disks are useful when the restoration extends onto the facial or lingual surface, thereby allowing access to the area. Some manufacturers produce a series of abrasive disks that are color-coded and gradually progress from coarse to fine. An example of a common disk system is Sof-Lex Discs (3M-ESPE, St. Paul, MN), shown in Figure 16.6. Use a smooth, deliberate, intermittent brush stroke. Starting from tooth structure, move over the surface of the restoration to smooth the surface and remove flash (see Fig. 36.4).

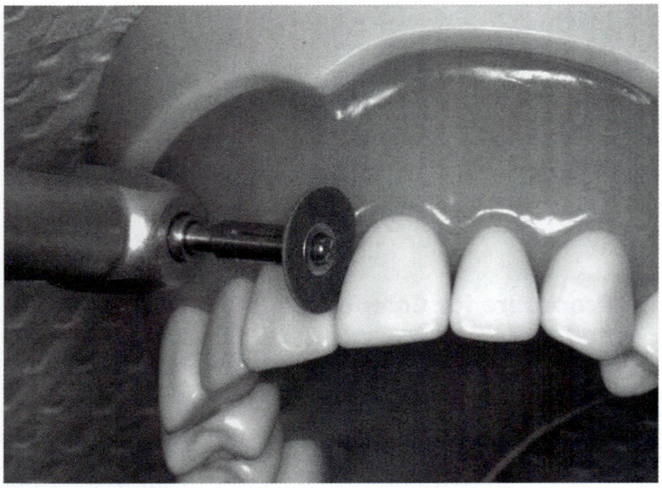

FIGURE 36.4 An abrasive disk used to finish the proximal area.

4. **Finishing Strips**

The center of the finishing strip contains no abrasives. Carefully pull or "floss" this portion of the strip through the proximal contact. Position the strip both on tooth structure and the restoration, and gently pull the strip over the surface or margin of the restoration, as pictured in Figure 36.5. Repeat this procedure as needed. Always confirm the finishing strip is situated gingival to the proximal contact to avoid opening the contact.

B. Occlusal Surfaces

Occlusal finishing includes smoothing of margins, refining anatomy, and removing flash.

1. **Egg or Football-shaped Finishing Burs**

Egg or football-shaped finishing burs can be used to complete practically all occlusal finishing. Use of a bur is shown in Figure 36.6. Existing tooth

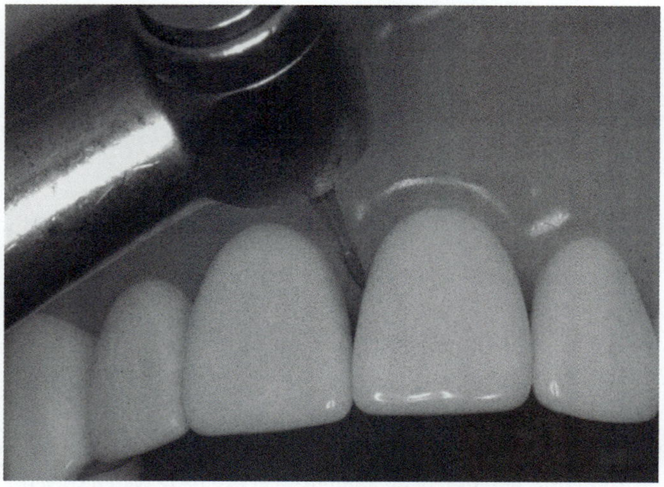

FIGURE 36.3 A flame shaped finishing bur used in the proximal area.

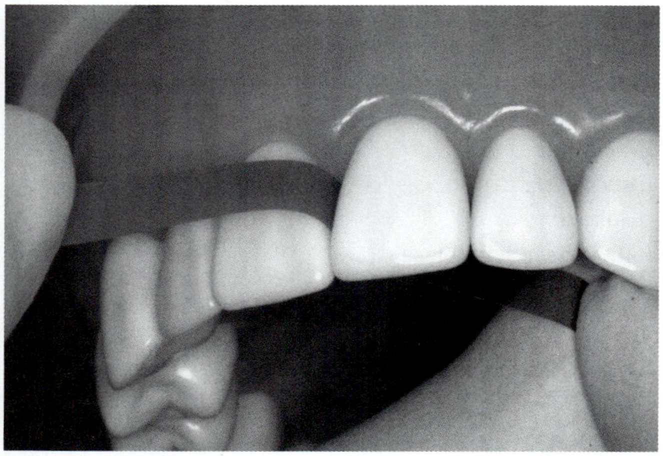

FIGURE 36.5 A finishing strip used to refine the proximal area.

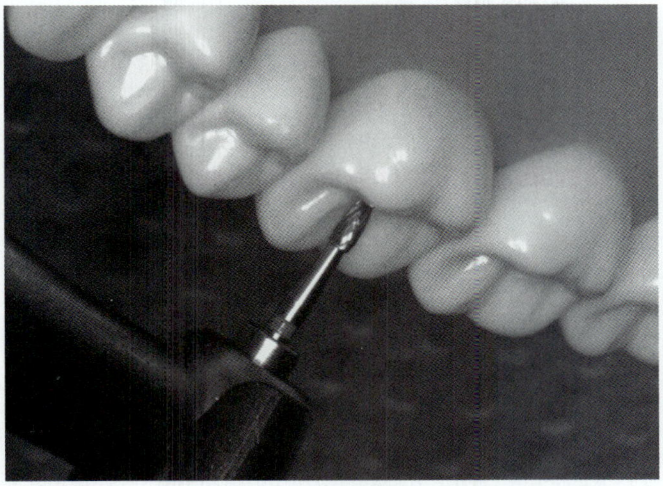

FIGURE 36.6 A finishing bur used to refine the occlusal surface.

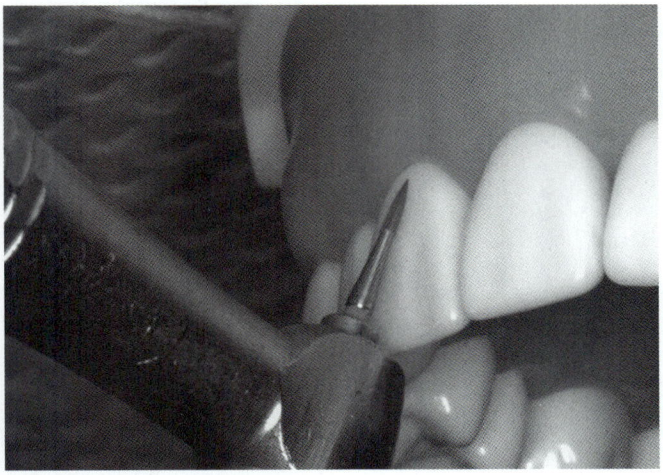

FIGURE 36.8 A finishing bur used to refine the contours of the facial surface.

structure is used to guide the bur over triangular ridges or the tip into grooves and fossae. Maintain smooth, intermittent brush strokes over the restored surface.

2. Finishing Points and Cups

Finishing points or cups are used to smooth the surface and grooves, such as those shown in Figure 36.7. Maintain smooth, intermittent brush-strokes over the restored surface.

C. Facial and Lingual Surfaces

Finishing of facial and lingual surfaces smooths margins, refines axial contours, removes flash, and eliminates surface stains.

1. Flame-shaped Finishing Burs

Flame-shaped finishing burs can be used to contour surfaces, smooth margins, and remove flash (see Fig. 36.8). As with other abrasives, move from tooth structure to restoration using smooth, deliberate, intermittent brush strokes. Stay in constant motion while engaging the surface to prevent gouging the restoration or tooth surfaces.

2. Egg or Football-shaped Finishing Burs

Egg or football-shaped finishing burs are often used on the lingual surfaces of anterior teeth. Their shape matches the lingual concavity of anterior teeth. Use existing tooth structure to guide the bur. Maintain smooth, intermittent brush strokes over the restored surface.

3. Finishing Disks, Points, and Cups

Finishing disks and cups (Figs. 36.9 and 36.10) are useful on the facial surfaces of anterior teeth while finishing points and cups are used on lingual surfaces of anterior teeth. A combination of disks, points, and cups is appropriate for posterior teeth. Use a smooth, deliberate, intermittent brush stroke. Starting from tooth structure, move over the surface of the restoration. Great care must be observed on the facial surfaces of anterior teeth, as esthetics are very important there.

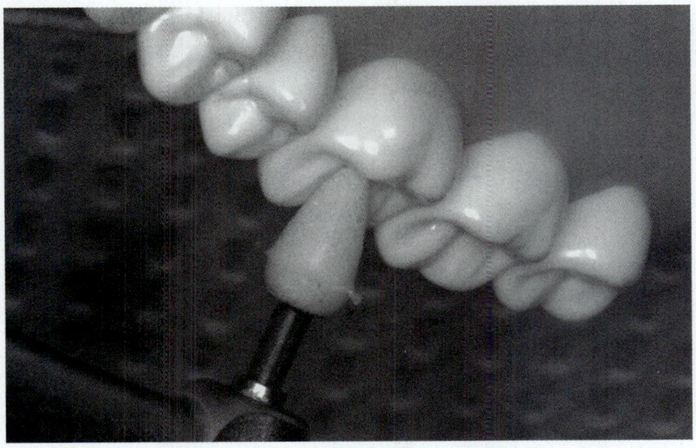

FIGURE 36.7 An abrasive point used to polish the occlusal surface.

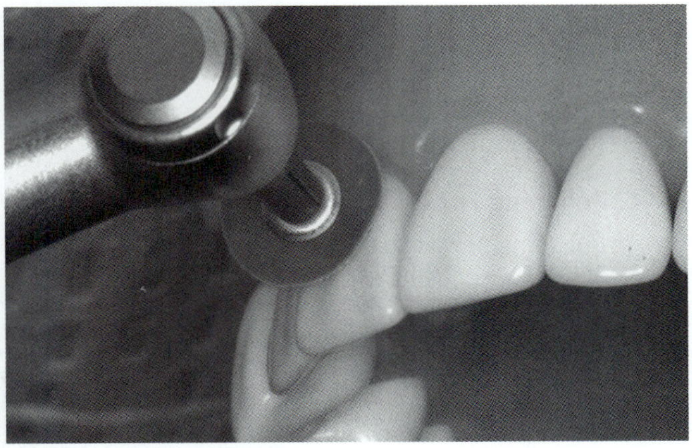

FIGURE 36.9 An abrasive disk used to finish the facial surface.

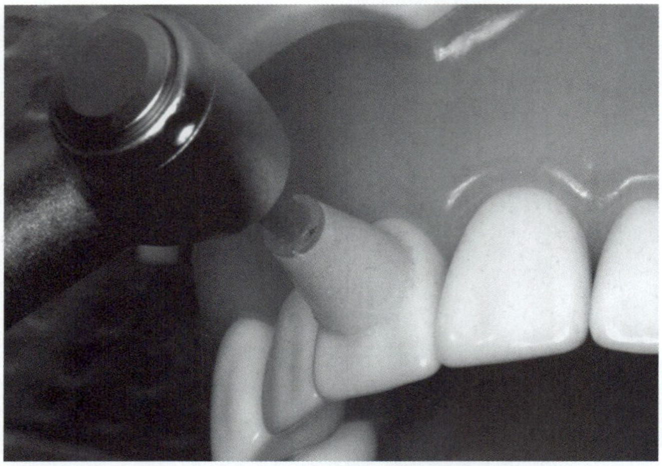

FIGURE 36.10 An abrasive cup used to polish the facial surface.

D. Evaluate the Finishing Procedure

Assess the finishing procedure by using the criteria listed in the Skill Performance Evaluation Sheet in Appendix 2. **Do not proceed to the polishing procedure until these criteria have been met. Polishing will not accomplish a smooth surface unless each step during the finishing process has been successfully accomplished.**

VI. Polish the Composite Restoration

The process of polishing composite restorations is very similar to the finishing process. The major differences include: fine abrasives are used, less material is removed and a lustrous surface results. Some abrasive devices are used to both finish and polish composites.

A. Polishing the Proximal Surfaces

Fine abrasive disks and strips or rubber polishing disks, points and cups are used in the polishing procedure. Use a smooth, deliberate, intermittent brush stroke. Starting from tooth structure, move over the surface of the restoration to produce a surface with a smooth, high luster.

B. Polishing Occlusal Surfaces

Polishing points or cups are used for the final polishing procedure. Again, keep moving across the surface using smooth and deliberate strokes.

C. Polishing Facial and Lingual Surfaces

Polishing points, disks, or cups are used for the final polishing procedure. Keep moving across the surface using smooth and deliberate strokes.

D. Composite Polishing Pastes

For some clinicians, the final polishing step uses a rubber cup with a polishing paste shown in as Figure 16.17.

E. Evaluate the Polishing Procedure

Assess the polished composite restoration using a mouth mirror, explorer, and the Skill Performance Evaluation Sheet in Appendix 2. The composite restoration should appear smooth and highly polished, and should have a lustrous shine. There should be no damage to the adjacent tooth structure.

VII. Conclusion

At each patient recall appointment, composite restorations should be evaluated for recurrent caries, voids and any need for refinishing and polishing. If indicated, this procedure may be performed during the recall visit, or scheduled as a separate appointment. When composite restorations are properly maintained, there will be less plaque retention, and subsequently, a lower incidence of periodontal disease and caries. In addition, finishing and polishing will increase the esthetics of the restoration and therefore patient satisfaction.

Summary of Composite Finishing and Polishing

Finishing

1. Evaluate restoration (margins, occlusion, proximal areas)
2. Discuss procedure with patient.
3. Isolate the area with cotton rolls or rubber dam.
4. Smooth proximal surfaces if necessary (with burs, disks, strips)
5. Remove occlusal excess and eliminate flash with burs
6. Define occlusal anatomy with burs
7. Smooth cavosurface margins and occlusal surface
8. Smooth facial and lingual surfaces

Polishing

1. Use fine abrasive disks, strips, cups, and points to polish occlusal, proximal, facial, and lingual surfaces.
2. Rinse, dry, and evacuate composite restoration.

Review Questions

1. The most effective method to prevent overheating of the pulp when polishing a composite is to:
a) Use light strokes
b) Maintain a moist tooth and composite
c) Lubricate with petroleum jelly
d) Use fine grit abrasives first

2. Ideally, composite restorations should be finished and polished:
a) After 1 week
b) After 24 hours
c) After 2 hours
d) At the placement appointment

3. During composite finishing and polishing, coarser abrasive disks should be followed by finer abrasive disks. This allows for initially more rapid removal of larger scratches in the composite surface followed by less aggressive removal of material containing the smaller scratches.
a) The first statement is true; the second statement is false.
b) The first statement is false; the second statement is true.
c) Both statements are true.
d) Both statement are false.

4. Finishing and polishing composite restorations improves all of the following *except* one. Which one is the EXCEPTION?
a) Surface luster
b) Gingival health
c) Marginal flash
d) Excessive corrosion

5. When finishing the lingual of a composite restoration in an anterior tooth, the most effect abrasive would be a?
a) Finishing disk
b) Finishing cup
c) Flame-shaped finishing bur
d) Egg/football-shaped finishing bur

Learning Activities

1. In the dental materials laboratory, observe existing composites in extracted teeth. Evaluate margins and contours.

2. During patient assessment, evaluate composite restorations with an explorer, mouth mirror, and floss.

3. In the dental materials laboratory, using a typodont tooth with an existing cavity prep, place a composite restoration. Finish and polish the restoration.

4. Make a 5×10 mm sample of composite material. Polish as described in the Learning Activities in Chapter 16, using medium, fine, and superfine Soflex Discs.

Supplemental Readings

Jefferies SR. The art and science of abrasive finishing and polishing in restorative dentistry. Dent Clin North Am 1998;42:613–627.

Wilkins EM. Clinical Practice of the Dental Hygienist. 10th ed. Baltimore: Williams & Wilkins, 2008, Chapter 42.

Yap AU, Wu SS, Chelvan S, Tan ES. Effect of hygiene maintenance procedures on surface roughness of composite restoratives. Oper Dent 2005;30:99–104.

37

Tips for the New Hygienist

John H. Tucker, D.M.D.

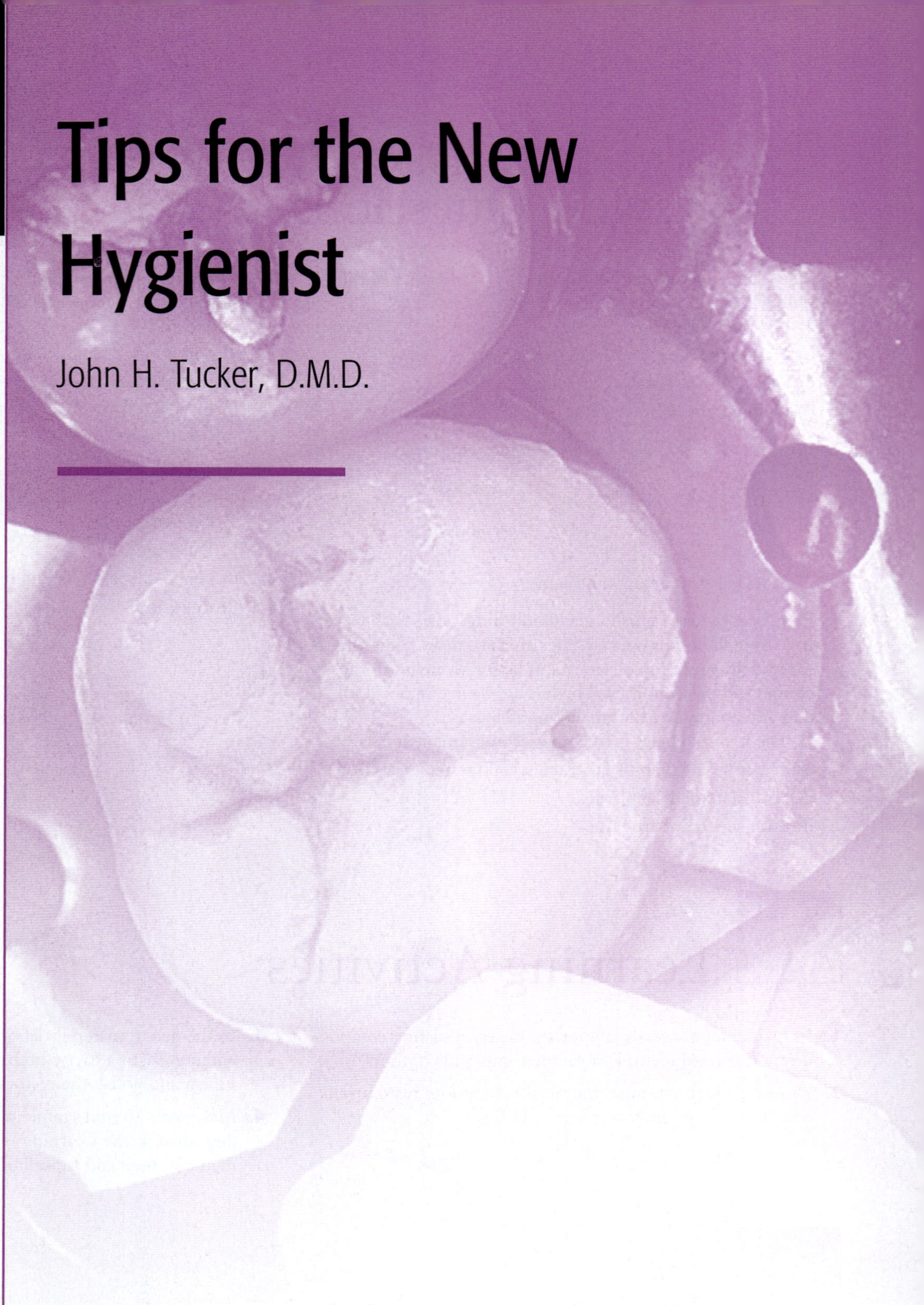

INTRODUCTION

A note from the authors: At this time, not many textbooks give tips to the graduate when entering dental hygiene practice. A contributing author who has practiced several years and has employed many dental hygienists has valuable information to share. And we, as authors of this text, wholeheartedly agree and have included his thoughts. Chances are, you have been presented the same messages in your practice management coursework.

I. The Philosophy of the Practice

The hygienist will need to know the philosophy of the dental practice in which he or she works. Many dental offices are owned and run by one practitioner. This philosophy would include the technology, techniques, and protocols currently favored and any changes planned to be incorporated in the future. What does the dentist believe and why does he believe it? What are his strengths and weaknesses? What procedures does he prefer to refer to specialists? What are his beliefs and attitudes about procedures such as orthodontics by a general dentist, implants, take-home and in-office whitening, laser treatment, all ceramic crowns, gold crowns, just to name a few?

If you know his dental practice philosophy (and hopefully agree) the hygienist can be a valuable asset in promoting the recommended treatment for the patient. If two people know what the other believes and are in agreement with these beliefs, isn't it easier to convey them to a third person? This is a very elementary principle, but in many cases the dentist does not make the philosophy of the practice clear to the hygienist, nor does the hygienist make a point of asking.

II. The Patient's Awareness of His Oral Condition

It is well accepted that patient education is one of the primary responsibilities of the dental hygienist. In most cases, this education is centered on the theme of oral hygiene home care procedures or disease prevention. When is the patient educated on his present oral condition? When is he given an update of his mouth? Does he know what kind of restorations he has and what material was used? Does he know the present condition of them? Are they worn, fractured, or ragged?

The use of the intra-oral camera is ideal to show the patient the areas of missing teeth, broken down restorations, cracked teeth, caries, and periodontal concerns. Take the time to educate the patient on the condition of his teeth, which must serve him for the rest of his life. I think you would be surprised at how many patients think that their teeth are fine and they are only worried about new cavities, when, in reality, the entire dentition may be in the process of breaking down. Deterioration can lead to arch collapse and possibly other more serious issues. There are a variety of multi-media patient education programs to have in the office to inform patients about the various treatments available. This now leads to the next bit of advice.

III. The Promotion of Dental Services

You must understand that patients often will trust the opinion of the assistant or the hygienist before that of the dentist. This comes from what the social psychologists call the Approach/Inhibition Theory of Power that suggests the patient may be more wary of the person "in power" (in this case the dentist) than the hygienist. The patient would act differently (their behavior would be more trusting) with the dental assistant or hygienist as compared to the dentist. Because you are a professional, but with less "power" than the dentist, they will place a great deal of trust in you. They know that you do not have a vested financial interest in the decision and they will readily ask, "What would you do if it were you?" This now sets the stage for the opportunity to promote dentistry in the sense of encouraging the best treatment plan for that particular patient. One of our ethical principles we abide by as professionals is beneficence, which is to promote good. We need to promote good restorative care as well as good oral hygiene care. At the same time, it must be made clear that we are *not* "selling" dental treatment, especially treatment that is not truly needed. Unfortunately there are a few dental practitioners out there that seem to engage in the unethical practice of convincing the patient to spend money on dental treatment that is unwarranted, solely for the dentist's financial gain.

The promotion of quality dentistry is actually more complicated. There are dental needs that should be addressed immediately, such as infections. Others are less urgent. The hygienist that understands the philosophy of the practice can counsel the patient when financial and other limitations place the entire treatment plan beyond the patient's resources. Often, the crown that a mom needs takes a back seat to the son's or daughter's braces. The hygienist can address the benefits of accepting the treatment plan (the crown for the mom) and the risks involved when treatment is delayed.

Our promotion of what is needed now opens the door to another debated issue, and that is the dental diagnosis by the hygienist. By no means do we advocate the hygienist be the professional in the office that informs the patient of a prescribed treatment plan on what they *think* the patient should have done. The majority of the state dental practice laws forbid dental diagnosis by the hygienist because it is obviously out of the scope of practice of the hygienist's education. However, the hygienist could reinforce and promote the prescribed treatment. An acceptable scenario could be: the dentist informs the patient of his diagnosis and treatment plan, and if the dentist leaves the room, the patient may turn to the hygienist for her opinion. This, then, is the golden opportunity in which the hygienist, because she agrees with the dentist's practice philosophy, can validate and encourage the patient to partake in the prescribed treatment.

IV. The Patient's Best Interest

As mentioned previously, the entire office personnel want the best treatment and care for the patient. The hygienist has now become the patient's advocate. This also extends to insurance companies. Most insurance companies have limits on the amount of money that will be paid for a procedure. It may not be enough to pay for that particular restoration. Dental hygienists should be able to explain what insurance will cover versus what it does not cover, and encourage the patient to make a personal financial investment in his restorative care. This investment may last a lifetime, or at least very many years.

V. Office Technology

The practice will be best served if all employees are familiar with all of the office technology. Know the computer system and software. This would include the software that not only you and the dentist may use, but the receptionist's too. It will make for a smooth, competent operation. Understand the use of all new, technologically advanced instruments and equipment that are utilized in the office. This knowledge and comfort with technology by all the employees will reflect in a very positive way in the eyes of the patients.

VI. A Member of the Dental Team

This has probably been presented to you before, in a variety of aspects. The entire practice should be revolving around the patient. "The patient is our first priority" may be a familiar motto that your program advocates. It takes ALL employees of the practice to fulfill this belief. Everyone in the office has their job responsibilities that contribute to making the patients the first priority. Once the patient's needs are met, the hygienist should be willing to help others when there is a cancellation in the schedule. He or she should not sit idle. Do not hesitate to ask others, such as the dental assistant or office manager, what you can do to contribute to office efficiency, organization, and cleanliness. Being a dental hygiene professional extends far beyond cleaning teeth. It is important to promote goodwill not only to patients but to other team members. A hygienist's poor attitude and laziness reflect negatively on the employer and other staff members. Certainly, patients will become aware of disharmony in the office. Doesn't the work day go by faster when you have been busy compared to one where there is idle time? And think of all the good you have done!

VII. Conclusion

Hopefully this short chapter has provided some insight for your future practice. Often it has been said that "experience is the best teacher," but having a few tips ahead of time can make your employment experiences more pleasurable.

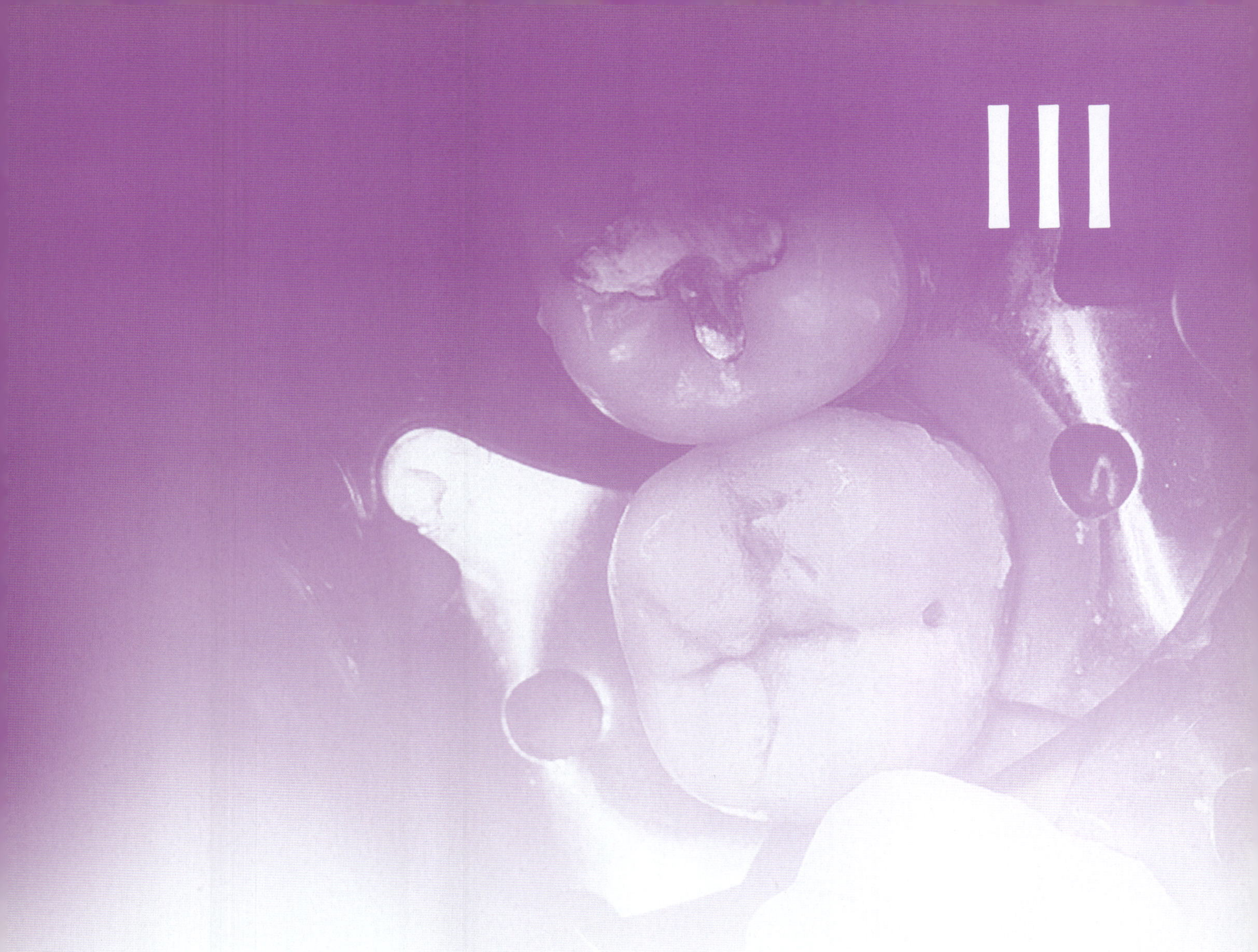

III

Case Studies

INTRODUCTION

The cases presented in this section are designed to stimulate discussion of the various dental materials that are used to restore or replace teeth. The questions involve not only dental materials but clinical dental hygiene as well. Maintenance of restorations, prostheses, and oral tissues should also be considered.

Case 1

The patient is a 63-year-old woman with a maxillary denture and the appliance presented in Figure CS1.1. She lives on a very limited income but visits the dental office yearly for a thorough dental examination, scaling, and polishing. At this visit, she presents with little plaque and stain but with a small amount of calculus on the supragingival, lingual surface of the remaining natural teeth.

QUESTIONS

1. The remaining natural teeth include:
   a) Teeth #18, #22, #27, and #28
   b) Teeth #19, #21, #25, and #26
   c) Teeth #19, #22, #27, and #28
   d) Teeth #18, #21, #26, and #27
2. The replacement prosthesis is correctly termed:
   a) A removable bridge
   b) A removable partial denture
   c) A partial
   d) A fixed partial denture
3. The clasps of the prosthesis encircle which of the following teeth?
   a) Teeth #19, #22, and #27
   b) Teeth #18, #21, and #26
   c) Teeth #18, #22, and #28
   d) Teeth #19, #22, and #28
4. The composition of the prosthesis may include as many as _____ dental materials.
   a) 2
   b) 3
   c) 4
   d) 5
5. The polishing agent of choice for the patient's natural teeth should be:
   a) A pumice slurry
   b) A coarse prophylaxis paste
   c) A fine prophylaxis paste for all teeth
   d) Selectively polish teeth with stain
6. After scaling and polishing the natural teeth, cleaning her dental prosthesis, and providing thorough patient education about calculus formation and removal, an appropriate recall recommendation for her particular situation would be:
   a) To continue the yearly recall date
   b) To change to a 6-month recall because of the calculus formation
   c) To keep the yearly recall but note in her record to closely assess the calculus formation and, if necessary, change the recall date accordingly
   d) To encourage the patient to accept a 4-month recall so that calculus formation can be closely monitored

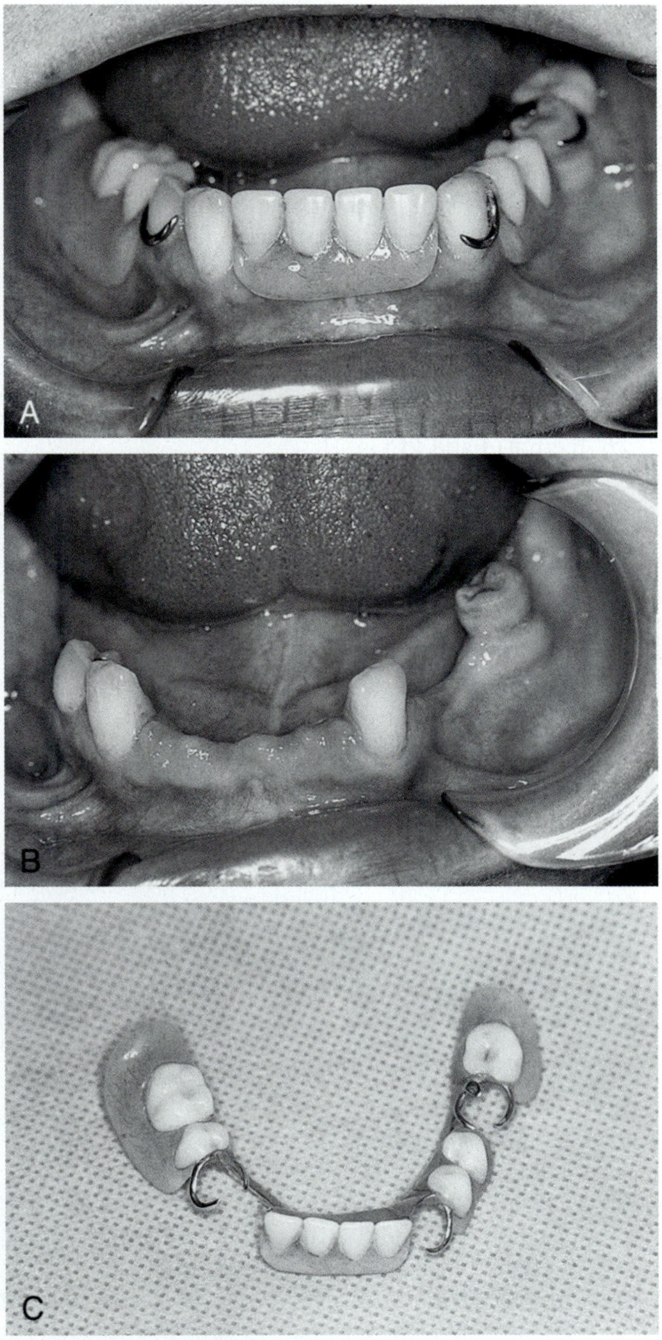

FIGURE CS1.1 **A.** Patient wearing dental appliance. **B.** Patient without appliance. **C.** Appliance.

Case 2

The photographs (Fig. CS2.1) show a 25-year-old man having three restorations placed during his appointment. His gums bleed easily, and the probing depths for this quadrant are noted on the charting in Figure CS2.2. His oral hygiene home care consists of brushing two or three times a week and swishing with Scope mouthwash on the days he does not brush. Flossing is not a part of his oral hygiene regimen.

QUESTIONS

1. The teeth being restored in the photographs below are:
   a) Teeth #2 and #3
   b) Teeth #14 and #15
   c) Teeth #13 and #14
   d) Teeth #1 and #2

2. In Figure CS2.1*A*, the "white" material on the floor of the preparation of the second tooth from the left is considered to be a ____________, and its purpose is ________________.
   a) Liner; to provide strength and thermal insulation
   b) Base; to provide strength and thermal insulation
   c) Liner; to protect the pulp from chemical irritation
   d) Base; to protect the pulp from chemical irritation

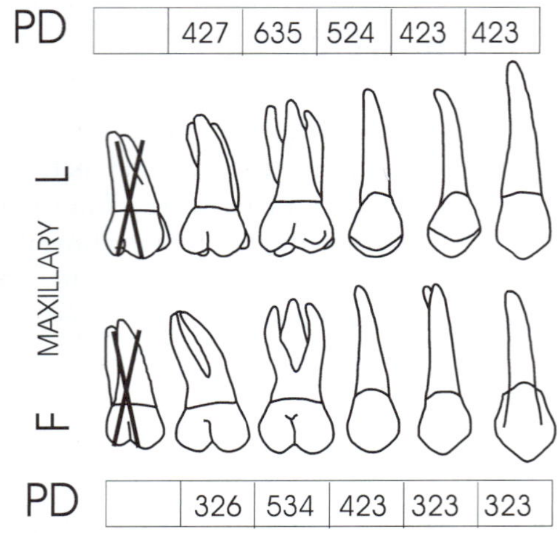

FIGURE CS2.2 Periodontal measurements of the teeth shown above.

3. From the most distal surface of the last tooth and moving mesially, the amalgam restorations would be named:
   a) Distocclusal (DO), mesiocclusal (MO), and disocclusolingual (DOL)
   b) Occlusal (O), MO, and DO
   c) O, MO, and DOL
   d) MO, DO, and DOL

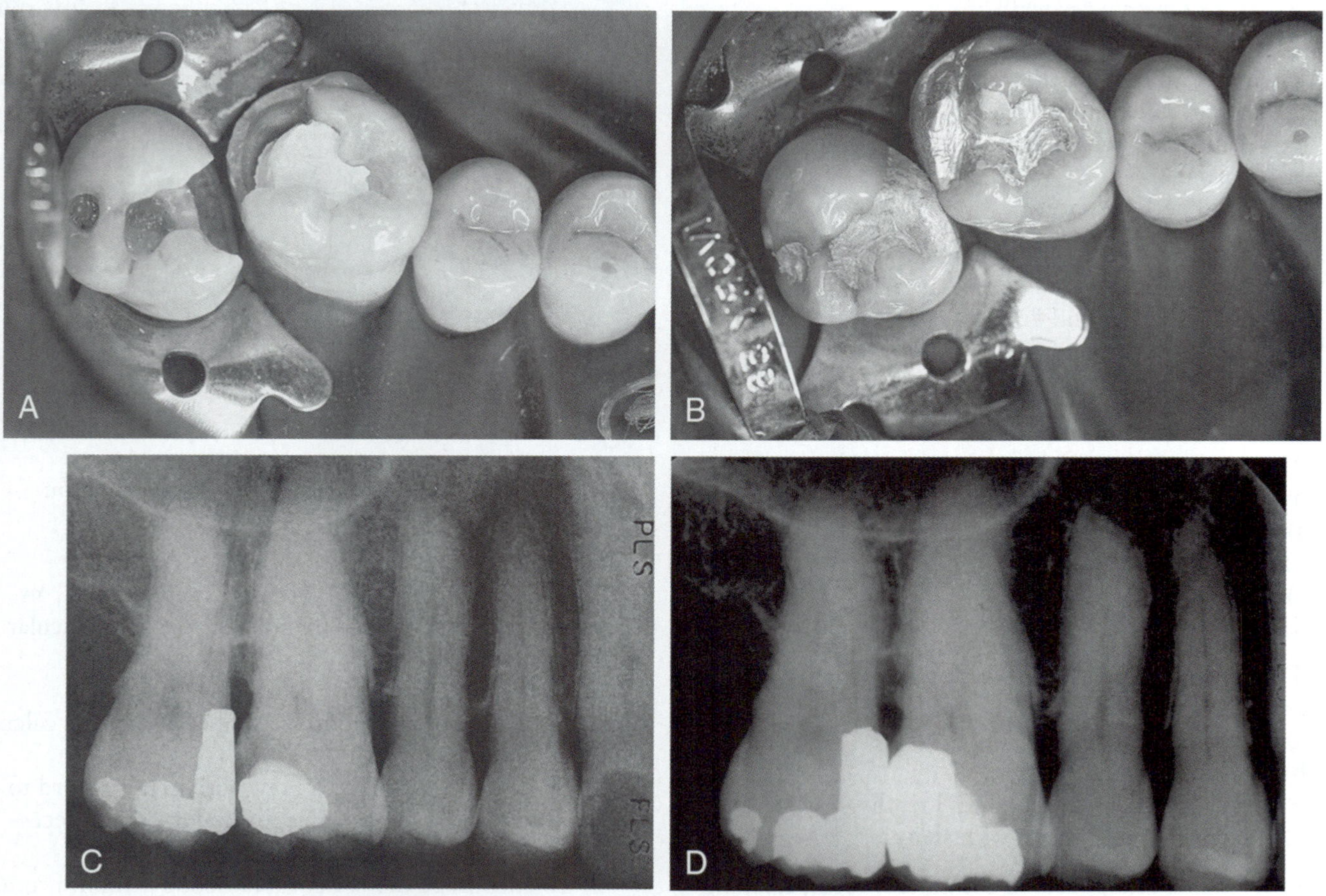

FIGURE CS2.1 **A** and **B.** Rubber dam isolation. **C.** Preoperative radiograph. **D.** Postoperative radiograph. (See color images.)

4. What two conditions also exist in this patient?
   a) Pulpal involvement and periodontal disease
   b) Premolar occlusal stain and gingivitis
   c) Root calculus and gingivitis
   d) Root calculus and periodontal disease

5. In between the patient's restorative appointments, he is appointed with you for the necessary dental hygiene care. Assuming that the dental and dental hygiene assessments and diagnoses have been made, implementation of the dental hygiene care would include:
   a) Scaling and polishing
   b) Scaling, root debridement, and polishing
   c) Radiographs, root debridement, and polishing
   d) Scaling, root debridement, polishing, and evaluation

6. The new amalgams could best be finished and polished with:
   a) Slurries of pumice and tin oxide
   b) A slurry of tin oxide
   c) Finishing burs, then slurries of pumice and whiting
   d) Coarse, and then fine prophylaxis pastes

7. Which of the following teeth should be closely "periodontally monitored"?
   a) #2
   b) #2 and #3
   c) #2, #3 and #4
   d) All teeth in the case presentation should be monitored in the same way.

Case 3

The patient is a 31-year-old woman who is very self conscious of a malformed tooth that everyone can see. She has yearly dental exams and also sees the hygienist during the same appointment. Her oral home care is excellent. She is most interested in having this tooth "look a lot better than it does." The procedure to restore this tooth is illustrated in Figure CS3.1.

QUESTIONS

1. Tooth #10 in Figure CS3.1*A* is commonly called:
   a) Fusion
   b) Traumatic injury
   c) Peg lateral
   d) Erosion

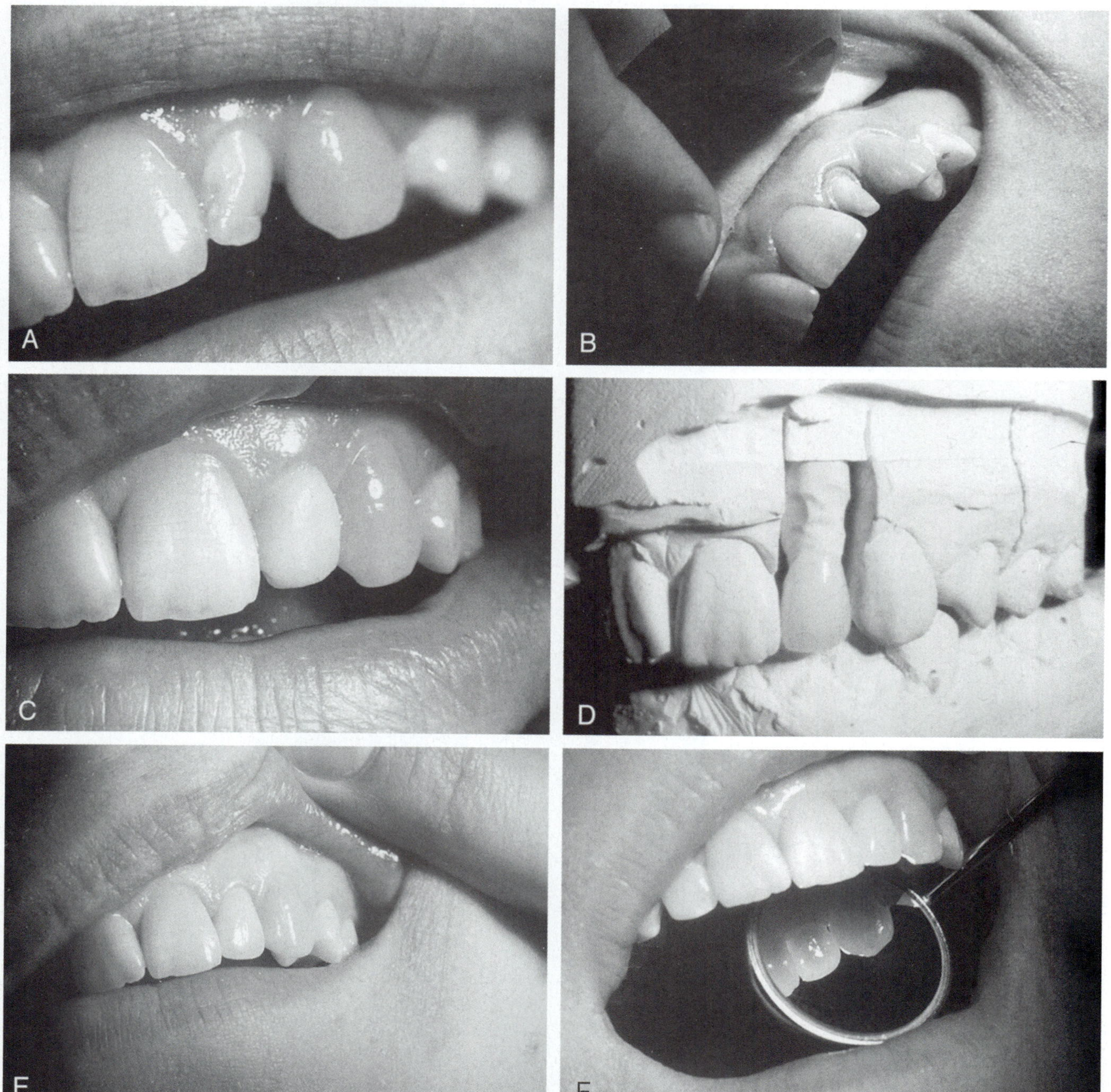

FIGURE CS3.1 **A.** Presentation of patient. **B.** Crown preparation. **C.** Temporary crown. **D.** Models with ceramic crown. **E.** Permanent crown placed (facial). **F.** Permanent crown placed (lingual). (See color images.)

2. The final restoration is said to be a _______ restoration, and the restorative procedure used to fabricate this particular restoration is called a(n) __________ technique.
   a) Removable; direct
   b) Fixed; indirect
   c) Removable; indirect
   d) Fixed; direct

3. After the crown preparation is made, the patient leaves with a restoration as the one shown in Figure CS3.1*C*. This is known as a __________ restoration.
   a) Interim
   b) Provisional
   c) Permanent
   d) Substitute

4. We can assume that the crown shown in Figure CS3.1*E* and *F* contains no metallic materials. Therefore, the dental material usually used in this technique is a:
   a) Cold-curing resin
   b) Special restorative cement
   c) Composite material
   d) Ceramic material

5. The "polishing agent of choice" for the dental material selected in question 4 is:
   a) Toothpaste only
   b) A "mild" prophy paste
   c) A slurry of whiting
   d) Any typical prophy paste

6. The most desirable characteristic of the dental material selected in question 4 is:
   a) Translucency
   b) Abrasion resistance (hardness)
   c) Fracture toughness
   d) Availability of many shades

7. If the patient in this case had discolored teeth and wanted to have them whitened besides having the new restoration fabricated, when should the whitening take place?
   a) Before the restoration is fabricated
   b) After the restoration is fabricated
   c) Between the fabrication appointments
   d) Whitening is contraindicated in this case

Case 4

Dr. Wesley Mullins, D.D.S.

This patient is a 43-year-old woman with an unremarkable medical history. The patient reports that she brushes and flosses two times each day. She says that her gums bleed sometimes and that she really wants to "get my teeth in good shape and keep them that way."

CLINICAL PHOTOGRAPHS

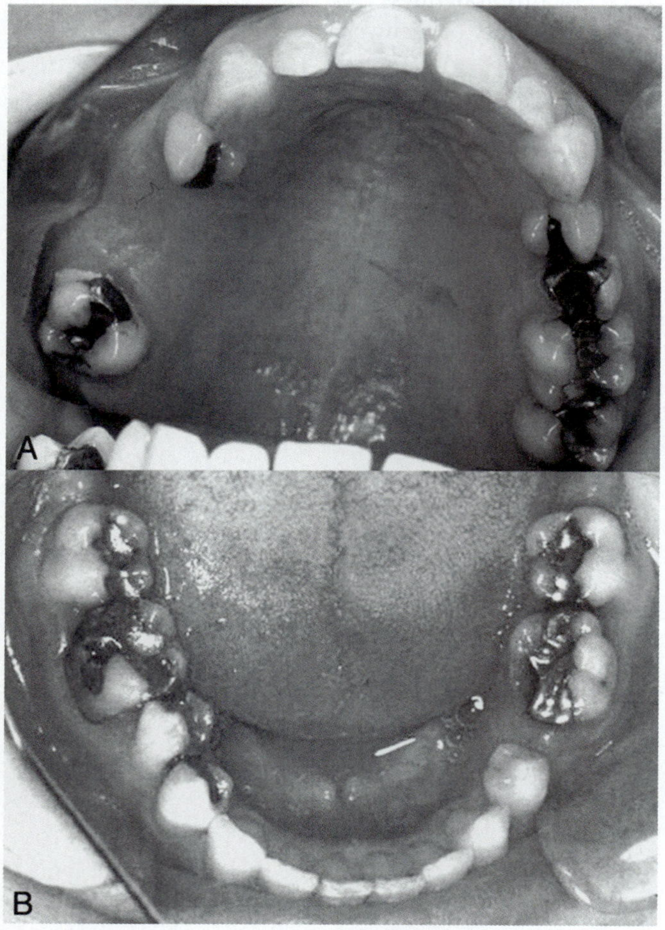

FIGURE CS4.1 Occlusal photographs of maxillary and mandibular arches. (Courtesy of Dr. Wes Mullins, Knoxville, TN.)

DENTAL AND PERIODONTAL CHARTING

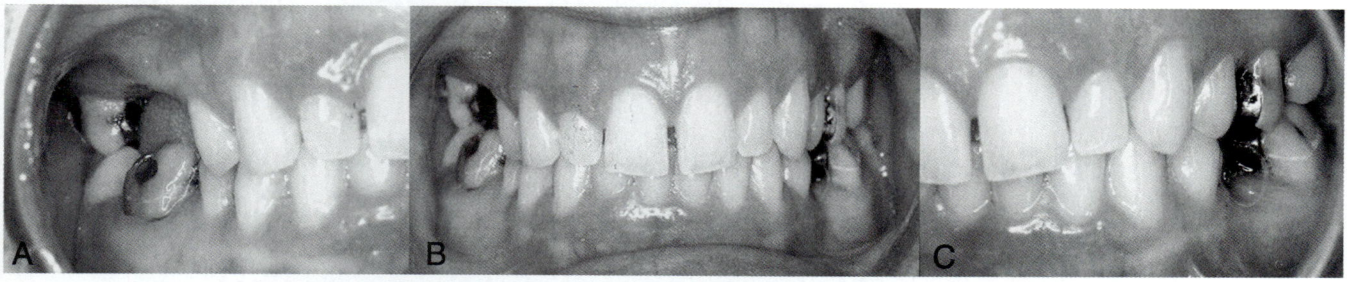

FIGURE CS4.2 Lateral and frontal photographs. (Courtesy of Wes Mullins, Knoxville, TN.)

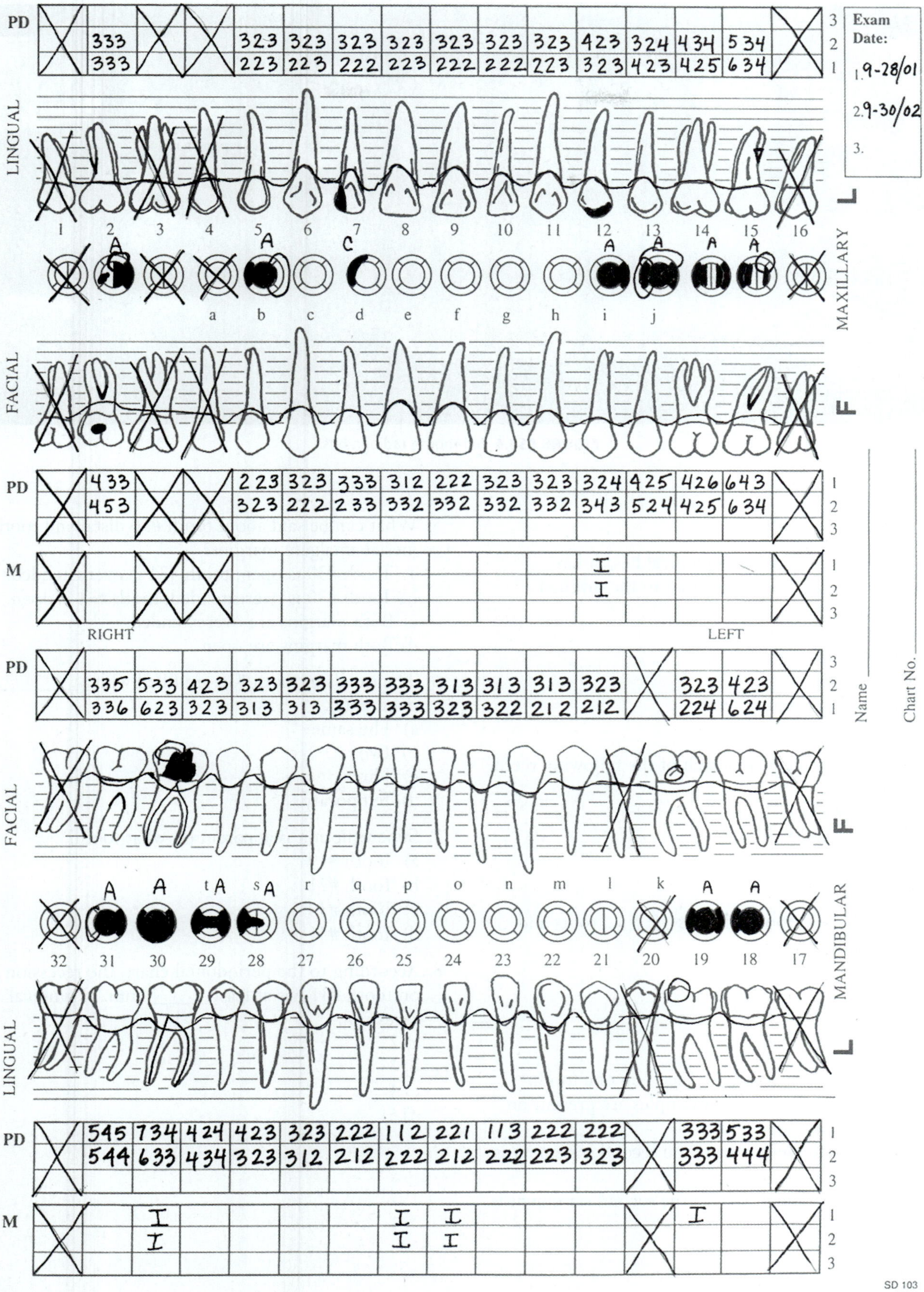

FIGURE CS4.3 Two appointments of dental and periodontal charting.

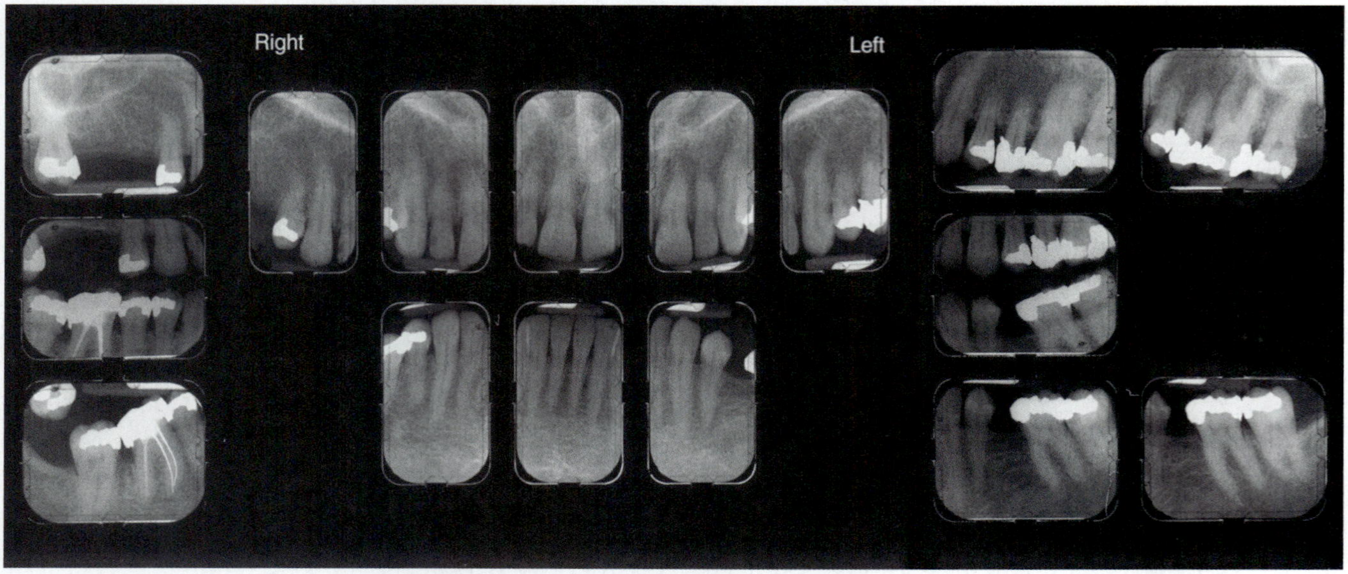

FIGURE CS4.4 Full-mouth radiographs.

QUESTIONS

1. Periodontally, the patient's gingival health has __________________ compared to the original baseline probing.
   a) Greatly improved
   b) Slightly improved
   c) Not changed
   d) Slightly deteriorated
   e) Greatly deteriorated
2. Fractures are evident on which of the following teeth?
   a) Tooth #19
   b) Teeth #19 and #31
   c) Teeth #13 and #19
   d) Teeth #19 and #30
   e) Teeth #13, #19, and #31
3. Radiographically, tooth #30 has ______ roots and ______ canals.
   a) 2; 2
   b) 3; 2
   c) 3; 3
   d) 2; 3
4. Multiple restorations can be placed on one tooth. From this patient's records, examples are present on teeth #2, #14, and #15.
   a) The first statement is true; the second statement is false.
   b) The first statement is false; the second statement is true.
   c) Both statements are true.
   d) Both statements are false.
5. What can be said about tooth #30 distal and tooth #31 mesial amalgam margins?
   a) Tooth #30 is open; tooth #31 is overextended.
   b) Tooth #30 is overextended; tooth #31 is open.
   c) Both margins are overextended.
   d) Both margins are open.
6. The canals in tooth #30 are filled with ____________ material(s).
   a) The same
   b) Two
   c) Three
   d) Temporary
7. Supereruption is apparent on what tooth?
   a) Tooth #19
   b) Tooth #21
   c) Tooth #30
   d) Tooth #31
8. According to the periodontal chart, the recession on tooth #31 has at least ______ mm. of gingival recession.
   a) 2
   b) 3
   c) 4
   d) 5

Case 5

This patient is a 73-year-old woman with controlled hypertension without dry mouth who takes medication for osteoporosis. She mentions she smokes 4 or 5 cigarettes a week because of anxiety. Her oral home care consists of brushing and flossing 2 times each day. She says her gums rarely bleed, she has no sensitivity, and she really wants to "keep my teeth in the best shape as possible." She is happy with her smile.

CLINICAL PHOTOGRAPHS

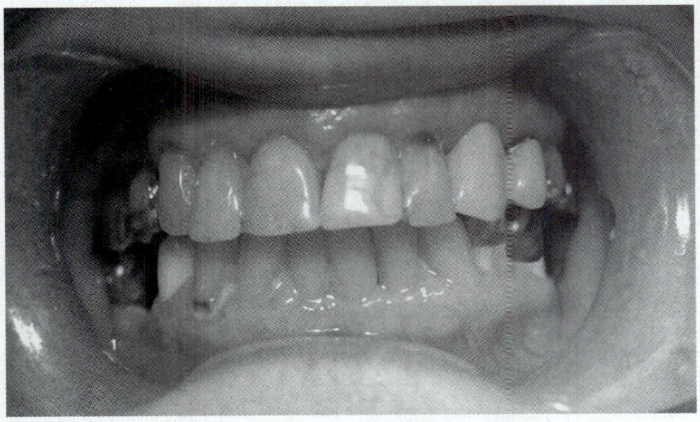

FIGURE CS5.1 Photograph of anterior teeth in occlusion.

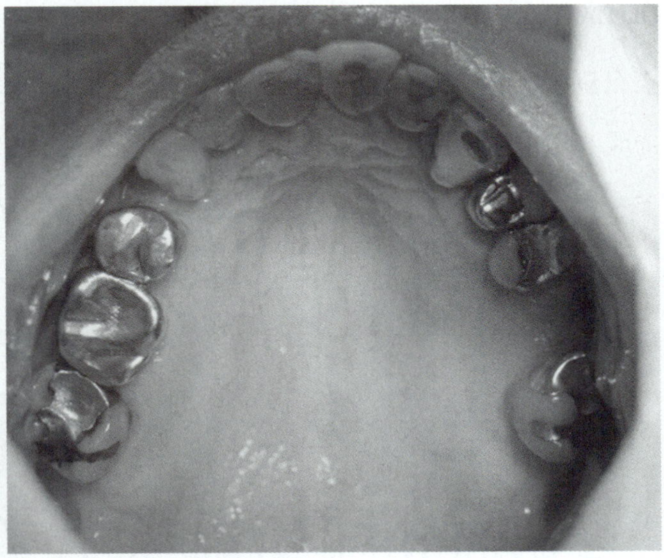

FIGURE CS5.3 Occlusal photograph of maxillary arch.

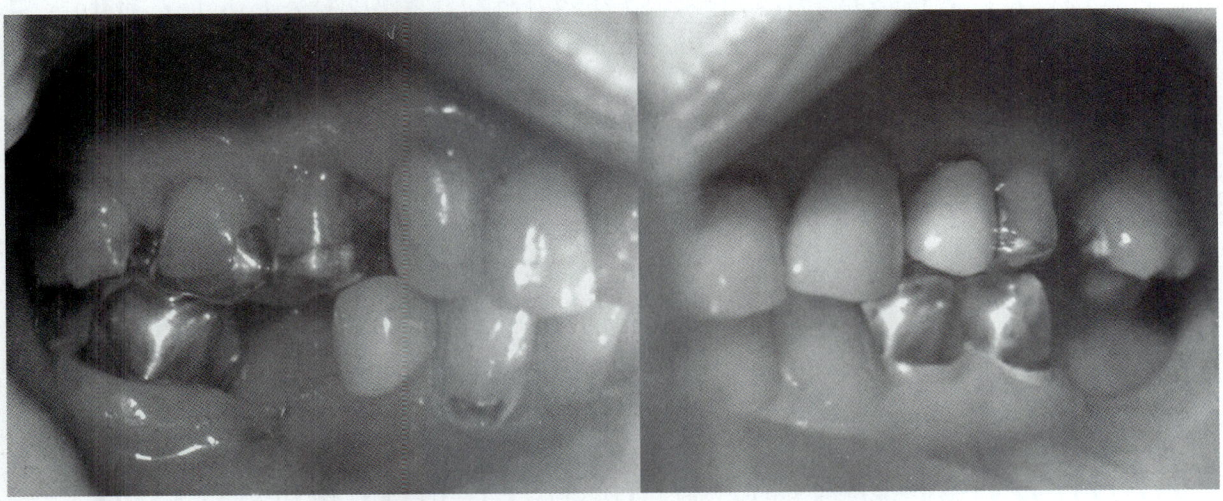

FIGURE CS5.2 Photograph of posterior teeth in occlusion.

DENTAL AND PERIODONTAL CHARTING

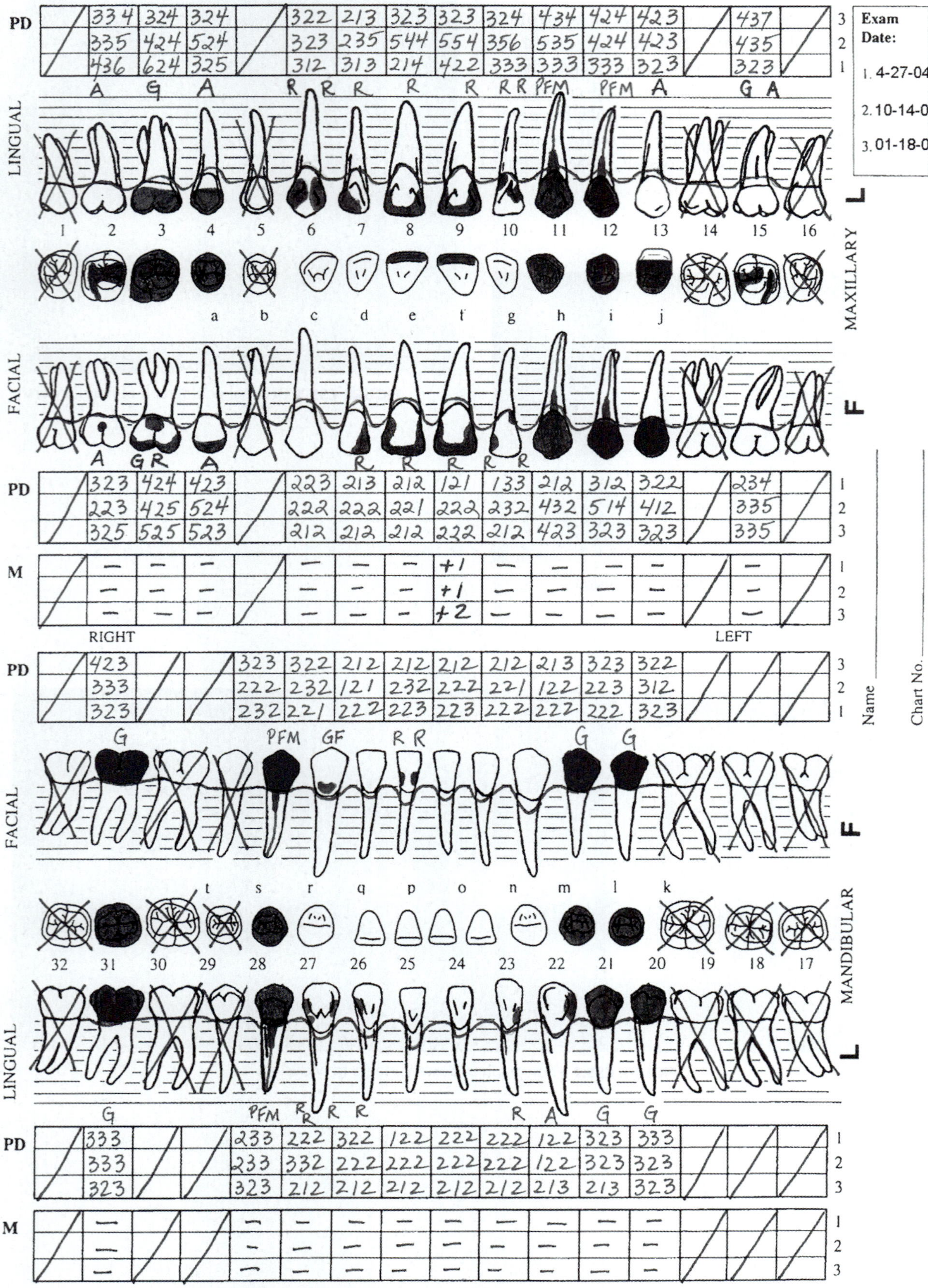

FIGURE CS5.4 Three appointments of dental and periodontal charting.

FULL MOUTH RADIOGRAPHS

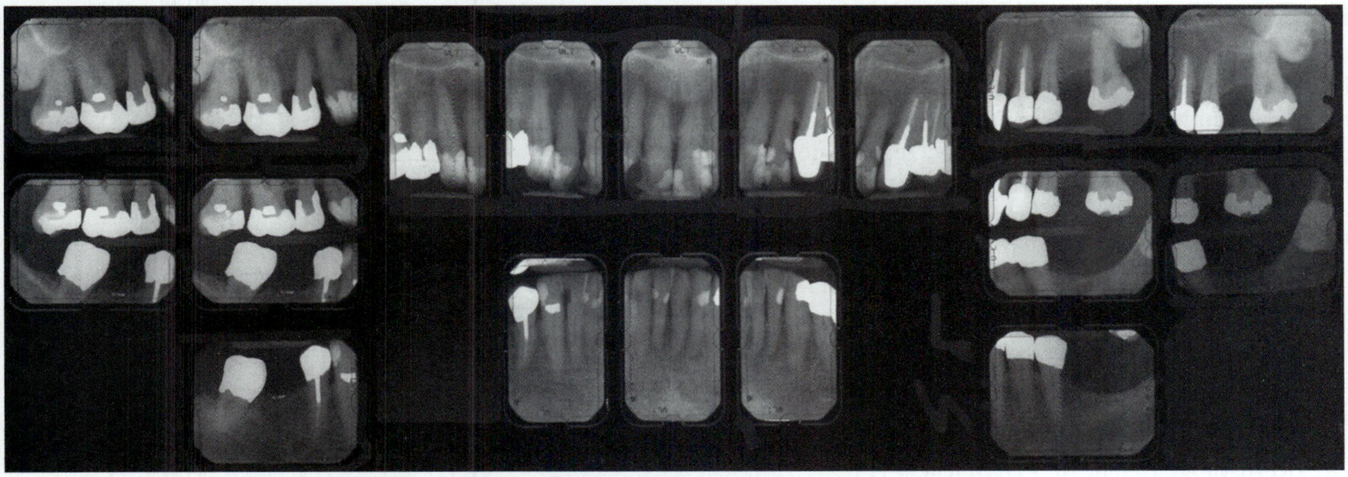

FIGURE CS5.5 Full mouth radiographs.

QUESTIONS

1. From the information presented, which arch of this patient is in better periodontal health?
   a) Maxillary
   b) Mandibular
   c) Both arches are in "periodontically identical health"
   d) Both arches are "periodontically unhealthy"
2. How many kinds of dental restorations have been placed in this patient's mouth?
   a) 2
   b) 3
   c) 4
   d) 5
3. When the patient reports she is on medication for osteoporosis, what possible oral ramifications come to mind?
   a) Necrotizing stomatitis
   b) Xerostomia
   c) Bisphosphonate-induced osteonecrosis (BON)
   d) Increased caries susceptibility
4. After learning the patient's medications, medical conditions, and habits, your chairside patient education should include information on:
   a) Nutritional counseling
   b) Pit and fissure sealants
   c) Tobacco cessation
   d) Tooth whitening
5. After performing an oral exam, reviewing the radiographs and dental history, an appropriate recommendation for this patient would be:
   a) Fluoride varnish on teeth #'s 9, 22, 25 and 26
   b) The use of patient applied fluoride
   c) Pit and fissure sealants
   d) The use of saliva substitutes
6. The largest restoration on tooth #15 is a (an):
   a) MO amalgam
   b) MO gold inlay
   c) DO amalgam
   d) Occlusal gold inlay
   e) DO gold inlay
7. Teeth #'s 11, 12, and 28 have:
   a) Root canals and post & cores
   b) Root canals and PFM crowns
   c) Post & cores and PFM crowns
   d) Root canals, post & cores, and PFM crowns

Case 6

Dr. John H. Tucker, D.M.D.

This patient is a 62-year-old woman with controlled type II diabetes. The patient reports she brushes in the morning and evening, but only flosses in the evening. She has excellent plaque control and has had regular dental care throughout the years. She is unhappy with her smile. The patient presents with a crown that fractured off of tooth #28 and shares with the dentist that she thought her "upper front teeth look fake" and her "lower front teeth look worn out." The photographs include pre-treatment, preparation, and post-treatment. The dental and periodontal charts were recorded before the upcoming restorative treatment.

PRETREATMENT CLINICAL PHOTOGRAPHS

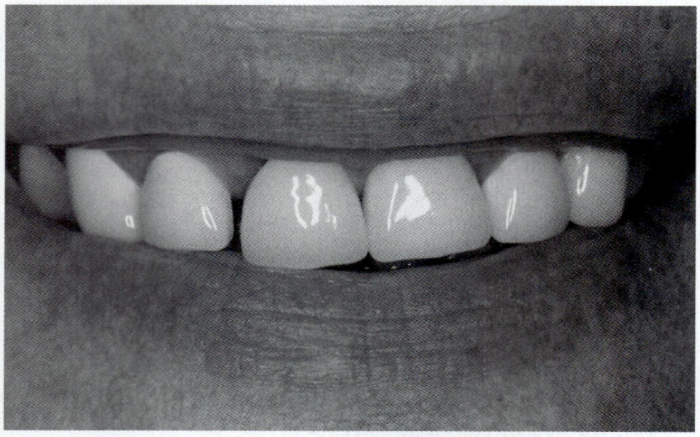

FIGURE CS6.1 Preoperative photograph of maxillary anterior teeth.

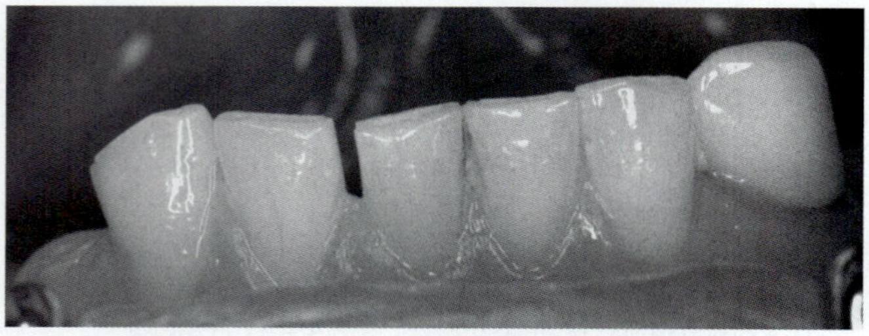

FIGURE CS6.2 Preoperative photograph of mandibular anterior teeth.

DENTAL AND PERIODONTAL CHARTING

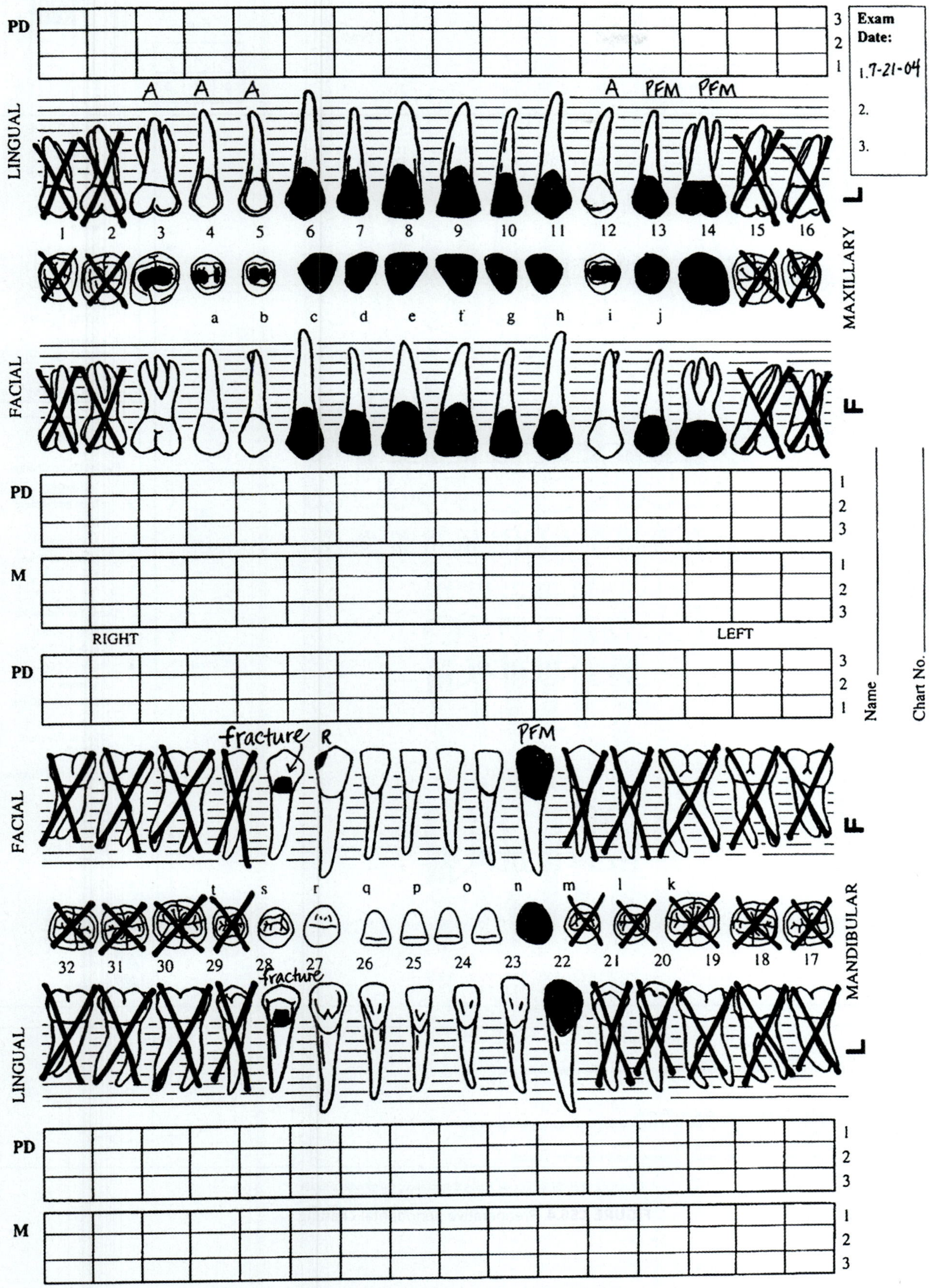

FIGURE CS6.3 Preoperative dental charting.

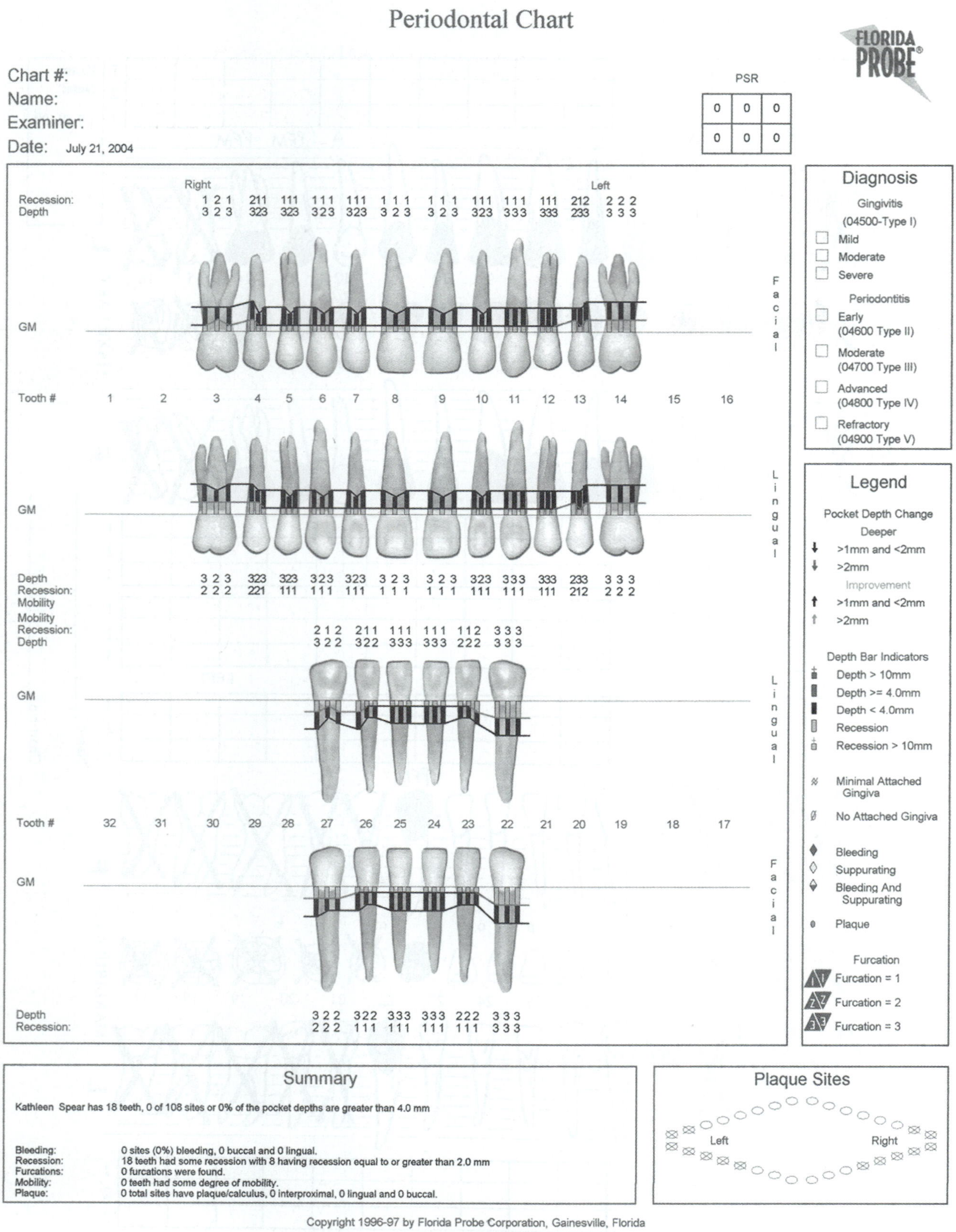

FIGURE CS6.4 Preoperative periodontal charting.

FULL MOUTH RADIOGRAPHS

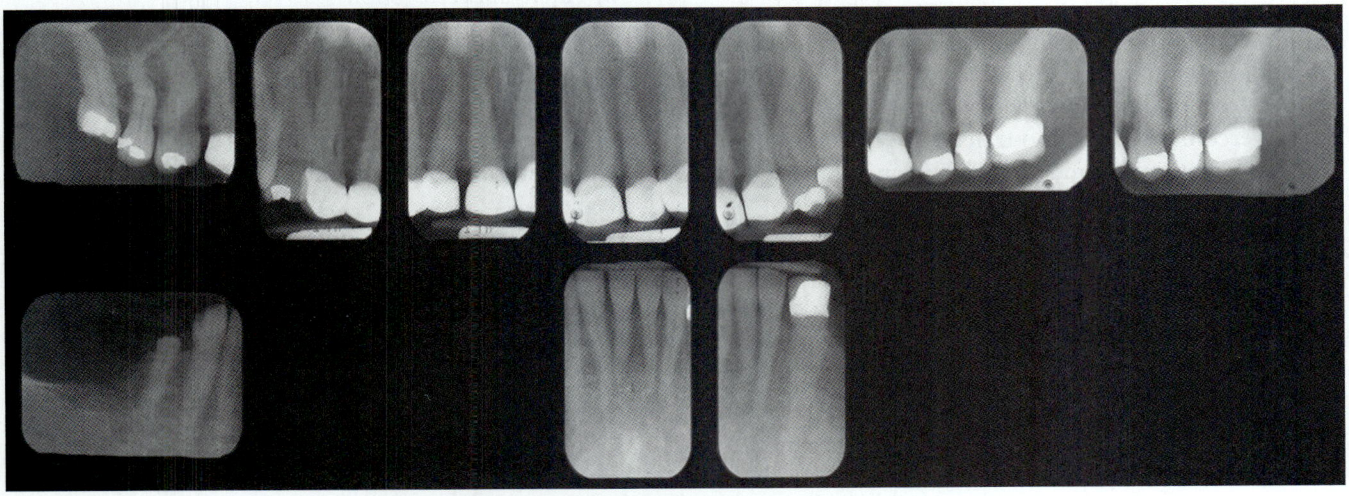

FIGURE CS6.5 Preoperative full mouth radiographs.

PREPARATIONS

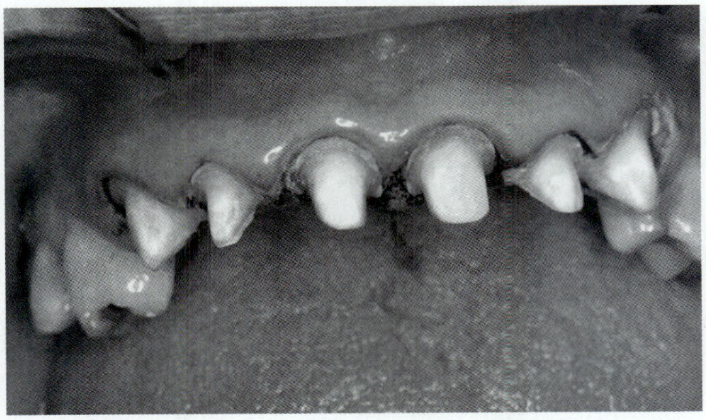

FIGURE CS6.6 Photograph of preparations of maxillary anterior teeth.

POST-TREATMENT CLINICAL PHOTOGRAPHS

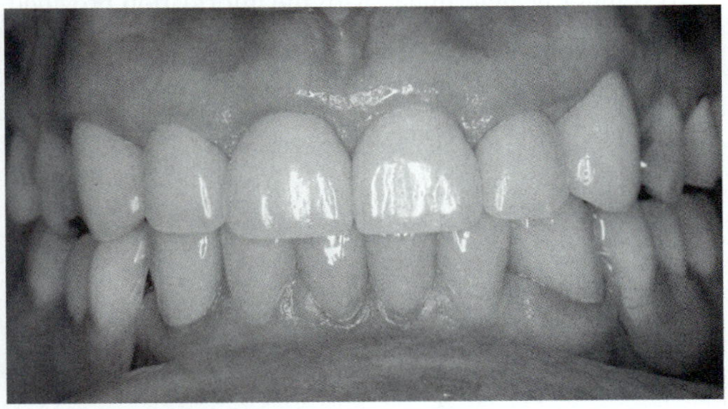

FIGURE CS6.7 Postoperative photograph of anterior teeth.

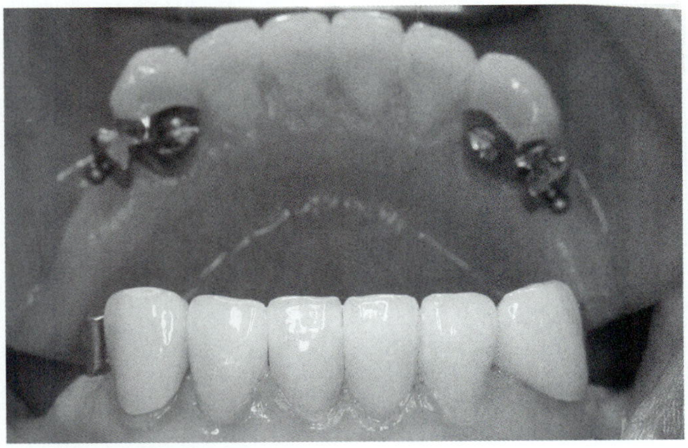

FIGURE CS6.8 Postoperative photograph of mandibular anterior teeth showing rest seats and precision attachments.

QUESTIONS

1. The patient said, "My upper front teeth look fake." This would professionally translate that her original maxillary ceramometal crowns are:
   a) Overcontoured and very opaque in color
   b) Overcontoured and too translucent in color
   c) Undercontoured and very opaque in color
   d) Undercontoured and too translucent in color
2. The treatment plan called for porcelain veneers on teeth 23, 24, 25, and 26. These would be recorded on the dental chart:
   a) The same way a porcelain crown is charted
   b) By outlining the lingual surface on these teeth
   c) By outlining the facial surface on these teeth
   d) By outlining the facial and lingual surfaces on these teeth
3. From the information provided in this case, the gingival health of this patient is considered to be:
   a) Poor
   b) Acceptable
   c) Very good
   d) Cannot be determined with the information provided
4. Which tooth exhibits the developmental condition of dilaceration?
   a) 3
   b) 4
   c) 5
   d) 6
5. The radiolucency on the distal of #27 is a(an):
   a) Amalgam restoration
   b) Gold inlay
   c) Carious lesion
   d) Composite restoration
6. The veneers that were placed on # 23–26 (Fig CS6-8 were most likely luted with a ____________ cement.
   a) Zinc-oxide and eugenol
   b) Polycarboxylate
   c) Glass ionomer
   d) Composite
   e) Zinc-oxide and eugenol
7. In the mandibular post-treatment photograph (Fig. CS6-8), teeth 22 and 27 have metallic projections extending from the distal surface. Their purpose is to attach to:
   a) Future implant restoration
   b) The provisional (temporary) temporary posterior teeth
   c) The new partial denture
   d) The orthodontic retainer

Appendix 1

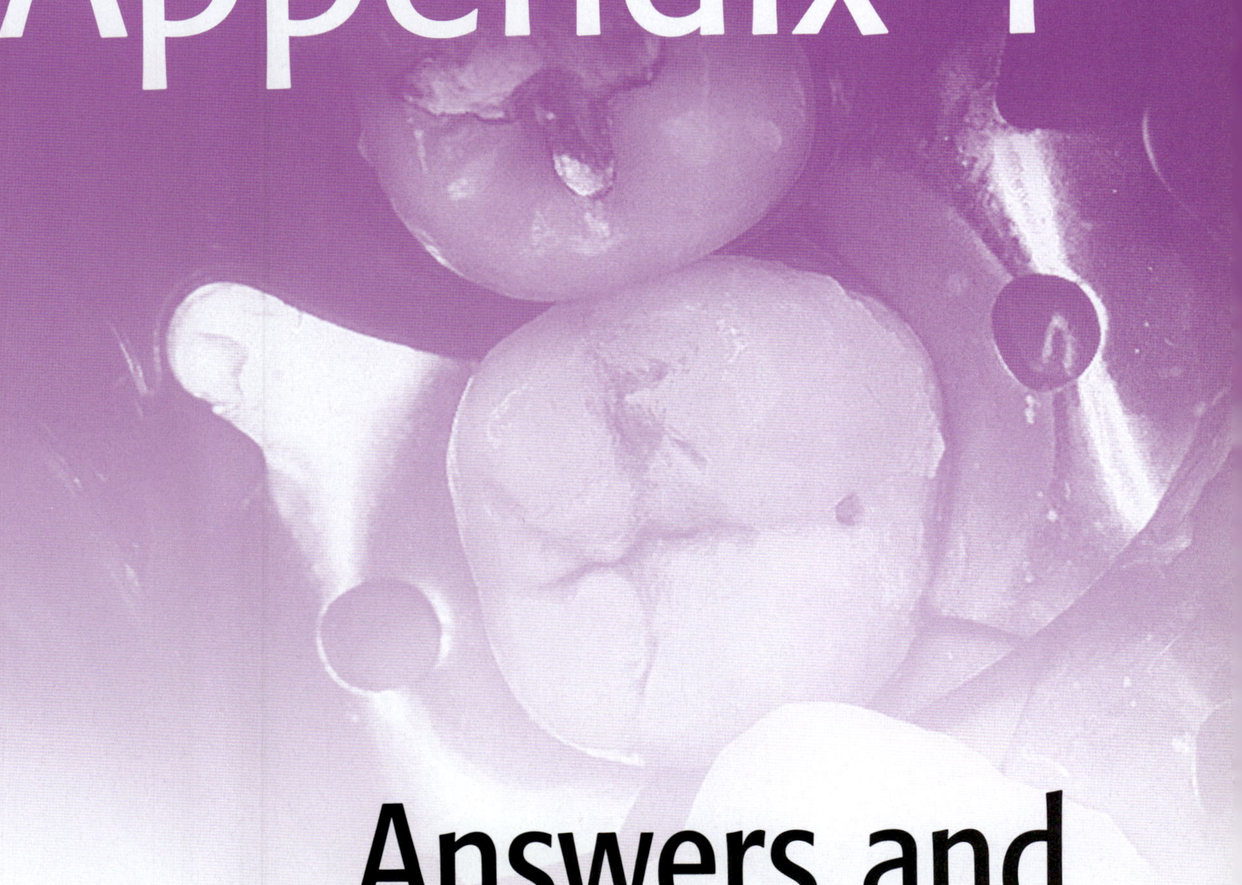

Answers and Justifications to Review Questions and Case Studies

Chapter 1

1. b. The FDA is the regulatory agency, whereas the ADA develops standards and administers those standards and guidelines. The AADR is a professional organization for dental researchers. The OSHA mandates the practice of standard (universal) precautions for bloodborne pathogens.
2. c. It is not within the scope of dental hygiene practice to choose the restorative material for the patient. This is the responsibility of the dentist. Understanding how dental materials behave, educating the patient, and assessing the patient are all patient care responsibilities of the hygienist.
3. e. Gingival third caries, anterior and posterior and both lingual and facial, are defined as Class V.
4. c. The degradation of teeth and dental materials, biocompatibility, biting forces, esthetic demands of the patient, and temperature changes are all restrictions that limit the use of dental materials.
5. d. When the temperature changes in the oral cavity, no dental material expands and contracts by exactly the same amount as the natural tooth structure. Over time, this expansion and contraction may cause leakage around the restoration and tooth sensitivity.
6. c. The periodontium supports the tooth in a stable condition and gives feedback on the forces being placed on the teeth. The gingival tissues seal out undesirable agents and attach to the teeth, forming a barrier. The pulp serves to respond to thermal stimuli, as it contains the nerve cells.
7. a. When a significant amount of tooth structure is missing from a particular tooth, a crown will encircle and support the remaining tooth structure. A pontic is the "false tooth" on a bridge, whereas an implant replaces the entire tooth, including the root. A fixed partial denture replaces teeth that may be missing in an arch and is cemented in place.
8. a. It is true that the cavity preparation design helps to secure the restoration in place. But because gold castings such as an inlay are cemented in place and must be first seated without cement as a "try-in," the walls must diverge so that it can be removed and then cemented. The converging walls of an amalgam preparation, as well as the added undercut areas, help to retain it in the cavity prep.
9. b. Technically, the only terms that would be interchangeable are study model and diagnostic cast. This replica is used to study the size and position of the oral tissues. If a restoration is constructed on the replica, it is called a cast.
10. d. Amalgam, composites and glass ionomers are all direct restorative materials. They are placed directly into the cavity preparation once all the decay is removed. Porcelain materials must be fabricated in a dental laboratory because they are fired in an oven at high temperatures. Temporary restorations are usually made for the patient to be used between appointments while indirect restorations are being fabricated.

Chapter 2

1. d. Window glass has strong atomic bonds but short-range order similar to that of liquids. The consistent spatial relationship between molecules is 5 to 10 neighbors apart. The short-range order is why glass sometimes flows; an example is a window in a very old house where the bottom half of the window may be slightly thicker than the top half.
2. b. Metallic bonds are formed when the electrons are shared by all the atoms. Covalent bonds result when two atoms share a pair of electrons. Ionic bonds occur when an electron is "given up" by one atom and then accepted by another. Secondary bonds involve the uneven distribution of electrons. Partial charges result.
3. a. The valence electrons in a metallic bond are shared between atoms. Metals have distinct properties, which are the result of their atomic bond. The "negative cloud" and the "positive core" result in many weak, multidirectional primary bonds. In turn, this results in a strong material. Secondary bonds are formed when a partial charge results from an uneven distribution of electrons around an atom or molecule. Covalent bonds result when two atoms share a pair of electrons. Ionic bonds occur when an electron is "given up" by one atom and then accepted by another.
4. b. Translucent materials are those that allow some light to pass through, such as the incisal third area of anterior teeth. Dental ceramics can be matched in translucency and color to replace the natural tooth structure. A ceramic dental restorative material is neither transparent (all light passes through) nor opaque (no light passes through). Brittleness is a disadvantage of ceramics as a dental restorative material.
5. c. The cross-linking not only adds strength, but the more cross-links that are present, the more rigid and stiff the material becomes. Polymers will stretch and recoil, similar to the movements of a "Slinky," if they have no or minimal cross-links.
6. d. Tin foil is a pure metal that has been compressed into a very thin film. The other materials listed are composed of two or more different materials. The

resulting material has improved properties compared with those of either individual material.

7. a. A permanent dipole is a bond that has a permanent partial charge. Permanent dipoles form weak secondary bonds. The bonds in a fluctuating dipole are the result of an intermittent, uneven distribution of electrons around the atoms or molecules. Hydrogen bonds are "special" permanent dipoles because of the single electron. Primary bonds are strong bonds between atoms that involve the transfer or sharing of electrons.

8. a. In a metal, each positive core is surrounded by an electron cloud, and the core "feels" little difference when an atom slides by another atom. Since the surroundings (atomic bonding) do not change, neither do the properties. Ceramics would fracture when bent because of the ionic bonding and the resulting electron repulsion if a negative ion slides "one over" to another negative ion. Polymers may bend easily or may fracture depending on the bonding between the chains.

9. b. A composite is a material that is made from two or more different solid materials. A colloid is a mixture of gases, liquids, or solids at a microscopic level, and is a suspension of one material in another. A solution is one material completely dissolved in another, whereas an emulsion is a type of colloid composed of two liquids that do not blend together to form one liquid. Their stability when mixed together is usually temporary.

10. c. A covalent bond results when two atoms share a pair of electrons, and is one of three types of primary bonds. An ionic bond results when an atom gives up an electron and another accepts it. A metallic bond is a primary bond in which valence electrons are shared, but by all the atoms in the object, not just two. Secondary bonds are the result of partial charges from an uneven distribution of electrons around an atom or molecule.

Chapter 3

1. c. Good wetting indicates that the adhesive is in very close contact with the adherend, forming a low contact angle. Poor wetting "stays as a drop," and a high contact angle is formed.

2. d. Tension is a pulling or stretching stress, which many times is referred to as tensile stress. Compression is a crushing or pushing force. Torsion is a twisting stress, and shear is a sliding stress.

3. c. The higher the modulus of elasticity, the stiffer the material. The modulus is a measure of flexibility. A rubber band has a low modulus; a mouth mirror has a high modulus. Resilience is the ability of a material to absorb energy without deforming, whereas toughness is the ability of a material to absorb energy up to and including failure or fracture.

4. c. Nearly all materials will contract (sometimes ever so slightly) when cooled and expand when heated. Measuring this change in size (volume) in relation to change in temperature is called the coefficient of thermal expansion. In dentistry, this property holds importance because, ideally, the tooth structure and the restorative material should expand and contract by the same amount.

5. b. Remember that you cannot have stress (load) without strain (change in length). They occur together. When they are proportional, as illustrated on a graph, it is a straight line. As we increase the load (by adding more monkey charms), eventually the spring will not go back to the original length. This stress is no longer proportional to the strain. We have reached the yield strength on the graph, and the line begins to curve.

6. a. The modulus of elasticity is defined as the stress divided by the strain in the linear portion of the stress–strain graph.

7. a. Other examples of physical properties are color and thermal conductivity. Strength and stiffness are mechanical properties, and setting reactions are chemical properties.

8. d. Torsion is a twisting stress, such as turning a doorknob. Shear stress occurs when parts of an object slide past each other. Tension is a pulling stress, and bending is a combination of compression, tension, and shear stresses.

9. c. Solubility is calculated as the amount of material that dissolves in a given time. Viscosity is the ability of a material to flow. Water sorption is the ability of a material to absorb water. Wetting is the interaction of a liquid with a surface.

10. b. Mechanical properties include stress, strain, resilience, toughness, fatigue and elasticity, to name a few. Physical properties include thermal conductivity, heat capacity, vapor pressure, viscosity, hardness, and many more. Chemical properties describe setting reactions and decay and degradation. Biologic properties are the effects materials have on living tissue.

11. d. Thermal conductivity is the rate of heat flow through a material. It is measured as heat flow over time. Heat capacity is a measure of the amount of thermal energy a material can hoard (like a microwave trivet), while heat of fusion is the amount of energy required to melt a material. The coefficient of thermal expansion is a measure of change in volume in relation to the temperature change.

12. b. The definitions of these four properties are described in #11 above. The composite resin restorative material expands and contracts at a different rate than enamel and dentin. Over time, a gap is created between the tooth and restoration when it contracts (from cold beverage) and then closes when the soup is eaten. This process is called percolation and may result in microleakage, tooth sensitivity and recurrent decay.
13. a. Those liquids that act as solvents and evaporate readily have a high vapor pressure. Materials with low vapor pressure do not evaporate quickly. All liquids have some degree of vapor pressure. A liquid's vapor pressure is a constant, and does not vary. Therefore, it cannot be "intermittent."
14. b. Compression is defined as "a pushing or crushing stress." The pressing of the plastic mass of amalgam by the amalgam condenser instrument is an example of compression.
15. a. Solubility is a measure of a materials' ability to dissolve in water. The dental cement has a low solubility and serves the patient well by not dissolving for a long period of time in the patient's mouth. Cements have the most demanding requirements of any material.
16. c. Stress concentration occurs near voids pits and cracks. Stress concentration may cause breaks and fractures at a much lower stress than if they were not present.

Chapter 4

1. a. The sticky material, or the bonding material that sticks the stamp to the envelope, is called the adhesive. The stamp and the envelope are referred to as adherends.
2. c. If the bracket breaks off cleanly between the bonding material and the enamel surface, it is called an adhesive failure. When the fracture or failure occurs within the bonding material, it is termed a cohesive failure. Residual bonding material may be present on both the bracket and the tooth surface.
3. The numbers for the correct sequence are: 2, 5, 7, 1, 3, 6, 8, and 4. The tooth surface must be cleaned and then rinsed and dried before the etchant can be placed. Next, the etchant is placed for 15 to 30 seconds. This, too, must be thoroughly rinsed and gently dried. The bonding resin is then applied, and it flows into the enamel micropores. The restorative material is applied last and bonds to the previously placed bonding resin.
4. c. A 37% concentration of ortho-phosphoric acid is commonly used. Lower concentrations have been tested but tend to be too weak. Higher concentrations are too aggressive.
5. d. The enamel rods are arranged less regularly than permanent teeth. The surface must be etched longer to assure a surface that has sufficient irregularities with which to retain a bonding (resin) material.
6. a. The micropores formed by the etchant are too small to be seen by the naked eye, so this bonding process is known as micromechanical bonding. Secondary, rather than primary, bonds are formed because the unset bonding resin flows around the decalcified collagen fibers and sets, thus entangling the two molecular chains together without primary bonds. Secondary bonds promote this entanglement.
7. b. This layer of "dentin debris" not only remains on the surface but also extends into the dentinal tubules. It is similar to sticky, sappy pinewood shavings, and it adheres to the newly cut surface. After the smear layer is removed with etchant, a primer layer is applied and flows into the open tubules of etched dentin. The adhesive (layer) is a low-viscosity resin and sets similarly to enamel-bonding resin.
8. b. The adhesion/bonding mechanism reduces microleakage, which decreases the likelihood of recurrent decay. Bonding agents seal off the space between the tooth and the restoration. This protects the interface area, not only from microleakage, but from postoperative sensitivity.
9. d. The hybrid layer is a combination of the resin adhesive and decalcified dentin. The dentin becomes decalcified during the etching process. A bond is formed when the collagen fibers (the organic component of the dentin) are surrounded by and become embedded in the resin adhesive material. Enamel tissue is not a part of the hybrid layer and the smear layer is actually "dentin debris" left by the dental bur.
10. c. It is a current belief that the smear layer is created when dentin tissue is cut during tooth preparation (see #7 above). Composites do not irritate the pulp; the microleakage of composites causes the irritation. Etching of dentin does not irritate the pulp tissue and the smear layer does not need to be preserved.

Chapter 5

1. d. The coefficient of thermal expansion for restorative resins can be 2 to 10 times greater than tooth structure. Repeated expansion and contraction can open and close the gaps at the margin of the restoration. Other problems with resins include polymerization shrinkage and lack of abrasion resistance.

2. c. The silane-coupling agent coats the filler particles of the composite and is chemically compatible with both the filler and the resin phases. It also transfers the stress from the weaker resin phase to the stronger filler phase. The matrix is composed of a soft resin, which has little strength and wears easily. The filler particles are made of "engineered" glass and add strength to the restoration. Polymers are another name for plastics, and adhesives are materials that will stick to a flat surface or bond two flat surfaces together. (These were discussed in Chapter 4.)
3. b. Because of the very small particle size, microfills finish and polish better than any other type of composite. They have, however, a high coefficient of thermal expansion, low strength, and a low percentage of filler (40–50%).
4. c. With chemical-cure materials, two pastes are mixed and set by a chemical reaction. This limits the operator's working time. There is also a possibility of incorporating air bubbles while mixing. Most contain more matrix material and less filler than light-cure products.
5. a. Depth of cure is the amount or increment of composite that can be successfully cured by a light source. Incremental addition refers to adding and curing small amounts of composite material in the cavity preparation.
6. d. The smaller the particle size of the filler, the better the clinician can finish and polish the surface of the restoration. Smaller particles are less likely to break down and fall out of the resin matrix, thus leaving a roughened surface to accumulate stain and debris. The size of the filler particle does not affect the polymerization reaction, the technique for adding increments, or the etching time.
7. c. A decreased filler content decreases the viscosity of the material and, therefore, increases the "flowability." This makes placement easier for the dentist. Flowable composites are usually placed under a hybrid composite material. Condensable composites aid in placement by inhibiting filler particles from sliding by one another. This makes them feel stiffer and thicker than the typical composites. Preventive resins use a dental bur, composite, and sealant material. Hybrid composites contain several particle sizes to create a material that has superior strength and that polishes well.
8. b. Hybrid composites are used in restorations undergoing moderate stress in which strength and wear resistance are more important than surface luster. For low-stress areas, high surface luster, and Class V restorations, microfill composites are used.
9. d. Preventive resin restorations combine a pit-and-fissure sealant and a composite restoration. The composite is placed first, with any remaining pits and fissures being covered by the sealant material. Compomers are a hybrid of glass ionomer and composite materials. Flowable composites will "flow" into the preparation because of lower viscosity. Condensable composites contain filler particles that inhibit them from sliding past each other for a "stiffer, thicker" feel. This consistency allows for easier placement.
10. d. Abrasion resistance for hybrid composites is very good compared to the other composite types. Abrasion resistance is poor for the older, macrofilled composites.
11. a. Thermal expansion is poor for microfill composites. For hybrid composites, thermal expansion is considered to be good.
12. b. Hybrid composites have 75% to 80% filler by weight. Microfills are 40% to 50%, and macrofills are 70% to 75%. Flowable composites are 50% filler by weight.
13. c. Light activated composites are supplied as a single paste, with no mixing required. Polymerization does not begin until the material is exposed to a very bright light. They are popular among dentists because they will "set on demand" (dentist has control of setting time). The chemically activated materials are usually a two-paste system that has to be mixed together to have the polymerization reaction begin. Once mixing begins, the reaction takes place until a set (hard) product forms.
14. c. Compomers bond and set like composite resins, but initially release fluoride like glass ionomers. Flowable composites are those that have a lower viscosity due to decreased filler content. Condensable composites are those that have a "thicker, stiffer feel," which possibly makes condensation easier. Preventive resin restorations are a combination of pit and fissure sealants and composite restorations; the composite is placed first, then the rest of the area is sealed.
15. d. Microfill composites have filler particles sized from .03 to .5 microns, low strength, good abrasion resistance and have very good polishability. Macrofill composites have 10–25 micron particle sizes, fair strength, poor abrasion resistance and poor polishability. Hybrid composites range in particle size from 0.5 to 1 micron, good strength, very good abrasion resistance and good polishability.

Chapter 6

1. d. Remember that the dental amalgam is comprised of mercury and amalgam alloy, approximately 50%

each. It was mentioned that silver (Ag) comprises 65% of the alloy, but this is 65% of the 50% of the alloy component of the dental amalgam. This reasoning is also true for copper (Cu) and tin (Sn). Aluminum (Al) is not found in dental amalgam.

2. c. Amalgam has a high compressive strength, but tensile and shear strengths are comparatively low. Bending strength is a combination of tensile and compression strengths and is low as well.

3. c. Tin–mercury comprises the gamma two phase of the setting reaction of low-copper (traditional) dental amalgams. "Gamma" is used to designate the silver–tin (Ag-Sn) phase. "Gamma-one" is used to designate the silver–mercury phase (Ag-Hg). There is no tin–tin compound in the setting reaction of amalgam.

4. b. Silver causes setting expansion and increases the strength and corrosion. Zinc will minimize oxidation. Tin will reduce strength and corrosion resistance and will maximize oxidation.

5. b. Lowering the mercury content increases the strength and results in less marginal breakdown. Increasing the mercury content decreases the strength and results in more marginal breakdown.

6. b. The marginal seal of corrosion products that forms over time, between the inner surface of the tooth and the restoration (interface), is the feature that makes amalgam a successful restorative material. The price and the ease of use are advantages, but they do not account for its success as a restorative material. Finishing and polishing can extend the service of the restoration, but the seal at the interface is the most important feature contributing to its success.

7. c. The proper trituration technique is controlled by the dentist, whereas the composition of the alloy, rate of the setting reaction, particle shape, and particle size of the alloy are controlled by the manufacturer.

8. f. An amalgam restoration that has been finished and polished reduces the ability for plaque to adhere, resists tarnish and corrosion, and is more likely to have continuous margins with tooth structure. Voids in the restoration are the result of the condensation technique of the clinician. They are not related to finishing and polishing.

9. b. In the high-copper amalgam reaction, tin reacts with copper rather than with mercury. This eliminates the undesirable gamma-two phase. Tin reacts with silver to form the gamma phase, an Ag-Sn compound. Tin reacts with mercury in the low-copper (traditional) setting reaction to form gamma-two. Zinc, if present, reduces oxidation of the other metals in the alloy.

10. a. The life expectancy of an amalgam restoration is indirectly related to the size of the restoration. As the restoration increases in size, so do the internal stresses, thus decreasing the life expectancy.

11. a. Amalgams using lathe-cut alloy particles require more force during condensation because these particles are rough and do not slide past each other easily. In contrast, spherical particles have a soft, "mushy" feel and a condenser may push through the mass easily. The blended, or admixed alloy particles would have an in-between consistency or "feel," that of spherical or lathe-cut.

12. b. Overtriturated amalgam is difficult to condense, exhibits a shortened working time, and will tend to crumble. Undertriturated amalgam has a mushy-grainy feel, and is difficult to properly condense. It may also appear soupy. Properly triturated amalgam is cohesive, smooth, and plastic. The mercury-alloy ratio is set and proportioned by the manufacturer and is usually not the cause of a poor consistency and decreased setting time.

13. d. Amalgam is a cost effective restorative material that provides good service over a reasonably long time. It is used for amalgam cores, tooth fractures, and cingulum pits on anterior teeth. It is commonly used for Class I, II, V, and VI caries. It is seldom used for Class III and IV caries because the "silver" color could be seen in the interproximal and facial areas.

14. c. One-tenth of 1% (0.1) of the population has a true allergy to mercury. Therefore, for the vast majority of patients, mercury toxicity is not a problem.

15. b. When properly placed, direct gold, or gold foil, is a long lasting restoration. It is placed by condensing it into the cavity preparation. Its cost is reasonable but the cost of labor to place it can be expensive. A disadvantage is the lack of strength when compared to other metallic restorations.

Chapter 7

1. d. Glass ionomer is the most common cement at this time that is supplied in capsule form and mixed in the amalgamator.

2. e. Glass ionomer and ZOE cements are used for caries control. Glass ionomer cements leach fluoride that inhibits caries. ZOE has an obtundent effect on the pulp; this is an advantage when caries are deep. Other cements do not have these advantages.

3. a. Only glass ionomer cements release fluoride. ZOE does, however, protect and soothe the pulp, but it is weak and lacks long-term strength compared to other cements.

4. c. In addition to its lack of strength, ZOE is the most soluble compared to glass ionomer, zinc phosphate, and polycarboxylate. Glass ionomer is the least soluble, with zinc phosphate and polycarboxylate ranking second and third, respectively, in their ability to resist solubility.

5. b. Glass ionomer must be mixed within 1 minute to achieve the correct consistency. It must also possess a shiny appearance on luting to maintain maximum adhesion.

6. a. In oral fluids, cements are much more soluble than gold alloy, porcelain, or porcelain-fused-to-metal restorations.

7. d. Because zinc phosphate produces an exothermic reaction during manipulation, it is important to release this heat during mixing. This is done by spreading the mix over the entire surface of the slab so that the heat can dissipate. This technique is not necessary for ZOE, polycarboxylate, or glass ionomer.

8. c. Calcium hydroxide promotes the formation of secondary dentin. Silicates, temporary cements, and composite cements do not promote the formation of secondary dentin.

9. b. Fluoride is added to the raw materials of certain cements to make manufacturing of the glass powder easier. An added clinical benefit is the leaching into enamel, which serves as a deterrent to secondary decay.

10. d. Composite cement would be the luting agent of choice because it would directly bond the ceramic restoration to tooth structure. It is assumed that a dentinal bonding system is used before the cement is applied. Composite cements are also called resin cements. Zinc phosphate, and polycarboxylate are more opaque and would tend to "defeat the purpose" of the esthetic, translucent properties of the ceramic. ZOE is also opaque, but could only serve as a temporary luting agent due to its low strength and high solubility.

11. a. The advantages of polycarboxylate cement are its ability to bond to tooth structure (one of the first) and its biocompatibility. It is usually used as a luting cement and an intermediate base. Its disadvantages are lack of strength and moderate solubility.

12. g. Zinc oxide and eugenol cement serves many purposes for the dental patient. Formulations of ZOE are used for luting temporary crowns, temporary restorations and intermediate bases under permanent restorations. It is soluble and lacks strength, so it is not recommended as a permanent restorative material or a luting agent for permanent crowns.

Chapter 8

1. b. A major advantage of alginate impression material is the ease of use. It is also fairly inexpensive. It is very much affected by the gain or loss of water. It should be poured as soon as possible because of its lack of stability.

2. b. Elastomeric impression materials, or elastomers, are flexible and may be deformed and then return to their original shape. Thermoplastic impression materials may be elastic or inelastic. They set by a physical change when cooled. Inelastic materials cannot be stretched; they also are rigid. Resins, by definition, are rigid polymers.

3. d. An increase in the water temperature will increase the rate of setting or shorten the gelation time. The mix is usable regardless of water temperature as long as there is adequate working time.

4. d. "Aqueous" refers to water. Therefore, the impression material must be water-based. In dentistry, there are two such materials: reversible and irreversible hydrocolloid. Irreversible was the only water-based choice. Polysulfides and addition silicones are elastomers. Impression compound is much like wax. ZOE impression material is an inelastic material and contains no water in its composition.

5. b. The brown paste in polysulfide impression material is the accelerator; the white paste is the base. Retarders are chemicals added to materials to decrease the setting rate. Fillers are added to the pastes to control the viscosity.

6. d. Dental impression compound is a thermoplastic material. It can be heated and softened repeatedly. Alginate is an example of an irreversible material. Once it has set, it cannot be resoftened. The other terms, chemoplastic and hydroelastic, are not used to describe impression materials.

7. b. ZOE impression paste sets into a hard, brittle mass. This makes it inelastic (or not elastic). Polysulfide and addition silicone are elastomers (they are elastic and will flex). Alginate also sets into an elastic material.

8. d. The hydrocolloids, alginate and agar, set by changing from a sol to a gel. This setting process is called gelation. Gypsum products (see Chapter 9) set by a crystallization process, and elastomeric impression materials set by polymerization. In dentistry, curing is another term for polymerization.

9. b. The use of agar impression material does require special equipment, but the impression material is very reasonably priced. The reproduction is excellent, and the impression is easy to pour compared to elastomeric impression material.

10. c. The shrinkage and exudation of water is syneresis. Imbibition occurs when the impression absorbs water, such as during long exposure to disinfecting solutions. Gelation is the term given to the setting process of hydrocolloid material. Hysteresis refers to a material's characteristic of having a melting temperature different from its gelling temperature.

11. a. Addition silicones are the most popular of the elastomeric impression materials, but cost is not the reason. They are expensive. Their ease of use and excellent characteristics and properties account for their popularity.

12. c. The accurate fit of the custom tray to the patient's oral tissues requires an existing model. Therefore, an alginate impression is usually taken and poured with a gypsum product (stone or plaster), and the tray is then made on the study model.

13. b. Alginate is the impression material of choice for these impressions They would be poured in dental stone and used for diagnosis and treatment planning. The accuracy of alginate is adequate for this purpose, but not for final impressions. Agar and elastomeric impression materials are final impression materials, meaning that casts and dies are made from these impressions on which restorations are fabricated. Dental impression compound is used for the fabrication of dentures.

14. c. With a triple tray, three "records" can be obtained: the prepared tooth, the bite registration and the impression of the opposing tooth. It is considered a special use tray. A custom tray is made on a model of the patient's arch with an acrylic resin. It is custom made by a dental professional. A stock tray is an "off the shelf" tray and can be purchased in a variety of shapes, sizes, and materials. Bite registration trays, another special use tray, record the occlusal surfaces of both arches.

15. a. ZOE, alginate, and addition silicone impression materials all set by a chemical reaction. Wax used as an impression material, agar, and impression compound set by a physical change, and will solidify or gel when cooled. These are said to be thermoplastic materials.

Chapter 9

1. a. The amount of water added to a gypsum product is directly related to its strength. The higher the W/P ratio, as in plaster, the softer and weaker the resulting gypsum product.

2. d. Potassium sulfate is a common accelerator for gypsum products, as is borax a retarder. Oleic acid, glycerin, and ethyl alcohol are not used to change the setting time of gypsum products.

3. d. High-strength stone may also be called die stone, improved stone, Type IV gypsum, Densite, or modified alpha-hemihydrate. Plaster is referred to as beta-hemihydrate or Type II gypsum. Dental stone may also be called Hydrocal, Type III gypsum, or alpha-hemihydrate.

4. b. As a standard setting time for gypsum products, 30 to 45 minutes for a final set is given. The Gillmore needle (or fingernail) should not leave indentations and can be used to determine a final setting time.

5. b. For 50 g of stone, 14 to 15 mL of water are required. For 100 g of stone, 28 to 30 mL of water are used. For 50 g of improved stone, 10 to 12 mL of water are used. For 100 g of plaster, 45 to 50 mL of water are needed.

6. c. Study models are used for observation, diagnosis, and treatment planning. Restorations or appliances are not made on them, as they are usually constructed from weaker gypsum products. Casts are replicas that are usually constructed with improved stone, and appliances and restorations are fabricated on them. A die is a working replica of a single tooth and is usually part of a cast.

7. a. Increasing the setting time would mean that it takes more time for a product to set. Thus, decreasing the setting time results in a product requiring less time to set. Manipulating the setting time does not enhance the properties of a gypsum product; in fact, it can be deleterious to them.

8. c. Because plaster requires the most water for a correct mix (proper W/P ratio), it would be the weakest, softest, and most porous of the three common gypsum products. Improved stone would be the most dense and the strongest, and dental stone would fall between plaster and improved stone.

9. b. Dry strength refers to the strength when excess water is not present. This may be two or three times the wet strength. The wet strength is measured at the final set (30–45 minutes). The initial strength occurs when loss of gloss is present and is an indication of the working time.

10. c. It is recommended to add first the water and then the powder to the mixing bowl. As a result, less air is incorporated into the mix. "Eyeballing" is not recommended because the W/P ratio will not be correct and inferior properties will result. Adding water to the powder or adding powder and water to the bowl simultaneously tend to increase the porosity of the resulting mix.

11. d. Final setting time can be determined by attempting to penetrate the material with a dull instrument or a fingernail. Initial setting time is said to occur when the material loses its shine, or "loss of gloss." Final setting time takes approximately 30–45 minutes. The change from wet to dry strength usually occurs after 8 hours.

12. a. When setting time is increased, it takes the material longer to set. A decreased setting time yields a faster setting material, or takes less time to set. If the setting reaction is decreased, the material will take longer to set, and if it is increased, it will take less time to set.

Chapter 10

1. c. The gypsum investment material that comprises the mold must be expanded to compensate exactly for the shrinkage of the metal casting. Otherwise, the cast restoration will not fit the preparation of the patient's tooth.

2. c. The mold (investment) must expand and provide compensation for the metal contraction during casting. The main, obvious purpose of the investment, however, is to create a mold from the wax pattern in the casting process.

3. c. Porcelain has outstanding esthetic properties, such as translucency and life-like appearance. It is very brittle, however, and may fracture when subjected to high occlusal forces. It is recommended for veneers and low-stress crowns for anterior teeth, such as maxillary lateral incisors.

4. b. The "crown" portion of a dental bridge is called a retainer. Joined to the retainers are the artificial, replacement teeth called pontics. The prepared teeth onto which the bridge is cemented are called abutments.

5. e. Inlay wax is used for casting procedures. It leaves no residue in the burnout process and has a higher melting temperature. It is also harder than other dental waxes. Sticky wax is also a hard wax that melts at a higher temperature, but this wax is used as an "attachment medium," such as attaching a sprue to a pattern. Boxing wax is used to pour impressions, and baseplate wax is used in the fabrication of dentures.

6. c. Burnout during casting is done to eliminate the wax pattern and create a mold space for the molten metal. Investment covers the wax pattern, which has been mounted within the casting ring, with a sprue. The crucible becomes heated when the solid casting metal is melted and turned into liquid, but it is an adjunct to the melting of the metal. Shrinkage compensation is necessary of the mold; it must expand the exact amount that the metal will shrink during casting.

7. a. Once the pattern is waxed, the sprue is gently attached with inlay or sticky wax. It is then placed into the crucible former (also called the sprue base). Next, a gypsum investment is usually vacuum mixed and poured into the casting ring that contains the wax pattern (investing process). After the casting ring is "burned out," the metal is melted and forced into the casting ring (casting).

8. c. 33% of 1,000 parts is 333. Fineness is described in parts per 1,000, so 33% would be 333 fine. A 33% gold alloy would be 8 carat. If the gold alloy is 50% gold, it would be 500 fine or 12 carat.

9. b. Changing porcelain powder to a solid is called sintering. The powder is not melted, so the shape of the restoration is maintained. Burnishing involves pushing the metal toward the tooth to close gaps between the casting and the tooth. Investing is covering a wax pattern mounted in a casting ring with a mixed gypsum product (investment).

10. a. It is true that castable glass is one type of all-ceramic restoration. It is not superior to ceramometal materials in the aspect of strength, however, and that makes the second statement false.

11. c. Amalgam, gold foil and composite restorations are direct restorations, meaning they are constructed directly in the oral cavity. It usually involves placing the restorative material "directly" into the cavity preparation. Other restorations, such as inlays, onlays, crowns, and bridges, are constructed outside of the oral cavity, in a dental laboratory. Hence, they are referred to as "indirect" restorations. The term "fixed" is used to designate that it is not removable because it is cemented, or luted, in place. A fixed restoration is not removable by the patient.

12. b. A veneer is a thin layer of material that covers another material. In dentistry, it is a restoration that is placed on the facial surface of anterior teeth to cover, or "veneer", esthetic problems. A buildup (core) is when a tooth is broken down to the point of needing "rebuilt" to hold the final restoration. A coping is the metal substructure that supports the porcelain layers in a ceramometal restoration. A pontic is a replacement tooth.

13. d. A provisional crown is the appropriate, professional name (especially used by prosthodontists) for a temporary crown.

14. c. Precious metals include the noble metals and silver. The noble metals are gold, platinum and palladium. Non-precious metals are those that do not

contain any noble elements. High-noble metals contain 60% or more gold and other noble elements.

15. a. Bonding porcelain to metal in a ceramometal restoration provides a precise fit to the prepared tooth structure. The disadvantage is the opacity, because of the metal. There is no difference between all ceramic or ceramometal crowns in the patient's ability to remove plaque.

Chapter 11

1. b. Once the denture teeth are set in the wax rims, it is called a denture setup. The other terms are not used to describe this step of denture fabrication and are listed as distracters.
2. a. A thin layer of material is ground away. The monomer is applied to dissolve some of the set material. One end of the dissolved polymer remains embedded in the acrylic denture resin. New material is then mixed and applied, and the new polymer chains entangle with the old dissolved chains. Applying monomer to the surface does not affect the setting reaction, finishing and polishing, or color of the denture.
3. d. The major difference between heat-activated and chemically activated resin systems is that no chemical activator is present in the liquid of the heat-activated resins. Heat-activated resins have more strength than chemically activated resins, and there is less, not more, inhibitor in the heat-activated liquid.
4. a. Today's denture teeth are usually acrylic rather than porcelain. Porcelain teeth are, however, harder than acrylic teeth and cause excessive wear to the natural opposing teeth.
5. c. Partial denture frameworks usually include clasps, connectors, and mesh. The denture base and teeth are not considered to be part of the framework, although they are a part of the removable partial denture.
6. b. Toughness is the ability of a material to absorb energy beyond the yield point, up to the failure point. Resilience is the ability to absorb energy and not become deformed until it reaches the yield point. Fatigue is the failure of an object after being stressed repeatedly for a long time. Creep is the small change in shape that results when an object is under continuous compression.
7. b. A maxillary denture is much easier to wear and a mandibular because of the extension of the borders of the denture (which helps to create the seal) and the larger surface bearing area. Saliva helps to achieve the seal and improve the suction.
8. d. The wax rims serve many purposes. They are used to determine the patient's midline, plane of occlusion, and the size of the denture teeth needed.
9. c. Partial dentures are processed the same way as a complete denture except that the acrylic resin must flow through and around the mesh of the framework. The finishing, polishing, and processing techniques take approximately the same amount of time.
10. 3, 6, 8, 5, 7, 1,10, 2, 9, and 4. After a master cast is made from patient impressions, a chemically activated resin baseplate and wax rims are constructed on it. These are tried in the patient's mouth and used to mount the master casts on an articulator. Next, the denture teeth are set in wax. This "wax denture" is called the denture setup and is inserted into the patient's mouth as the "wax try-in." Once the dentist and patient are satisfied with the fit, occlusion, function, esthetics, and phonetics, the master cast and denture setup are embedded in stone within the denture flask. The flask is heated in hot water and the wax is flushed out, creating a mold space. The denture teeth remain embedded in stone. The acrylic resin is mixed and placed in the mold, and the mold is then compressed. The closed mold is heated in a water bath to activate the resin. After processing, the denture is removed from the mold, finished, polished, and disinfected.

Chapter 12

1. d. Endosseous or tooth form implants are screwed or pressed into a cut hole in the bone. Transosseous or staple implants include a plate and bolts that transverse the anterior mandibular region. Subperiosteal implants involve two surgeries, an impression, cast, and a metal framework.
2. c. A healing cap is placed on the implant during the second surgery. It extends out of the mucosa into the oral cavity. Once this heals and epithelial tissues form, the healing cap is removed, and an abutment is placed. Impressions may be necessary before treatment is completed, but they are not taken during the second surgery. Osseointegration is not measured during either surgery.
3. b. The patient must maintain excellent plaque control and practice frequent and effective oral hygiene to ensure longevity of the implant. The dentist would adjust and monitor the occlusion of the implant with the opposing teeth. Fluoride applications at home are not typical for maintenance of implants.
4. d. The temperature of the bone must not be greater than 117°F or 47°C when the surgical handpiece is being used. The bone can be heated a little past body temperature, or 98.6°F. The temperature of 117°C is

equivalent to 243°F and would definitely damage the bone tissue.

5. a. Patients with systemic diseases, such as diabetes, are contraindicated for dental implants. Smokers and patients practicing poor oral hygiene are also poor candidates for implants. Recurrent caries are not associated with contraindications for dental implants.

6. c. It is true that titanium is very difficult to cast and does not have high strength compared to other metals. The strength of titanium is adequate for implants, however, and it will osseointegrate with bone.

7. b. An alveolar ridge having no teeth is said to be edentulous. In most cases, when the mandibular arch atrophies, it becomes smaller in size due to aging. An atrophic edentulous mandible is one that has no teeth, is very "low" and small, and would not be adequate to support a denture. The word "iatrogenic" means "caused by a professional by accident" and the word "dentulous" means "with, or having, teeth."

8. c. The patient's home care regimen may consist of only a toothbrush and floss, or a variety of many auxiliary aids. The hygienist will work with the patient to select the proper aids and instruct in their use to accomplish the necessary removal of plaque. Many appointments may be needed to accomplish this. Plaque removal by the patient is critical for the health and longevity of the implant. Without excellent homecare maintenance by the patient, the implant may fail over time.

9. d. In the first surgery, an implant is placed. In the next surgery, a healing cap is placed, which is exposed to the oral cavity. Later, the healing cap is removed and an abutment is placed on the implant. It acts as an abutment of a bridge and supports the prosthesis. A cylinder is then placed on the abutment, and then a crown is placed on the cylinder. All of these attachments are depicted in Figure 12.4.

10. c. The scope of practice of a dental hygienist does not include selecting restorative materials for tooth restoration. However, a very important role of the hygienist is patient education, determining the time between dental hygiene visits and selecting the best auxiliary aids for the patient to achieve optimal plaque removal.

Chapter 13

1. b. Obturate refers to the filling and sealing of the root canal once the pulp tissue is removed. Accessing the canal means to create an opening through the tooth to the pulp chamber. This is done with a handpiece and bur.

2. b. Macrofilled composite resins have large filler particles compared to microfills and hybrids. A metal instrument drawn across residual composite will result in a gray line. The filler particles in the resin are harder than the metal explorer and will abrade the metal tip, thus leaving a metal residue (gray line) on the remaining composite. The filler particles in microfill and hybrid composites are much smaller than the macrofill particles, and they may not leave a gray line.

3. d. An apicoectomy surgically removes 1 to 3 mm of the root apex. A retrofill is preparing, filling, and sealing of the apical end of the root. A root resection, another surgical procedure, is removal of an entire root of a multirooted tooth. Retreatment is root canal therapy performed a second time.

4. c. Irrigants are aqueous solutions used to disinfect the canal system. Common irrigants are sodium hypochlorite, saline, and chlorohexidine gluconate. Paper points are used to dry the root canal. Sealers are a type of cement used to coat the canal and to fill in voids between the canal wall and gutta percha. Gutta percha is a polymeric material with zinc oxide and barium sulfate added.

5. d. A retainer is a fixed (bonded) or removable appliance to prevent relapse after active orthodontic treatment is completed. A bracket is a small metal, ceramic, or polymer material that has a centered, horizontal slot. The archwire fits into the slot of each bracket, usually across the entire arch. A ligature, either wire or elastic, secures the archwire into the bracket slot.

6. a. Brackets are secured to the tooth surface by acid etching and composite resin. Dental cements may be used to secure bands to the tooth (molars). Chemically activated resins are used to make custom trays and denture fabrication and repairs. Ligatures secure the archwire into the bracket slot.

7. d. Lateral condensation is used to fill the root canal with gutta percha. Condensation is a term used in dentistry to describe the method of compressing and filling a small area in a tooth, such as a preparation or root canal. Of all the answers, this one is most appropriate.

8. a. For permanent molars, a pulpotomy is a temporary procedure and is followed by root canal therapy. For primary molars, it is a permanent procedure and is restored with a stainless-steel crown. This will maintain space and function until the permanent molar takes its place.

9. b. Orthodontic brackets are bonded onto the facial surfaces and hold an arch wire in place on each tooth in the arch. The brackets transfer the forces of the wire, springs and elastics to the teeth. Bands encircle the crown, and are used on molars because they

require more force to move compared to other teeth. Retainers are used to prevent relapse after treatment. Composite resin is used to attach the bracket to the tooth surface.

10. c. Surgical silk suture is nonabsorbable and must be removed at a later appointment. Absorbable sutures are usually placed on the inside of the body, and since the body resorbs them, a later appointment for removal is not necessary. Surgical gut suture is one type of absorbable suture.

Chapter 14

1. c. Glass ionomers, porcelain, and composite are the restorative materials that could be adversely affected by acidulated phosphate fluoride (APF). Because glass is a component of each of these materials, the APF could etch the surface of these restorative materials and result in a dull appearance and diminished luster.
2. c. When scalers and curettes are used around cast gold margins, use of a horizontal or oblique stroke, rather than a vertical one, is recommended. Vertical strokes have a tendency to "lift" the tightly adapted gold margins next to tooth structure. Posterior instruments are recommended for posterior teeth. Sonic and ultrasonic scalers are not recommended for use on cemented castings because they could fracture the cement underneath.
3. d. A dull sound would be heard from an explorer on composites and glass ionomers. Sharp sounds would be heard from gold foil, base metal alloys, enamel, dentin, amalgam, and cast gold.
4. d. Tactile sensitivity is derived from the sense of touch. When the clinician *lightly* holds an instrument, such as an explorer, the character of a surface is transmitted from the tip through the shank and then through the handle and into the clinician's fingertips. Therefore, the clinician would be distinguishing rough from smooth surfaces. Distinguishing dull sounds from sharp addresses auditory capabilities, or the sense of hearing; glossy from dull is a visual determination; and opaque from translucent are characteristics pertaining to radiographs.
5. b. When high heat is created during amalgam polishing, surface characteristics will be altered when temperatures reach or exceed 140°F. At high temperatures, mercury is released from the amalgam, which causes accelerated (not arrested) corrosion and marginal breakdown. Surfaces should be smoother, not rougher, after finishing and polishing. Tactile, rather than auditory, sensitivity is the criterion that best describes polishing (from rough surface to smooth), rather than a "dull" compared to a "sharp" sound.
6. a. The agents of choice for a final polish of a gold crown intraorally are silex and tin oxide. Brown and green polishing points are used for the initial steps. Aluminum oxide discs are used on composites, and prophylaxis pastes are used for porcelain.
7. a. There is much less heat production when a wet or moist abrasive or polishing agent is used compared to when it is dry. Swallowing and rinsing does not play a major role when using a moist polishing agent. In actuality, a dry polishing agent would remove stain faster than a moist one.
8. b. When the margins of a cast gold restoration have been marginated, it means the dentist has used hand instruments to adapt the edges of the restoration tightly to the preparation. The term "try-in" is used to describe if a casting fits precisely into the preparation before cementation. Margination and marginal ridges have very little in common. Marginal ridges are the mesial and distal boundaries of the occlusal surface. The gingival margin is the edge of the gingiva nearest the incisal or occlusal surface.
9. b. Because gold and/or gold foil are metallic restorations, like amalgam, they may be polished in a similar manner. The surface hardness of glass ionomer and composite are softer and the abrasives used on gold would be too abrasive for these materials. The porcelain on a PFM restoration could essentially be polished with anything; the metal portion, similar to amalgam or gold.
10. d. Because glass ionomer, porcelain and composite are made of glass particles or particles very similar to glass, the acidulated fluoride will etch the outer surface and cause a loss of reflection or possibly dull the appearance of the restoration.

Chapter 15

1. b. Dental hygienists must be competent to collect and assess data to formulate a dental hygiene diagnosis and to recognize anatomy, landmarks, and restorations to identify normal from abnormal, both clinically and radiographically. Dental hygienists do not legally provide a definitive diagnosis to the patient or prescribe radiographs.
2. c. The radiographic appearance for contrast of different objects in the mouth depends on the thickness and composition of the object/material. Very dense (compact) objects/materials absorb or attenuate more of the x-rays, thus allowing less of the primary beam to hit the film emulsion and fewer silver halide crystals to be exposed.

3. d. Less dense (compact) objects/materials absorb fewer x-rays and appear radiolucent on the radiograph. More dense objects appear radiopaque.

4. a. Gutta percha, although not a dense material, has fillers added to make it more dense and radiopaque.

5. a. Porcelain is radiolucent, and metal is radiopaque. When the two materials are combined in the fabrication of a crown (PFM), both the opacity and the lucency can be viewed. This is because of the density of the metal and the less-compact porcelain materials.

6. c. Amalgam is radiopaque because of its very compact/dense properties. A ZOE base is also more radiolucent (less radiopaque) than the adjacent amalgam restoration. Carious lesions appear more radiolucent compared to a ZOE base.

7. b. Orthodontic bands are metal and are radiographically opaque. Because the band encircles the entire tooth, it prohibits the practitioner from viewing the proximal or occlusal surfaces of the tooth on a radiographic film. Whether the band is bonded or cemented on the tooth would not make the difference. Fogging would appear radiolucent, not radiopaque.

8. c. A resorbable periodontal material used to heal and/or repair is not dense or compact enough to be viewed on a radiograph. The loss of periodontal bone that was radiolucent can be viewed, however. In the healing or repairing process, the alveolar bone "fills in" with new bone, which will be viewed as radiopaque.

9. a. Because the crestal bone is compact bone, it is radiographically opaque. When vertical or horizontal bone loss occurs, the opaque area of crestal bone becomes a radiolucent proximal space. The amalgam overhang is a radiopaque projection in the proximal space between the mesial of tooth #14 and the distal of tooth #13.

10. c. A base is somewhat dense because it is radiographically visible. Yet, the base is not as dense as the metal restoration. As a result, some x-rays pass through the base material to expose the silver halide crystals in the gelatin. This is not true of the metal restoration because the x-rays are absorbed (attenuated) by the metal, not allowing x-rays to pass through, thus resulting in an opaque image. If an object is translucent, it means you can see through it, as light will pass through. If an object is opaque, you are not able to see through it.

11. c. It is important to be able to distinguish dental materials from tooth tissues. Therefore, the shape of materials placed on, and in the tooth should be somewhat different from the expected anatomy of the tooth. The composition, the size or the amount of the restorative material is NOT a radiographically distinguishing critical feature when differentiating a radiopaque dental material from tooth tissues."

12. c. The composition and the amount of filler particles add density to the material when viewed radiographically. This density makes them more radiopaque, which distinguishes them from carious lesions. Compressive strength, elasticity, and coefficients of thermal expansion have nothing to do with the radiographic appearance of the restoration.

Chapter 16

1. d. Emery is the abrasive that is sometimes referred to as corundum. It is a natural form of aluminum oxide and appears as grayish-black sand. Tin oxide and pumice are abrasive powders, and garnet is a dark-red abrasive that is usually found on coated disks.

2. b. Pumice is a silica-like volcanic glass that is used to polish enamel, gold foil, amalgam, and acrylic denture bases. Aluminum oxide is another name for emery. Sand is a form of quartz, may be of various colors, and is bonded to paper disks for grinding metals and plastics. Zirconium silicate is a common abrasive in dentifrices.

3. b. Calcium carbonate is also called chalk, or whiting. It is a mild abrasive, usually supplied in powder form, and mixed with a "vehicle" (liquid) to produce a slurry. Silex and pumice are used in the same manner. Aluminum oxide is an abrasive that is found in many grits, bonded onto disks and strips, and impregnated into rubber wheels and points.

4. a. The abrasive particle must be harder than the surface being abraded to achieve the desired result. If it is softer, the surface meant to be abraded will not be, and instead, the abrasive will be worn away.

5. d. Hardness of the abrasive particle, particle size, particle shape, pressure, speed, and lubrication used all affect the rate of abrasion. Bonded and coated abrasives encompass a wide variety of agents. They are usually bonded, impregnated, or coated onto disks, strips, points, rubber wheels, burs, or stones.

6. d. Finishing is the term used when producing the final shape and contour of a restoration. Polishing is the abrasion of a surface to reduce the size of the scratches until the surface appears shiny. Abrasion is the wearing away of a surface. Cutting is removing material by a shearing-off process. Examples of cutting are milling, machining, or drilling.

7. c. "Vehicles," usually liquids, are used with powders to create a slurry. Examples of vehicles used with powders include water, glycerin, alcohol, and mouthwash.

Rubber cups and brushes as well as felt cones are devices used in polishing teeth and dental appliances.

8. c. Both statements are true. Abrasives are used in a series (most abrasive to least abrasive) during polishing. The same agent (from larger grit to smaller grit) or different agents (from most abrasive to least abrasive) may be used. The size of the scratches becomes smaller as the chosen abrasive becomes finer, until the scratches finally are smaller than the wavelength of visible light. When the scratches are this size, the surface appears shiny.

9. b. It has been documented in the literature that up to 3 to 4 μm of enamel may be removed when polishing with pumice. This coronal portion of the tooth is the fluoride-rich layer of enamel that has been absorbing fluoride from various sources, including food, water, dentifrices, and topical fluoride applications.

10. d. Ideal prophylaxis pastes should possess the characteristics of high polish and low abrasion. A high polish produces the shiny, smooth surface as a result of polishing, and low abrasion refers to the grit of the abrasive within the paste and the resulting "scratches" that it leaves on the surface after "polishing."

11. a. Looking at Table 16.1, restorative materials, abrasives, and tooth tissues are listed in order of hardness. Pumice is harder than enamel, but amalgam, composite, and gold alloy are all softer than enamel.

12. b. Air powder polishing is designed to remove plaque, biofilm (soft deposits), and stain. This equipment is unlike a sonic or ultrasonic scaler that would remove calculus. It is designed as a "polisher" combining air, water, and an abrasive agent under pressure.

13. c. Silica is the most frequently used abrasive in dentifrices. The other two dentifrices used in recent years are phosphates and carbonates.

14. c. A finely ground diamond powder would be used to polish esthetic restorations. Calcium carbonate and pumice would be found in specific traditional prophylaxis pastes. Emery is an abrasive that is mostly used in dental laboratory procedures.

15. a. The traditional prophy paste would be used on the stain on the natural teeth. The tin oxide is recommended for the gold, and the polishing agent for the esthetic restorations would be used on the composite restorations. Pumice and silex have been used to remove heavy stains on natural teeth in the past, and are also used for polishing amalgams. In the selection of polishing agents for restorations and natural teeth, it is important remove the deposit with the least abrasive agent.

Chapter 17

1. d. A nonvital tooth is one that does not have a live (vital) pulp. The pulp may be present but necrotic, missing, or replaced with a root canal filling material.

2. b. Tooth structure must be removed to obtain an opening into the pulp chamber of a nonvital tooth. A facial veneer requires removal of facial tooth structure, and a porcelain-bonded-to-metal crown requires removal of tooth structure from all surfaces.

3. c. Carbamide peroxide is more stable than hydrogen peroxide. It is used only in the vital tooth whitening technique. It decomposes into hydrogen peroxide and is used in concentrations from 10% to 20%. Hydrogen peroxide decomposes into water and oxygen radicals.

4. a. Any number of teeth can be treated at the same time. A full arch of teeth can be treated in the same time as one tooth in the same arch.

5. d. Extrinsic stains are more effectively treated than intrinsic stains and discolorations. Tetracycline-stained teeth and teeth with fluorosis are difficult to treat.

6. b. Tooth sensitivity, the most common side effect associated with tooth whitening, is usually reversible. After the treatment is discontinued, it should be absent in a few days. Potassium nitrate and neutral sodium fluoride are common topical agents used in the active treatment of tooth sensitivity. A tray made of rigid material frequently produces pressure on one or more teeth to cause sensitivity.

7. d. Esthetic dental procedures are increasing in popularity, but the procedure most commonly used today is tooth whitening.

8. a. Brushing with a potassium nitrate containing dentifrice will aid in reducing tooth sensitivity that may occur during/after whitening. Anesthesia should not be used during power bleaching so that a patient could respond to any painful stimuli possibly produced by excessive heat created during the procedure.

9. d. The restoration should not be placed sooner than 1–2 weeks, preferably 2 weeks. The bonding capabilities of composite are initially weaker post bleaching and usually return after 1 week. The tooth initially lightens but tends to darken and remains a stable color around 2 weeks post treatment. Any sooner placement will result in a composite that may not match or may not adhere to tooth structure.

10. d. All of the conditions except previous use of night guard bleaching system is contraindicated. Patients

using photosensitive drugs, undergoing chemotherapy or radiation therapy, or having a history of melanoma are all at additional risks of medical complications with light-activated bleaching systems. Many patients move from the use of night guard tray systems to the light activated systems in search of better and quicker whitening results.

Chapter 18

1. d. The goal of oral appliance therapy is to enlarge the airway and to reduce its collapsibility to maintain an adequate airway during sleep. Reducing the airway would make it more difficult to maintain adequate breathing.
2. d. According to published research, patients wearing an oral appliance during sleep have demonstrated no changes in their periodontal health. There have been no increases in periodontal conditions or diseases reported with use of the oral appliance.
3. c. Athletic mouthguards, when worn correctly and consistently, may prevent a concussion by aiding absorption of the dynamic pressures of head trauma.
4. b. Nightguards are worn to alleviate tooth surface wear by absorbing occlusal pressure that occurs from grinding of teeth during sleep. Nightguards have not been reported to decrease dental caries. Orthodontic appliances may be worn to provide minor tooth movement or teeth stabilization. Space maintainers temporarily hold teeth in position.
5. d. Stock mouthguards are premade, in various sizes, and may be purchased at athletic and department stores. Custom mouthguards are fabricated by dental professionals to fit the patient's arch; they require an impression and cast.
6. a. Thermoplastic material will soften on heating and reharden on cooling. This makes them ideal for adapting to an individual's dentition.
7. a. Wet, soft-bristled toothbrushes are recommended to clean oral appliances. Commercial liquid cleaners are also available for soaking. Hot water is not recommended because of possible distortion of the appliance.
8. d. Mouth protectors can be custom-made by the dental professional, bought at a store in a presized selection (stock mouthguard), and prepared through the "boil-n-bite" method by the individual.
9. c. Space maintainers are used to temporarily hold teeth in position. For example, if a deciduous molar is prematurely lost, a space maintainer may be used to keep the adjacent teeth from moving into that area where the tooth is missing. Nightguards are worn to alleviate bruxism. Custom bleaching trays are designed to hold bleaching solutions. Sleep apnea is alleviated by an appliance that enlarges the airway.
10. a. It is vital that the athletic mouthguard be compatible with the athlete's dentition, so that the force can be absorbed by the appliance and the athlete will be more likely to wear the appliance when needed. In most cases, athletic mouthguards are fabricated for maxillary teeth.
11. c. The gingival contours of teeth should be detailed, or replicated in an oral appliance because they are needed to help the appliance fit properly and aid with retention. The sulcus and periodontal ligament are essentially subgingival and do not aid in retention of the appliance. The soft palate is located posterior to the hard palate, and is not adjacent to the teeth, so it would not help to retain the appliance.
12. c. An adult patient undergoing radiation for head or neck cancer is at increased risk for dental caries. The radiation damages the salivary glands, resulting in xerostomia, which in turn contributes to caries. Fluoride will not aid in the treatment of halitosis or periodontal disease. A 3 year old may not be compliant in the use of custom trays and there is an increased risk of ingesting fluoride.

Chapter 19

1. b. Tarnish is a corrosive attack that produces a film or layer on a metal surface. Corrosion is a process in which a metal is changed to a metal oxide. Electrochemical corrosion is a combination of a chemical reaction and the flow of an electric current. Galvanic corrosion is an electrochemical process in a wet environment. Two dissimilar metals and an electrolyte solution cause a current to flow, which results in corrosion.
2. c. Passivation is done in the manufacture of instruments and creates a layer of chromium oxide on the instrument surface to protect it from corrosion. Tarnish is a corrosive attack that produces a film or layer on a metal surface. Electropolishing produces a smooth, highly polished finish that is less likely to corrode. Alloys are made by combining two or more metals in a molten state.
3. d. The standard protocol for chemical vapor sterilization is 270°F, 20 to 40 psi, for at least 20 minutes (not 10 minutes, as in choice "c"). Steam autoclaving occurs at 270°F, 27 psi, for at least 6 minutes. Dry heat sterilization involves 2 hours and a temperature of 320°F.

4. a. Risks are involved when retipping instruments, but frequent breakage between the shank and tip is not listed as one of the many risks. These risks include detachment, contamination, imbalance, and wear rates.
5. b. Three questions need to be asked to determine when instruments should be sharpened: First, "How many times a day did I, or will I, use that instrument?" Second, "What degree of difficulty did I, or will I, encounter while using this instrument?" Third, "For what procedures did I use, or will I be using, the instrument?"
6. d. The major components of stainless-steel alloy are iron, chromium, and nickel.
7. a. The disadvantage of using noble metals in the fabrication of instruments is cost. They are very expensive compared to stainless steel or carbon steel. Pitting and corrosion would not occur with noble metals and would be ideal for instrument composition. A faster wear rate may occur with "noble metal instruments" compared to carbon-steel and stainless-steel instruments, but it is not the major disadvantage.
8. c. Dry heat sterilization is used when items to be sterilized cannot withstand compressed steam conditions. Unsaturated chemical vapor sterilization is recommended for carbon steel instruments, but disadvantages include odor and a need for ventilation. The temperature for steam autoclaving is 270° F and for dry heat it is 320° F, therefore materials that could not withstand these heat sterilization processes should be sterilized with chemical solutions.
9. c. The correct sequence in the instrument maintenance cycle is to use sterile instruments, inspect them after use, clean them appropriately, sterilize them, and then sharpen sterile instruments. The safest time to sharpen instruments is after sterilization, immediately before use.
10. b. Electropolishing is the procedure that produces a highly polished finish. Passivation is the creation of a corrosion resistant chromium oxide layer. Cryogenics is the science of very low temperatures, far below the freezing point of water. Heat treatment is a combination of heating and cooling operations timed and applied to a metal or alloy, that result in desired mechanical properties.

Chapter 20

1. c. PPE must not be worn out of the treatment area because it is contaminated from splatter and aerosol and, thus, is a source of infection.
2. b. Nonsterile exam gloves are sufficient for most dental procedures. Sterile surgeon's gloves are necessary only during invasive (surgical) procedures. Neither copolymer gloves nor utility gloves are acceptable for any intraoral procedure.
3. c. Because of the potential for leakage of gloves, hands should be washed before donning and after removing them. In October 2002, the CDC endorsed the use of alcohol-based products for hand cleaning as long as the hands are not visibly contaminated.
4. c. Utility gloves are the thickest glove and would afford more protection against potential injury from a sharp instrument.
5. c. If a patient with a highly infectious disease spread by aerosol is treated, a HEPA mask must be worn to filter out microbes. Standard masks do not have a high-enough filtration capability. Use of surgeon's gloves does not protect against aerosol, and a face shield allows for suction of aerosol up under the shield.
6. a. Sharp objects must be disposed of in hard, puncture-resistant containers and not in cardboard boxes or plastic bags.
7. e. Glutaraldehydes are high-level disinfectants in which items must be immersed. They are too toxic to be sprayed.
8. c. Both statements are true. An acceptable disinfectant must kill both hydrophilic and lipophilic viruses. The protein coating on hydrophilic viruses makes them much more difficult to kill compared to lipophilic viruses.
9. a. According to Spalding's classification, any item with the potential to penetrate soft tissue or bone is considered to be a "critical" item and must be heat sterilized only.
10. c. Neither disinfection nor sterilization will occur if bioburden is not first removed from the object being disinfected or sterilized.
11. c. Steel-toed shoes will protect the feet from falling objects but are not common in dental offices. Fire extinguishers, GFCI outlets, neoprene (rubber) gloves, and eye protection are common.
12. e. Mercury, disinfectants, latex gloves, and nitrous oxide have all caused problems to health care workers. Fluorescent lighting has not.
13. c. A variety of chemicals in the dental office can penetrate latex gloves. Information regarding the proper protective gloves is found in the materials safety data sheet.
14. c. Poor lighting, poor posture, and repetitive motions contribute to musculoskeletal problems. Use of indirect vision contributes to proper posture and lower strain on the back and neck.

15. a. Mercury (Hg) vapor is the most hazardous form of Hg encountered in a dental office. It is readily absorbed by the lungs. Liquid Hg is also hazardous because it has a high vapor pressure. Dental amalgam is safe, however, because the Hg is bound in a metallic compound. The same is true for amalgam scrap.

Chapter 21

1. c. All blood and saliva must be cleaned from any item before application of a disinfectant because they inhibit disinfection.
2. a. Unlike the other impression materials, alginate may be adversely affected by disinfectants. The process of imbibition, or uptake of water, may occur and result in a distorted impression. Therefore, full immersion time should be limited to 10 minutes.
3. c. Disinfecting appliances is not indicated when adjustments at chairside are performed as long as sterile handpieces, burs, and rag wheels are used.
4. b. 10 minutes. Less than 10 minutes is not adequate for disinfection to occur, and longer than 10 minutes may adversely affect the metal.
5. b. Do not clean ultrasonically by placing appliances directly into solution in the ultrasonic holding tank. All other statements must be followed. When cleaning the appliance in an ultrasonic unit, however, the appliance must be placed in a leak-proof, zippered bag or sterile glass beaker that contains fresh ultrasonic solution. Then, the bag or beaker is placed in the solution in the holding tank. This will prevent cross-contamination during cleaning.
6. b. Neither statement nor reason is correct. Even though a dental prosthesis is disinfected before making adjustments with a rag wheel in the laboratory and before returning the prosthesis to the patient, there is the potential for cross-contamination between patients if a sterile rag wheel is not used for each patient's prosthesis.
7. c. A zippered plastic bag containing mouthwash and water is the recommended storage method. Water is needed for hydration and to prevent distortion. The mouthwash provides a pleasant taste for the patient. The patient's stone cast would not be clean. An individualized, closed container (denture cup) must have a liquid in it to prevent distortion of the prostheses.
8. c. Iodophors are suitable for all impression materials. The impression materials and the recommended disinfectants are listed in Table 21.1. Glutaraldehydes should not be sprayed because they are toxic as aerosols, and sodium hypochlorite could bleach out the pink, gingival tissue color in the appliance.
9. c. The primary goal is to prevent cross-contamination. This includes protecting the patient, laboratory personnel from each other, as well as the dental office staff and laboratory equipment.
10. c. When using a spray, constant contact with all the surfaces cannot be assured. Spraying twice is not a recommended method, and only the aerosol of glutaraldehydes are considered toxic.

Chapter 22

1. c. The tubes of paste/paste materials have openings sized to dispense the proper ratio of pastes when equal lengths are utilized.
2. c. It is important to read, understand, and follow directions. Understanding the procedures involved when using a material will reduce the likelihood of an error.

Chapter 23

1. c. Both calcium hydroxide and ZOE are significantly accelerated by humidity as water increases ionization of the components and thus setting.
2. b. ZOE has an sedative or obtundent effect on the dental pulp. Calcium hydroxide and glass ionomer are fairly neutral while zinc phosphate is initially irritating.
3. c. Zinc phosphate cement is mixed slowly to dissipate the heat of the setting reaction. ZOE takes time to mix because of the effort required to incorporate sufficient powder. Calcium hydroxide and glass ionomer cements are mixed quickly.
4. d. Glass ionomer cements should be used before they lose their glossy appearance. If the cement is dull, the setting reaction may have progressed to the point where adhesion is decreased.
5. c. Set dental cements are insoluble in water and therefore not soluble with soap and water. Cleaning is much easier before these materials set as they can be wiped off instruments and are soluble in soap and water before setting.

Chapter 24

1. b. 6×6 inch square is the most common pre-cut size of rubber dam material. The 5×5 inch square is used for primary dentition or anterior teeth.

2. e. All of the above are used on the removal of the rubber dam, see Table 24.2.
3. c. The treatment tooth is mesial to the anchor to allow access without interference by the clamp.
4. c. The rubber dam is contraindicated for patients with severe asthma.
5. c. The butterfly-shaped clamp is used to isolate the facial surfaces of anterior and some posterior teeth and retracts the adjacent gingiva.

Chapter 25

1. c. Dental sealants are effective in preventing dental caries by eliminating sites difficult to clean with normal patient oral hygiene. They do not contribute to remineralization of tooth structure, so they do not reverse decay or restore enamel integrity.
2. b. Enamel appears chalky white when properly etched because the surface is microscopically rough. The etched surface scatters light like ground glass rather than reflecting it like a smooth mirror.
3. c. After placing, the sealant should be checked for both high occlusal contacts with articulating paper and open interproximal contracts with floss

Chapter 26

1. b. Tin oxide is used as a polishing agent to produce a high luster on amalgam restoration surfaces.
2. d. Excessive heat generation may produce an increased susceptibility to breakdown and corrosion.
3. b. The surface is discolored. Tarnish is a removable surface film or discoloration on the amalgam. It does not affect the internal integrity of the restoration.
4. c. Both statements are true. It is important to begin with coarser abrasives and progress to less abrasive materials. Coarse abrasives produce larger scratches and as the operator progresses to smaller abrasives, the larger scratches become less defined.
5. b. Ideally, all amalgam restorations should be finished and polished 24 hours after placement. This allows for correction of problems or conditions incurred during placement, thereby reducing plaque accumulation.
6. a. The primary purpose of finishing and polishing amalgams is to produce a smooth surface, free of voids, that is less likely to tarnish or corrode.
7. a. A submarginal area is a term used when an internal wall of the preparation is exposed, most likely due to an overcarved amalgam.
8. c. During the finishing of amalgam restorations, it is important to maintain the original anatomy of the restoration to assure functional anatomy.
9. d. Corrosion is a surface or subsurface chemical deterioration that occurs on or within the amalgam restoration. Finishing and polishing are unable to improve the excessive corrosion defects within the amalgam alloy.
10. c. Green and brown points and cups are used to produce a smooth satin and shiny surface to the amalgam restoration. They are used only for polishing and not for finishing.

Chapter 27

1. f. All of these procedures should be accomplished before the impression is taken. Clothing should be protected with a napkin and the patient should be upright to minimize gagging. Appliances should be removed so they are not captured in the impression. The mouthwash will reduce organism count for the operator and dental lab technicians.
2. c. The 11:00 position for the maxillary impression gives the operator the best access and control over the patient and helps to ensure the best results. The operator would be at 7:00 for the mandibular arch. For the left handed operator, the maxillary impression would be taken at the 1:00 position, and the mandibular at the 5:00 position.
3. b. Add the powder to the water to ensure the proper mix and best result. It has been thought that adding water to powder would increase the chance of incorporating air bubbles into the mix.
4. d. It is true that the cooler water will increase, or lengthen, the time the operator has to work with the material. Conversely, warmer water will decrease, or shorten, the working time. Working time begins when the powder and water come in contact with each other.
5. b. The mixing time is usually one minute to mix the material, fill the tray and seat the impression. For regular set, the setting time is usually 3 to 4 minutes.

Chapter 28

1. b. The first pour will have initially set before the second pour is done, which helps to prevent distortion. It may take longer than a single-pour or boxing wax technique. There is no difference in reproduction quality among the different types of pours.
2. a. Loss of gloss (the cast or model is no longer shiny) is an indication that the initial setting time is near,

usually 10 minutes after the initial pour. Resilience and elasticity are characteristics that do not apply to gypsum products. As a gypsum product sets, the compressive strength would increase, rather than decrease.

3. a. This combined height is most esthetically pleasing while maintaining the integrity of the oral structures. Choices a and b would mean that the models have no, or very little base; the last choice, an overall height of 3.0–3.5 inches would indicate models with extremely thick bases.

4. Answer: 3, 5, 1, 6, 7, 2, 4 is the correct sequence for the steps in model trimming.

Chapter 29

1. b. As mentioned in the reading, one of the main advantages of using custom trays for impressions is that the operator has complete control of every dimension of the impression tray. By customizing the shape of the tray during fabrication, anatomic anomalies can readily be accommodated.

2. c. The accuracy of the final impression is influenced by the thickness of impression material. To ensure the proper thickness of impression material, there should be 2 mm to 3 mm of space between the impression tray and the cast during fabrication.

3. b. The extension of the custom tray resin 3 mm to 4 mm beyond the gingival margin onto the tissues is adequate to capture all of the anatomy of the teeth and supporting gingiva. A tray that is too short will not control the flow of the impression material. The resulting impression could lack all of the anatomic features necessary to fabricate the final prosthesis.

4. a. When taking the final impression, occlusal stops allow the dentist to confirm the tray has been fully seated and stable in the mouth. This, in turn, allows a consistent and proper thickness of impression material for an accurate impression.

5. a. Custom tray borders should always be checked with your fingers to verify the borders are smooth, continuous and rounded. Remember, these borders will be engaging the soft tissues of the patient's mouth. Sharp edges can traumatize the soft tissues.

Chapter 30

1. c. The impression tray must be held in place for 5 to 7 minutes so that the tray material and the syringe material can join and set properly. It is very important to follow the manufacturer's directions.

2. d. The benefits of using this material are that it is stable, accurate, is easy to clean up and the impression can be poured at a later time. Even though it is more expensive than other impression materials, many dentists feel the advantages outweigh the cost.

3. b. Two people should be involved in preparing addition silicone impression material. One person fills the tray, while the other is working with the syringe material. Once the syringe material is injected around the area of interest, the tray material is immediately seated on top of it.

4. c. The warmer temperature of the palm will accelerate, or decrease the setting time of the impression material. Using the fingertips allows for proper working and setting time. The material does not stain the operator's hands, nor is it difficult to remove from the surface of the skin.

5. d. In most instances, the tray adhesive will dry in the impression tray in 10 minutes.

Chapter 31

1. c. The power (light/heat activated) whitening agent is the professionally applied whitening material. The night guard whitening agents may be professionally supervised but are patient applied. Dentifrices and mouthrinses are over the counter and patient applied materials.

2. c. The custom vinyl tray would be used to apply night guard whitening. Boil and bite and athletic mouth guards would be too bulky. Fluoride trays would not fit snugly for the whitening material.

3. d. Using a scalloped tray and using a small dot of whitening in the facial surfaces of tray will help keep the material from leaching onto gingival tissues. There is no evidence that rinsing prior to whitening would eliminate gingival irritation. Mouthrinses containing alcohol may cause gingival irritation.

4. d. All of the above. To observe results and record them accurately, a photograph is necessary with a shade guide, both initially and after bleaching has been completed.

5. a. Teeth must be isolated to limit the whitening agent to tooth surfaces only. The gingival tissue must also be protected from irritation by the whitening agents. The whitening agent is activated by light or heat. Teeth and tissue are not hydrated but actually dehydrated during the procedure. There are no known nutrients in the resin dam material.

Chapter 32

1. b. The recommended bur is the tapered plain-cut finishing bur. It should be used with a low speed handpiece for better access and control. In addition, in most state practice acts, use of high speed handpieces is not permitted by hygienists. There are no tapered cross-cut finishing burs. Straight fissure plain-cut and cross-cut burs are designed to take away much more surface than finishing burs and therefore, would not be indicated for debonding.
2. c. It is true that all debonding methods remove some enamel. Some methods remove much more than others. It is the responsibility of the hygienist to select the least damaging method for resin removal.
3. d. The stroke of the debonding bur should be toward the incisal or occlusal surface to avoid accidental trauma to the gingiva. One would not intentionally use the bur in the gingival direction because of the possibility of tissue injury. It is not recommended to use the bur toward the interproximal/ embrasure surface. It may be efficient in one direction (i.e., toward the mesial), but it may not be in the other direction (toward the distal).
4. a. All composite resin material should be removed to avoid gingival inflammation, stain, plaque, poor esthetics, decalcification/caries formation, and mucosal response from rough resin. Resin left from the bonding of orthodontic brackets should not affect the patient's occlusion.
5. b. Compressed air should be applied frequently and the surface examined visually to determine if the surface is free of resin. Having the patient rub his or her tongue over the surface will also aid in residual resin detection. The bur should be used in brush-like strokes and there is no determined time limit in its use. In most cases burs do not need to be changed before one patient is completed. In heavy cases though, a new bur may be needed for each patient.

Chapter 33

1. c. Post-surgical healing proceeds at a normal rate with or without a dressing. Antimicrobials can be added to some dressings to decrease likelihood of an infection, but the healing rate is not influenced. Bleeding of the surgical site is stopped before the dressing is placed. The dressing will help control post-surgical bleeding, however, by holding the initial clot in place. Also, a surgical dressing cannot "sterilize" the surgical site. Bacteria and food particles will find their way under the dressing, although a smooth surface will make the dressing less plaque retentive. The presence of the dressing does provide a physical barrier to friction during eating and speaking, thus providing comfort for the patient. This also helps to hold tissues in place during healing, which is particularly important in graft and flap surgeries. The rigidity of the noneugenol mineral oxide packs supports mobile teeth during healing, also.
2. a. As the dressing is being placed, pressure is applied in the interdental spaces to help force dressing between the teeth, providing physical or mechanical retention. The dressing can also be forced interdentally by use of an instrument, or by molding small pieces of dressing into the interproximal spaces.
3. d. The surgical site should be covered, but extending a surgical pack to the occlusal surface is not necessary. This over extension will likely be in the way of movements of the mandible, which would be disconcerting to the patient and may jeopardize the integrity of the dressing. Extension to the depth of the vestibule would also cause discomfort. The noneugenol metallic oxide dressing is maintained in place by mechanical retention, thus interlocking in the interdental embrasures is needed for retention rather than easy removal. The properly placed dressing should be smooth with tapered edges and have just enough bulk to provide rigidity.
4. d. Saltwater rinses alone may not provide adequate comfort for the patient. The noneugenol zinc oxide dressing would be too bulky, and aesthetics would be of concern. Although the visible light-activated surgical dressing may be aesthetically acceptable, the dressing would need to be removed at a follow-up appointment. The cyanoacrylate dressing gives esthetically acceptable coverage without bulk and is biodegradable.
5. b. Exposing the dressing to warm liquids or warm foods may soften the dressing. Smoking also exposes the dressing to heat. (It also delays healing.) If a small piece of dressing crumbles off, it is usually of no consequence and can simply be discarded. If a piece of the dressing is broken away, one needs to return to the office for care only when this causes discomfort.

Chapter 34

1. a. Surgical pack removal is done by inserting a sturdy, blunt instrument under the edge of the dressing and applying steady controlled movement. The surface of the instrument that is against the friable soft tissue should be smooth. The pressure applied to the dressing should be steady and controlled in case suture material has become incorporated into the

dressing material. These sutures will need to be cut to allow dressing removal.

2. c. Healing is not compromised by age alone, nor is it compromised when diabetes is well controlled. Retained calculus would most likely cause overgrowth of beady granulation tissue. The cause is most likely due to a suture that was overlooked in the posterior of the maxillary vestibule.
3. d. Areas of residual calculus are removed at the post-surgical appointment to allow for healing of the tissues.
4. c. Care should be taken not to cut the knot away from the submerged suture material. This could result in suture material that is completely submerged and not retrievable. One blade of the scissors is inserted into the opening created under the knot, and only one end of the suture is cut.
5. c. Chromic gut and polylactic suture materials are absorbable. Looking for a "smaller" sized suture material, one would look for more 0s. A 3-0 sized suture material would be larger than the 4-0 suture material asked for.

Chapter 35

1. b. An alternative term used to describe a temporary crown is provisional restoration. Temporary crowns are custom fit to the tooth. They are made with suck-down molds and acrylic resins materials.
2. c. Proper occlusal and interproximal contacts of a temporary crown are important. If the occlusal contacts are high, the patient will likely return with a sore tooth from hyperocclusion. If they are low, the tooth may drift up (down) into occlusion and the permanent crown will need a great deal of adjustment. The interproximal contacts need to be properly adjusted so the tooth does not move mesial or distal which will result in excessively tight or open contacts for the permanent crown.
3. d. A well-constructed temporary crown will improve patient comfort, esthetics, and function. A tooth prepared for a crown will likely feel very odd to the tongue, appear very small or malformed, and must function well for eating.

Chapter 36

1. b. The most effective method to prevent overheating of the pulp when polishing a composite is to keep the tooth and composite moist with water spray or irrigation. Light strokes will help but overheating can occur rapidly with abrasive rubber points. Petroleum jelly is not as effective as water. Fine grit abrasives are used last, not first.
2. d. Ideally, composite restorations should be finished and polished at the placement appointment. Composites obtain the great majority of their strength when polymerized. Therefore, there is no need to wait before finishing and polishing. Delaying finishing and polishing could negatively affect plaque retention and esthetics.
3. c. Coarser abrasive disks should be followed by finer abrasive disks to initially remove material containing the larger scratches and defects in the composite surface. Less aggressive removal of material is needed to remove the materials containing the remaining smaller scratches.
4. d. Composite materials are made of a polymer filled with a ceramic material. Neither component corrodes as metals do. Finishing and polishing composites does improve the surface luster, marginal contours and thus gingival health.
5. d. The egg/football-shaped finishing bur most closely matches the desired shape of the anatomy of the lingual surface of an anterior tooth and therefore, is the most effective abrasive to use.

Case 1

1. c. The remaining natural teeth are the mandibular right first (tooth #28) and second (tooth #29) premolars, the right canine (tooth #22), and the left first molar (tooth #19). It is easiest to see this tooth arrangement if you look at the removable appliance in Photo C.
2. b. The correct terminology for this appliance is "removable partial denture." Bridges are usually a fixed appliance. "Partial" is a commonly used name, shortened from the correct term. It is not a fixed partial denture, however, because the patient can remove it.
3. d. The clasps on this appliance encircle the mandibular right second premolar (tooth #28), the left canine (tooth #22), and the left first molar (tooth #19).
4. b. If the appliance contains porcelain teeth, it would have three materials: porcelain, the metal framework, and the resin base. If the teeth are resin (somewhat different than the denture base resin), the appliance could still be said to be composed of three materials.
5. d. The information presented in the case states that the patient has very little plaque and stain. The patient will be best served by closely examining the

teeth after scaling to determine which teeth warrant polishing because they are extrinsically stained. The other agents contain an abrasive (even the fine paste) that is more than the patient would need to clean the surfaces of the teeth.

6. c. Keeping the patient's limited income in mind and making thorough notes in the chart, you could see if the patient education resulted in a lower deposit accumulation at the next recall. If it did, keep the recall date at 1 year; if it did not, change the recall date to 6 months.

Case 2

1. a. The prepared teeth in the photographs are the maxillary right second (tooth #2) and first (tooth #3) molars. The dental anatomy, as well as the radiographs, help the observer to identify these teeth. The roots and the sinus cavity help to determine the arch, and the narrowed occlusal outline helps to distinguish left from right.
2. b. Base materials are usually thick in dimension so that they can provide strength and thermal insulation from hot and cold foods and liquids. Liners are usually thin and protect the pulp from chemical irritation, such as that from acid etching.
3. c. From the most distal surface going mesially, the names of the cavity preparations are: occlusal (O), mesiocclusal (MO), and distocclusolingual (DOL). The most distal prep (the occlusal) is not a DO, even though it may appear that way. The marginal ridge has not been prepared—hence, an occlusal preparation.
4. d. Besides the restorative needs, the patient also exhibits root calculus on the distal of tooth #2 and significant bone loss. The bone loss and deposits are evidence of periodontal disease. The patient may have gingivitis as well. The Photographs A and B are only black and white, but the patient is wearing a rubber dam; therefore, evidence of gingivitis cannot be seen. Gingivitis is never evident on a radiograph.
5. d. The root calculus indicates the need for root planing. This may need to be done with local anesthesia in several appointments. Ideally, a reevaluation appointment is scheduled after all the scaling is complete to check the tissue, presence of deposits, and the patient's home care regimen. Polishing is also performed in this appointment if indicated.
6. c. The use of a finishing bur, polishing first with a slurry of pumice, and then one of tin oxide, is a typical technique used in polishing amalgams. Using finishing burs will provide a smooth finished surface before polishing. Using tin oxide alone is not an adequate abrasive and prophylaxis pastes are designed to remove stain on natural teeth rather than provide a smooth surface and a high shine that we hope to achieve for amalgam restorations.
7. c. Monitoring all the teeth would not necessarily be an incorrect approach to take, but knowing that the probing depths on teeth #s 2, 3, and 4 range from 5 to 7 mm, it would seem logical to monitor these very closely with frequent baseline recordings and prescribed radiographs. As we know, teeth with measurements of 4 mm or less can be successfully managed by the patient's oral home care regimen.

Case 3

1. c. The lateral incisors are usually the teeth that develop in a "peg" shape. Fusion is the joining of two teeth into one during development. Erosion is a result of acidic substances wearing away the enamel, such as occurs in a person who frequently sucks on lemons.
2. b. When a permanent crown is cemented in place, it is said to be "fixed" (or not removable). The indirect technique is the method of fabrication involving an impression, stone casts or dies, and a casting or firing process. The fabrication is done "indirectly," meaning the patient is not in the chair. The patient must have a temporary restoration when this technique is used. Examples of the direct technique are those restorations such as amalgam and composites, in which the restoration is "made" (or placed) directly in the patient's mouth, usually in one appointment.
3. b. A provisional (or temporary) restoration is one that is planned to be replaced in a short time. An interim restoration is a "long-term" temporary restoration. After an existing condition is resolved, a permanent restoration is placed. Permanent restorations are those that are not planned to be replaced in a particular time period.
4. d. In this case, the lingual aspect of the crown is visible (with use of the mouth mirror). Looking closely, translucency is evident. When metal is not included as part of an anterior crown, one can assume that the material used is a ceramic material.
5. d. Because porcelain is "fired" at very high temperatures, it results in a very hard surface. It can tolerate most grits of prophy pastes. This is not the case for other tooth-colored restorative materials, such as composite resins and glass ionomer. For those materials, mild abrasive and polishing agents should be used.
6. a. The most desirable characteristic of porcelain is its esthetic properties, specifically the translucency, like that of tooth enamel. True, many shades are

available, but other tooth-colored restorative materials have a wide shade selection as well. The hardness and low fracture toughness of porcelain are undesirable characteristics. In fact, porcelain is so hard that it will wear away the opposing natural enamel, and it is so brittle that it will fracture quite easily.

7. a. Whitening procedures should be done before the restoration is fabricated so that the color of the porcelain will match the natural teeth. Whitening is contraindicated for situations such as root sensitivity, unrealistic expectations, pregnancy, patients younger than the age of 18, and heavy smokers. From time to time, the patient will have to use the whitening agent again so that the color will be maintained.

Case 4

1. b. As seen on the periodontal charting, the areas of 5, 6, and 7 mm on the first visit have slightly improved or stayed the same. These are the areas a clinician would look at first to determine the progression of the periodontal condition.
2. c. As seen on the intraoral photographs, the maxillary left second premolar and the mandibular left first molar both have cuspal fractures on the lingual surface.
3. d. Tooth #30, the mandibular right first molar, has two roots. The mesial root has two canals. The mesial canals are filled with a different material (silver points) than the distal canal (gutta percha). The two materials appear radiopaque; the silver points appear more radiopaque than the gutta percha. Maxillary molars usually have three roots.
4. c. It is not uncommon for a single tooth to have multiple restorations. As indicated on the patient's record, especially the dental charting, teeth #2, #14, and #15 have two restorations. Remember that on maxillary molars, attempts will be made to preserve the transverse ridge. This ridge provides strength to the tooth. Therefore, you would most likely see a MO and a DO rather than a MOD restoration.
5. c. Both amalgam margins are overextended in the interproximal area. These are commonly termed "amalgam overhangs." An open margin may be described as a gap between the tooth and the restoration in which the explorer catches in both directions, from tooth to restoration and restoration to tooth. A submarginal area exists when the preparation is underfilled and the explorer catches from restoration to tooth.
6. b. Two different filling materials were used to fill the three root canals. This is evident by the different radiopacity of the materials in the canals for tooth #30 on the radiographs. Both materials are permanent root canal filling materials.
7. c. Supereruption occurs when a tooth does not have an opposing tooth in the opposite arch. The tooth will erupt above the occlusal plane. This patient does not have teeth #3 and #4. Therefore, tooth #30 has no opposing contact. The radiographs illustrate the obvious extent of the supereruption of tooth #30.
8. b. Each line in the apical section of this periodontal chart is marked off in increments of 2 mm. The line drawn over tooth #31 goes just past the first line, meaning that it is at least 3 mm. You may have "read up" to the next increment and answered 4, but drawings on a chart should be made as exact as possible.

Case 5

1. b. From the periodontal chart, one can see the 7mm pocket on #15 and the increased mobility on #9. Both arches have gingival recession. The probing depths on the mandibular arch are all within normal limits. Therefore, the mandibular arch is "periodontally healthier" than the maxillary.
2. d. Five kinds of dental restorations are present in this patient. They are: amalgam, gold, composite resin, gold foil (or cohesive gold) and porcelain (fused to metal).
3. c. The patient may be prone to bisphosphonate induced osteo-necrosis especially if she has procedures done such as periodontal surgery, extractions, or implant placement. The hygienist should perform thorough dental exams, have the patient in the best periodontal health as possible, evaluate oral hard and soft tissues every 3 to 6 months, and evaluate the fit of all oral prostheses.
4. c. The patient shared her habit of cigarette smoking. Your oral hygiene home care instruction should include information on tobacco cessation. Tooth whitening, pit and fissure sealants, and nutritional counseling are not indicated for this patient.
5. b. Looking at the patient's dental charting, one can see a multitude of restorations. Of the choices listed, the patient would benefit most from patient-applied fluoride. Even though the gingiva on #s 9, 22, 25 and 26 is recessed, the patient reports no sensitivity, so fluoride varnish is not indicated. No dry mouth is reported, so salivary substitutes are not needed. The patient would not need sealants because all posterior occlusal surfaces are either restored or missing.
6. b. The large restoration on #15 is a mesio-occlusal gold inlay. It is labeled "G" on the chart and the restoration drawn on the occlusal view of the chart is drawn to the outside line on the left side, indicating a

mesio-occlusal restoration. This "MO" can also be viewed in the photograph. The amalgam restoration extends from the occlusal to the lingual.

7. d. Teeth #s 11, 12, and 28 all have had root canal therapy, post and cores placed, and have been restored with porcelain-fused-to-metal crowns. "PFM" is labeled on the dental chart. The apical portions of these root canals have had gutta percha (less radiolucent) and the post (more radiopaque) fills the remainder of the canal.

Case 6

1. a. Ceramometal crowns tend to look "fake" or unnatural when they are overcontoured and very opaque in color. This happens because the lab may have had to add many layers of porcelain in order to sufficiently cover the metal coping underneath. The result is a "bulky looking" tooth and with all the porcelain layers, the translucent properties are lost, and thus the tooth becomes opaque.
2. c. In most dental and dental hygiene educational curriculums, esthetic veneers are charted by only outlining the facial surface on the tooth on the chart.
3. c. From the case information, we learn the patient is 62 years old. We see from the periodontal chart that there is a limited amount of recession. However, the probing depths are very much within normal limits. It is well accepted that gingival recession is a common oral finding in older individuals. Therefore, taking all the aforementioned into consideration, the patient's gingival health may be considered as being "very good."
4. b. The root of tooth #4 is dilacerated. This can be seen radiographically and is quite obvious. As you may recall, dilaceration is a developmental disturbance in the shape of teeth. It refers to an angulation, or a sharp bend or curve, in the root of a formed tooth.
5. d. The radiolucency on the distal of #27 is a composite resin. As you can see from these cases, the radiographic appearance of composite resins can vary greatly depending on the composition of the resin material. Some are quite radiopaque while others are very radiolucent. Metals, such as amalgam or gold will always appear opaque. The radiographic appearance of composites when compared to caries is that composite restorations will have a more defined outline.
6. d. Composite cements are usually used to attach ceramic veneers to the tooth surface. They employ the acid etch technique and have the property of translucency when set as compared to polycarboxylate and zinc phosphate. Glass ionomers can be used, but do not have the benefits of acid etching.
7. c. The projections on the distal surface of teeth 22 and 27 are precision attachments designed to retain the new removable partial denture to the natural teeth. These attachments do not have a retention arm that can be visible on the facial surfaces of the canines. Neither an orthodontic retainer nor dental implants use these types of retention.

Appendix 2

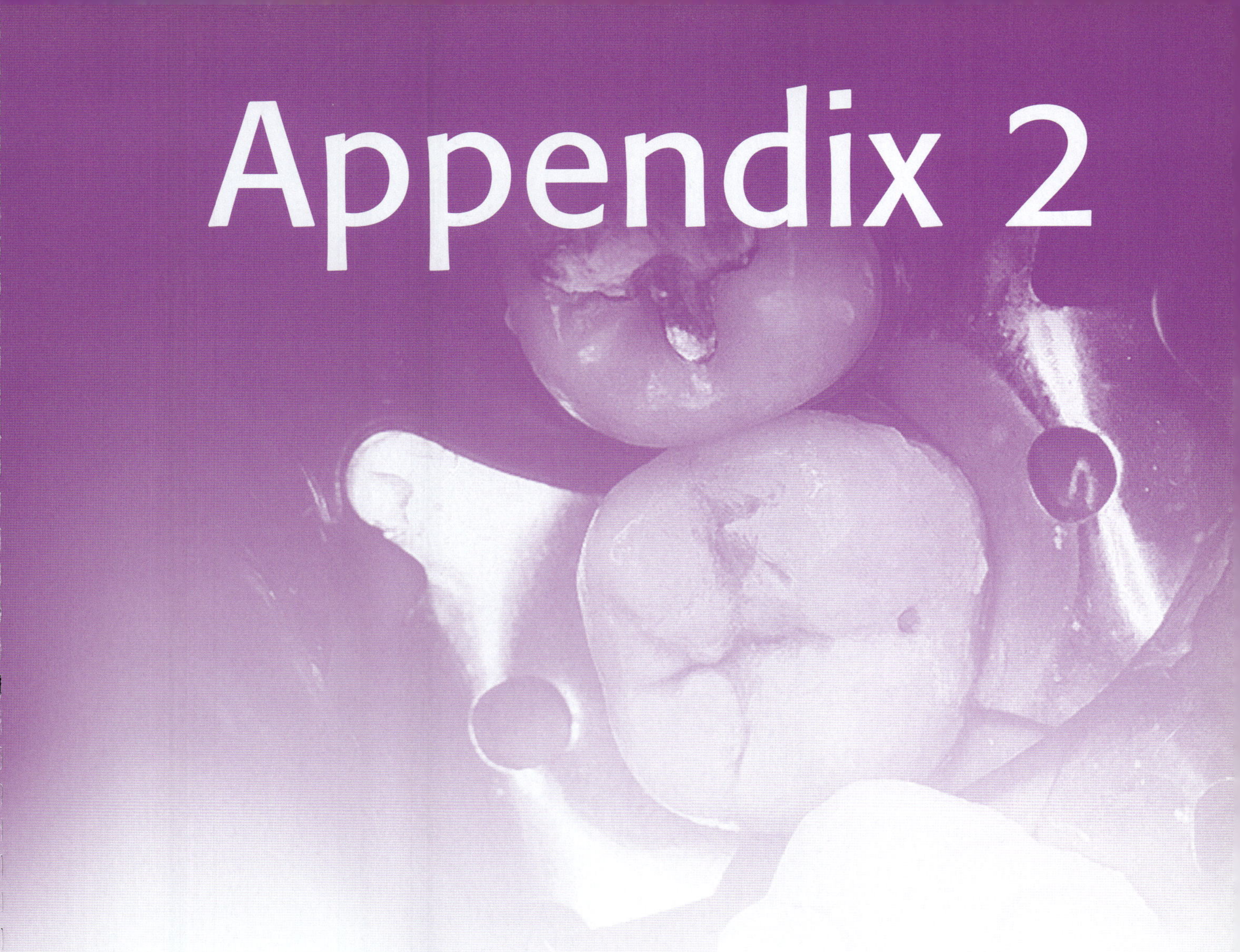

Skill Performance Evaluations

Student Name:______________________________ Date:______________

Chapter 23: Mixing Zinc Phosphate Cement for Luting and as a Base

Satisfactory performance of this lab/clinical skill is expected. The student is to self-evaluate using the designated column. After faculty evaluation, the skill performance is to be discussed based on both evaluations.

If satisfactory, the skill evaluation is complete. If unsatisfactory, remediation will occur until criteria are performed satisfactorily.

CRITERIA	INSTRUCTOR		STUDENT	
	S	U	S	U
1. Luting Consistency:				
a. Powder is properly incorporated into the liquid.				
b. Mix is completed within the specified mixing time.				
c. Mix will form a "1 inch string" between the spatula and slab.				
2. Base Consistency:				
a. Powder is properly incorporated into the liquid.				
b. Mix is completed within specified mixing time.				
c. Mix is thick, putty-like, and shaped into a ball.				

(Fold)

Faculty, please identify minimum lab and clinical competency levels:

Laboratory: #______ criteria must be performed satisfactorily

Clinical: #______ criteria must be performed satisfactorily

Time Started: ___________ Time Completed: ___________

Instructor: ______________________________________

Suggestions/Comments:

____

____

____

Student Name:______________________________ Date:______________

Chapter 23: Mixing Glass Ionomer Cement—Luting Consistency

Satisfactory performance of this lab/clinical skill is expected. The student is to self-evaluate using the designated column. After faculty evaluation, the skill performance is to be discussed based on both evaluations.

If satisfactory, the skill evaluation is complete. If unsatisfactory, remediation will occur until criteria are performed satisfactorily.

	INSTRUCTOR		STUDENT	
CRITERIA	S	U	S	U
1. The powder is incorporated into the liquid in one portion.				
2. The mix is completed within the specified time.				
3. The completed mix will stretch at least a half-inch.				

(Fold)

Faculty, please identify minimum lab and clinical competency levels:

Laboratory: #______ criteria must be performed satisfactorily

Clinical: #______ criteria must be performed satisfactorily

Time Started: ____________ Time Completed: ___________

Instructor: ____

Suggestions/Comments:

____

____

____

Student Name:______________________________ Date:_______________

Chapter 23: Mixing Zinc Oxide-Eugenol as a Base or Temporary Restorative Material

Satisfactory performance of this lab/clinical skill is expected. The student is to self-evaluate using the designated column. After faculty evaluation, the skill performance is to be discussed based on both evaluations.

If satisfactory, the skill evaluation is complete. If unsatisfactory, remediation will occur until criteria are performed satisfactorily.

	INSTRUCTOR		STUDENT	
CRITERIA	S	U	S	U
1. Powder and liquid are properly incorporated into the mix.				
2. Mix is consistent and has a putty-like appearance.				
3. Mix is completed within 1.5 minutes.				

(Fold)

Faculty, please identify minimum lab and clinical competency levels:

Laboratory: #______ criteria must be performed satisfactorily

Clinical: #______ criteria must be performed satisfactorily

Time Started: ____________ Time Completed: ___________

Instructor: ____

Suggestions/Comments:

____

____

____

Student Name: ______________________________ Date: __________

Chapter 24: Rubber Dam Application and Removal

Satisfactory performance of this lab/clinical skill is expected. The student is to self-evaluate using the designated column. After faculty evaluation, the skill performance is to be discussed based on both evaluations.

If satisfactory, the skill evaluation is complete. If unsatisfactory, remediation will occur until criteria are performed satisfactorily.

	INSTRUCTOR		STUDENT	
CRITERIA	S	U	S	U
1. Rubber dam is punched correctly.				
2. Clamp is ligated and seated properly.				
3. Rubber dam is inverted around isolated teeth.				
4. Rubber dam is smooth and tear-free.				
5. Frame is properly placed and centered.				
Removal				
1. Dam material and frame are removed as one unit.				
2. Interproximals are free of rubber dam remnants.				

(Fold)

Faculty, please identify minimum lab and clinical competency levels:

Laboratory: #______ criteria must be performed satisfactorily

Clinical: #______ criteria must be performed satisfactorily

Time Started: ___________ Time Completed: ___________

Instructor: ____

Suggestions/Comments:

____

____

____

Student Name: ______________________________ Date: __________

Chapter 25: Pit and Fissure Sealants

Satisfactory performance of this lab/clinical skill is expected. The student is to self-evaluate using the designated column. After faculty evaluation, the skill performance is to be discussed based on both evaluations.

If satisfactory, the skill evaluation is complete. If unsatisfactory, remediation will occur until criteria are performed satisfactorily.

	INSTRUCTOR		STUDENT	
CRITERIA	S	U	S	U
1. Tooth surface is plaque-free.				
2. Tooth is adequately isolated.				
3. Etched surfaces appear chalky white.				
4. Sealant covers all areas indicated for placement.				
5. Bubbles, voids, and defects are not present.				
6. Interproximal areas remain open and "unsealed."				
7. Sealant does not interfere with occlusion.				

(Fold)

Faculty, please identify minimum lab and clinical competency levels:

Laboratory: #______ criteria must be performed satisfactorily

Clinical: #______ criteria must be performed satisfactorily

Time Started: __________ Time Completed: __________

Instructor: ______________________________

Suggestions/Comments:

____

____

____

Student Name: ______________________________ Date: ________________

Chapter 26: Amalgam Finishing and Polishing

Satisfactory performance of this lab/clinical skill is expected. The student is to self-evaluate using the designated column. After faculty evaluation, the skill performance is to be discussed based on both evaluations.

If satisfactory, the skill evaluation is complete. If unsatisfactory, remediation will occur until criteria are performed satisfactorily.

	INSTRUCTOR		STUDENT	
CRITERIA	S	U	S	U
Finishing				
1. Excessive amalgam has been removed from cavosurface margins.				
2. Amalgam appears smooth.				
3. Occlusion registers properly with articulating paper.				
4. Occlusal and marginal anatomy well defined.				
5. Porosity and pits have been removed.				
6. Contour of the restoration approximates the original contour of the tooth.				
7. Adjacent tooth structure is left undamaged.				
Polishing				
1. Amalgam is void of scratches and appears smooth.				
2. Amalgam has a high polish and lustrous shine.				
3. Adjacent tooth structure is left undamaged.				
4. Time utilization is satisfactory.				

(Fold)

Faculty, please identify minimum lab and clinical competency levels:

Laboratory: #______ criteria must be performed satisfactorily

Clinical: #______ criteria must be performed satisfactorily

Time Started: ___________ Time Completed: ___________

Instructor: ____

Suggestions/Comments:

____

____

____

Student Name: ______________________________ Date: ________________

Chapter 27: Alginate Impressions

Satisfactory performance of this lab/clinical skill is expected. The student is to self-evaluate using the designated column. After faculty evaluation, the skill performance is to be discussed based on both evaluations.

If satisfactory, the skill evaluation is complete. If unsatisfactory, remediation will occur until criteria are performed satisfactorily.

	INSTRUCTOR		STUDENT	
CRITERIA	S	U	S	U
1. All teeth are present without voids and air bubbles.				
2. All edentulous ridge/spaces are present.				
3. All vestibular areas are present and intact.				
4. All frena and muscle attachments are present and intact.				
5. All interpapillary spaces are present with minimal tearing.				
6. No voids in critical areas: palate, floor of mouth, vestibular areas, tray showing through impression.				
7. Impression is stable; alginate is attached to the tray.				
8. Adequately extended; retromolar area included.				
9. Appropriate infection control procedures: bowls, spatula, impression.				

(Fold)

Faculty, please identify minimum lab and clinical competency levels:

Laboratory: #______ criteria must be performed satisfactorily

Clinical: #______ criteria must be performed satisfactorily

Time Started: ___________ Time Completed: ___________

Instructor: ____

Suggestions/Comments:

____

____

____

Student Name:______________________________ Date:______________

Chapter 28: Trimming and Finishing Study Models

STUDENT		Study Models		**FACULTY**
MAX	MAND		MAX	MAND
		OVERALL		
		1. All teeth and anatomy are preserved (none removed through trimming; no broken or chipped teeth).		
		2. Stone is smooth; no voids or blebs >1 mm; cleared of dust and trimming debris.		
		BASES		
		3. Occluded models and occlusal plane are parallel to the benchtop (height does not differ by >1/8 inch).		
		4. Bases are smooth and flat; no bevels; does not rock (a nail file will not slide under).		
		5. Height of occluded models is 2.5 to 2.75 inches.		
		6. Bases are 1/3 of height; anatomy is 2/3 of height in the anterior region.		
		BORDERS		
		7. Posterior borders are flat and bite will not open when occluded models are placed on their backs (<1 mm).		
		8. Arch length extends at least 0.25 inch beyond most posterior teeth, not removing maxillary tuberosity, hamular notch, or mandibular retromolar areas.		
		9. Back of maxillary model is perpendicular to median line (<3°).		
		10. The vestibule is not removed by trimming.		
		11. Sides are flush, flat, and smooth.		
		OTHER		
		12. Tongue area is flat and smooth without removing any anatomy.		
		13. Models are labeled with student's (or patient's) name and date.		

(Fold)

Laboratory: #______ criteria must be performed satisfactorily

Instructor: ____

Student Name: ______________________________ Date: ________________

Chapter 29: Custom Impression Tray

Satisfactory performance of this lab/clinical skill is expected. The student is to self-evaluate using the designated column. After faculty evaluation, the skill performance is to be discussed based on both evaluations.

If satisfactory, the skill evaluation is complete. If unsatisfactory, remediation will occur until criteria are performed satisfactorily.

	INSTRUCTOR		STUDENT	
CRITERIA	S	U	S	U
1. Tray has uniform thickness.				
2. Tray is smooth.				
3. Placements of stops are appropriate.				
4. Sizes of stops are adequate.				
5. Handle size is acceptable.				
6. Handle location is acceptable.				

(Fold)

Faculty, please identify minimum lab and clinical competency levels:

Laboratory: #______ criteria must be performed satisfactorily

Clinical: #______ criteria must be performed satisfactorily

Time Started: ____________ Time Completed: ___________

Instructor: ____

Suggestions/Comments:

____

____

____

Student Name:______________________________ Date:_______________

Chapter 30: Elastomeric Impressions

Satisfactory performance of this lab/clinical skill is expected. The student is to self-evaluate using the designated column. After faculty evaluation, the skill performance is to be discussed based on both evaluations.

If satisfactory, the skill evaluation is complete. If unsatisfactory, remediation will occur until criteria are performed satisfactorily.

	INSTRUCTOR		STUDENT	
CRITERIA	S	U	S	U
1. No bubbles or voids are present in critical areas.				
2. Impression is not distorted.				
3. All critical areas are reproduced.				
4. No critical areas are torn.				

(Fold)

Faculty, please identify minimum lab and clinical competency levels:

Laboratory: #______ criteria must be performed satisfactorily

Clinical: #______ criteria must be performed satisfactorily

Time Started: ___________ Time Completed: ___________

Instructor: ____

Suggestions/Comments:

____

____

____

Student Name: ______________________________ Date: ________________

Chapter 31: Bleaching Tray Construction—Clinical Procedure

Satisfactory performance of this lab/clinical skill is expected. The student is to self-evaluate using the designated column. After faculty evaluation, the skill performance is to be discussed based on both evaluations.

If satisfactory, the skill evaluation is complete. If unsatisfactory, remediation will occur until criteria are performed satisfactorily.

	INSTRUCTOR		STUDENT	
CRITERIA	S	U	S	U
1. Medical history is completed.				
2. Informed consent is explained to and signed by patient.				
3. Pretreatment intraoral examination is completed.				
4. Prophylaxis is completed.				
5. Intraoral photography is completed with matching shade guide tab in place.				
6. Full-arch alginate impression is taken.				
7. Gypsum casts are produced and trimmed.				
8. Block-out resin is applied and cured to facial surfaces of teeth to be whitened.				
9. Resin tray is constructed and trimmed to specification.				
10. Patient is instructed in use of tray to apply whitening agent.				
11. Follow-up examination is completed and retreatment assigned as necessary.				
12. Posttreatment intraoral photography is completed with matching shade guide tab in place				

(Fold)

Faculty, please identify minimum lab and clinical competency levels:

Laboratory: #______ criteria must be performed satisfactorily

Clinical: #______ criteria must be performed satisfactorily

Time Started: ____________ Time Completed: ___________

Instructor: ____

Suggestions/Comments:

____

____

____

Student Name: ______________________________ Date: ________________

Chapter 32: Debonding Orthodontic Resins

Satisfactory performance of this lab/clinical skill is expected. The student is to self-evaluate using the designated column. After faculty evaluation, the skill performance is to be discussed based on both evaluations.

If satisfactory, the skill evaluation is complete. If unsatisfactory, remediation will occur until criteria are performed satisfactorily.

	INSTRUCTOR		STUDENT	
CRITERIA	S	U	S	U
1. The enamel contains no gouges or scarring.				
2. No resin remains on the tooth.				
3. The enamel appears glossy when dried with air.				
4. The enamel feels smooth and glass-like with the explorer.				
5. Disclosing solution does not adhere to the remaining resin.				
6. Patient reports a smooth enamel feel with their tongue.				

(Fold)

Faculty, please identify minimum lab and clinical competency levels:

Laboratory: #______ criteria must be performed satisfactorily

Clinical: #______ criteria must be performed satisfactorily

Time Started: ____________ Time Completed: ____________

Instructor: ____

Suggestions/Comments:

____

____

____

Student Name:____________________________ Date:______________

Chapter 33: Placement of the Periodontal Dressing

Satisfactory performance of this lab/clinical skill is expected. The student is to self-evaluate using the designated column. After faculty evaluation, the skill performance is to be discussed based on both evaluations.

If satisfactory, the skill evaluation is complete. If unsatisfactory, remediation will occur until criteria are performed satisfactorily.

	INSTRUCTOR		STUDENT	
CRITERIA	S	U	S	U
1. Dressing material is dispensed and mixed until uniform in color.				
2. Dressing has set sufficiently to allow for easy manipulation.				
3. Dressing is 3 to 4 mm at its thickest area.				
4. Dressing is 8 to 10 mm wide.				
5. Surface of the dressing is smooth with tapered edges (i.e., no slices or cracks).				
6. Dressing is placed with interproximal retention.				
7. Dressing does not interfere with muscle attachments.				
8. Dressing does not extend beyond the cervical 1/3 of the crown (height of contour).				
9. At least four teeth are incorporated in the dressed area.				

(Fold)

Faculty, please identify minimum lab and clinical competency levels:

Laboratory: #______ criteria must be performed satisfactorily

Clinical: #______ criteria must be performed satisfactorily

Time Started: ___________ Time Completed: ___________

Instructor: ____

Suggestions/Comments:

____

____

____

Student Name:______________________________ Date:______________

Chapter 34: Periodontal Dressing Removal

Satisfactory performance of this lab/clinical skill is expected. The student is to self-evaluate using the designated column. After faculty evaluation, the skill performance is to be discussed based on both evaluations.

If satisfactory, the skill evaluation is complete. If unsatisfactory, remediation will occur until criteria are performed satisfactorily.

	INSTRUCTOR		STUDENT	
CRITERIA	S	U	S	U
1. Dressing material is removed by applying constant, controlled lateral pressure until the dressing is released from the dentoform/patient.				
2. Dressing material is thoroughly removed from the dentoform/patient.				

(Fold)

Faculty, please identify minimum lab and clinical competency levels:

Laboratory: #______ criteria must be performed satisfactorily

Clinical: #______ criteria must be performed satisfactorily

Time Started: ____________ Time Completed: ___________

Instructor: ____

Suggestions/Comments:

____

____

____

Student Name:______________________________ Date:_______________

Chapter 34: Suture Removal

Satisfactory performance of this lab/clinical skill is expected. The student is to self-evaluate using the designated column. After faculty evaluation, the skill performance is to be discussed based on both evaluations.

If satisfactory, the skill evaluation is complete. If unsatisfactory, remediation will occur until criteria are performed satisfactorily.

	INSTRUCTOR		STUDENT	
CRITERIA	S	U	S	U
1. The suture is retracted from the tissue by grasping the knot by forceps in the nondominant hand.				
2. A fulcrum or rest is used when cutting the suture.				
3. Only one "end" of the suture is cut.				
4. The suture is cut close to the tissue, in the area previously submerged, without tissue damage.				
5. The suture is removed with a smooth, continuous motion.				
6. Removed sutures are placed on a gauze square and counted. Number of removed sutures is recorded in the chart.				

(Fold)

Faculty, please identify minimum lab and clinical competency levels:

Laboratory: #______ criteria must be performed satisfactorily

Clinical: #______ criteria must be performed satisfactorily

Time Started: ____________ Time Completed: ___________

Instructor: ____

Suggestions/Comments:

____

____

____

Student Name:______________________________ Date:_______________

Chapter 35: Constructing a Temporary Crown

Satisfactory performance of this lab/clinical skill is expected. The student is to self-evaluate using the designated column. After faculty evaluation, the skill performance is to be discussed based on both evaluations.

If satisfactory, the skill evaluation is complete. If unsatisfactory, remediation will occur until criteria are performed satisfactorily.

	INSTRUCTOR		STUDENT	
CRITERIA	S	U	S	U
1. Mesial and distal contacts are not open. Cannot see light through the contacts.				
2. Shape approximates that of the unprepared tooth.				
3. All margins are closed.				
4. No voids >1 mm are present.				
5. Optional—Occlusal contacts are similar to adjacent teeth.				

(Fold)

Faculty, please identify minimum lab and clinical competency levels:

Laboratory: #______ criteria must be performed satisfactorily

Clinical: #______ criteria must be performed satisfactorily

Time Started: ___________ Time Completed: ___________

Instructor: ____

Suggestions/Comments:

____

____

____

Student Name: ______________________________ Date: ______________

Chapter 36: Composite Finishing and Polishing

Satisfactory performance of this lab/clinical skill is expected. The student is to self-evaluate using the designated column. After faculty evaluation, the skill performance is discussed based on both evaluations.

If satisfactory, the skill evaluation is complete. If unsatisfactory, remediation will occur until criteria are performed satisfactorily.

	INSTRUCTOR		STUDENT	
CRITERIA	S	U	S	U
Finishing:				
1. Excessive composite has been removed from cavosurface margins.				
2. Composite appears to be smooth.				
3. Occlusion registers properly with articulating paper.				
4. Occlusal and marginal anatomy is well defined.				
5. Porosity and pits have been removed.				
6. Contour of the restoration approximates the original contour of the tooth.				
7. Adjacent tooth structure is left undamaged.				
Polishing				
1. Composite is void of scratches and appears smooth.				
2. Composite has a lustrous shine.				
3. Adjacent tooth structure is left undamaged.				
4. Time utilization is satisfactory.				

(Fold)

Faculty, please identify minimum lab and clinical competency levels:

Laboratory: #______ criteria must be performed satisfactorily

Clinical: #______ criteria must be performed satisfactorily

Time Started: ___________ Time Completed: ___________

Instructor: ______________________________________

Suggestions/Comments:

____

____

____

Index

Pages numbers in *italics* indicate figure. Page numbers followed by a t indicate table.